Culture and Occupation:
Effectiveness for Occupational Therapy Practice, Education, and Research, 3rd Edition

Edited by **Shirley A. Wells, DrPH, OTR, FAOTA;**
Roxie M. Black, PhD, OTR/L, FAOTA;
and **Jyothi Gupta, PhD, OTR/L, FAOTA**

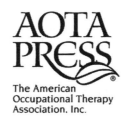

AOTA PRESS
The American
Occupational Therapy
Association, Inc.

AOTA Vision 2025
Occupational therapy maximizes health, well-being, and quality of life for all people, populations, and communities through effective solutions that facilitate participation in everyday living.

Mission Statement
The American Occupational Therapy Association advances the quality, availability, use, and support of occupational therapy through standard-setting, advocacy, education, and research on behalf of its members and the public.

AOTA Staff
Frederick P. Somers, *Executive Director*
Christopher M. Bluhm, *Chief Operating Officer*

Chris Davis, *Director, AOTA Press*
Caroline Polk, *Digital Manager and* AJOT *Managing Editor*
Ashley Hofmann, *Development Editor*
Barbara Dickson, *Production Editor*

Rebecca Rutberg, *Director, Marketing*
Amanda Goldman, *Marketing Manager*
Jennifer Folden, *Marketing Specialist*

American Occupational Therapy Association, Inc.
4720 Montgomery Lane
Bethesda, MD 20814
Phone: 301-652-AOTA (2682)
TDD: 800-377-8555
Fax: 301-652-7711
www.aota.org
To order: 1-877-404-AOTA or store.aota.org

Disclaimers
This publication is designed to provide accurate and authoritative information in regard to the subject matter covered. It is sold or distributed with the understanding that the publisher is not engaged in rendering legal, accounting, or other professional service. If legal advice or other expert assistance is required, the services of a competent professional person should be sought.
—*From the Declaration of Principles jointly adopted by the American Bar Association and a Committee of Publishers and Associations*

It is the objective of the American Occupational Therapy Association to be a forum for free expression and interchange of ideas. The opinions expressed by the contributors to this work are their own and not necessarily those of the American Occupational Therapy Association.

ISBN: 978-1-56900-371-8
Library of Congress Control Number: 2016955020

Cover Design by Debra Naylor, Naylor Design Inc., Washington, DC
Composition by Manila Typesetting Company, Philippines
Printed by Automated Graphic Systems, Inc., White Plains, MD

CONTENTS

DEDICATION

SHIRLEY A. WELLS dedicates this book to her four-legged girls, Foxxy, Sandy, and Sarah, who aided me in understanding that diversity in people, just like in dogs, makes life interesting.

ROXIE M. BLACK dedicates this book to the memory of her mother, Faylene Alice Perkins, who taught me to view the world with wonder.

JYOTHI GUPTA dedicates this work to Diwakar, Nikhil, and Divya, who inspire me on a daily basis to fight the good fight for diversity and social inclusion.

ACTIONS, APPENDIXES, CASE EXAMPLES, EXHIBITS, FIGURES, REFLECTIONS, AND TABLES

Figures

Reflections

Tables

CONTRIBUTORS

ROXIE M. BLACK, PhD, OTR/L, FAOTA
Professor Emerita
Department of Occupational Therapy
University of Southern Maine
Lewiston

CORA J. BRUNS, MS, OTR/L
Academic Fieldwork Coordinator
Department of Occupational Therapy
Utica College
Utica, NY

ANNE CRONIN, PhD, OTR/L, FAOTA
Professor
Division of Occupational Therapy
West Virginia University
Morgantown

JAMI E. FLICK, MS, OTR/L
Academic Fieldwork Coordinator and Assistant Professor
Department of Occupational Therapy
University of Tennessee Health Science Center,
    College of Health Professions
Memphis

JYOTHI GUPTA, PhD, OTR/L, FAOTA
Professor and Chair
Department of Occupational Therapy
Arizona School of Health Sciences
A.T. Still University
Mesa

CHERYL J. HICKEY, EdD, MPT
Associate Professor
Department of Physical Therapy
College of Health and Human Services
California State University
Fresno

NANCY L. HOLLINS, PhD, OTR/L
Professor and Program Director, Occupational Therapy
Utica College
Utica, NY

ROSALIE M. KING, DHS, OTR/L
Retired Associate Professor
The University of Findlay
Findlay, OH

THERESA LETO, DHS, OTR/L
Associate Professor
College of Health Professions
Davenport University
Grand Rapids, MI

PEGGY M. MARTIN, PhD, OTR/L
Assistant Professor and Program Director,
    Occupational Therapy
Department of Rehabilitation Medicine
University of Minnesota
Minneapolis

DIANNA MICHELLE MEDINA, OTD, MOT, OTR/L
Adjunct Faculty
Occupational Therapy Assistant Program
The Alamo Colleges
San Antonio, TX

VICTORIA L. NACKLEY, MS, OTR/L
Professor of Practice
Department of Occupational Therapy
Utica College
Utica, NY

NINA ROBINS, PhD, OTR/L
Occupational Therapist, Gerontology Program
Health Pro Rehab
Chicago

JULEEN RODAKOWSKI, OTD, OTR/L
Assistant Professor
Department of Occupational Therapy
University of Pittsburgh
Pittsburgh

LESLIE K. ROUNDTREE, DHS, MBA, OTR/L
Dean, College of Health Sciences
Chairperson, Department of Occupational Therapy
Chicago State University
Chicago

ANGELA E. SCOGGIN, PhD, OTR, FAOTA
Professor, Occupational Therapy Department
The University of Texas Rio Grande Valley
Edinburg

REGINA T. SMITH, DHS, OTR/L
Assistant Professor
Department of Occupational Therapy
Chicago State University
Chicago

YDA J. SMITH, PhD, OTR/L
Assistant Professor/Lecturer
Department of Occupational Therapy
University of Utah
Salt Lake City

YOLANDA SUAREZ-BALCAZAR, PhD
Professor and Department Head,
    Department of Occupational Therapy
University of Illinois at Chicago
Chicago

TONI THOMPSON, MA, OTR/L, C/NDT
Doctoral Candidate
Nova Southeastern University
Senior Instructor
TherapyEd
Tampa

JACQUELINE THRASH, MS, OTR
Occupational Therapist Certified Fieldwork Educator
    PAMS
Intergro Rehab
Glendale, CA

ELIZABETH WANKA, DrOT, OTR/L
Assistant Professor
Department of Occupational Therapy
Governors State University
University Park

SHIRLEY A. WELLS, DrPH, OTR, FAOTA
Associate Professor and Chair
Department of Occupational Therapy
University of Texas Rio Grande Valley
Edinburg

LEANNE YINUSA-NYAHKOON, ScD, OTR/L
Lecturer, Department of Occupational Therapy
Research Associate, Department of Family Medicine
Boston University
Boston

HON K. YUEN, PhD, OTR/L
Professor and Director of Research
Department of Occupational Therapy
University of Alabama at Birmingham
Birmingham

PREFACE

Today, as the American population is becoming more multiracial, multicultural, and multilingual, people seeking and providing health care are increasingly from diverse groups. The modern health care system also is influenced by differences in the age, sexual identity, educational background, and occupation of health care providers and consumers. It is clear that culture matters in clinical practice.

Culture is not static but rather is dynamic and fluid. Culture is inseparable from economic, political, religious, psychological, and biological conditions. It is manifested through ordinary activities and can take an emotional tone and meaning for people. It can differ within and among the same racial and ethnic, social, and cultural groups.

Cultural factors are not always central to a health care case but can hinder a deeper understanding of a patient's condition. Therefore, the need for culturally effective health care providers is more important now than ever.

Culturally effective health care providers are able to communicate with people of cultures different from their own in a way that earns their patients' and clients' respect and trust. These clinicians have the capacity to adapt their professional skills (both technical and managerial) to fit local conditions and constraints and are content and at ease working with individuals from diverse backgrounds. Therapists who integrate and transform knowledge about themselves, individuals, and groups of people into specific standards, practices, and attitudes used in appropriate settings to increase quality of services produce better outcomes and practice culturally effective care. Culturally effective services are respectful of and responsive to the beliefs, practices, and linguistic needs of diverse populations. Being culturally effective is a multifaceted process for both individuals and organizational systems that evolves over an extended period of time.

In this third installment in the *Culture and Occupation* series, we continue to expand on the concepts that health care students and professionals will need on their journey to becoming culturally competent. The first book in 2000, *Cultural Competency for Health Professionals*, introduced the importance of culture and diversity to occupational therapy. The second book in 2007, *Culture and Occupation: A Model of Empowerment in Occupational Therapy*, illustrated the dynamic connection between cultural exchanges and therapeutic outcomes. This latest publication, *Culture and Occupation: Effectiveness for Occupational Therapy Practice, Education, and Research*, is designed to assist occupational therapy practitioners in answering the question "Is it possible to deliver culturally effective care?" in the affirmative. Clinicians need to understand what matters most to others in their experience of illness and treatment—what is really at stake for clients, their families, and their communities and for themselves. Then clinicians can use that information in thinking through treatment decisions, negotiating with clients, and reflecting on the process.

What Is New in This Edition

The book has been organized around culture effectiveness in occupational therapy practice, education, and research. The chapters include core information and evidence, as well as clinical findings and thoughtful analysis. Section I, "Culture and Occupation" (Chapters 1–4), provides the foundation and explains the need for cultural effectiveness by addressing the sociocultural and sociopolitical aspects of occupation. The concluding chapter in this section describes the transition to cultural effectiveness in language and terms used to describe cross-cultural practice.

Section II, "Characteristics of Cultural Effectiveness" (Chapters 5–12), focuses on the Model for Cultural Effectiveness and presents a road map for providing culturally effective care. It addresses the areas of changes—self-awareness, cultural knowledge, cultural skills, and reflection—necessary for becoming culturally effective. Section III, "Culture and Clinical Practice" (Chapters 14–21), helps readers incorporate cultural effectiveness in clinical practice. It emphasizes the effect of ethical decision making related to culture. Several evidence-based chapters include the influence of culture on food in occupational therapy intervention; cultural values and lifestyles; the cultural essence of patient encounters; and the integration of health promotion, culture, and occupational therapy.

Section IV, "Culture and Education" (Chapters 22–26) addresses issues related to educating students to be culturally effective practitioners. It examines occupational therapy educational program curricula and pedagogies used to teach culture effectiveness. These chapters explore experiential and reflective educational strategies that bridge classroom and community, foster positive fieldwork experiences, and build an inclusive educational environment to support diversity. Section V, "Culture and Community, Population-Based Practice" (Chapters 27–29), provides examples of the integration of culture effectiveness in community practice through a handwriting program for adults learning English as a second language and a wellness program for elderly persons. Section VI, "Culture and Research" (Chapters 30–31), expounds on the issues of culture and diversity in the research process and includes a research study on Mexican American older adults. Section VII, "Evaluating Cultural Effectiveness" (Chapters 32–33), examines cultural competence and cross-cultural interactions and critical reflection. It discusses strategies and tools used to assess cultural competence, including some currently available assessment tools.

Throughout the book, readers are provided with cases and questions that occupational therapy practitioners can use to reflect on and examine their own cultural effectiveness and the cultural effectiveness of their practice setting.

Outcome

Not being culturally effective in the provision of health care is no longer an option in an increasingly diverse society. Caring for patients and clients from cultures different than one's own can present a variety of challenges. The relationship between culture and health-related behaviors is inherently complex. Cultural effectiveness is not about lists of cultural characteristics but instead is about investing in an environment that celebrates and respects cultural differences. It is about understanding and appreciating these differences and planning for them in the delivery of care. The more occupational therapy practitioners examine and articulate culturally effective interventions, the more we can adapt, negotiate, collaborate, and deliver quality health care in a multicultural environment.

—Shirley A. Wells, DrPH, OTR, FAOTA;
Roxie M. Black, PhD, OTR/L, FAOTA;
and Jyothi Gupta, PhD, OTR/L, FAOTA

Section I.

CULTURE AND OCCUPATION

Chapter 1.

EXPLORING CULTURE

Jyothi Gupta, PhD, OTR/L, FAOTA

If we are to achieve a richer culture, rich in contrasting values, we must recognize the whole gamut of human potentialities, and so weave a less arbitrary social fabric, one in which each diverse human gift will find a fitting place.
Margaret Mead (1935, p. 322)

Chapter Highlights

- What Is Culture?
- Theoretical Concepts in Culture
- Culture and the Individual
- Culture and Values
- Culture and Attitudes
- Culture in the United States
- Globalization and Technology
- The Culture of Occupational Therapy

Key Terms and Concepts

- ✧ Acculturation
- ✧ Attitudes
- ✧ Attitudinal barriers
- ✧ Autonomy
- ✧ Biomedical culture
- ✧ Biopsychosocial paradigm
- ✧ Client-centered practice
- ✧ Code switching
- ✧ Cultural globalization
- ✧ Cultural imperialism
- ✧ Cultural pluralism
- ✧ Culture
- ✧ Culture as external
- ✧ Culture as internal
- ✧ Culture codes
- ✧ Culture group
- ✧ Culture-specific values

- ✧ Cyber imperialism
- ✧ Emic knowledge
- ✧ Ethnogenesis
- ✧ Etic knowledge
- ✧ Evidence-based practice
- ✧ Globalization
- ✧ High-context culture
- ✧ Hybrid culture
- ✧ *ICF* model
- ✧ Individualism
- ✧ Intersection Framework
- ✧ Kawa Model
- ✧ Low-context culture
- ✧ Masculinity
- ✧ Melting pot
- ✧ National identity
- ✧ Occupational justice

✧ Occupational science
✧ Othering
✧ Power distance
✧ Salad bowl
✧ Socialization

✧ Time orientation
✧ Transactionalism
✧ Uncertainty avoidance
✧ Values
✧ World shrink

Culture influences all aspects of human life. Human social organization, the institutions that form the foundation of societies, and even individual behaviors, including the habits and routines that set the rhythms of everyday life, provide evidence of the pervasive influence of culture in the everyday lives of individuals, communities, and society.

This chapter explores definitions, theoretical concepts, and dimensions of culture and discusses general implications of culture for occupational therapy practitioners. The chapter aims to introduce some basic fundamental theoretical perspectives and concepts associated with culture to help occupational therapy practitioners understand the role of culture in habits, routines, behaviors, and traditions that influence both how clients experience daily life and how occupational therapy is practiced.

What Is Culture?

Culture is a complex system of multiple universal elements, such as language, values, traditions, and behaviors, that coalesce, in different combinations akin to a kaleidoscope, to create a whole. Culture may be defined from different perspectives, such as historical, behavioral, symbolic, structural, and normative.

From a *historical perspective,* culture encompasses traditions that are passed on from one generation to the next. From a *behavioral perspective,* culture constitutes the learned and accepted ways of behaving or conducting oneself. The *symbolic perspective* of culture is the shared subjective meanings of a group or society. Symbols include shared meanings for language, objects, and gestures. For example, a band worn on the left ring finger symbolizes the marital status of a person in many cultures. Similarly wearing silver toe rings, a specific type of chain called the *mangalsutra,* and/or coloring one's hair parting in vermillion red symbolizes a married woman in many Indian communities.

The *structural perspective* of culture includes "patterns and interrelated ideas, symbols, or behaviors" (Jandt, 2004a, p. 1). Examples of this include

family organization (e.g., head of household, how major decisions are made in a family) and social institutions such as education and health care systems. Finally, from a *normative perspective,* culture comprises the prescribed ideals, values, and rules for belonging to a group (Jandt, 2004a). Regardless of the perspective on culture in use, it is always understood that culture is learned, not inherited, which speaks to its evolving and dynamic nature.

Culture has attributes that are both external and internal to the individual (Jahoda, 2012). **Culture as external** is visible and observable and provides evidence of human development through interactions with and transformation of the environment (Cole & Parker, 2011). Some examples include foods, arts, literature, festival celebrations, and traditional clothes.

Culture as internal refers to aspects of culture that are expressed in individual lives, particularly the ways people behave in certain situations. Human behaviors are elicited and influenced by knowledge that is shared and transmitted among culture groups (Hong, 2009). Examples are gestures, facial expressions, and behavioral norms.

A **culture group** is any group whose members agree on symbolic elements that are essential to the group's core identity (Wan & Chiu, 2009). Symbolic elements are embedded in shared meanings that create a group identity and membership. Flags, the peace sign, and a blue and yellow equal sign logo communicate a message that requires insider knowledge. Through the process of socialization, culture groups transmit shared networks of beliefs, values, and attitudes, which are modified over time by individuals' experiences in novel contexts (Oyserman & Sorensen, 2009). People are born into a culture, but they morph over their lifetimes shaped by their experiences and exposure to different cultures. For this reason it is important to perceive each individual person as a unique cultural being.

Culture can be conceived of as a process that is learned, localized, patterned, value based, and adaptive (Bonder & Martin, 2013). In this sense, culture can be viewed as a cumulative product of human endeavors that is by no means monolithic and that evolves over time. Culture can also be thought of as luggage that we carry around throughout our lives (Spector, 2004).

Theoretical Concepts in Culture

Anthropologist Edward T. Hall (1976) conceptualized high-context and low-context cultures to describe differing communication styles across cultures. People from a *high-context culture* know more about others in their cultural group implicitly and thus can understand the meaning of what is said without it being stated explicitly. Fewer words convey greater nuance because the parties share a consistent context, and the individual is firmly part of the group.

In *low-context cultures*, communication is clear and transparent even to those outside the cultural group. Communication is explicit, specific, and detailed to ensure that meaning is understood by people of diverse backgrounds or contexts, and the individual sees himself or herself as distinct from the group.

People from low-context cultures may miss the implied meaning in communication by people from high-context cultures unless they have a deep understanding of the high-context culture. Body language, tone of voice, and nonverbal communication are important in high-context communication. Because communication is based on relationships and degrees of trust, high-context communication varies depending on the situation and person.

Asian, Latin American, and Mediterranean countries are high context (Jandt, 2004b). Subcultures within these countries, however, may vary considerably. In general, the United States and northern European nations are low context; communication is literal, and words communicate the message in its entirety.

A popular and longstanding framework for understanding the culture of countries, organizations, and groups has five major dimensions (Hofstede, 2001):

1. *Power distance* refers to one's social position relative to the distribution of power in society.
2. *Individualism* versus *collectivism* refers to the degree of the individual's dependence or interdependence on others. The manner in which the social framework is loosely knit versus tightly knit.

3. *Uncertainty avoidance* involves the degree to which a society is able to tolerate an uncertain and ambiguous future.
4. *Masculinity* versus *femininity* refers to cultures that value masculine traits such as competition, assertion, bravado, and material rewards for success versus feminine attributes of cooperation, consensus, quality of life, and caring in society.
5. *Time orientation* refers to the relative degree to which a society values the past, present, and future.

All cultures contain aspects of these core concepts and differ in where they fall between the extremes in each dimension. It is best not to think of these concepts in an either/or manner but rather as a continuum, where cultures differ in the degree to which they value the two ends.

Table 1.1 summarizes the opposite ends of the continuum for each of the five major cultural dimensions. It is important to remember that people from the same culture are not all alike; intracultural diversity often exceeds intercultural diversity (Jandt, 2004b). So knowing a person's cultural identity does not tell his or her complete story. Rather, a given person's beliefs and behaviors reflect a specific point on a continuum and a blend of different attributes.

The cultural domains described in Table 1.1 influence the social organization of a society and behavioral attributes of people's interpersonal interactions, communication, and daily habits and routines. Certain behaviors and concepts fit better with each other. Individualism, for example, meshes well with a strong sense of self, control over context, a present orientation, and competition over resources to accomplish goals that advance the individual. Similarly, collectivism blends with group identity, hierarchy, harmony, cooperation, cyclical or past orientation, and individual goals that serve the common good of the collective.

Reflection 1.1. Cultural Domains

Consider the cultural domains and the continuum of attributes outlined in Table 1.1.

- Where do you place yourself along each continuum?
- What are the reasons for your choices?
- Are some of your choices more stable than others that may be situation dependent?

Table 1.1. Summary of the Continuum of the Major Cultural Domains

Cultural Domain	Continuum of Characteristics	
	One End--**Other End**	
Power	Equality is valued. Individual freedoms and choices are valued.	Hierarchy is valued. Status, kinship, and age determine one's position and importance in the hierarchy.
	Relationships are informal despite power differences.	Duty and obligations are formally established and respected.
	Relationships are oriented toward the individual.	Relationships are collateral or hierarchical.
	Confrontation is accepted.	Harmony is valued.
Sense of Self	*Individualist:* The "I" supersedes the "we."	*Collectivist:* The "we" supersedes the "I."
	Individual goals, achievement, and decision making are valued.	Collective goals, achievement, and decision making are valued. Members draw support from and are loyal to the group.
	Individual identity stems from individual attributes.	Individual identity stems from the group identity.
	Individual achievement, rights, self-esteem, and fulfillment are valued.	Group goals and solidarity, family duty, and social obligations are valued.
	The individual is the focus and is dominant over nature.	The environment is the focus, and the individual is in harmony with or subordinate to nature.
	Focus is on doing.	Focus is on becoming or being.
	Morality is defined by individuals and guided by individual motivations.	Morality is defined by the collective and guided by a sense of duty.
	Behavior reflects the individual's personality and attitudes.	Behavior is influenced by social norms and roles.
	The individual perceives control over reality.	The individual has an attitude of acceptance of reality.
	People have many and casual relationships.	People have few and enduring relationships.
Human–Nature Relationship	Humans dominant over Nature.	Humans in Harmony with Nature.
	Individuals are the focus.	Individuals and Environment are both in focus.
Human Activity	Doing is valued and is means to Being, Becoming, and Belonging.	Belonging is valued and influences Doing, Being, and Becoming.
Communication Style	Low degree of internalization or low context.	High degree of internalization or high context.
	Communication is explicit, specific, and detailed to the extent of redundancy.	Communication is implicit, does not need details, as context is consistent, shared, and internalized by the person.
Morality	Defined by individuals.	Defined by the collective.
	Guided by individual motivations.	Guided by sense of duty to the group.
Behavioral Flexibility	*Weak or low:* Attitudes toward behaviors are relaxed.	*Strong:* Behavioral codes are rigid.
	A certain degree of risk taking is tolerated.	Risk taking is generally not tolerated.
Preferred Gender Traits	*High masculinity:* Competition, achievement, and success are valued.	*High femininity:* Caring for others, quality of life, harmony, sharing, and cooperation are valued.
	Standing ahead of and apart from the crowd is admired.	One's standing among others is important.
Sense of Time	*Short term:* Focus is on the present.	*Long term:* Focus is on the past and future.
	Immediate gratification, current social standing, and ability to meet social obligations are valued.	Persistence, delayed gratification, thrift, and willingness to adapt are valued.
	Time is perceived as linear.	Time is perceived as cyclical.

Note. A culture, country, or individual does not necessarily occupy either end of the continuum but may fall at any point between the two extremes.
Sources. Gallagher, 2000, 2001; Hall, 1976; Hofstede, 2001; Jandt, 2004b; Kohls & Knight, 1994; Myers, 2013.

Culture and the Individual

Figure 1.1 depicts the nested cultural affiliations and allegiances people typically have. The level of influence most proximal to the individual is family and friends, and the more distal are the greater social contexts of community, nation, and world. Each level of influence confers a sense of belonging and identity while influencing a person's ways of knowing, doing, and being.

People acquire knowledge about their own culture from the inside. Cultural knowledge acquired early in life through socialization is called **emic knowledge.** Emic knowledge forms a view of how the world operates that, unless called into question, is taken for granted. When exposed to another culture, people have to learn **etic knowledge**—that is, information acquired explicitly in theoretical ways (e.g., by reading) or through observation (e.g., of people from that culture; Jandt, 2004b).

Socialization: Acquiring Emic Knowledge

A person's first cultural encounter is within the family context, and from parents in particular, through socialization that family values and attitudes are transmitted. **Socialization** is the process by which people acquire the characteristics of a culture group: Family members teach a child situation-appropriate behaviors initially, and as the child's circle expands,

community institutions such as the school system also contribute to socialization into the dominant cultural norms of the community and society. Socialization into multiple cultural groups occurs throughout the lifespan, and these experiences, which occur in various combinations and permutations, create the unique cultural mosaic of an individual.

Rapaille (2007) explored the idea that people acquire a silent and invisible system of coded communication as they grow up within a sociocultural milieu. **Culture codes** are "symbols and systems of meaning that are relevant to members of a particular culture or society" (Hyatt & Simons, 1999, p. 23). They influence how people process information, conduct their social lives, and assign hidden meanings to things. Culture codes work subconsciously, shaping behaviors that make a people distinctly American or French or Japanese. Hidden meanings are understood by those inside the culture group and are not available to those outside the group. However, with enough interactions over time and an understanding of nuanced cultural subtexts, outsiders can understand hidden meanings and thus acquire etic knowledge.

Membership in a group comes with the expectation that the individual accepts group values and norms, so deviation from normative behaviors can be a source of cultural conflict when emic knowledge contributes to bias, stereotypes, and attitudinal intolerances (Schneider & Ingram, 1993). Although people are socialized into their cultural group affiliations and environment, for most people

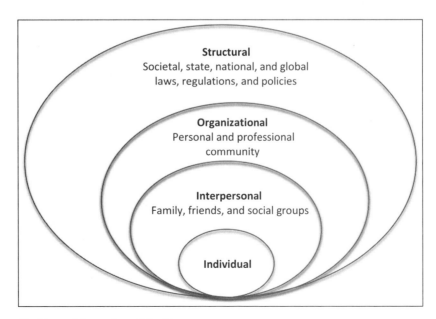

Figure 1.1. Cultural levels of influence.

neither the affiliations nor the environment are stable throughout their lifetime.

Migration: Acquiring Etic Knowledge

Migration patterns are highly varied, complex, and specific to migrants' local-level social, economic, and political contexts. Migration is also a consequence of the larger global economic and social processes of development and globalization (Collinson, 2009). Regardless of why migration occurs, successful integration in the new context is essential for occupational participation by the individual (see Chapter 2 for an expanded discussion of sociocultural influences on occupation).

Recent patterns of global migration include movement of people from less-industrialized nations to Western democracies such as the United States. People migrate for various reasons; some migrate by choice (e.g., to study or work), whereas others are forcefully displaced for reasons such as civil wars, natural disasters, and refugee resettlement. Some migrate with the intention of a temporary stay in the host country, some with the intention of relocating permanently.

The majority of recent immigrants in the United States are from Latin America and Asian countries (Zong & Batalova, 2015). Immigrants from these countries strive to balance the value of individualism they encounter in the larger American context with collectivism of their home countries within the family context. *Ethnogenesis* is a term coined by Flannery, Reise, and Yu (2001) to describe the "hybrid" culture that evolves through the blending of home or heritage culture and host or receiving culture. Again, although a group may generally behave in a communal way, individuals within the group vary in their degree of conformity to expected behaviors.

Acculturation occurs when people encounter and experience cultures that are different from their original culture; these transformative experiences shape and alter people, their occupations, and their environments. The United States is a nation of immigrants from many different parts of the world that illustrates *cultural pluralism,* a society in which individuals from different cultural groups coexist, enjoy the freedom to retain their cultural practices, and participate in the larger society. Acculturation is the process of cultural transformation that happens over time when individuals from different cultures interact continuously.

Linguists use the term *code switching* to describe the mixing of languages that happens with bilingual or multilingual speakers (Heredia & Altarriba, 2001). The idea of code switching can be expanded to include mixing behaviors and attitudes as adaptive strategies to cope with the stress of navigating different cultural spaces. For example, when I visit India, where I was born and spent my formative years into early adulthood, patterned cultural behaviors and mannerisms reemerge, such as how I greet elders or how I serve food during mealtimes, without my making any conscious effort. Even in the United States, when I am among people from the South Asian community, I speak and act differently without any effort. It is like I get back into my formative cultural self. Code switching is used by members of all cultural groups to fit in, to stand apart, or to communicate in a tacit manner in a context different from their most proximal or familiar context (Thompson, 2013).

Intersection Framework

A critique of focusing on culture to define an individual is that "it ignores the various social categories, such as social class, sexuality, gender, and age, that influence the health experiences and outcomes of minority patients" (Sears, 2012, p. 546). An individual belongs to different social subcultures that create a cultural mosaic unique to that particular individual. According to the *Intersection Framework,* popularized by critical scholars of identity politics across many disciplines, individuals occupy multiple social locations on the basis of their gender, social class, education, citizenship, sexual orientation, ability, age, and race and ethnicity (Collins, 1993; Rogers & Kelly, 2011). Some factors may be socially advantageous, whereas others may be a disadvantage. The Intersection Framework has two unique perspectives: (1) It considers the intersections among multiple issues (e.g., race, gender, class), and (2) it takes into account the social and political institutional inequities and power differentials that lead to and perpetuate cumulative disadvantages of certain disenfranchised groups.

The Intersection Framework draws attention to the assumptions held by dominant or privileged groups about the experiences of marginalized groups that are excluded from the mainstream social context of politics, culture, education, and economics on the basis of gender, sexuality, ability, race, or ethnicity. *Othering* is described as "a process that identifies those that are thought to be different from oneself or the mainstream, and it can reinforce and reproduce positions of domination and subordination" (Johnson et al., 2004, p. 253). Othering is a manifestation of power relations in society that creates a us-versus-them mentality as a way of differentiating a superior self from the perceived inferiority of those who are different (Dervin, 2011).

Culture and Values

Values, which exist at the core of any culture, are integral to cultural identity. Broadly, *values* are the principles or beliefs that people hold about what is fundamentally important in life. These beliefs influence behavioral standards and action and prescribe what is deemed as appropriate behavior given a particular situation.

Culture-specific values are beliefs, assumptions, attitudes, motivations, and behaviors adhered to by a specific culture group. They also are the lenses group members use to view themselves, the world, and outsiders. These values are often unconsciously taken for granted as self-evident by individual members of the culture group.

Schwartz (2012) identified six characteristics that all values share:

1. Values are beliefs that are related to emotions.
2. Values are concerned with desirable actions or goals.
3. Values transcend specific situations and actions.
4. Values set the norms or standards.
5. Values have a rank order of importance.
6. The relative importance of values is situation dependent and guides the course of action or behavior. (p. 3)

According to Schwartz, what distinguishes one value from another is "the type of goal or motivation it expresses" (p. 4). For example, the defining goal for the value of achievement is personal accomplishment through meeting the competencies and normative standards of the culture group, and the defining goal for the value of power is social status, prestige, dominance, and control over resources.

In diverse cultural terrains, values serve as anchors and guideposts, but they can also be a source of tension. For example, values related to conservation of tradition may contradict those related to openness to change, as illustrated by tension between first-generation immigrants and their children who desire to adopt the behaviors of their American peers to fit in and be accepted. Although the parents understand the importance of integrating into their adopted country, they also fear losing their original culture and their ability to transmit their cultural values (Gupta & Sullivan, 2013). Similarly, values that enhance self or the individual may contradict those aligned with interdependence that favor the common or collective good over the individual. Behaviors that stem from value systems thus are contextual, and people constantly evaluate the relative importance of their values in a given situation.

As important as values and beliefs are in explaining cultural dispositions, it must be reiterated that culture is complex and is a composite of other additional "interrelated orientations" (Qingxue, 2003, p. 22). Cultural values exist on a continuum, and their relative importance may vary across subcultures, subgroups, and situations.

Culture and Attitudes

Values serve as the basis for culturally motivated, appropriate behaviors and also for judgmental attitudes toward behaviors that do not fit a cultural way of doing. *Attitudes* are products of values and guide interpersonal behaviors and relationships. Jandt (2004b) observed that values define "[the] good or bad, beautiful or ugly, normal or abnormal, that are present in a majority of members of a culture or at least in those that occupy pivotal positions" (p. 7).

Theorists from multiple disciplines believe that values affect attitudes because they are the "criteria people use to evaluate actions, people and events" (Schwartz, 2012, p. 1). They also guide the organization of people's daily occupational lives in cultural groups to successfully enact socially patterned roles and responsibilities.

The *International Classification of Functioning, Disability and Health* ([ICF]; World Health Organization, 2001) identified attitudinal barriers as an environmental factor that can affect health and participation. Attitudes influence how people who look and act differently are treated in the dominant culture and judged in terms of their worth and value as human beings. *Attitudinal barriers* are prevailing negative ways of feeling or thinking in any society that affect interpersonal interactions, social inclusion, and participation for certain groups (e.g., racism). For example, people with disabilities experience multiple disadvantages in participation, work, and community integration because of the negative attitudes of people who are not disabled (Gupta, 2012; Pereira, 2013; Reiter & Bryen, 2010; Robert & Harlan, 2006; Shaw, Chan, & McMahon, 2012; Ward & Baker, 2005).

A person's place of birth and childhood socialization are very influential in cultural programming and exert influence on the attitudes held by insiders of a culture group toward outsiders. But throughout their lives, people learn, unlearn, and relearn concepts and ideas: Attitudes, like culture, are not static and can change over time.

Attitudes can affect therapeutic encounters and rehabilitation (Reiter & Bryen, 2010). Clients whose lifestyle choices, daily habits and routines, and ways of doing occupations deviate from practitioners' ideas of what is normative or desirable may challenge practitioners to adopt a nonjudgmental attitudes toward clients.

Culture in the United States

The United States is a complex society with many subcultures within the dominant culture that are based on social class, ethnicity, race, and geography (Jandt, 2004b). The larger cultural context of the United States, characterized by both great diversity and an identifiable national identity, permeates and influences all levels that it encompasses (see Figure 1.1).

Diversity

The United States is a nation of immigrants, and there have been four great waves of immigration. The first wave, from northern and western Europe, came during the frontier expansion phase, between 1820 and 1880. Between 1880 and 1920, during industrialization, the second wave of immigrants came primarily from southern and eastern Europe. Western Europe immigrants dominated during the immigration pause phase that extended from 1920 to 1960. The most recent great wave of immigrants, which began in 1965 and is ongoing, has come predominantly from Asia and Latin America (Martin & Midgley, 2006; Zong & Batalova, 2015).

Immigrants have adapted to the dominant culture through acculturation, and they have influenced the dominant culture in turn by exposing Americans to other cultures. The metaphors of a melting pot and a salad bowl are frequently used in describing American culture. The ***melting pot*** metaphor came into use very early in the 20th century and refers to the notion of a single American cultural identity in which immigrants forsake their original culture and adopt the dominant cultural values to assimilate into mainstream American culture. The ***salad bowl,*** a metaphor of more recent preference, captures the idea of immigrants' retaining their own culture while adopting aspects of mainstream culture to better participate in everyday life.

Cultural diversity in the United States resulting from the presence of many racial and ethnic groups has created a social milieu in which many people are naturally exposed to diverse worldviews and values. Over time, the original culture has been altered through this interaction with people of other cultures, and aspects of their cultures have been integrated with the original culture to create a ***hybrid culture*** (Berry, 1997). Societies in which people of different cultural groups live together, preserve their cultural heritage, and participate in broader national life are characterized by ***cultural pluralism.*** Within mainstream American culture, diverse cultural groups retain certain aspects of their own culture, which is a feature of a culturally pluralistic society. The presence of a Chinatown or Little Italy in many large cities, for example, has made Italian and Chinese cuisine a part of everyday food choices for many Americans.

National Identity

Since the first three great waves of immigrants came from Europe, European values have strongly influenced the dominant U.S. cultural values (Martin & Midgley, 2006). ***National identity*** is belief in a set of common core values and is essential for society to function.

Americans typically are perceived as religious, humanitarian, patriotic, informal, and direct (low-context) communicators. Other cultural values consistently associated with the United States include freedom of speech, individual rights, equal opportunity, achievement through hard work, and social mobility (Spindler, Spindler, Trueba, & Williams, 1990).

These values are not absolute or universal to all parts of the country. Values, traditions, and communication style vary between regions and individuals within the United States (Lun, Mesquita, & Smith, 2011). A valid question is, given the level of cultural pluralism in the United States, if there are cultural values and attributes that are uniquely American, that provide a national identity (Hing, 1993). In his first inaugural address, President Bill Clinton stated, "Each generation of Americans must define what it means to be an American" (Clinton, 1993, para. 1). This remark further illustrates that culture and cultural identity are dynamic concepts.

The degree to which a given culture group values the collectivist or individualist mentality varies; all groups harbor aspects of both extremes. In addition, individuals within a group vary in their acceptance of the dominant group values. For example, individual Americans vary in how much they accept the notions of rugged individualism and self-reliance that are the hallmark of the general American ethos. From a regional perspective, collectivist tendencies are strongest in the Deep South, whereas individualist tendencies are greatest in the Great Plains and Mountain West (Vandello & Cohen, 1999). Exhibit 1.1 summarizes some additional generally accepted American values (Jandt, 2004b; Kohls, 1984).

Globalization and Technology

Since the mid-20th century, globalization and technology have been drivers of the phenomenon of *world shrink*, which is the increased connectivity of all societies around the globe. Social media is a great example of global connectivity; in a matter of seconds, one can be aware of events occurring, in real time, across the world. World shrink has heightened people's awareness of the outer level of cultural influence (see Figure 1.1) and increased their sense of responsibility for those beyond their families, local communities, and nations. The need for corporate

Exhibit 1.1. Dominant U.S. Values

Dominion over nature and personal control over the environment	The individual and nature are separate, and human life is worth more than nature.
Science and technology	Faith in the ability of science and technology to solve societal problems is strong.
Progress and change, future orientation	Faith in the future and willingness to accept change are high. Change is good, including change in social values.
Perception of time	Time is a commodity and resource and hence must be managed, controlled, and used responsibly. Time is linear, and past, present, and future are clearly delineated.
Human nature	Humans are rational beings, are born with the potential for both good and evil, and are capable of being changed by society.
Interpersonal relationships	People define themselves by their occupation rather than relationships. Individuals maintain a separate self-concept that is not strongly tied to their family, make decisions independently, solve their own problems, and view the world from the point of the self.
Self-reliance and motivation	People are responsible for making the best of their lives by setting and pursuing goals.
Class	American class structure is based on power, money, and membership in influential social groups.
Equality and egalitarianism	All people are equal and have equal opportunities to build their lives.
Action and work orientation	Value is placed on doing. Work is part of one's primary identity and is taken very seriously. People define themselves by their productive occupation.
Competition and free enterprise	Achievement and success are valued. Freedom from government influence and regulations is desirable.
Practicality and efficiency	Life is organized to be productive in the most efficient manner possible. Short-term goals are favored as being more practical than long-term ones. The focus is on the here and now, and delayed gratification is not favored.
Materialism and acquisitiveness	Regarding possessions, the new is preferable to the old.

Sources. Jandt, 2004b; Kohls, 1984.

global connectivity, economic development in the developing world, the ease of global travel, and the Internet have routinized cross-cultural encounters and interactions. Advances in technology have made global communication cost-effective and accessible, and globalization has ushered in the free movement of people, goods, and services.

Globalization is the phenomenon of global economic cooperation and integration that has facilitated the easy movement of people, goods, services, ideas, and culture across nations. It also has been defined as "a process that encompasses the causes, course, and consequences of transnational and transcultural integration of human and non-human activities" (Al-Rodan & Stoudmann, 2006, p. 5).

Globalization and technology have enhanced the interrelated nature of nations, making it necessary for them to work together. Political and economic disruptions and the spread of infectious diseases in one part of the world reverberate around the globe and affect the entire global community, often in real time.

Globalization and Culture

The twin forces of globalization and technology have triggered a diffusion of culture across nations. Although definitions of globalization predominantly focus on the economic and technological characteristics, the social and cultural aspects of this phenomenon cannot be ignored. Changes in everyday cultural life brought about by the introduction of goods, ideas, and values from around the world is termed *cultural globalization* (Sanagavarapu, 2010).

The presence of American and European corporations and commodities in the developing world is transforming traditional cultures, habits, and routines. Concern about the erosion of traditional cultural values and integration of Western cultural perspectives and lifestyles has been raised as globalization ushers in the integration and uniformity of commerce, technology, and language around the world.

Cultural imperialism is "the economic, technological and cultural hegemony of the industrialized nations, which determines the direction of both economic and social progress, defines cultural values, and standardizes the civilization and cultural environment throughout the world" (Sarmela, 1977, p. 13). Western ideologies, beliefs, moral concepts, sexual symbols and ideals of beauty, working methods and leisure activities, foods, and pop idols have often been construed as the "best" norms to emulate, resulting in the dilution of traditional culture and sometimes even a backlash against Western influence.

Technology and Culture

Technology and culture influence each other reciprocally; as culture evolves, so does technology and vice versa. Technology changes the beliefs and behaviors of individuals in any society, altering their ways of doing and being. Digital communication has revolutionized connectivity, albeit paradoxically: People are more connected than ever in the digital space, whereas interpersonal interactions and face-to-face conversations in real time are increasingly rare (Turkle, 2012). The influences of globalization and telecommunications have not only fostered integration of national economies but also increased the flow of information and movement of people and goods across national borders.

The term *cyber imperialism* has recently emerged to describe cultural imperialism via the Internet (Gittinger, 2014). Few societies are beyond the reach of technology and globalization. Cyber imperialism's influences are bidirectional, however, in that American society is influenced and transformed by different cultures just as American and European influences are changing non-Western cultures.

The Culture of Occupational Therapy

Every profession has a unique culture that influences its practitioners' ways of thinking and doing. The profession's values, beliefs, and attitudes shape the behaviors and traditions accepted by members of the profession. The areas of expertise and specialization that develop around the core focus of the profession determine the contexts of practice (Hall, 2005). In the process of professional education, students are socialized into their profession's culture and become acculturated into the professional identity.

Occupational therapy has its own understanding of culture, and it has its own culture. Diversity in American society has made multiculturalism increasingly relevant to and imperative for occupational therapy research, theory, and practice. The profession is challenged to make its traditional approach to promoting participation in occupations responsive to a critical approach to culture. Attention to the role of culture in occupation will benefit the profession as the need for multicultural practice increases (Castro, Dahlin-Ivanoff, & Mårtensson, 2014).

The occupational therapy profession's unique culture is based on its foundational values and beliefs. This section discusses occupational therapy values, the culture of the health care system in which many occupational therapists practice, and sources of tension caused by differences in these two value systems.

Occupational Therapy Values

Occupational therapy, like all others, is a value-laden profession. Several of occupational therapy's most important values are the centrality of occupation, client-centered practice, autonomy, and individualism. Taken together, occupational therapy's values constitute a professional cultural bias that practitioners must keep in mind in multicultural practice.

Centrality of Occupation

Since the genesis of the occupational therapy profession a century ago, occupation has remained its foundational construct. Practitioners have always used occupation as the vehicle to promote the health and well-being of disadvantaged people through enabling participation in activities they found meaningful (Gordon, 2009; Head & Friedland, 2011). Participation in occupation thus is the most representative value of the profession (Drolet, 2014), the profession's cultural identity or essence (Watson, 2006) that distinguishes occupational therapy from other health professions.

The occupational therapy profession's philosophy of occupation as the means and ends to health, well-being, and quality of life uniquely situates it to empower people of diverse cultures to participate in their everyday occupational roles and responsibilities. The profession's practice is configured around occupation, and the occupational lens is used to view the client, the environment, and occupation (Yerxa, 1998). Prominent occupational therapy conceptual practice models, such as the Person–Environment–Occupation Model (Law et al., 1996), the Model of Human Occupation (Kielhofner, 2009), and Occupational Adaptation (Schkade & Schultz, 1992; Schultz & Schkade, 1992), support the transactional relationship among the person, occupation, and environment to guide holistic practice.

Client-Centered Practice

What distinguishes authentic occupational therapy is its emphasis on ***client-centered practice,*** which is aimed at facilitating occupational performance in natural contexts (Gupta & Taff, 2015; Hammell, 2013; Sumsion & Law, 2006). Client-centered practice is a philosophical approach to the therapist–client relationship that is grounded in the values of respect, autonomy, dignity, and empowerment (Canadian Association of Occupational Therapists [CAOT], 2013; Sumison & Law, 2006) and essentially recognizes clients as the experts on their occupational lives (Gupta & Taff, 2015).

The occupational therapy profession was founded on the belief that engaging clients in meaningful and purposeful occupations has the potential to heal and restore health and that using occupations clients identify as important and meaningful promotes their motivation to actively engage in the therapy process. Client-centered practice, introduced in occupational therapy nearly 30 years ago in Canada (CAOT, 2002, 2013), has come to be accepted as the way occupational therapy should be practiced. By focusing on clients' strengths and soliciting their input during the therapy process, practitioners collaborate and share their power and responsibility with clients (Hammell, 2013; Sumsion & Law, 2006).

Autonomy

The need for autonomy is universal across cultures and is associated with well-being. ***Autonomy*** refers to people's capacity to be their own authentic self and to live according to their personal motivations and not just externally imposed standards and expectations (Christman, 2015). Autonomy is often used to connote independence or individualism, but autonomy is primarily concerned with one's freedom and ability to act. Therefore, autonomy is valued by all cultural groups, including those that value interdependence over independence and collectivism over individualism (Chirkov, Ryan, Kim, & Kaplan, 2003).

Individualism

The relative degree of individualism varies across Western nations, and both the United States and the occupational therapy profession in general are considered to highly value individual freedoms and personal responsibility. Scholars have critiqued the individualistic view of occupation in occupational science, to the point that context is in the background (Fogelberg & Frauwirth, 2010; Laliberte Rudman, 2015). Similarly, Dickie, Cutchin, and Humphry (2006) critiqued the prevailing tendency to conceptualize occupation as residing within the individual and to view the person and context as distinct from each other, arguing that this tendency limits the understanding of occupation and of the relationship of person and context.

Some occupational therapy scholars have suggested another perspective that combines the individual and context. *Transactionalism* views the person and the environment in a confluent, uninterrupted manner in which occupation transforms the environment, and occupation is shaped by both the person doing it and the environment in which it is being done (Aldrich, 2008; Cutchin, 2004; Cutchin & Dickie, 2012; Kuo, 2011). For instance, the *Kawa Model* reflects a transactional relationship from the Eastern worldview of the person and environment as existing in harmony when they are whole and seamless (Iwama, 2009). Using nature to capture the essential belief of human–environment harmony as essential to life, the Kawa Model uses the image or metaphor of a river as a representation of life course and of the ease and hardships one encounters in daily life.

Recognizing Professional Cultural Bias

Occupational therapy practitioners are cultural beings who are products of their own sociocultural milieu. Professional education socializes them to the profession's values and worldview. It is important for practitioners to recognize these values and worldview and to be aware of their personal and professional biases regarding occupations and health (Whiteford & Wilcock, 2000).

Scholars have critiqued the focus on the individual in the study of occupation and practice, arguing that the profession's Eurocentric origins reflect the sociocultural context in which they practice (Iwama, 2003). Consider how little racial and ethnic diversity is represented in the profession: In 2014, 85.3% of occupational therapy practitioners were White, whereas 3.1% were African American or Black, 3.2% were Hispanic or Latino, 4.4% were Asian or Pacific Islander, and 1.4% were multiethnic (American Occupational Therapy Association [AOTA], 2015, p. 10). Thus, for the majority of occupational therapy practitioners, their cultural ancestry is European.

Awareness of their professional bias is important to enable occupational therapy practitioners to practice from an empowered stance and in a culturally effective manner. As Hammell (2009) asserted, "assumptions underpinning occupational therapy's theories of occupation are culturally specific, class-bound, ableist, and lacking in supportive evidence" (p. 107). The profession's view of the relationship between occupations and health and well-being may not resonate with all clients (Iwama, 2003). Therefore, occupational therapy practitioners must think critically and question the relevance of the profession's beliefs and tenets in practice with clients of diverse cultural origins.

Biomedical Culture of the Health Care System

As a health profession, occupational therapy culture is affected by the *biomedical culture* of the health care system, which views the purview of health care as treating impairments in body systems (e.g., nervous system) caused by pathology (e.g., cerebrovascular accident), trauma (e.g., traumatic brain injury from a motor vehicle accident), and other health conditions (e.g., infection such as meningitis). In 2014, the majority of occupational therapy practitioners (65.8%) worked in medical settings: 25.8% worked in long-term care or skilled nursing facilities, 23.9% in hospital settings, 9.8% in freestanding outpatient rehabilitation settings, and 6.3% in home health care (AOTA, 2015, p. 16). The predominantly biomedical paradigm of the health care context has important implications for occupational therapy practice within medical settings.

Current Paradigms of Health and Well-Being

The dominant paradigms of health and well-being in the literature offer contrasting perspectives on how health is viewed with respect to the person and the environment (Stewart & Law, 2003; World Health Organization [WHO], 2001). As Table 1.2 shows, the medical and social paradigms form two extremes that lay responsibility for health and well-being on either the individual (medical paradigm) or society (social paradigm). Neither captures the complexity of health, participation in social life, or disability as well as the *biopsychosocial paradigm,* which holds that biological, psychological, and social factors play an equally significant role in human functioning

Table 1.2. Contrasting Paradigms of Health and Well-Being

Concept	Medical Paradigm	Biopsychosocial Paradigm	Social Paradigm
Locus of the problem	Individual	Individual and society	Society
Assumptions about health	Biomedical	Biomedical, psychosocial, and sociocultural	Sociocultural
	Health as the absence of disease	Health and well-being as more than the absence of disease	Health and well-being as more than the absence of disease
	Disease as caused by malfunctioning of body systems and processes	Interactions of personal factors and contextual factors as contributing to health and ill health through activity limitations	Interactions of factors within and outside of the person as contributing to health and ill health
View of disability	Deviation from normative biomedical functioning resulting from disease, trauma, and so forth	Interaction of personal factors and environmental factors to produce activity limitations that affect participation	Social construct that results from the built environment
View of the environment	Person and environment as separate	Person and environment as interactive	Person and environment as interactive
	Environmental factors as contributing to disease (e.g., infectious agents)	Interaction between a person's body systems and body functions and contextual factors as determining health condition	Broad environmental factors as influencing health, including physical, social, cultural, societal, and institutional factors
Context of intervention	Medical care	Context-specific care Medical care setting in acute and subacute stages Community setting for non–life-threatening stages	Sociopolitical activism for rights and integration
Who intervenes	Health professionals and experts	Health professionals in partnership with the individual Individual and collective social responsibility	Individual and collective social responsibility
Target of intervention	Individual: Change individual behaviors to adapt to environment	Both individual and environmental: Eliminate micro-level, meso-level, and macro-level barriers to enable participation	Environmental: Manipulate meso-level and macro-level environment to enable participation
Desired outcome	Cure or functional restoration of the person	Health and well-being through participation and social integration	Health promotion and social integration
	Change in individual behavior	Change in individual and social behaviors and attitudes	Change in individual and social behaviors and attitudes
Mediatory mechanisms	Health insurance	Health insurance, social policies, and legislation	Social policies and legislations

(WHO, 2001). This paradigm best matches occupational therapy's culture and values.

Global adoption of the biopsychosocial paradigm (AOTA, 2014; CAOT, 2013; World Federation of Occupational Therapists, 2005) supports the profession in addressing contextual factors and their contributions to occupational issues, health, and well-being and in embracing an ideological shift from the biomedical paradigm to the biopsychosocial paradigm more consistent with the profession's culture. Occupational therapy practitioners also must advocate for the biopsychosocial paradigm to promote occupational justice, including access to services and inclusive sociocultural conditions that support health-sustaining occupations and equitable participation for all members of society. Occupational justice is the topic of Chapter 3 of this volume.

Role of Evidence

The scientific protocols and methodology that are suitable for medicine may not be optimal for occupational therapy. Practitioners must critically evaluate the compatibility of research evidence with the philosophy of occupational therapy practice before applying the evidence in practice (Gustafsson, Molineux, & Bennett, 2014). The ethics of clinical reasoning must take into account not only evidence and reimbursement policies but also client need as a matter of justice: "When [resource] allocation decisions are linked to the availability of evidence, matters of justice are at stake" (Vos, Willems, & Houtepen, 2004, p. 166).

Kielhofner (2004) identified three periods of paradigm shift in the culture of the profession. In its early years, from 1900 to 1950, there was general consensus in the occupational underpinnings of the profession. In the 1960s, the profession adopted the mechanistic paradigm of medicine. Since the 1980s, the profession has been reclaiming its roots in occupation. During this time, the language surrounding evidence-based practice percolated into the medical landscape (Sackett, Strauss, Richardson, Rosenberg, & Haynes, 2000), and recognition of the need to ground medicine in scientific evidence in health care put pressure on other health professions, including occupational therapy.

In the United States, the occupational therapy profession responded by developing the field of occupational science as a knowledge base for occupational therapy (Clark et al., 1991, 1993; Pierce, 2014). *Occupational science* is the study of humans as occupational beings and the occupational meanings, experiences, and contextual aspects that enrich the health, well-being, and quality of human lives.

A parallel development occurred in Australia under the leadership of Wilcock (1998). There, however, occupational science was conceptualized very differently, going beyond traditional occupational therapy practice to align with interdisciplinary population health (Wilcock, 1998). The Australian view focuses on population health and contextual and social factors that contribute to occupational justice and influence policy.

Occupational justice (the subject of Chapter 3 of this volume) refers to the right of people to engage in occupations to sustain their health and well-being (Townsend & Wilcock, 2004). In contrast, the American perspective of occupational science is to produce knowledge that will support the effectiveness of occupational therapy practice (Pierce, 2014).

Occupational therapy practitioners must uphold the values of the profession and use the definition of *evidence-based practice* in its entirety: "the integration of best research evidence with clinical expertise and patient values" (Sackett et al., 2000, p. 1). Although Sackett and colleagues provided a hierarchy of levels of evidence, it does not appear that they proposed using any particular level to the exclusion of all others. Use of information from multiple and diverse sources to obtain a holistic understanding of the clinical scenario is required of practitioners.

Cultural Tension Between Occupational Therapy and the Health Care System

Occupational therapy practice in environments that do not share the profession's worldview of participation is culturally conflicted, which affects practitioners' professional identity and creates dissonance in the being and doing of occupational therapy. The value of client centeredness, for example, conflicts with the focus on disease and impairments in medical settings, in which health professionals are the experts on curing and fixing clients' problems. Time and resources have been cited as common barriers to client-centered practice (Sumsion & Smyth, 2000).

The biomedical culture of health care has been critiqued for its focus on disease and illness and impairments (Stewart & Law, 2003). The biomedical culture's reductionist perspective of health as the absence of disease and its focus on treating disease and other impairments is suitable for medicine but is incongruent with occupational therapy's holistic view of health.

The **ICF** *model* includes both personal and environmental factors among the influences on health, and medicine is increasingly adopting this biopsychosocial model (WHO, 2001). Despite this progress, many aspects of the medical context remain philosophically incongruent with the paradigms of occupational therapy (Kielhofner, 2004; Molineux & Baptiste, 2011).

Holistic practice, a fundamental tenet of the occupational therapy profession, is challenged by reimbursement, scope of practice issues, billing codes, and organizational role delineation. The health care industry culture and norms influence practitioners' behaviors and services. However, the health care system is not the client's natural environment, and the very purpose of medical settings constrains and compromises occupation-based practice (Gupta & Taff, 2015).

Recent calls for a return to the roots of the profession support the need for occupational therapy practitioners to "return occupation to the center of occupational therapy practice" (Molineaux, 2010, p. 361). It is widely accepted that occupation-based interventions are capable of promoting health, well-being, and quality of life and that occupational participation itself is a determinant of health and well-being (CAOT, 2013; Stadnyk, Townsend, & Wilcock, 2010). Maintaining a focus on occupation will guide practitioners in aligning their practice with the profession's foundational philosophy, values, and beliefs when they experience conflict with the culture of the health care system.

Reflection 1.2. Culture and Occupational Therapy

- Why is culture relevant to occupational therapy?
- As American society becomes increasingly diverse, what challenges and opportunities will occupational therapy practitioners encounter in managing multiple cultures: the culture of health care, the profession, society, the client, and themselves?

Summary

Culture is an incredibly relevant personal and contextual factor contributing to human occupation, identity, and health. Client-centered practice requires seeing people as unique occupational beings whose identity is informed by the multiple cultural affiliations they hold. Cultural influences, including community, organizations, professions, and society as a whole, are important because they determine social arrangements, policy and politics, resource allocation, opportunities, and access to occupation and participation.

Although people can be seen as cultural beings, it is not helpful to consider culture in isolation, apart from human–human and human–environment interactions. Occupational therapy practitioners should work to perceive individuals in a dynamic process of negotiating and enacting occupational behaviors depending on their context.

References

Aldrich, R. M. (2008). From complexity theory to transactionalism: Moving occupational science forward in theorizing the complexities of behavior. *Journal of Occupational Science, 15,* 147–156. http://dx.doi.org/10.1080/14427591.2008.9686624

Al-Rodan, N. R. F., & Stoudmann, G. (2006). *Definitions of globalization: A comprehensive overview.* Geneva: Geneva Center for Security Policy.

American Occupational Therapy Association. (2015). *2015 AOTA salary and workforce study.* Bethesda, MD: AOTA Press.

Berry, J. W. (1997). Immigration, acculturation and adaptation. *Applied Psychology: An International Review, 46,* 5–34. http://dx.doi.org/10.1111/j.1464-0597.1997.tb01087.x

Bonder, B., & Martin, L. (2013). *Culture in clinical care: Strategies for competence* (2nd ed.). Thorofare, NJ: Slack.

Canadian Association of Occupational Therapists (CAOT). (2002). *Enabling occupation: An occupational therapy perspective* (2nd ed.). Ottawa, ON: Author.

Canadian Association of Occupational Therapists (CAOT). (2013). *Enabling occupation II: Advancing an occupational therapy vision for health, well-being, and justice through occupation* (2nd ed.). Ottawa, ON: Author.

Castro, D., Dahlin-Ivanoff, S., & Mårtensson, L. (2014). Occupational therapy and culture: A literature review. *Scandinavian Journal of Occupational Therapy, 21*(6), 401–414. http://dx.doi.org/10.3109/11038128.2014.898086

Chirkov, V., Ryan, R. M., Kim, Y., & Kaplan, U. (2003). Differentiating autonomy from individualism and independence: A self-determination theory perspective on internalization of cultural orientations and well-being. *Journal of Personality and Social Psychology, 84*(1), 97. http://dx.doi.org/10.1037//0022-3514.84.1.97

Christman, J. (2015). Autonomy in moral and political philosophy. In E. N. Zalta (Ed.), *The Stanford encyclopedia of philosophy.* Stanford, CA: Stanford University. Retrieved from http://plato.stanford.edu/archives/spr2015/entries/autonomy-moral

Clark, F., Parham, D., Carlson, M. E., Frank, G., Jackson, J., Pierce, D., & Zemke, R. (1991). Occupational science: Academic innovation in the service of occupational therapy's future. *American Journal of Occupational Therapy, 45*, 300–310. http://dx.doi.org/10.5014/ajot.45.4.300

Clark, F., Zemke, R., Frank, G., Parham, D., Neville-Ian, A., Hendricks, C., . . . Abreu, B. (1993). Dangers inherent in the partition of occupational therapy and occupational science. *American Journal of Occupational Therapy, 47*, 184–186. http://dx.doi.org/10.5014/ajot.47.2.184

Clinton, W. J. (1993). *Inaugural address, January 20, 1993*. Online by Gerhard Peters and John T. Woolley, *The American Presidency Project*. http://www.presidency.ucsb.edu/ws/index.php?pid=46366

Cole, M., & Parker, M. (2011). Culture and cognition. In K. D. Keith (Ed.), *Cross-cultural psychology: Contemporary themes and perspectives* (pp. 133–159). Chichester, England: Wiley-Blackwell.

Collins, P. H. (1993). Toward a new vision: Race, class, and gender as categories of analysis and connection. *Race, Sex and Class*, 25–45. http://www.jstor.org/stable/41680038

Collinson, S. (2009). *The political economy of migration processes: An agenda for migration research analysis*. Oxford, England: International Migration Institute. Retrieved from http://www.imi.ox.ac.uk/pdfs/wp/wp-12-09.pdf

Cutchin, M. P. (2004). Using Deweyan philosophy to rename and reframe adaptation-to-environment. *American Journal of Occupational Therapy, 58*, 303–312. http://dx.doi.org/10.5014/ajot.58.3.303

Cutchin, M. P., & Dickie, V. (2012). Transactionalism: Occupational science and pragmatic attitude. In G. E. Whiteford & C. Hocking (Eds.), *Occupational science: Society, inclusion, participation* (pp. 23–37). Hoboken, NJ: Wiley-Blackwell.

Dervin, F. (2011). Cultural identity, representation, and othering. In J. Jackson (Ed.), *Routledge handbook of intercultural communication*. London: Routledge.

Dickie, V., Cutchin, M. P., & Humphry, R. (2006). Occupation as transactional experience: A critique of individualism in occupational science. *Journal of Occupational Science, 13*, 83–93. http://dx.doi.org/10.1080/14427591.2006.9686573

Drolet, M.-J. (2014). The axiological ontology of occupational therapy: A philosophical analysis. *Scandinavian Journal of Occupational Therapy, 21*, 2–10. http://dx.doi.org/10.3109/11038128.2013.831118

Flannery, W. P., Reise, S. P., & Yu, J. (2001). An empirical comparison of acculturation models. *Personality and Social Psychology Bulletin, 27*, 1035–1045. http://dx.doi.org/10.1177/0146167201278010

Fogelberg, D., & Frauwirth, S. (2010). A complexity science approach to occupation: Moving beyond the individual. *Journal of Occupational Science, 17*, 131–139. http://dx.doi.org/10.1080/14427591.2010.9686687

Gallagher, T. J. (2000). Value orientations and conflict resolution: Using the Kluckhohn Value Orientations Model. In K. W. Russo (Ed.), *Finding the middle ground: Insight and applications of the value orientations method* (pp. 185–194). Yarmouth, ME: Intercultural Press.

Gallagher, T. J. (2001). The value orientations method: A tool to help understand cultural differences. *Journal of Extension, 39*(6). Retrieved from http://www.joe.org/joe/2001december/tt1.php

Gittinger, J. L. (2014). Is there such a thing as "cyberimperialism"? *Continuum: Journal of Media and Cultural Studies, 28*, 509–519. http://dx.doi.org/10.1080/10304312.2014.907873

Gordon, D. (2009). The history of occupational therapy. In E. B. Crepeau, E. Cohn, & B. A. B. Schell (Eds.), *Willard and Spackman's occupational therapy* (11th ed., pp. 202–215). Philadelphia: Lippincott Williams & Wilkins.

Gupta, J. (2012). An issue of occupational (in)justice: A case study. *Disability Studies Quarterly, 32*(3). http://dx.doi.org/10.18061/dsq.v32i3.3280

Gupta, J., & Sullivan, C. (2013). The central role of occupation in the doing, being and belonging of immigrant women. *Journal of Occupational Science, 20*, 23–35. http://dx.doi.org/10.1080/14427591.2012.717499

Gupta, J., & Taff, S. (2015). The illusion of client-centred practice. *Scandanavian Journal of Occupational Therapy, 22*, 244–251. http://dx.doi.org/10.3109/11038128.2015.1020866

Gustafsson, L., Molineux, M., & Bennett, S. (2014). Contemporary occupational therapy practice: The challenges of being evidence based and philosophically congruent. *Australian Occupational Therapy Journal, 61*, 121–123. http://dx.doi.org/10.1111/1440-1630.12110

Hall, E. T. (1976). *Beyond culture*. New York: Anchor Books.

Hall, P. (2005). Interprofessional teamwork: Professional cultures as barriers. *Journal of Interprofessional Care, 19*(Suppl. 1), 188–196. http://dx.doi.org/10.1080/13561820500081745

Hammell, K. W. (2009). Sacred texts: A sceptical exploration of the assumptions underpinning theories of occupation. *Canadian Journal of Occupational Therapy, 76*, 6–13. http://dx.doi.org/10.1177/000841740907600105

Hammell, K. W. (2013). Client-centred occupational therapy in Canada: Refocusing on core values. *Canadian Journal of Occupational Therapy, 80*, 141–149. http://dx.doi.org/10.1177/0008417413497906

Head, B., & Friedland, J. (2011). Jessie Luther: A pioneer of social justice. *Occupational Therapy Now, 13*(1), 17–18. Retrieved from http://www.caot.ca/otnow/jan11/luther.pdf

Heredia, R. R., & Altarriba, J. (2001). Bilingual language mixing: Why do bilinguals code-switch? *Current Directions in Psychological Science, 10*, 164–168. http://dx.doi.org/10.1111/1467-8721.00140

Hing, B. O. (1993). Beyond the rhetoric of assimilation and cultural pluralism: Addressing the tension of separatism and conflict in an immigration-driven multiracial society. *California Law Review, 81,* 863–925. http://dx.doi.org/doi:10.15779/ Z38NM8Q

Hofstede, G. (2001). *Culture's consequences: Comparing values, behaviors, institutions, and organizations across nations.* Thousand Oaks, CA: Sage.

Hong, Y.-Y. (2009). A dynamic constructivist approach to culture: Moving from describing culture to explaining culture. In R. S. Wyer, C.-Y. Chiu, & Y.-Y. Hong (Eds.), *Understanding culture: Theory, research and application* (pp. 3–23). New York: Psychology Press.

Hyatt, J., & Simons, H. (1999). Cultural codes—Who holds the key? The concept and conduct of evaluation in Central and Eastern Europe. *Evaluation, 5*(1), 23–41. http://dx.doi.org /10.1177/13563899922208805

Iwama, M. (2003). The issue is—Toward culturally relevant epistemologies in occupational therapy. *American Journal of Occupational Therapy, 57,* 582–588. http://dx.doi.org/10.5014 /ajot.57.5.582

Iwama, M. K., Thomson, N. A., & Macdonald, R. M. (2009). The Kawa model: The power of culturally responsive occupational therapy. *Disability and Rehabilitation, 31*(14), 1125–1135. http://dx.doi.org/10.1080/09638280902773711

Jahoda, G. (2012). Critical reflections on some recent definitions of "culture." *Cultural Psychology, 18,* 289–303. http://dx.doi .org/10.1177/1354067X12446229

Johnson, J. L., Botorff, J. L., & Browne, A. J., Grewal, S., Hilton, B. A., & Clarke, H. (2004). Othering and being othered in the context of health care services. *Health Communication, 16*(2), 255–271. http://dx.doi.org/10.1207/S15327027 HC1602_7

Jandt, F. E. (2004a). *Intercultural communication: A global reader.* Thousand Oaks, CA: Sage.

Jandt, F. E. (2004b). *An introduction to cultural communication: Identities in a global community* (4th ed.). Thousand Oaks, CA: Sage.

Kielhofner, G. (2004). *Conceptual foundations of occupational therapy practice.* Philadelphia: F. A. Davis.

Kielhofner, G. (2009). The model of human occupation. In *Conceptual foundations of occupational therapy practice* (4th ed., pp. 147–174). Philadelphia: F. A. Davis.

Kohls, L. R. (1984). *The values Americans live by.* New York: Meridian House International.

Kohls, L. R., & Knight, J. M. (1994). *Developing intercultural awareness: A cross-cultural training handbook* (2nd ed.). Yarmouth, ME: Intercultural Press.

Kuo, A. (2011). A transactional view: Occupation as a means to create experiences that matter. *Journal of Occupational Science, 18,* 131–138. http://dx.doi.org/10.1080/14427591 .2011.575759

Laliberte Rudman, D. (2013). Enacting the critical potential of occupational science: problematizing the 'individualizing of occupation.' *Journal of Occupational Science, 20*(4), 298–313. http://dx.doi.org/10.1080/14427591.2013.803434

Law, M., Cooper, B., Strong, S., Stewart, D., Rigby, P., & Letts, L. (1996). The Person–Environment–Occupation Model: A transactive approach to occupational performance. *Canadian Journal of Occupational Therapy, 63,* 9–23. http://dx .doi.org/10.1177/000841749606300103

Lun, J., Mesquita, B., & Smith, B. (2011). Self- and Other-presentational styles in the Southern and Northern United States: An analysis of personal ads. *European Journal of Social Psychology, 41*(4), 435–445. http://dx.doi.org/10.1002 /ejsp.804

Martin, P., & Midgley, E. (2006). *Immigration: Shaping and reshaping America* (2nd ed.). Washington, DC: Population Reference Bureau. Retrieved from http://www.prb.org/pdf06 /61.4USMigration.pdf

Mead, M. (1935). *Sex and temperament in three primitive societies.* New York: William Morrow.

Molineux, M. (2010). Occupational science and occupational therapy: Occupation at centre stage. In C. Christiansen & E. Townsend (Eds.), *Introduction to occupation: The art and science of living* (2nd ed., pp. 359–383). Upper Saddle River, NJ: Prentice Hall.

Molineux, M., & Baptiste, S. (2011). Emerging occupational therapy practice: Building on the foundations and seizing the opportunities. In M. Thew, M. Edwards, S. Baptiste, & M. Molineux (Eds.), *Role emerging occupational therapy: Maximising occupation-focused practice* (pp. 3–14). West Sussex, England: Wiley-Blackwell.

Myers, D. G. (2013). *Psychology* (10th ed.). New York: Worth Publishers.

Oyserman, D., & Sorensen, N. (2009). Understanding cultural syndrome effects on what and how we think. In R. S. Wyer, C.-Y. Chiu, & Y.-Y. Hong (Eds.), *Understanding culture: Theory, research and application* (pp. 25–52). New York: Psychology Press.

Pereira, R. (2013). *The politics of participation: A critical occupational science analysis of social inclusion policy and entrenched disadvantage.* Unpublished doctoral dissertation, Macquarie University, Sydney, Australia.

Pierce, D. (2014). *Occupational science for occupational therapy.* Thorofare, NJ: Slack.

Qingxue, L. (2003). Understanding different cultural patterns or orientations between East and West. *Investigationes Linguisticae, 9,* 21–30. Retrieved from http://www.staff.amu .edu.pl/~inveling/pdf/liu_quingxue_inve9.pdf

Rapaille, C. (2007). *The culture code: An ingenious way to understand why people around the world live and buy as they do.* New York: Broadway Books.

Reiter, S., & Bryen, D. N. (2010). Attitudinal barriers to rehabilitation. In J. H. Stone & M. Blouin (Eds.), *International encyclopedia of rehabilitation*. Buffalo, NY: Center for International Rehabilitation Research Information and Exchange, University at Buffalo SUNY. Retrieved from http://cirrie.buffalo.edu/encyclopedia/en/article/297/

Robert, P. M., & Harlan, S. L. (2006). Mechanisms of disability discrimination in large bureaucratic organizations: Ascriptive inequalities in the workplace. *Sociological Quarterly, 47,* 599–630. http://dx.doi.org/10.1111/j.1533-8525.2006.00060.x

Rogers, J., & Kelly, U. A. (2011). Feminist intersectionality: Bringing social justice to health disparities research. *Nursing Ethics, 18*(3), 397–407. http://dx.doi.org/10.1177/0969733011398094

Sackett, D. L., Strauss, S. E., Richardson, W. S., Rosenberg, W., & Haynes, R. B. (2000). *Evidence-based medicine: How to practice and teach EBM* (2nd ed.). Edinburgh, Scotland: Churchill Livingstone.

Sanagavarapu, P. (2010). What does cultural globalisation mean for parenting in immigrant families in the 21st century? *Australasian Journal of Early Childhood, 35*(2), 36–42.

Sarmela, M. (1977). What is cultural imperialism? In C. Sandbacka (Ed.), *Cultural imperialism and cultural identity* (pp. 13–36). Helsinki: Finnish Anthropological Society. Retrieved from http://www.kotikone.fi/matti.sarmela/culturimperialism.pdf

Schkade, J. K., & Schultz, S. (1992). Occupational adaptation: Toward a holistic approach to contemporary practice, Part 1. *American Journal of Occupational Therapy, 46,* 829–837. http://dx.doi.org/10.5014/ajot.46.9.829

Schneider, A., & Ingram, H. (1993). Social construction of target populations: Implications for politics and policy. *American Political Science Review, 87,* 334–347. http://dx.doi.org/10.2307/2939044

Schultz, S., & Schkade, J. K. (1992). Occupational adaptation: Toward a holistic approach to contemporary practice, Part 2. *American Journal of Occupational Therapy, 46,* 829–837. http://dx.doi.org/10.5014/ajot.46.10.917

Schwartz, S. H. (2012). An overview of the Schwartz theory of basic values. *Online Readings in Psychology and Culture, 2*(1). Retrieved from http://dx.doi.org/10.9707/2307-0919.1116

Sears, K. P. (2012). Improving cultural competence education: The utility of an intersectional framework. *Medical Education, 46,* 545–551. http://dx.doi.org/10.1111/j.1365-2923.2011.04199.x

Shaw, L. R., Chan, F., & McMahon, B. T. (2012). Intersectionality and disability harassment: The interactive effects of disability, race, age, and gender. *Rehabilitation Counseling Bulletin, 55*(2), 82–91. http://dx.doi.org/10.1177/0034355211431167

Spector, R. E. (2004). *Cultural diversity in health and illness* (6th ed.). Upper Saddle River, NJ: Prentice Hall.

Spindler, G. D., Spindler, L., Trueba, H., & Williams, M. D. (1990). *The American cultural dialogue and its transmission.* New York: Farmer Press.

Stadnyk, R., Townsend, E., & Wilcock, A. (2010). Occupational justice. In C. Christiansen & E. Townsend (Eds.), *Introduction to occupation: The art and science of living* (pp. 329–358). Upper Saddle River, NJ: Pearson Education.

Stewart, D., & Law, M. (2003). The environment: Paradigms and practice in health, occupational therapy, and inquiry. In L. Letts, P. Rigby, & D. Stewart (Eds.), *Using environments to enable occupational performance* (pp. 3–15). Thorofare, NJ: Slack.

Sumsion, T., & Law, M. (2006). A review of evidence on the conceptual elements informing client-centred practice. *Canadian Journal of Occupational Therapy, 73,* 153–162. http://dx.doi.org/10.1177/000841740607300303

Sumsion, T., & Smyth, G. (2000). Barriers to client-centredness and their resolution. *Canadian Journal of Occupational Therapy, 67,* 15–21. http://dx.doi.org/10.1177/000841740006700104

Thompson, M. (2013). *Five reasons why people code-switch* [Blog post]. Retrieved from http://www.npr.org/blogs/codeswitch/2013/04/13/177126294/five-reasons-why-people-code-switch

Turkle, S. (2012). *Alone together: Why we expect more from technology and less from each other.* New York: Basic Books.

Vandello, J., & Cohen, D. (1999). Patterns of individualism and collectivism across the United States. *Journal of Personality and Social Psychology, 77,* 277–292. http://dx.doi.org/10.1037/0022-3514.77.2.279

Vos, R., Willems, D., & Houtepen, R. (2004). Coordinating the norms and values of medical research, medical practice and patient worlds—The ethics of evidence based medicine in orphaned fields of medicine. *Journal of Medical Ethics, 30,* 166–170. http://dx.doi.org/10.1136/jme.2003.007153

Wan, C., & Chiu, C. (2009). An intersubjective consensus approach to culture: The role of intersubjective norms versus cultural self in cultural processes. In R. S. Wyer, C.-Y. Chiu, & Y.-Y. Hong (Eds.), *Understanding culture: Theory, research and application* (pp. 79–91). New York: Psychology Press.

Ward, A. C., & Baker, P. M. A. (2005). Disabilities and impairments: Strategies for workplace integration. *Behavioral Sciences and the Law, 23,* 143–160. http://dx.doi.org/10.1002/bsl.631

Watson, R. M. (2006). Being before doing: The cultural identity (essence) of occupational therapy. *Australian Occupational Therapy Journal, 53,* 151–158. http://dx.doi.org/10.1111/j.1440-1630.2006.00598.x

Whiteford, G. E., & Wilcock, A. A. (2000). Cultural relativism: Occupation and independence reconsidered. *Canadian Journal of Occupational Therapy, 67,* 324–336. http://dx.doi.org/10.1177/000841740006700505

Wilcock, A. A. (1998). Reflections on doing, being and becoming. *Canadian Journal of Occupational Therapy, 65,* 248–257. http://dx.doi.org/10.1177/000841749806500501

World Federation of Occupational Therapists. (2005). *World Federation of Occupational Therapists (WFOT) code of ethics.* Forrestfield, Western Australia: Author.

World Health Organization. (2001). *International classification of functioning, disability and health.* Geneva: Author.

Yerxa, E. J. (1998). Occupation: The keystone of a curriculum for a self-defined profession. *American Journal of Occupational Therapy, 52,* 365–372. http://dx.doi.org/10.5014/ajot.52.5.365

Zong, J., & Batalova, J. (2015). *Frequently requested statistics on immigrants and immigration in the United States.* Washington, DC: Migration Policy Institute. Retrieved from http://www.migrationpolicy.org/article/frequently-requested-statistics-immigrants-and-immigration-united-states

Chapter 2.

SOCIOCULTURAL ASPECTS OF OCCUPATION

Jyothi Gupta, PhD, OTR/L, FAOTA

Culture makes people understand each other better. And if they understand each other better in their soul, it is easier to overcome the economic and political barriers. But first they have to understand that their neighbor is, in the end, just like them, with the same problems, the same questions.
Paulo Coelho (2010, para. 10)

Chapter Highlights

- Sociocultural Aspects of Occupation
- Sociocultural Ways of Doing
- Sociocultural Ways of Being
- Sociocultural Ways of Belonging

Key Terms and Concepts

✧ Being in place
✧ Cultural distance
✧ Habitus
✧ Individual identity
✧ Integrated identity
✧ Intersectionality theory

✧ Occupation
✧ Occupational identity
✧ Performance
✧ Society
✧ Sociocultural influences
✧ Vertical mosaic

Culture shapes *occupation,* or the everyday activities people do to occupy their time, take care of themselves, enjoy life, and contribute to society. "Occupations are various kinds of life activities in which individuals, groups, or populations engage, including activities of daily living, instrumental activities of daily living, rest and sleep, education, work, play, leisure, and social participation" (American Occupational Therapy Association [AOTA], 2014, p. S19). These everyday activities are named, organized, and given value and meaning by people and their culture (Canadian Association of Occupational Therapists & Health Services Directorate, 2013).

Culture and occupations mutually influence and shape each other. Because culture and occupations both exist in a social context, they are subject to social influences. Consider these questions:

- How do social and cultural factors influence occupation?
- How do interpersonal interactions affect everyday occupational choices?
- How does the social position of different cultural groups shape occupational choices and opportunities?

These questions are complex and have no easy answers, but they are relevant to untangling the intricate relationships among culture, human occupations, and social conditions in a culturally diverse society. This chapter examines sociocultural aspects of occupation and the ways of doing, ways of being, and ways of belonging that contribute to how people experience occupation.

Sociocultural Aspects of Occupation

Humans are social beings. Neither culture nor occupation exists in a vacuum, so human occupation might best be understood in terms of a combination of cultural and social factors—that is, *sociocultural influences*—because it is impossible to tease the cultural from the social. An understanding of occupations and daily life patterning as socially constructed, particular, and context specific is necessary to appreciate the diversity of beliefs and attitudes that motivate individuals and groups to organize their daily occupations to support their notions of what constitutes a good and healthy life. Occupational performance, experiences, meaning, and identity are based on values upheld in a particular sociocultural context.

Differing Perspectives on Occupation

Western social institutions have had a profound influence on the occupational therapy profession's conceptualization of occupation, health, and what constitutes a good life (Kantartzis & Molineux, 2011). The profession's view of occupation as active, purposeful, temporal, and meaningful derives from Western Anglophone perspectives. Classification of

occupations into categories such as self-care and productive activity has been described as value laden and decontextualized and as failing to capture the subjective perspectives of the doer (Aldrich, McCarty, Boyd, Bunch, & Balentine, 2014; Hammell, 2009).

The occupational therapy profession's focus on functional ability and independence has been critiqued as not resonating with many interdependent societies (Whiteford & Wilcock, 2000). Japanese occupational therapists, for example, are socialized differently by their cultural context, which is characterized by dependence or interdependence, one's position in the hierarchy, a dynamic location of power, hard work and enduring hardship as virtues, and the values of obligation, responsibility, and situatedness (Kondo, 2004). These values, in turn, may not resonate with those of other collectivist societies around the world.

Reflection 2.1. Values and Beliefs

- Which of the profession's values and beliefs about human occupation resonate with your personal values and beliefs?
- Are there some aspects of the profession's values and beliefs that you do not agree with or have difficulty accepting?
- How do you explain the fit or lack of fit with your own personal values and beliefs?

Occupation, Place, and Identity

Occupational scientists have researched the reciprocal relationship of place and occupation to identity. Conceptual models such as the Person–Environment–Occupation model (Law et al., 1996) and AOTA's (2014) *Occupational Therapy Practice Framework: Domain and Process* view the person–environment–occupation relationship as transactional.

The meaning that people associate with a particular space and particular activity transforms space into place and activity into occupation. Huot and Rudman (2010) used the sociological concepts of *habitus* (i.e., lifestyle, values, and disposition) and *performance* (i.e., everyday life activities that are observable by others) to show the interconnectedness of occupation, place, and identity. The performance or doing of daily occupations is how habits and routines are developed and performed in sociocultural contexts.

The *doing* of occupation in turn influences a person's *being* by contributing to his or her sense of self and identity. Doing also is a means for the person's *becoming*, that is, a life-long process of growth, self-actualization, and reaching one's full potential (Wilcock, 1998). Finally, through doing and being, people also gain a sense of *belonging* (Rebeiro, 2004), a concept that is positively correlated with well-being and resonates with people from diverse cultures (Hammell, 2014). Humans as occupational beings enact their everyday lives not just to meet their individual basic needs, but to exercise their capabilities to create meaning, satisfaction, and contributions to benefit self, community, society, and humanity.

Reflection 2.2. Occupation, Place, and Identity

- How have occupations and place contributed to your identities?
- Have you ever experienced the loss of occupational identity or the loss of meaning of a particular occupation?
- What factors contributed to this loss?

Reflection 2.3. Sociocultural Environment

- How has your sociocultural environment influenced your occupations in terms of choices, meaning, interest, and opportunities?

Sociocultural Ways of Doing

Culture influences people's choice of occupations (Kondo, 2004). Culture also influences the organization of everyday life occupations and how they are performed. Customs, rituals, routines, and behaviors are dictated by cultural norms and expectations. Cultural and social values influence the relative importance of certain occupations over others, the meanings attached to occupations, and how occupations are orchestrated.

Orchestration of Daily Occupations

Occupations are culturally and socially sanctioned, and they help structure how time and resources are organized and used. Habits and routines evolve over time and change depending on context-specific attributes (Bonder, 2007). Temporal and spatial organization of occupations also depend on the

economy (Kantartzis & Molineux, 2011; Larson & Zemke, 2003). In rural areas of developing nations, artisan-based economies, typical of the preindustrialization era of Western nations, persist in which the place of dwelling and work are not spatially separate. This arrangement makes personal and productive occupations spatially seamless.

With industrialization and the need for mass production, factories were built that physically separated one's place of living from the workplace and also compartmentalized time into work time and personal time for self-care, home, and leisure occupations (Kantartzis & Molineux, 2011). Specialization and the rise of professionals further fragmented society into multiple subcultures and classes (Sarmela, 1977). Interestingly, technology has again made it possible for people to work from home. The orchestration of daily occupations varies across cultures, is shaped by the nature of the economy, and structures people's day and pace of life.

The ongoing American Time Use Survey captures the average time spent on various daily activities, such as work, child care, socializing, household work, and so on (U.S. Bureau of Labor Statistics [BLS], 2013). Time-use data have been collected by the BLS since 2003 and provide a snapshot of how much time people allocate to different aspects of their lives. This survey is useful both in informing public policy (e.g., policies concerning maternity leave and benefits) and as a measure of well-being. American culture is frequently described as fast paced and action oriented, and generally people want to do as much as they can in any given day (Brown, 2014). The Centers for Disease Control and Prevention (2015) has reported that sleep deprivation is a national epidemic.

Schulte (2014) captured the American fixation on time management and staying busy and the perception that leisure is inconsequential and a waste of time. The United States is the only industrialized country that does not have a vacation policy for all its workers; nearly 25% of Americans do not get paid vacation, and 40% of those who get paid vacation do not take it (Ray, Sanes, & Schmitt, 2013).

Occupational Experiences of Immigrants

The occupational challenges experienced by immigrants illustrate how a change in the sociocultural environment alters occupational lives by changing the way everyday occupations are performed. A change in context alters the meaning of some occupations. Losing collective occupations and interdependence that perhaps characterized the original culture can render meaningful occupations merely functional activities (Gupta & Sullivan, 2013).

Because it is difficult to bring to conscious awareness the taken-for-granted acceptance of dominant cultural ways of doing, the occupational experiences of immigrants are valuable in making visible the invisible and enabling one to "see" American and Western culture. Occupational scientists' research on immigrants and refugees provides good examples that illustrate the interwoven relationships between the sociocultural context and occupation. The process of integration for immigrants is the means for creating meaning in daily occupational lives in an unfamiliar and challenging sociocultural environment. Understanding these challenges makes visible and highlights dominant sociocultural behaviors, expectations, and ways of doing.

Cultural Distance and Adjustment

All people experience the tug between the cultural values of the place in which they were socialized during their formative years and other places they visit for short periods or take up residence in, on either a temporary or more permanent basis. In the case of long-term residence, adjustment is complex, and integration requires a recalibration of values, beliefs, traditions, habits, and routines. This is also true for the dominant group; the host environment is changed through interactions among culturally diverse inhabitants.

Cultural distance refers to the degree to which two cultures are similar or different (Hofstede, 2001). It appears intuitive that adjustment may be easier across cultures that are similar, but studies have shown that people who perceive the other culture as similar to their own do not expect to adjust very much. So when unanticipated differences are encountered, the adjustment process is experienced as difficult (Selmer, 2007). People's mindset and personal characteristics, such as level of education, age, and gender, affect the adjustment and integration process (Jenkins & Mockaitis, 2010).

The process of integration is complex, posing multiple challenges that people must overcome to reconstruct their lives in a new context. The meaning of places, like occupations, is socially constructed, so the same place may have different meanings for different people. Meaning making of place is based on its purpose, memory of meaningful shared experiences associated with the place, and familiarity (Hamilton, 2010). When, over time, a familiar place or environment becomes subsumed as part of the self, a sense of *being in place* is established (Rowles, 1991, 2000).

Relocation to a new place necessitates establishing a sense of place. Immigrants' integration into a different sociocultural environment entails successful orchestration of daily occupations that over time enables their being in place. Nayar (2009) described how Indian immigrants in New Zealand performed occupations that reflected either the Indian or New Zealand cultures, or a combination of both cultures, to create a place where they could be Indian in the New Zealand context. Immigrants create *being in place* by retaining cultural habits, routines, rituals, and behaviors while incorporating new behaviors of new cultural environment. Examples include celebrating festivals, preparing culture-specific meals, women working outside of home or driving, men helping out with family chores, communicating in a new language, adopting new ways of dressing, and incorporating exercise in daily routine.

Daily Occupation in Identity (Re)Construction

A special thematic issue on occupation, immigration, and well-being of the *Journal of Occupational Science* illustrates the recent interest of occupational scientists in understanding how displacement and migration affect the occupational lives and well-being of immigrants and refugees (Gupta, 2013b). A theme across articles describing studies situated in many different immigrant-receiving Western nations was "the centrality of daily occupations in immigrant identity reconstruction, health and well-being, and the complexity of the process of social integration" (Gupta, 2013a, p. 1).

A scoping review of the immigrant literature identified how immigration involves changes in roles, work, identity, health, and well-being (Bennett, Scornaiencki, Brzozowski, Denis, & Magalhães, 2012). For immigrants from a less modern, industrialized, and technology-based society, it can be overwhelming to navigate in an unfamiliar context that is markedly different from their home country. Immigrants have to contend with disruption to their established occupational lives; roles, habits, and routines established in their home country must be reconfigured to meet the demands of the new context, and new occupational and cultural identities need to be constructed.

Occupation is the vehicle for adjustment and integration, and the use of occupations to adapt, adjust, and integrate into a new sociocultural context has been reported (Gupta & Sullivan, 2008; Nayar, Hocking, & Giddings, 2012). Table 2.1 provides examples showing that almost all aspects of daily occupational life—parenting, mealtime

Table 2.1. Occupational Experiences of Immigrants: Themes From the Occupational Science Literature

Occupational Experience	Theme
Change in the meaning of occupation	Schedules, productivity, and efficiency at the workplace may alter the meaning of work for people from free-flowing or rigid work environments. Busy lifestyles and conflicting schedules may lead to loss of collective family occupations. Lack of time and isolation can change meaningful occupations into functional activities. Assertive communication adopted by children may challenge traditional parenting practices. Inability to own a car or drive may create barriers to participation; when they become possible, acquiring a car and learning to drive can be empowering (Gupta & Sullivan, 2013).
Productive occupation (work)	Government and official documents consider "economic productivity as the occupation-based marker of integration," influencing the process of integration in complex ways (Huot, Rudman, Dodson, & Magalhães, 2013, p. 6). Downward economic mobility and underemployment affect many immigrants because of the devaluation of foreign credentials, lack of work experience in the host country, loss of social capital, lack of fit in gendered occupations, and time required for the resettlement process (Gupta & Sullivan, 2008; Mpofu & Hocking, 2013; Suto, 2013).
Meal preparation and routines	Meal preparation as a collective and social occupation may be lost. In Western societies, where meals are prepared in isolation for the nuclear family, cooking becomes "shortened, chunked and functional" (Gupta & Sullivan, 2013, p. 28) and thus is not the same occupation (Torp, Berggren, & Erlandsson, 2013). Family members may be unable to eat their meals together because of schedule conflicts, which may be viewed as a loss of culture (Gupta & Sullivan, 2013). Altered sensory experiences of grocery shopping and the taste of food may create a sense of alienation (Bailliard, 2013; Torp et al., 2013). Mealtime occupations can be a site for the enactment of cultural rituals and behaviors that connect past to present and keep original culture alive (Farias & Asaba, 2013).
Gendered occupational roles	Traditional roles and gendered occupations may have to be renegotiated; for example, men who traditionally did not do housework may have to begin to contribute (Torp et al., 2013; Gupta & Sullivan, 2008, 2013). Immigrant women may prioritize their time toward family obligations (e.g., aiding others in the resettlement process, helping those left behind) and learning the dominant language over their vocational aspirations (Gupta & Sullivan, 2013; Heigl, Kinébanian, & Josephsson, 2011). For women from more traditional cultures, paid employment may be empowering and liberating (Gupta & Sullivan, 2008, 2013).
Community mobility	Driving a car can be a novel and liberating occupation (Gupta & Sullivan, 2008, 2013).
Child rearing	Mealtimes can be a source of contention when children reject traditional food in favor of foods preferred in the host culture. Gupta and Sullivan (2008) found that "immigrants may change their eating habits and traditions out of a desire to fit in" (p. 30). Tensions may arise between children wanting to assimilate and parents wanting to impart traditional cultural values (Gupta & Sullivan, 2008, 2013; Vang, 2005).

(Continued)

Table 2.1. Occupational Experiences of Immigrants: Themes From the Occupational Science Literature (Cont.)

Occupational Experience	Theme
Leisure and social belonging	Immigrant children often develop bicultural occupational repertoires to belong in the blended environment (Lencucha, Davis, & Polatajko, 2013). Lack of time and unfamiliarity with local leisure occupations may mean that immigrants consider playing with their children, talking to extended family during free time, and talking to their spouse at the end of the day to be leisure activities (Suto, 2013). Traditional occupations, such as weaving by Karen women from Myanmar living in Utah, can be a vehicle for cultural identity maintenance, socialization, and economic benefits (Stephenson, Smith, Gibson, & Watson, 2013). Music making can be used to integrate and create a sense of place and belonging (Adrian, 2013). People who are not allowed to work because of visa restrictions (Syverson, 2005) and who are seeking asylum (Burchett & Matheson, 2010) may feel an intense unmet need for belonging.
Health and well-being	Immigrants may experience threats to their occupational identity and efficacy because of occupational losses. The cultural meaning of occupations can be altered in the new context (Gupta & Sullivan, 2013; Krishnagiri, Fuller, Ruda, & Diwan, 2013; Suto, 2013). Many immigrants experience occupational challenges and disruptions (Bailliard, 2013; Farias & Asaba, 2013; Gupta & Sullivan, 2008, 2013; Johansson et al., 2013; Krishnagiri et al., 2013; Mpofu & Hocking, 2013; Suto, 2013). Occupational deprivation through restrictions on use of one's skills can make it difficult to fill the day (Morville & Erlandsson, 2013).

routines, home management, community mobility, and social participation—have to be reconfigured in the new cultural environment.

Many immigrant families and communities continue to celebrate traditional festivals as a way to transmit the cultural heritage to the next generation and build community with others of the ethnic diaspora. For some, however, celebrating traditional cultural events does not hold much meaning and value because such events are decontextualized and lack the essential elements of a collective occupation: shared experience with extended family, community, and the larger social context. Doing occupation or not doing occupation shapes the being and identity of the person.

Reflection 2.4. Ways of Doing

- What are some of the ways of doing occupations that you take for granted and assume that others do in the same way?
- Have you ever been challenged when you traveled to another cultural context to continue to perform occupations in your typical ways?

Sociocultural Ways of Being

Internalization of sociocultural values and behaviors is an important aspect of identity formation (Erikson, 1968). The term *occupational identity* was coined by Kielhofner (2002), who defined it as the identity as an occupational being that is forged through participation in occupations. Christiansen (1999) was among the first to explicitly link occupation to an individual's personal and social identity. It is not just *doing* occupations that contributes to occupational identity; *being* also encompasses the total expression of the physical, cognitive, affective, and spiritual aspects of human nature in various environments across the lifespan during engagement in various occupations (Unruh, Versnel, & Kerr, 2002).

The social environment and participation in socially sanctioned occupations influence occupational identity. Phelan and Kinsella (2009), citing theorists on the social construction of identity, identified the need for occupational therapy practitioners to move beyond the individual and doing to consider the ways in which involvement in society, culture, and social relationships may actually shape, form, or even produce occupational identity.

Because the United States is considered a multicultural society, is there such a thing as a shared American culture that all those who reside in this country are socialized into? According to Appiah (1994), a *society* is a group of people with shared geography, social institutions, and culture. Therefore, by this definition, "unless Americans also share a culture, there is no American society" (p. 2). There is little doubt, however, that the mainstream culture and worldview in the United States is the Euro-American worldview that has historically valued rugged individualism, mastery and control over nature, competition, and religion based on Christianity. These elements continue to influence social organizations, arrangements, and institutions to the present day.

Individual Identity

Psychology and sociology describe *individual identity* as a person's sense of self—the conception and expression of one's own individual identity, referred to as *self-identity*, and other identities shared through group affiliations, such as national identity and cultural identity (Adams & Marshall, 1996; Deaux, 2006). Thus, although people hold a unique self-identity, they simultaneously hold multiple social group identities.

When dealing with social identities that are based on race, ethnicity, ability, and so forth, occupational therapy practitioners must exercise caution not to assume that all members who share a collective identity form a homogenous group (Appiah, 1994). This perception of members of a group as identical or alike is what leads to stereotyping, bias, and attitudinal issues, which are covered in more depth in Chapter 6, "Cultural Self-Awareness, Critical Reflection, and Transforming Attitudes."

Integrated Identity

Liu (2014), a second-generation immigrant and author, pointed out that his identity includes "American-ness" that is completely infused with "Chinese-ness." He refers to himself as *Chinese American,* without a hyphen. *"American* is the noun, *Chinese* the adjective. Or, rather, Chinese is one adjective. I am many kinds of American, after all: a politically active American, a short American, an earnest American, an educated American" (Liu,

2014, para. 5). The idea of an *integrated identity* resonates with a majority of long-term residents as well as more recent immigrants (Berry, 1997, 2008; Gupta & Sullivan, 2008) and speaks to the multiple cultural identities (through affiliation with subcultures) that all Americans hold.

Social Status

Social stratification, or groups' social position on the basis of certain characteristics, occurs in all societies, including the United States (Coburn, 2010; Reeves, 2014). For example, socioeconomic status confers class status, and groups may be upper class, middle class, or lower class. The *vertical mosaic* locates different cultural groups in different class positions in society, with White Anglo-Saxon people at the top and Black or Native people at the bottom (Porter, 1965). Location along the vertical dimension determines access to resources, power, and privilege that, in turn, influence access to occupational opportunities. Complex and intersecting pathways of sociopolitical and sociocultural influences determine a group's position in the social hierarchy and their occupational context, choices, resources, and access to participation.

In sociology, *intersectionality theory* includes the idea that people hold multiple social locations or statuses based on characteristics such as gender, age, sexual orientation, disability, nationality, ethnicity, and race (Castiello Jones, Misra, & McCurley, 2013). *Social status* or *location* is important in determining one's life trajectory because the availability of and access to opportunities and resources are dependent on social status. Personal factors alone, such as self-determination and motivation, are insufficient to achieve one's occupational potential if the living context is impoverished. Achievement of occupational potential requires the social context to convey the necessary resources, security, stability, and access to occupational opportunities.

Current social location and social attitudes toward any group are influenced by historical legacy and relationships. Marginalized and oppressed groups "live under an umbrella of individual, institutional, and cultural forces that often demean them, disadvantage them, and deny them access and opportunity" (Sue, 2006, p. 48).

Often, the visible, a person's tip-of-the-iceberg characteristic such as external appearance (e.g., skin color, attire, accent, behaviors that are contrary to expected norms) is used as the basis for assumptions, stereotyping, and bias. The submerged part of the iceberg represents the underlying cultural values, assumptions, and thought processes that motivate behaviors and attitudes that may be different from what are deemed the norm. Submerged attitudes are unknown or not obvious to outsiders until they invest the time and effort to interact with and understand people of different cultural groups.

Although a person may be discriminated against on the basis of external observable traits, these traits may or may not define who they are as a person. For example, a person who looks Asian or African may be more American in worldview than Asian or African. Social status is generally affiliated with higher levels of education, which has the potential to change how people think and perceive life situations, and higher earnings, both of which increase the individual's access and exposure to resources.

Perceived cultural differences are the main basis for treating people differently (Sears, 2012). Results of a landmark study reported 83,000 excess deaths per year (i.e., above deaths among White Americans) in the African American community (Satcher et al., 2005). One of this study's authors, Troutman, stated in the documentary *Unnatural Causes* (California Newsreel, 2008) that being positioned high on the socioeconomic gradient did not insulate him from attitudinal issues:

> I'm highly educated. I have a medical degree. I have several other degrees. I make good money. I live in a good neighborhood. But I know that according to the research, if you're an African American, no matter what your social status, your socioeconomic status, your health outcomes are going to be worse than your white counterpart. (p. 14)

Although Troutman's identity and social location placed him in a privileged bracket (on the basis of education, class, and the social status of a medical doctor), prevailing social attitudes toward African Americans put him at risk for poor health outcomes. How an individual is perceived in society affects his or her being, identity, health, and social inclusion.

Sociocultural Ways of Belonging

The need to belong is a basic human need, and occupations are vehicles for bringing people together and conferring a sense of belonging. This process is easier in an open community that values diversity, inclusion, and equitable distribution of resources.

People live and participate in individual and collective occupations in personal and public spaces in their communities. With time, social connections are established through shared interests or beliefs (Christiansen & Townsend, 2010). The experience of shared occupations is key to creating social identity, building social networks, and building a cohesive community. These social connections are forged in places of work, worship, volunteerism, neighborhood parks and community centers, and more.

Social groups can be an informal or formal arrangement for coming together for a common purpose. Membership in groups generally is based on some criteria and expectations. For example, people who are interested in birds, wildlife, conservation of habitats, and ecosystems and want a shared and collective experience might seek membership in the local chapter of the National Audubon Society. A popular occupation for book lovers is participating in book clubs in their local communities or in virtual communities.

Every culture has examples of social groups from all areas of occupation, including leisure, sports, art, and music, to mention a few. Even in a fast-paced, individualistic society like the United States, people belong to multiple social groups in pursuit of collective occupations that are of interest and benefit them personally or professionally.

The social media have revolutionized how people connect temporally and spatially. A quick search on the Internet easily identifies multiple options for finding a group based on any occupation of interest. Groups that are organized around shared beliefs, values, interests, and purpose are basically cultural and social microcosms. Everyday interaction is a multicultural social environment that profoundly affects perception of self in relation to others (Harris, 2009).

Summary

The sociocultural aspects of occupation influence the occupations people engage in, the ways they perform occupations across contexts, and the sense of belonging they gain from participation in social occupations. Immigrants' occupational experiences make explicit many aspects of the implicit dominant culture. Occupational therapy practitioners are encouraged to be aware of the profession's cultural view of occupation as they work with their clients, who may have other views on occupation.

References

Adams, G. R., & Marshall, S. K. (1996). A developmental social psychology of identity: Understanding the person-in-context. *Journal of Adolescence, 19,* 429–442.

Adrian, A. (2013). An exploration of Lutheran music-making among US immigrant and refugee populations. *Journal of Occupational Science, 20,* 160–172. http://dx.doi.org/10.1080/14427591.2013.775690

Aldrich, R. M., McCarty, C. H., Boyd, B. A., Bunch, C. E., & Balentine, C. B. (2014). Empirical lessons about occupational categorization from case studies of unemployment. *Canadian Journal of Occupational Therapy, 81,* 289–297. http://dx.doi.org/10.1177/0008417414540129

American Occupational Therapy Association. (2014). Occupational therapy practice framework: Domain and process (3rd ed.). *American Journal of Occupational Therapy, 68*(Suppl. 1), S1–S48. http://dx.doi.org/10.5014/ajot.2014.682006

Appiah, K. A. (1994). *Identity against culture: Understandings of multiculturalism.* Berkeley, CA: Doreen B. Townsend Center for the Humanities. Retrieved from http://townsendcenter.berkeley.edu/sites/default/files/publications/OP01_Appiah.pdf

Bailliard, A. L. (2013). The embodied sensory experiences of Latino migrants to Smalltown, North Carolina. *Journal of Occupational Science, 20,* 120–130. http://dx.doi.org/10.1080/14427591.2013.774931

Bennett, K. M., Scornaiencki, J. M., Brzozowski, J., Denis, S., & Magalhães, L. (2012). Immigration and its impact on daily occupations: A scoping review. *Occupational Therapy International, 19,* 185–203. http://dx.doi.org/10.1002/oti.1336

Berry, J. (1997). Immigration, acculturation and adaptation. *Applied Psychology, 46,* 5–34. http://dx.doi.org/10.1111/j.1464-0597.1997.tb01087.x

Berry, J. (2008). Globalisation and acculturation. *International Journal of Intercultural Relations, 32,* 328–336. http://dx.doi.org/10.1016/j.ijintrel.2008.04.001

Bonder, B. R. (2007). An occupational perspective on cultural evolution. *Journal of Occupational Science, 14,* 16–20. http://dx.doi.org/10.1080/14427591.2007.9686579

Brown, S. (2014). *Speed: Facing our addiction to fast and faster and overcoming our fear of slowing down.* New York: Berkley Books.

Burchett, N., & Matheson, R. (2010). The need for belonging: The impact of restrictions on working on the well-being of an asylum seeker. *Journal of Occupational Science, 17,* 85–91. http://dx.doi.org/10.1080/14427591.2010.9686679

California Newsreel. (2008). *Unnatural causes: Is inequality making us sick? In sickness and in wealth.* Retrieved from http://www-tc.pbs.org/unnaturalcauses/assets/resources/in_sickness_and_wealth_transcript.pdf

Canadian Association of Occupational Therapists & Health Services Directorate. (1983). *Guidelines for the client-centred practice of occupational therapy.* Ottawa: Health Services Directorate.

Castiello Jones, K., Misra, J., & McCurley, K. (2013). *Intersectionality in sociology.* Lawrence, KS: Sociologists for Women in Society. Retrieved from http://www.socwomen.org/wp-content/uploads/swsfactsheet_intersectionality.pdf

Centers for Disease Control and Prevention. (2015). *Insufficient sleep is a public health epidemic.* Retrieved from http://www.cdc.gov/features/dssleep/

Christiansen, C. H. (1999). Defining lives: Occupation as identity: An essay on competence, coherence, and the creation of meaning (Eleanor Clarke Slagle Lecture). *American Journal of Occupational Therapy, 53,* 547–558. http://dx.doi.org/10.5014/ajot.53.6.547

Christiansen, C. H., & Townsend, E. (2010). *Introduction to occupation: The art of science and living* (2nd ed.). Upper Saddle River, NJ: Prentice Hall.

Coburn, D. (2010). Health and health care: A political economy perspective. In T. Bryant, D. Raphael, & M. Rioux (Eds.), *Staying alive: Critical perspectives on health, illness and healthcare* (2nd ed., pp. 65–90). Toronto: Canadian Scholars Press.

Coelho, P. (2010). *Interview with Paulo Coelho, UN messenger of peace.* Geneva: UN News Center. Retrieved from http://www.un.org/apps/news/newsmakers.asp?NewsID=27

Deaux, K. (2006). *To be an immigrant.* New York: Russell Sage Foundation.

Erikson, E. H. (1968). *Identity, youth, and crisis.* New York: Norton.

Farias, L., & Asaba, E. (2013). "The family knot": Negotiating identities and cultural values through the everyday occupations of an immigrant family in Sweden. *Journal of Occupational Science, 20,* 36–47. http://dx.doi.org/10.1080/14427591.2013.764580

Gupta, J. (2013a). Occupation, well-being and immigration [Editorial]. *Journal of Occupational Science, 20,* 1–2. http://dx.doi.org/10.1080/14427591.2013.774683

Gupta, J. (Ed.). (2013b). Occupation, well-being and immigration [Special issue]. *Journal of Occupational Science, 20*(1). http://dx.doi.org/10.1080/14427591.2013.792316

Gupta, J., & Sullivan, C. (2008). Enabling immigrants to overcome participation challenges. *OT Practice, 13*(5), 25–32.

Gupta, J., & Sullivan, C. (2013). The central role of occupation in the doing, being and belonging of immigrant women. *Journal of Occupational Science, 20,* 23–C. http://dx.doi.org/10.1080 /14427591.2012.717499

Hamilton, L. B. (2010). Occupation and places. In Christensen and E. Townsend (Eds.), *Introduction to occupation: The art and science of living* (pp. 251–279). Upper Saddle, NJ: Pearson Education.

Hammell, K. W. (2009). Sacred texts: A skeptical exploration of the assumptions underpinning theories of occupation. *Canadian Journal of Occupational Therapy, 76,* 6–13. http://dx.doi .org/10.1177/000841740907600105

Hammell, K. W. (2014). Belonging, occupation, and human well-being: An exploration. *Canadian Journal of Occupational Therapy, 81,* 39–50. http://dx.doi.org/10.1177 /0008417413520489

Harris, A. (2009). Shifting the boundaries of cultural spaces: Young people and everyday multiculturalism. *Social Identities, 15,* 187–205. http://dx.doi.org/10.1080/13504630902778602

Heigl, F., Kinébanian, A., & Josephsson, S. (2011). I think of my family, therefore I am: Perceptions of daily occupations of some Albanians in Switzerland. *Scandinavian Journal of Occupational Therapy, 18*(1), 36–48. http://dx.doi.org/10.3109 /11038120903552648

Hofstede, G. (2001). *Culture's consequences: Comparing values, behaviors, institutions, and organizations across nations.* Thousand Oaks, CA: Sage.

Huot, S., & Rudman, D. L. (2010). The performances and places of identity: Conceptualizing intersections of occupation, identity and place in the process of migration. *Journal of Occupational Science, 17,* 68–77. http://dx.doi.org/10.10 80/14427591.2010.9686677

Huot, S., Rudman, D. L., Dodson, B., & Magalhães, L. (2013). Expanding policy-based conceptualizations of "successful integration": Negotiating integration through occupation following international migration. *Journal of Occupational Science, 20,* 6–22. http://dx.doi.org/10.1080/14427591.2012.717497

Jenkins, E. M., & Mockaitis, A. I. (2010). You're from where? The influence of distance factors on New Zealand expatriates' cross-cultural adjustment. *International Journal of Human Resource Management, 21,* 2694–2715. Retrieved from http:// www.anzam.org/wp-content/uploads/pdf-manager/996 _ANZAM2009-149.PDF

Johansson, K., Rudman, D. L., Mondaca, M., Park, M., Luborsky, M., Josephsson, S., & Asaba, E. (2013). Moving beyond 'aging in place' to understand migration and aging: Place making and the centrality of occupation. *Journal of Occupational Science, 20*(2), 108–119. http://dx.doi.org/10 .1080/14427591.2012.735613

Kantartzis, S., & Molineux, M. (2011). The influence of Western society's construction of a healthy daily life on the conceptualisation of occupation. *Journal of Occupational Science, 18,* 62–80. http://dx.doi.org/10.1080/14427591.2011 .566917

Kielhofner, G. (2002). *A Model of Human Occupation: Theory and application.* Baltimore: Lippincott Williams & Wilkins.

Kondo, T. (2004). Cultural tensions in occupational therapy practice: Considerations from a Japanese vantage point. *American Journal of Occupational Therapy, 58,* 174–184. http://dx .doi.org/10.5014/ajot.58.2.174

Krishnagiri, S. S., Fuller, E., Ruda, L., & Diwan, S. (2013). Occupational engagement and health in older South Asian immigrants. *Journal of Occupational Science, 20,* 87–102. http://dx.doi.org/10.1080/14427591.2012.735614

Larson, E. A., & Zemke, R. (2003). Shaping the temporal patterns of our lives: The social coordination of occupation. *Journal of Occupational Science, 10,* 80–89. http://dx.doi.org/10 .1080/14427591.2003.9686514

Law, M., Cooper, B., Strong, S., Stewart, D., Rigby, P., & Letts, L. (1996). The Person–Environment–Occupation Model: A transactive approach to occupational performance. *Canadian Journal of Occupational Therapy, 63,* 186–192. http://dx.doi.org/10.1177/000841749606300103

Lencucha, J. C., Davis, J. A., & Polatajko, H. J. (2013). Living in a blended world: The occupational lives of children of immigrants to Canada. *Journal of Occupational Science, 20,* 185–200. http://dx.doi.org/10.1080/14427591.2013.786799

Liu, E. (2014). Why I don't hyphenate Chinese American. *CNN Opinion.* Retrieved from http://www.cnn.com/2014/07/11 /opinion/liu-chinese-american/

Morville, A. L., & Erlandsson, L. K. (2013). The experience of occupational deprivation in an asylum centre: The narratives of three men. *Journal of Occupational Science, 20,* 212–223. http://dx.doi.org/10.1080/14427591.2013.808976

Mpofu, C., & Hocking, C. (2013). "Not made here": Occupational deprivation of non-English speaking background immigrant health professionals in New Zealand. *Journal of Occupational Science, 20,* 131–145. http://dx.doi.org/10.10 80/14427591.2012.729500

Nayar, S. C. (2009). *The theory of navigating cultural spaces* (Doctoral dissertation, Auckland University of Technology). http://dx.doi.org/10.1080/14427591.2011.602628

Nayar, S., Hocking, C., & Giddings, L. (2012). Using occupation to navigate cultural spaces: Indian immigrant women settling in New Zealand. *Journal of Occupational Science, 19,* 62–75. Retrieved from http://hdl.handle.net/10292/733

Phelan, S., & Kinsella, E. A. (2009). Occupational identity: Engaging socio-cultural perspectives. *Journal of Occupational Science, 16,* 85–91. http://dx.doi.org/10.1080/14427591.2009 .9686647

Porter, J. (1965). *Vertical mosaic: An analysis of social class and power in Canada.* Toronto: Toronto University Press.

Ray, R., Sanes, M., & Schmitt, J. (2013). *No-vacation nation revisited.* Washington, DC: Center for Economic and Policy Research. Retrieved from http://www.cepr.net/documents/no-vacation-update-2014-04.pdf

Rebeiro, K. (2004). How qualitative research can inform and challenge occupational therapy practice. In K. W. Hammell & C. Carpenter (Eds.), *Qualitative research in evidence-based rehabilitation* (pp. 89–102). Edinburgh: Churchill Livingstone.

Reeves, R. (2014). *Saving Horatio Alger: Equality opportunity, and the American dream.* Washington, DC: The Brookings Institution. Retrieved from http://www.brookings.edu/research/essays/2014/saving-horatio-alger

Rowles, G. D. (1991). Beyond performance: Being in place as a component of occupational therapy. *American Journal of Occupational Therapy, 45,* 265–271. http://dx.doi.org/10.5014/ajot.45.3.265

Rowles, G. D. (2000). Habituation and being in place. *Occupational Therapy Journal of Research, 20,* 52S–67S. http://dx.doi.org/10.1177/15394492000200S105

Sarmela, M. (1977). What is cultural imperialism? In C. Sandbacka (Ed.), *Cultural imperialism and cultural identity: Transactions of the Finnish Anthropological Society* (Vol. 2, pp. 13–36). Retrieved from http://www.kotikone.fi/matti.sarmela/culturimperialism.pdf

Satcher, D., Fryer, G. E., Jr., McCann, J., Troutman, A., Woolf, S. H., & Rust, G. (2005). What if we were equal? A comparison of the Black–White mortality gap in 1960–2000. *Health Affairs, 24,* 459–464. http://dx.doi.org/10.1377/hlthaff.24.2.459

Schulte, B. (2014). *Overwhelmed: Work, love, and play when no one has the time.* New York: Farrar, Strauss, & Giroux.

Sears, K. P. (2012). Improving cultural competence education: The utility of an intersectional framework. *Medical Education, 46,* 545–551. http://dx.doi.org/10.1111/j.1365-2923.2011.04199.x

Selmer, J. (2007). Which is easier: Adjusting to a similar or to a dissimilar culture? American business expatriates in Canada and Germany. *International Journal of Cross Cultural Management, 7*(2), 185–201. http://dx.doi.org/10.1177/1470595807079385

Stephenson, S. M., Smith, Y. J., Gibson, M., & Watson, V. (2013). Traditional weaving as an occupation of Karen refugee women. *Journal of Occupational Science, 20,* 224–235. http://dx.doi.org/10.1080/14427591.2013.789150

Suto, M. J. (2013). Leisure participation and well-being of immigrant women in Canada. *Journal of Occupational Science, 20,* 48–61. http://dx.doi.org/10.1080/14427591.2012.732914

Syverson, T. (2005). *Occupational adjustment of immigrant women: The importance of paid employment.* Unpublished Master's thesis, St. Catherine University, St. Paul, MN.

Torp, J. A., Berggren, V., & Erlandsson, L.-K. (2013). Somali women's experiences of cooking and meals after immigration to Sweden. *Journal of Occupational Science, 20,* 146–159. http://dx.doi.org/10.1080/14427591.2012.734426

Unruh, A. M., Versnel, J., & Kerr, N. (2002). Spirituality unplugged: A review of commonalities and contentions, and a resolution. *Canadian Journal of Occupational Therapy, 69,* 5–19. Retrieved from http://www.pubpdf.com/pub/11852691/Spirituality-unplugged-a-review-of-commonalities-and-contentions-and-a-resolution

U.S. Bureau of Labor Statistics. (2013). *American time use survey—2013 results* [News release]. Retrieved from http://www.bls.gov/news.release/archives/atus_06182014.pdf

Vang, N. (2005). *Cross cultural adjustment to immigration in the first and second generation Hmong women immigrants.* Unpublished Master's thesis, St. Catherine University, St. Paul, MN.

Whiteford, G. E., & Wilcock, A. A. (2000). Cultural relativism: Occupation and independence reconsidered. *Canadian Journal of Occupational Therapy, 67,* 324–336. http://dx.doi.org/10.1177/000841740006700505

Wilcock, A. A. (1998). Reflections on doing, being and becoming. *Canadian Journal of Occupational Therapy, 65,* 248–257. http://dx.doi.org/10.1177/000841749806500501

Chapter 3.

SOCIOPOLITICAL DIMENSIONS OF PARTICIPATION: OCCUPATIONAL JUSTICE

Jyothi Gupta, PhD, OTR/L, FAOTA

It is not our differences that divide us. It is our inability to recognize, accept, and celebrate those differences.
Audre Lorde (1994, p. 121)

Chapter Highlights

- Sociopolitical Context of Occupation
- Health Inequity and Occupation
- Occupational Justice
- Implications for Occupational Therapy Practice

Key Terms and Concepts

- ✧ Accountability–Well-Being–Ethics Framework
- ✧ Distributive justice
- ✧ Framework of Occupational Justice
- ✧ Health inequity
- ✧ Imbalance
- ✧ Interactional justice
- ✧ Occupational alienation
- ✧ Occupational apartheid
- ✧ Occupational deprivation
- ✧ Occupational imbalance
- ✧ Occupational justice
- ✧ Occupational marginalization
- ✧ Participatory Occupational Justice Framework
- ✧ Procedural justice
- ✧ Social determinants of health
- ✧ Social justice
- ✧ Social stratification
- ✧ Sociopolitical context

Occupations are fundamental to human survival and to the development of self and society. People perform daily occupations to take care of themselves and their families, contribute to society, and meet societal expectations. Occupations are shaped by the environment, and human occupational activities in turn shape and transform the environment. Therefore, the relationship between occupations and environment is reciprocal and transactional (Dickie, Cutchin, & Humphrey, 2006; Law et al., 1996).

As noted in Chapter 1, "Exploring Culture," an important aspect of the environment is the institutions society is founded on, and social and political institutions are heavily influenced by culture. This chapter focuses on social and political factors, collectively termed the *sociopolitical context,* that influence occupation and participation in social life; the relationship between health inequity and occupation; principles of occupational justice, and implications for occupational therapy practice. This chapter addresses the question, To what extent do all humans have a right and responsibility to participate in occupations?

Sociopolitical Context of Occupation

The fundamental premise of occupational therapy is that people's health and well-being are determined by their ability to engage in occupations that are culturally and personally meaningful to them (American Occupational Therapy Association [AOTA], 2014; Canadian Association of Occupational Therapists [CAOT], 2013; Townsend, 2002; Wilcock, 2006). Occupational therapy's practice models portray occupational performance and participation as dependent on context (AOTA, 2014; Law et al., 1996; Whiteford & Townsend, 2011); thus, sociopolitical contexts influence occupational performance and participation. Understanding the context of clients' everyday occupational experiences is necessary to holistically understand their life context.

Humans have an innate need to engage in occupations, but the question of who decides which occupations are valuable and meaningful and the "normative" ways of doing occupations is often political. Politics are present in every aspect of daily life and interpersonal interactions in society; they create the tension in conflict and cooperation (Pollard, Sakellariou, & Kronenberg, 2008).

Social and political forces at the micro, meso, and macro level affect the occupations of individuals and populations. Sociopolitical influences "generate, configure, and maintain social hierarchies . . . [and] generate stratification and social class divisions" with differential access to "power, prestige and access to resources" (World Health Organization [WHO], 2010, p. 5). Income, education, occupation, social class, gender, and race or ethnicity

determine one's social position, and consequently one's culture and identity (Powell-Sears, 2012).

Occupational therapy's historical roots are grounded in the community; its founders sought to alleviate the hardships of people who were poor, immigrants, mentally ill, and disabled. From the start, occupational therapy practitioners have recognized the importance of contextual factors and believed that "complex social, economic, and biological reasons caused disease, not single microbes" (Quiroga, 1995, p. 14). The biopsychosocial model of the *International Classification of Functioning, Disability and Health* (WHO, 2001) delineates the role of both personal and environmental factors, including cultural and sociopolitical context, as contributing to health.

The occupational therapy profession's focus has traditionally been on locating occupation with the individual rather than viewing the occupational experience as a whole in a larger context and on perceiving the individual and occupation as separate from each other and the environment as a container within which occupations occur. This focus has been called into question because it ignores the complex transactional and relational aspects of the person, the occupation, and the context (Dickie et al., 2006). The person–occupation–environment interaction is seamless, and each mutually influences the other.

Reflection 3.1. Context

- What elements in your context (e.g., family, community) influenced your occupational choices and opportunities for social participation?

Health Inequity and Occupation

Health inequity refers to unjust differences and disparities in health interventions and outcomes between groups of people (WHO, 2010). Health inequity is a moral perspective on health disparities that result from unjust or unfair social practices and policies (Kawachi, Subramanian, & Almeida-Filho, 2002).

Discussions concerning health and health inequity in the United States have focused on health care access and individual behavior and lifestyle choices as the reasons for poor health (Adelman,

2010; Centers for Disease Control and Prevention [CDC], 2014; Smedley, Stith, & Nelson, 2002; Lynch, Kaplan, & Salonen, 1997). The emphasis on health care access as the primary contributor to health has been critiqued; the accepted definition of *health* involves more than the mere absence of disease or infirmity but rather a state of physical, mental, and social well-being (WHO, 2001).

Social and economic factors have a far greater influence on individual and population health and lifestyle choices than access to health care (Hofrichter & Bhatia, 2010). Some authors prefer to use the term *health inequity* rather than *health disparity* because *inequity* captures the idea that differences in health are a consequence of social injustice, political imbalance, and historical factors (e.g., Braveman, 2006).

Structural Influences on Health

The complex interactions among social structures and their relationships to individual health behaviors and lifestyle have been well established. Social position based on one's income and location in society or at an organization determines the degree of control, choices, and resources available to manage life stressors and health (Marmot et al., 2008; Marmot & Wilkinson, 2006). Health is much more than access to health services; it is about everyday life conditions that include access to health services. The conceptual framework of the WHO Commission on Determinants of Social Health (2008) identifies the relationships among the individual and structural influences on health. *Individual influences* are genetics, behaviors, and psychosocial abilities. *Structural influences* include the greater sociopolitical context, governance, economy, policy, and cultural values and beliefs. These factors influence opportunities, access, and quality of everyday life circumstances, such as affordable housing, education, transportation, health services, and social cohesion.

Health inequity may be addressed by

- Improving the conditions of daily life—where people live, grow, work, play, and age;
- Challenging the structural factors that contribute to the inequitable distribution of power, money, and resources and their influences on everyday life at local, national, and global levels; and
- Educating the public and the health workforce about the social determinants of health.

In large part, the recipe for the elimination of health inequity is to improve and enhance the context of everyday occupations.

These principles resonate with occupational therapy's conceptual models that emphasize the centrality of context and its transactional relationship with individuals, occupations, occupational performance, and participation (AOTA, 2014; CAOT, 2013; Law et al., 1996). Although these models are helpful in thinking about occupations contextually, they do not address the moral and ethical aspects of participation. There is clearly a gap between the view of occupation as context based and the necessity of occupational participation as a fundamental right and moral imperative.

Reflection 3.2. Occupational Opportunity

Reflect on your life achievements so far and think about how much of it was personal effort alone, how much was your life context (e.g., your family, community), and how much was a combination of both personal and context.

- Do you believe that individuals on their own can reach their full occupational potential?
- What responsibility does society have to create a context with rich and diverse occupational opportunities that enable full social participation for all citizens (e.g, the role of government to create conditions for a healthy economy, good public schools, basic health care, public transportation, safe neighborhoods)?
- Do we, as individuals, have a right and obligation to fully participate in the occupations and contribute to society?

Social Determinants of Health

The economic and social conditions in which people are born, grow, live, work, and age are referred to as the ***social determinants of health*** because they influence how people live their daily lives and whether or not they experience good health (CDC, 2014; Hofrichter, 2003; Hofrichter & Bhatia, 2010; Iton et al., 2010; Marmot & Wilkinson, 2006). The U.S. Department of Health and Human Services (2010) identified the following social determinants of health:

- Socioeconomic conditions
- Culture

- Social support
- Social norms and attitudes
- Community resources to support health lifestyles, including recreational opportunities
- Access to education, economic, and employment opportunities and transportation (CDC, 2014).

Social Stratification and Health

Complex societies are characterized by *social stratification*, a hierarchical organization that differentially distributes power, privilege, and access to resources and opportunities on the basis of socioeconomic conditions. In all countries, a continuous health–wealth gradient parallels social stratification, all the way from the top to the bottom, and occurs irrespective of universal access (or not) to health care and whether society acknowledges the presence of a class structure (Marmot & Wilkinson, 2006). In the United States, socioeconomic stratification accounts for 60% of health inequity, as follows: behaviors (40%), social circumstances (15%), and environment (5%). Access to health care accounts for only 10% and biology 30% (Tarlov, 1999).

Residential zip code is a strong indicator of health (Cummins, Curtis, Diez-Roux, & Macintyre, 2007; Williams & Collins, 2001), attesting to the importance of contextual factors in enhancing or constraining occupational choices, opportunities, and behaviors. For example, a study compared a measure of greenness across urban neighborhoods in one city and found greenness to be directly related to body mass index in child and youth residents (Bell, Wilson, & Liu, 2008). The researchers found 19 times more green space in White neighborhoods than Black and Latino neighborhoods, affecting play and other leisure occupations for children and adults who reside in them. Poor neighborhoods are also more likely to:

- Be "food deserts," with a preponderance of fast food and limited or no access to fresh food;
- Have higher crime rates, lowering neighborhood safety (Larson, Story, & Nelson, 2009); and
- Have low-performing schools with limited resources (Ainsworth, 2002; Goldsmith, 2004).

Such conditions constrict the occupational lives of the children and adults living in such neighborhoods and have a detrimental effect on health and quality of life.

Sociopolitical Barriers to Participation

Negative social attitudes affect health through social exclusion and barriers to participation that certain individuals and groups experience as restricted access, choices, and opportunities to engage in occupations. These barriers are relevant to occupational therapy practice for the following reasons:

- Client-centered practice entails viewing the client holistically as a unique occupational being.
- People confer their own meaning and purpose on their daily occupational repertoire.
- Context matters for occupational participation.

Location in the social hierarchy determines access to the resources and opportunities that are necessary for participation, occupational engagement, and health. If occupational therapy assessment and intervention are directed mainly at individual or person factors, the contextual or environmental factors that influence participation, health, and well-being can easily be ignored or minimized (WHO, 2001).

Overwhelming evidence shows how social determinants shape the health outcomes of people and communities (CDC, 2014; Hofrichter & Bhatia, 2010). Health inequity correlates with wealth, education, and residential segregation along income lines (Williams & Collins, 2002).

Satcher and colleagues (2005) provided evidence of population-specific health inequity. Their study found the Black–White mortality gap to account for 83,570 excess deaths of Black Americans each year, where *excess death* refers to the number of deaths for a given population, in a given time frame, that exceeds the predictable numbers based on epidemiology in comparison to another group. As Krieger puts it, "We all will die. But the question is: At what age? With what degree of suffering? With what degree of preventable illness?" (Adelman, 2008, 01:04:54). Chronic disease takes a major toll on Black lives. A recent study estimates that 1 in 3 Black deaths counts as excess death. These researchers noted that excess death had political implications, as essentially 1 million Black voters are missing from the political process (Rodriguez, Geronimus, Bound, & Dorling, 2015).

Despite improvements in access to quality health care, Black Americans continue to receive worse care than White Americans for about one-third of quality measures. The need for culturally appropriate services is clearly urgent (Agency for Healthcare Research and Quality, 2015).

Historical experiences of marginalization, segregation, and oppression and current institutional racism affect interactions between people, including health service providers and clients. For example, psychological barriers between minority service recipients and White American service providers influence interactions in health care settings and, consequently, health outcomes (Sue, 2006). Practitioners must be aware of this fact when seeking to establish trust and provide culturally effective services.

Reflection 3.3. Personal and Contextual Factors

- Identify some personal and contextual factors and influences in your life that have contributed to the development of your physical, mental, and emotional health and well-being.

Sociopolitical Influences on Access to Health Care

The larger societal ethos regarding health and access to health care illustrates how social and cultural attitudes affect the occupational therapy profession and its clients. For most Americans (65%), health insurance is linked to employment as private health insurance coverage, and 35% are covered through government programs for people who are older and low income. In 2014, the first year of implementation of the major health insurance reform the Patient Protection and Affordable Care Act of 2010 (Pub. L. 111–148), known as the Affordable Care Act, the number of uninsured Americans declined by 2.9%, with 8.8 million more nonelderly adults receiving insurance coverage. However, about 10.4% of the population, or 33 million, still remain uninsured (Smith & Medalia, 2015). Occupational therapy practitioners now have an opportunity to provide cost-effective occupation-based care focused on health promotion and prevention to a large underserved population.

The Affordable Care Act was passed to alleviate high costs and provide greater access to health care. This legislation has been deemed radical, and its constitutionality has been called into question. At the heart of the debate is the question of how

Americans view health and health care. The U.S. cultural and political landscape is dominated by the ethics of market justice based on individualism: self-determination, individual effort, personal responsibility, limited government intervention, and little concern for the collective good (Dorfman, Wallack, & Woodruff, 2005). In this society, health care is a commodity that is sold by competing vendors in the marketplace (Budetti, 2008).

In contrast, societies that value collective well-being over individual well-being, cooperation, and shared responsibility view government intervention as necessary for basic social goods (Dorfman et al., 2005). Some societies view health as a necessary asset and an essential requisite for participation in social life. Such places have universal access to health care that is based upon the ethics of social justice and collective responsibility. Among industrialized Western nations, the United States is unique in that it does not provide universal access to health care, reflecting its cultural values and illustrating how social and cultural values influence social attitudes and social policies.

Occupational therapy's humanistic roots and notions of occupational rights and occupational justice may seem incongruent not only with the larger current sociocultural ethos but also most certainly with the culture of the health care industry. Health depends on factors outside of health care. How individuals live their daily lives, the choices they make, access to opportunities and resources, and social inclusion are examples of factors outside of health care that contribute far more to good health than health care (Adelman, 2008; Marmot & Wilkinson, 2006).

Occupational therapy can significantly contribute to improving society's health and occupational needs both within and outside of health care. Being present in communities, the natural contexts where daily occupations occur, and influencing policies that create environments that promote life-sustaining occupations and living conditions are two ways occupational therapy practitioners can enact the values of the profession to fulfill its social vision (Townsend, 1993).

Occupational Justice

During the past decade, the concept of *occupational justice* has developed and proliferated in the occupational science and occupational therapy literature.

Occupational justice refers to people's right to engage in meaningful occupations (Townsend & Wilcock, 2004). Its rationale is that because occupation is a health determinant, people must be able to partake in daily occupation to optimally support their health and well-being.

Occupational justice is an evolving concept that emerged in the literature in 2000 (Wilcock & Townsend, 2000). Ideas of occupational justice rest on the belief that humans are occupational beings (Wilcock, 2006; Yerxa et al., 1990), that occupations are necessary for survival (Wilcock, 2006) and give meaning to life (Hasselkus, 2011), and that occupations are a determinant of health (CAOT, 2013; Townsend, 2002) and well-being (Hammell, 2008; Hammell & Iwama, 2012; Law, Steinwender, & Leclair, 1998).

Townsend and Wilcock (2004) coined the term *occupational justice* and contended that because occupation is a fundamental aspect of human existence, all people should have the right to access and opportunities to participate in daily occupations. Although they did not explicitly state this, it is clear that enacting occupational justice is dependent upon supportive contexts for participation.

Occupational Justice and Social Justice

In 1993, Townsend noted that the values, beliefs, and language of the occupational therapy profession resonate with those of other social movements, such as civil rights and feminism, and that the profession, like these movements, is grounded in principles of social justice. *Social justice,* a characteristic of social systems, in a general sense refers to

- The distribution of societal benefits and burdens;
- Laws and social institutions, policies, and procedures that preserve the liberty, rights, and entitlements of all people; and
- The obligation of social policies and institutions, as well as fellow citizens, to confer the same dignity and fair treatment to all members of society.

The profession has espoused a vision to "promote social justice by enabling people to participate as valued members of society despite diverse or limited occupational potential" (Townsend, 1993, p. 176). Townsend and Wilcock (2004) identified occupational rights that they viewed as an extension of social justice:

the right to experience meaning and enrichment in one's occupations; to participate in a range of occupations for health and social inclusion; make choices and share decision-making power in daily life; and receive equal privileges for diverse participation in occupations. (p. 80)

These occupational rights allow all people to fully participate in social life through equitable access to opportunities and resources.

Contention arises over specific ways to put social justice into action through fair and equitable allocation of resources. Three major social justice paradigms are distributive, procedural, and interactional (Jost & Kay, 2010), described in the sections that follow.

Distributive Justice

Townsend and Polatajko (2013) described occupational injustice that stems from lack of social and public resources, such as transportation, recreational facilities, and work opportunities in poor neighborhoods. Poverty is a social condition that decreases the ability of people and communities to participate equitably. Social justice and occupational justice are complementary, and both involve the belief in working for a just society governed by principles of "fairness, empowerment, equitable access to resources, and sharing of rights and responsibilities" (Wilcock & Townsend, 2000, p. 84).

The paradigm of *distributive justice* has dominated notions of social justice and concerns the equitable distribution of resources and goods in society so that all members share both benefits and burdens. Within this paradigm, basic social structures or institutions have the responsibility to allocate rights, opportunities, and resources. The challenge for health has been that health is not considered a primary social good, and most philosophers do not give health the same moral consideration they do to health care (Ruger, 2004).

The oppression Young (1990) referred to is the disadvantage and injustice some people experience in their everyday experiences through unquestioned norms, habits, unconscious assumptions, and cultural stereotypes. The *five faces of oppression,* as identified by Young, are exploitation, marginalization, powerlessness, violence, and cultural imperialism (p. 39). The first three—exploitation, marginalization, and powerlessness—are primarily a result of the social division of labor.

Stemming from identity politics, the *recognition paradigm* targets cultural injustices presumed "to be rooted in social patterns of representation, interpretation and communication" (Fraser, 1998, p. 7). Fraser (1998) and Young (1990, 2002) contended that social justice based solely on the distributive paradigm is insufficient. For Young (1990), social justice must address the elimination of systemic domination and oppression and address the "institutional conditions necessary for the development of individual capacities and collective communication and cooperation" (p. 39).

Cultural imperialism refers to the universalization of the dominant group's culture and experiences, rendering invisible other cultures. Cultural minority groups internalize the "othering" oppressive experiences of invisibility and stereotyping. Fraser (1998) proposed *parity of participation* as an integrated perspective of the redistribution and recognition paradigms. This requires that all individuals must have equal opportunity for social equity, independence, and voice in order to fully participate in society. In other words, people are not excluded from participation because of their social position or other criteria. Fraser's approach fits well with the *capability approach* of economist Sen (1999) and philosopher Nussbaum (2004) that has human functioning as a means to being free and flourishing. This approach draws attention to the social conditions necessary for human functioning and capabilities (i.e., choices) to live and thrive. According to the capability approach, health capability is a moral imperative because health is an essential asset for human development, and society is morally obligated to create conditions that support human functioning (Ruger, 2004). The capability approach has been introduced into the profession's literature and aligns with the conceptualization of humans as occupational beings (Taff, Bakhshi, & Babulal, 2014; Whiteford & Pereira, 2012).

Procedural Justice

Procedural justice refers to fairness in the methods and procedures used to make decisions. Procedures are considered as *fair* when they are consistent (applies to all), neutral (not biased against one group or other), ethical (based on principles), based on factual information (accuracy in data or evidence being used), and consider interests of all relevant parties (Jost & Kay, 2010). In other words, the processes are egalitarian and do not distinguish between individuals based on their position in the organizational hierarchy.

Interactional Justice

Social interactions or interpersonal exchanges also have aspects of justice that are important in any social group or society. Individuals treating each other in a fair and equitable manner that affirms human dignity in all members of a society, regardless of differences, embodies ***interactional justice*** (Jost & Kay, 2010). Interpersonal relations free of bias and stereotypes toward individuals who are different is an example of interactional justice. A hallmark of client-centered practice is that all clients, regardless of differences, be treated with dignity and respect (Townsend & Polatajko, 2013). When therapists are client-centered, they are performing interactional justice.

Forms of Occupational Injustice

Occupational justice focuses on the inequality, unfairness, discrimination, and other injustices that prevent people from participating in meaningful occupations: "Occupational injustices exist when, for example, participation is barred, confined, segregated, prohibited, undeveloped, disrupted, alienated, marginalized, exploited, or otherwise devalued" (Townsend & Whiteford, 2005, p. 112). Table 3.1 summarizes the definitions of various forms of occupational injustice.

Occupational Alienation

Chronic illness, poverty, and economic and social forces, as well as paid work that does not enrich the worker and is meaningless and boring, may result in ***occupational alienation.*** People deprived of occupational choices and opportunities are essentially denied full social participation. Consequently, they are socially excluded and thus alienated from experiencing the meaning, purpose, and enrichment in their lives other members of society experience (Townsend & Wilcock, 2004).

Underemployment, a source of occupational alienation, occurs when there is a mismatch between job demands (low) and worker skills (high). Gupta (2008) described stress and alienation in the workplace from a mismatch between job demands, employee control, and reward. A worker under pressure to meet deadlines, for example, is better served by

Table 3.1. Forms of Occupational Injustice

Form of Injustice	Definition
Occupational alienation	Lack of choices and opportunities to experience meaningful and enriching occupations owing to extrinsic factors outside the control of the individual. Alienation is experienced as "disconnectedness, isolation, emptiness, lack of a sense of identity, a limited or confined expression of spirit, or a sense of meaninglessness" (Townsend & Wilcock, 2004, p. 80).
Occupational deprivation	"State of prolonged preclusion from engagement in occupations of necessity and/or meaning due to factors that stand outside the control of the individual" (Whiteford, 2004, p. 222).
Occupational marginalization	Inability of individuals and populations to exert micro, everyday choices and exercise the decision-making power to participate in occupations; imposition of "normative standardization of expectations of how, when and where people 'should' participate" (Townsend & Wilcock, 2004, p. 81).
Occupational imbalance	Inability of individuals and populations to share in both the labor and the benefits of economic production; terms used in describing this concept include *unoccupied, underoccupied,* and *overoccupied* (Townsend & Wilcock, 2004).
Occupational apartheid	"Segregation of groups of people through restriction or denial of access to dignified and meaningful participation in occupations of daily life on the basis of race, color, disability, national origin, age, gender, sexual preference, religion, political beliefs, status in society or other characteristics. Occasioned by political forces, its systematic and pervasive social, cultural and economic consequences jeopardize health and well being as experienced by individuals, communities, and societies" (Kronenberg & Pollard, 2005, p. 67; originally coined by Steinberg, 1991, to address work-related injustices).

having greater autonomy in choosing ways to get the job done on time. Lack of control over getting the job done causes the stress, rather than the actual job demand (Gupta, 2008). An imbalance between the efforts of the worker (e.g., diligence, motivation) and the reward for the work (e.g., salary, promotion, recognition) also causes stress and leads to job dissatisfaction, resentment, and health issues.

Lack of control, choice, freedom, recognition, and fairness in the workplace creates worker alienation and inherently pertains to justice. In alienating situations, workers do not feel empowered, enjoy the doing of their occupation, or experience a sense of belonging. The documentary *Unnatural Causes* demonstrated that although all workers experience stress, those higher up the social ladder have more control and resources to deal with stress (Adelman, 2008).

Bryant, Craik, and McKay (2004) studied people with mental illness and noted the importance of a sense of belonging, which they felt "can be achieved through the sustained provision of a safe place and meaningful occupation in a social context" (p. 288). The stigma and stereotypes of disability often prevent access to occupational choices and opportunities. People with disabilities, barred from participation, experience social exclusion and are alienated; despite legislation, they experience a variety of workplace occupational injustices, including alienation (Gupta, 2012).

Occupational Deprivation

Occupational deprivation results from complex interactions among social, economic, environmental, geographic, historic, cultural, or political factors and often are beyond the individual's control (Whiteford, 2004). Among the groups who experience occupational deprivation are indigenous people; prisoners of war; ethnic, religious, and cultural minority groups; refugees; women; and child laborers (Cockburn, 2005; Fiddler & Peerla, 2009; Molineux & Whiteford, 1999; Whiteford, 2000, 2004; Zeldenryk & Yalmambirra, 2006).

Whiteford (1997) found that inmates she interviewed in New Zealand experienced "sustained occupational deprivation" (p. 129), and an absence of tools limited their opportunities for engagement in occupation. In addition, the inmates' time use was impaired; few activities, with the exception of mealtimes, helped them mark time. The lack of orientation to time also disrupted typical activity, and many inmates slept throughout large portions of the day. The New Zealand minister of corrections stated that "unless they [inmates] learn the value of an honest day's work, they will find it hard to get a job upon release and may reoffend" and that "the government wants inmates to . . . work hard towards self improvement" (quoted in Whiteford, 1997, p. 130). Whiteford concluded, however, that her observations of the lack of access to meaningful and productive occupations indicated "a substantive gap between rhetoric and practice" (p. 130). People cannot understand what "an honest day's work" means if they have no opportunity to engage in an honest day's daily activities, including productive work.

Incarceration is a consequence of retributive justice: Society's punishment for criminal acts is to restrict the privilege of social inclusion. Although an argument can be made for the fairness of this approach, denying prisoners their humanity through occupational deprivation will not help them reintegrate into society when released.

Occupational Marginalization

Marginalization is manifested as social exclusion of certain groups or individuals, often on the basis of nonconformity or differences. For example, individuals with disability experience workplace exclusion and feel socially excluded by their able-bodied coworkers (Gupta, 2012). Individuals with spinal cord injury who were denied their sexuality and sexual identity reported marginalization (Sakellariou, 2006). In another study, transgendered persons felt marginalized when they had to conform to gender-normative occupational expectations in order to survive and in the process felt that they were not living a full life as they envisioned it to be (Beagan et al., 2012).

Occupational Imbalance

A balance of occupations is thought to be important for health and well-being (Backman, 2004). *Imbalance* occurs when people spend too much time in paid labor to the detriment of other aspects of their lives or, conversely, spend so much time in a caregiver role for a child or aging parent with a disability that they cannot work outside the home. *Occupational imbalance* occurs when a person has an insufficient repertoire of daily occupations that are necessary for health and well-being.

Occupational balance is a social construct that is influenced by culture, class privilege, life circumstances, and availability of resources, including time. For instance, a single mother who holds more than one minimum-wage job to make ends meet and who juggles work and family responsibilities with no social support may not have the means or the time for balance. Workaholism, another example of an occupational imbalance, has a negative effect

on life balance and personal and family well-being (Matuska, 2010). Research has documented the adverse effects of chronic stress on children's mental and physical health (Gronski et al., 2013).

Occupational Apartheid

Steinberg (1991), a sociologist, first described **occupational apartheid** as "a system of occupational segregation that relegates most Blacks to the least desirable jobs or that excludes them altogether from legitimate job markets" (p. 744). Steinberg (1991) limited his ideas to the occupation of paid labor, arguing that racism's legacy and current reality in the United States maintain the myth that African Americans are "inefficient and unproductive workers, deficient in the work habits and moral qualities that have delivered other groups from poverty" (p. 745).

Occupational apartheid's root causes are structural and political, and policies and negative attitudes lead to differences in the ability of certain individuals and groups to engage in the full range of occupational choices and opportunities (Kronenberg, Pollard, & Sakellariou, 2005). Critics of the term *occupational apartheid* have noted that "it is too strong, emotional and politically charged," but Kronenberg and Pollard (2005) contended that it is an evolving idea, a work in progress (p. 58).

Multiple Forms of Injustice

The different forms of occupational injustice described in this section are not mutually exclusive; a particular situation may involve more than one type of injustice. For example, for the residents of Appalachia, lack of access to necessary resources, such as clean water, creates occupational deprivation, alienation, and imbalance (Blakeney & Marshall, 2009). Older adults experience the occupational injustices of alienation, deprivation, and marginalization when participation is prevented because of disability (e.g., physical, social, economic, cultural, personal) attributable to old age (Häggblom-Kronlöf & Sonn, 2006). People with a disability experience multiple forms of injustices at the workplace (Gupta, 2012). What makes these situations unjust is that they result from forces beyond a person's control and preventable social issues. Occupational therapy practitioners can play an important role in working to alleviate situations that result in occupational injustice.

Slow Acceptance in the United States

Most of the influential scholars on occupational justice are from outside the United States (Kronenberg, Algado, & Pollard, 2005; Kronenberg, Pollard, & Sakellariou, 2011; Whiteford & Hocking, 2012). Occupational justice–related literature and ideas have started to take root in the United States, but they have yet to gain widespread acceptance in the larger professional community.

Many probable reasons exist for this lukewarm response. The occupational therapy profession is composed predominantly of members of the dominant society, and many practitioners may not fully comprehend the causal factors for health disparities and social inequities that affect so many vulnerable populations in the United States. The tendency of the dominant group to take for granted its own reality as a given is well documented in literature (Tatum, 2000; Whiteford & Pereira, 2012).

Practitioners' resistance or hesitancy to embrace ideas of occupational justice may stem from the idea that dealing with issues of oppression is "too political." Understanding that oppression persists for certain social groups is hard emotional work. It requires authentic examination of one's beliefs, attitudes, and biases, as well as the understanding that the historical legacy of colonization and slavery influences present-day social attitudes toward people of color.

In addition, most occupational therapy practitioners practice in a health care system that is essentially biomedical and driven by reimbursement by third-party insurance. These settings prioritize medical issues and provision of interventions in the most cost-effective manner. In this context of high productivity and reimbursable services, few practitioners have reason to think beyond traditional health services provision.

Furthermore, many practitioners may not have the competence to analyze health inequity in relation to systemic issues and political activism, seeing health as largely a biomedical issue. People are socially conditioned to their values, beliefs, and worldview, which operate at the subconscious level (Sue, 2006).

Cultural values shape society and social policies. The United States has lagged behind other countries in championing economic, social, and cultural rights and, in fact, has not ratified the International Covenant on Economic, Social, and Cultural Rights, which frames health as a human right (McGill,

2012). Social justice is also a contentious issue in the U.S. occupational therapy professional community. Recently, the professional community eliminated social justice as one of the key principles in its code of ethics (AOTA, 2014).

Implications for Occupational Therapy Practice

A scoping review by Durocher, Gibson, and Rappolt (2014) found a lack of conceptual clarity in the concept of occupational justice, which would benefit from further refinement and elaboration to facilitate its use in practice. They also reported that further research is needed to build evidence for the profession's claims of causal linkages between occupation and health (Durocher, Rappolt, & Gibson, 2014).

Gupta and Garber (2014) conducted a systematic mapping review of justice in the occupational science and occupational therapy literature that examined historical and evolving justice-based values to better understand the existing tensions in current practice. They identified four major themes:

1. The health and well-being of individuals and groups are at risk when socially constructed barriers prevent their participation in occupation.
2. Contextual and social conditions are determined by the dominant group.
3. Tensions exist between the practice contexts and values of the profession, creating a crisis in professional identity.
4. Occupational therapy practitioners are called on to be true to the profession's core values.

Practice that incorporates occupational justice addresses individual and contextual factors that impede occupational participation. Although occupational therapy models include sociocultural contexts, the profession still focuses far more on individual factors and on adapting the person to the environment. Advocacy for clients in line with frameworks put forth by the profession can guide practitioners in addressing occupational justice and facilitating participation.

Practitioners are bound by their code of ethics (AOTA, 2014) to advocate for their clients in ways that go beyond ensuring access to occupational therapy services to include advocating for healthy and inclusive environments that enable individuals and communities to flourish. Whiteford and Townsend's (2011) ***Participatory Occupational Justice Framework (POJF)*** entails the use of six interrelated processes to identify and address injustices experienced by individuals and communities who are restricted from participation in everyday life:

1. Raising awareness of occupational injustice
2. Engaging in collaboration with community partners
3. Mediating agreement on a course of action
4. Strategizing on funding for sustainability
5. Supporting implementation of the action plan and continuous evaluation
6. Inspiring advocacy for sustainability or closure.

The POJF is based on concepts of *occupation, enablement,* and *justice.* This conceptual tool focuses on enabling occupation, promoting participation, and doing justice in everyday practice (Whiteford & Townsend, 2011). The POJF is specifically focused on the policy, funding, and legal aspects of the contexts of everyday living, participation, and health.

Stadnyk, Townsend, and Wilcock's (2010) ***Framework of Occupational Justice*** addresses the relationship of structural factors to personal, historical, or spatial contextual factors of individuals and communities to identify occupational outcomes of occupational justice or injustice. It can be used to identify macrolevel occupational determinants, such as the type of economy, policies, values underlying policies, and cultural values, that shape the occupational injustices that, in turn, contribute to health inequity.

The ***Accountability–Well-Being–Ethics Framework*** offers a balanced and holistic view of health and the profession's responsibility in addressing social issues such as health inequity, disability, and so forth. This sociocultural framework resonates with occupational justice ideas in its focus on well-being, empowerment, hope, capabilities, and social and occupational justice (Taff et al., 2014). This framework not only expands occupational therapy to include community-based practice with underserved or vulnerable populations but also enhances the profession's "commitment to human rights principles, understanding collectivistic values, such as choice and meaning" (Taff et al., 2014, p. 327). This framework thus promotes ethical, context-specific,

occupation-based, and culturally responsive occupational therapy practice.

Summary

Occupational therapy rests on the fundamental belief that occupations influence health. Social health determinants that produce health inequity also create inequities in occupational experiences and social participation. The profession has a social responsibility to advocate for health policies that improve societal health by changing contexts to promote and sustain a healthy repertoire of occupations that will enhance the quality of life and improve the overall well-being of society.

Reflection 3.4. Social Responsibility

- Does occupational therapy have a social responsibility to address occupational inequities at the societal level? Why or why not?
- How can the profession attain its articulated vision of meeting society's occupational needs?

References

Adelman, L. (2008). Unnatural causes.[Documentary]. *San Francisco: California Newsreel.* Retrieved from http://www-tc.pbs.org/unnaturalcauses/assets/resources/in_sickness_and_wealth_transcript.pdf

Adelman, L. (2010). Unnatural Causes: Using media to build a constituency for health equity. In R. Hofrichter & R. Bhatia (Eds.), *Tackling health inequities through public health practice: Theory to action* (pp. 477–494). New York: Oxford University Press.

Agency for Healthcare Research and Quality. (2015). *2014 national healthcare quality and disparities report.* Rockville, MD: Author. Retrieved from http://www.ahrq.gov/research/findings/nhqrdr/nhqdr14/index.html

Ainsworth, J. W. (2002). Why does it take a village? The mediation of neighborhood effects on educational achievement. *Social Forces, 81,* 117–152. http://dx.doi.org/10.1353/sof.2002.0038

American Occupational Therapy Association. (2014). Occupational therapy practice framework: Domain and process (3rd ed.). *American Journal of Occupational Therapy, 68*(Suppl. 1), S1–S48. http://dx.doi.org/10.5014/ajot.2014.682006

Backman, C. L. (2004). Occupational balance: Exploring the relationships among daily occupations and their influence on well-being. *Canadian Journal of Occupational Therapy, 71*(4), 202–209. http://dx.doi.org/10.1177/000841740407100404

Bell, J. F., Wilson, J. S., & Liu, G. C. (2008). Neighborhood greenness and 2-year changes in body mass index of children and youth. *American Journal of Preventive Medicine, 35,* 547–553. http://dx.doi.org/10.1016/j.amepre.2008.07.006

Blakeney, A. B., & Marshall, A. (2009). Water quality, health, and human occupations. *American Journal of Occupational Therapy, 63,* 46–57. http://dx.doi.org/10.5014/ajot.63.1.46

Braveman, P. (2006). Health disparities and health equity: Concepts and measurement. *Annual Review of Public Health, 27,* 167–194. http://dx.doi.org/10.1146/annurev.publhealth.27.021405.102103

Bryant, W., Craik, C., & McKay, E. A. (2004). Living in a glasshouse: Exploring occupational alienation. *Canadian Journal of Occupational Therapy, 71,* 282–289. http://dx.doi.org/10.1177/000841740407100507

Budetti, P. P. (2008). Market justice and US health care. *JAMA, 299*(1), 92–94. http://dx.doi.org/10.1001/jama.2007.27

Canadian Association of Occupational Therapists. (2013). *Enabling occupation II: Advancing an occupational therapy vision for health, well-being, and justice through occupation* (2nd ed.). Ottawa: Author.

Centers for Disease Control and Prevention. (2014). *Social determinants of health.* http://www.cdc.gov/socialdeterminants/FAQ.html#a

Cockburn, L. (2005). Canadian occupational therapists' contributions to prisoners of war in World War II. *Canadian Journal of Occupational Therapy, 72,* 183–188. Retrieved from http://www.pubpdf.com/pub/15988965/Canadian-occupational-therapists-contributions-to-prisoners-of-war-in-World-War-II

Cummins, S., Curtis, S., Diez-Roux, A. V., & Macintyre, S. (2007). Understanding and representing "place" in health research: A relational approach. *Social Science and Medicine, 65,* 1825–1838. http://dx.doi.org/10.1016/j.socscimed.2007.05.036

Dickie, V., Cutchin, M. P., & Humphry, R. (2006). Occupation as transactional experience: A critique of individualism in occupational science. *Journal of Occupational Science, 13,* 83–93. http://dx.doi.org/10.1080/14427591.2006.9686573

Dorfman, L., Wallack, L., & Woodruff, K. (2005). More than a message: Framing public health advocacy to change corporate practices. *Health Education and Behavior, 32*(3), 320–336. http://dx.doi.org/10.1177/1090198105275046

Durocher, E., Gibson, B. E., & Rappolt, S. (2014). Occupational justice: A conceptual review. *Journal of Occupational Science, 21,* 418–430. http://dx.doi.org/10.1080/14427591.2013.775692

Durocher, E., Rappolt, S., & Gibson, B. E. (2014). Occupational justice: Future directions. *Journal of Occupational Science, 21,* 431–442. http://dx.doi.org/10.1080/14427591.2013.775693

Fiddler, A., & Peerla, D. (2009). The Kitchenuhmaykoosib Inninuwug and the struggle for the right to say no. *Journal of Occupational Science, 16,* 10–11. http://dx.doi.org/10.1080/14427591.2009.9686635

Fraser, N. (1998). *Social justice in an age of identity politics: Redistribution, recognition, and participation.* Berkeley, CA: Doreen B. Townsend Center for the Humanities. Retrieved from http://tannerlectures.utah.edu/_documents/a-to-z/f/Fraser98.pdf

Goldsmith, P. A. (2004). Schools' racial mix, students' optimism, and the Black–White and Latino–White achievement gaps. *Sociology of Education, 77,* 121–147. http://dx.doi.org/10.1177/003804070407700202

Gronski, M. P., Bogan, K. E., Kloeckner, J., Russell-Thomas, D., Taff, S. D., Walker, K. A., & Berg, C. (2013). Childhood toxic stress: A community role in health promotion for occupational therapists. *American Journal of Occupational Therapy, 67,* e148–e153. http://dx.doi.org/10.5014/ajot.2013.008755

Gupta, J. (2008). Promoting wellness at the workplace. *Work and Industry Special Interest Section Quarterly, 22*(2), 1–4.

Gupta, J. (2012). An issue of occupational (in)justice: A case study. *Disability Studies Quarterly, 32*(3). Retrieved from http://dsq-sds.org/article/view/3280/3114

Gupta, J., & Garber, T. (2014, October). *A systematic mapping review of justice notions in occupational science and occupational therapy literature.* Poster session presented at the conference of the Society for the Study of Occupation USA, Canadian Society of Occupational Scientists, & International Society for Occupational Science, Minneapolis.

Häggblom-Kronlöf, G., & Sonn, U. (2006). Interests that occupy 86-year-old persons living at home: Associations with functional ability, self-rated health and sociodemographic characteristics. *Australian Occupational Therapy Journal, 53,* 196–204. http://dx.doi.org/10.1111/j.1440-1630.2005.00526.x

Hammell, K. W. (2008). Reflections on well-being and occupational rights. *Canadian Journal of Occupational Therapy, 75,* 61–64. http://dx.doi.org/10.2182/cjot.07.007

Hammell, K. R. W., & Iwama, M. K. (2012). Well-being and occupational rights: An imperative for critical occupational therapy. *Scandinavian Journal of Occupational Therapy, 19,* 385–394. http://dx.doi.org/10.3109/11038128.2011.611821

Hasselkus, B. R. (2011). *The meaning of everyday occupation.* Thoroghfare, NJ: Slack.

Hofrichter, R. (2003). *Health and social justice: Politics, ideology, and inequity in the distribution of disease* (Vol. 11). San Francisco: Jossey-Bass.

Hofrichter, R., & Bhatia, R. (Eds.). (2010). *Tackling health inequities through public health practice: Theory to action.* New York: Oxford University Press.

Iton, A., Witt, S., Desautels, A., Schaff, K., Luduquisen, M., Maker, L., . . . Beyers, M. (2010). Tackling the root causes of health disparities through community capacity building. In R. Hofrichter & R. Bhatia (Eds.), *Tackling health inequities through public health practice: Theory to action* (pp. 370–403). New York: Oxford University Press.

Jost, J. T., & Kay, A. C. (2010). Social justice: History, theory, and research. In S. T. Fiske, D. Gilbert, & G. Lindzey (Eds.), *Handbook of social psychology* (5th ed., Vol. 2, pp. 1122–1165). Hoboken, NJ: Wiley.

Kawachi, I., Subramanian, S. V., & Almeida-Filho, N. (2002). A glossary for health inequalities. *Journal of Epidemiology and Community Health, 56*(9), 647–652. http://dx.doi .org/10.1136/jech.56.9.647

Kronenberg, F., Algado, S. S., & Pollard, N. (2005). *Occupational therapy without borders: Learning from the spirit of survivors*. Edinburgh: Elsevier/Churchill Livingstone.

Kronenberg, F., & Pollard, N. (2005). Overcoming occupational apartheid: A preliminary exploration of the political nature of occupational therapy. In F. Kronenberg., S. S. Algado, & N. Pollard (Eds.), *Occupational therapy without borders: Learning from the spirit of survivors* (pp. 58–86). Edinburgh: Elsevier/ Churchill Livingstone.

Kronenberg, F., Pollard, N., & Sakellariou, D. (Eds.). (2011). *Occupational therapies without borders: Vol. 2. Towards an ecology of occupation-based practices*. Edinburgh: Elsevier Health Sciences.

Larson, N. I., Story, M. T., & Nelson, M. C. (2009). Neighborhood environments: Disparities in access to healthy foods in the U.S. *American Journal of Preventive Medicine, 36,* 74–81. http://dx.doi.org/10.1016/j.amepre.2008.09.025

Law, M., Cooper, B., Strong, S., Stewart, D., Rigby, P., & Letts, L. (1996). The Person–Environment–Occupation Model: A transactive approach to occupational performance. *Canadian Journal of Occupational Therapy, 63,* 9–23. http://dx.doi.org/10.1177/000841749606300103

Law, M., Steinwender, S., & Leclair, L. (1998). Occupation, health and well-being. *Canadian Journal of Occupational Therapy, 65,* 81–91. http://dx.doi.org/10.1177/000841749806500204

Lorde, A. (1994). *Our dead behind us: Poems*. New York: Norton.

Lynch, J. W., Kaplan, G. A., & Salonen, J. T. (1997). Why do poor people behave poorly? Variation in adult health behaviours and psychosocial characteristics by stages of the socioeconomic lifecourse. *Social Science and Medicine, 44,* 809–819. http://dx.doi.org/10.1016/S0277-9536(96)00191-8

Marmot, M., Friel, S., Bell, R., Houweling, T. A., Taylor, S., & Commission on Social Determinants of Health. (2008). Closing the gap in a generation: Health equity through action on the social determinants of health. *Lancet, 372*(9650), 1661–1669. http://dx.doi.org/10.1016/S0140-6736(08)61690-6

Marmot, M., & Wilkinson, R. (Eds.). (2006). *Social determinants of health*. Oxford, England: Oxford University Press.

Matuska, K. M. (2010). Workaholism, life balance, and well-being: A comparative analysis. *Journal of Occupational Science, 17,* 104–111. http://dx.doi.org/10.1080/14427591.2010 .9686681

McGill, M. (2012). Human rights from the grassroots up: Vermont's campaign for universal health care. *Health and Human Rights, 14,* E106–E118. Retrieved from https://cdn2 .sph.harvard.edu/wp-content/uploads/sites/13/2013/06 /McGill-FINAL2.pdf

Molineux, M. L., & Whiteford, G. E. (1999). Prisons: From occupational deprivation to occupational enrichment. *Journal of Occupational Science, 6,* 124–130. http://dx.doi.org/10.1080 /14427591.1999.9686457

Nussbaum, M. C. (2004). Beyond the social contract: Capabilities and global justice. *Oxford Development Studies, 32,* 3–18. http://dx.doi.org/10.1017/CBO9780511614743.014

Patient Protection and Affordable Care Act, Pub. L. 111–148, 42 U.S.C. §§ 18001–18121 (2010).

Pollard, N., Sakellariou, D., & Kronenberg, F. (2008). *A political practice of occupational therapy*. Philadelphia: Elsevier Health Sciences.

Powell-Sears, K. (2012). Improving cultural competence education: The utility of an intersectional framewoek. *Medical Education, 46*(6), 545–551. http://dx.doi.org/10.1111/j.1365 -2923.2011.04199.x

Quiroga, V. A. (1995). *Occupational therapy history: The first 30 years, 1900 to 1930*. Bethesda, MD: American Occupational Therapy Association.

Rodriguez, J. M., Geronimus, A. T., Bound, J., & Dorling, D. (2015). Black lives matter: Differential mortality and the racial composition of the US electorate, 1970–2004. *Social Science & Medicine, 136,* 193–199. http://dx.doi.org/10.1016 /j.socscimed.2015.04.014

Ruger, J. P. (2004). Health and social justice. *Lancet, 364*(9439), 1075–1080. http://dx.doi.org/10.1016/S0140-6736(04) 17064-5

Satcher, D., Fryer, G. E., McCann, J., Troutman, A., Woolf, S. H., & Rust, G. (2005). What if we were equal? A comparison of the Black–White mortality gap in 1960 and 2000. *Health Affairs, 24,* 459–464. http://dx.doi.org/10.1377 /hlthaff.24.2.459

Sen, A. (1999). *Development as freedom*. Oxford, England: Oxford University Press.

Smedley, B. D., Stith, A. Y., & Nelson, A. R. (Eds.). (2002). *Unequal treatment: Confronting racial and ethnic disparities in health care*. Washington, DC: National Academies Press.

Smith, J. C., & Medalia, C. (2015). *Health insurance coverage in the United States: 2014*. U.S. Department of Commerce, Economics and Statistics Administration, U.S. Census Bureau,

Current Population Reports, P60-253. Washington, DC: U.S. Government Printing Office. Retrieved from https://www.census.gov/content/dam/Census/library/publications/2015/demo/p60-253.pdf

Stadnyk, R. L., Townsend, E. A., & Wilcock, A. A. (2010). Occupational justice. In C. H. Christiansen & E. A. Townsend (Eds.), *Introduction to occupation: The art and science of living* (pp. 329–358). Upper Saddle River, NJ: Prentice Hall.

Steinberg, S. (1991, December 9). Occupational apartheid. *Nation*, pp. 744–746.

Sue, D. W. (2006). *Multicultural social work practice*. Hoboken, NJ: Wiley.

Taff, S. D., Bakhshi, P., & Babulal, G. M. (2014). The Accountability–Well-Being–Ethics Framework: A new philosophical foundation for occupational therapy. *Canadian Journal of Occupational Therapy, 81*, 320–329. http://dx.doi.org/10.1177/0008417414546742

Tarlov, A. R. (1999). Public policy frameworks for improving population health. *Annals of the New York Academy of Sciences, 896*, 281–293. http://dx.doi.org/10.1111/j.1749-6632.1999.tb08123.x

Tatum, B. D. (2000). The complexity of identity: "Who Am I?" In M. Adams, W. J. Blumenfeld, H. W. Hackman, X. Zúñiga, & M. L. Peters (Eds.), *Readings for diversity and social justice: An anthology on racism, sexism, anti-semitism, heterosexism, ableism, and classism* (pp. 9–14). New York: Routledge.

Townsend, E. (1993). Occupational therapy's social vision. *Canadian Journal of Occupational Therapy, 60*, 174–184. http://dx.doi.org/10.1177/000841749306000403

Townsend, E. (2002). *Preface 2002 to Enabling Occupation: An occupational therapy perspective*. Ottawa: Canadian Association of Occupational Therapists.

Townsend, E. & Polatajko, H. (2013). *Enabling occupation II: Advancing an occupational therapy vision for health, well-being, & justice through occupations* (2nd ed.). Ottawa: CAOT Publications ACE.

Townsend, E., & Wilcock, A. A. (2004). Occupational justice and client-centred practice: A dialogue in progress. *Canadian Journal of Occupational Therapy, 71*, 75–87. http://dx.doi.org/10.1177/000841740407100203

U.S. Department of Health and Human Services, & Office of Disease Prevention and Health Promotion. (2010). *Healthy people 2020*. Retrieved from https://www.healthypeople.gov/2020/leading-health-indicators/Leading-Health-Indicators-Development-and-Framework

Whiteford, G. (1997). Occupational deprivation and incarceration. *Journal of Occupational Science, 4*, 126–130. http://dx.doi.org/10.1080/14427591.1997.9686429

Whiteford, G. (2000). Occupational deprivation: Global challenge in the new millennium. *British Journal of Occupational Therapy, 63*, 200–204. http://dx.doi.org/10.1177/030802260006300503

Whiteford, G. (2004). When people cannot participate: Occupational deprivation. In C. H. Christensen & E. Townsend (Eds.), *Introduction to occupation: The art and science of living* (pp. 221–242). Upper Saddle River, NJ: Prentice Hall.

Whiteford, G. E., & Hocking, C. (Eds.). (2012). *Occupational science: Society, inclusion, participation*. Chichester, West Sussex, England: Wiley.

Whiteford, G. E., & Pereira, R. B. (2012). Occupation, inclusion and participation. In G. Whiteford & C. Hocking (Eds.), *Occupational science: Society, inclusion, participation* (pp. 185–207). Chichester, West Sussex, England: Wiley.

Whiteford, G., & Townsend, E. (2011). Participatory Occupational Justice Framework (POJF 2010): Enabling occupational participation and inclusion. In F. Kronenberg, N. Pollard, & D. Sakellariou (Eds.), *Occupational therapies without borders: Vol. 2. Towards an ecology of occupation-based practices* (pp. 65–84). Edinburgh, Scotland: Elsevier Health Sciences.

Wilcock, A. A. (2006). *An occupational perspective of health*. Thorofare, NJ: Slack.

Wilcock, A., & Townsend, E. (2000). Occupational terminology interactive dialogue: Occupational justice. *Journal of Occupational Science, 7*, 84–86. http://dx.doi.org/10.1080/14427591.2000.9686470

Williams, D. R., & Collins, C. A. (2001). Racial residential segregation: A fundamental cause of racial disparities in health. *Public Health Reports, 116*, 404–416. http://dx.doi.org/10.1016/S0033-3549(04)50068-7

Williams, D. R., & Collins, C. (2002). U.S. socioeconomic and racial differences in health: Patterns and explanations. In T. A. LaVeist (Ed.), *Race, ethnicity and health: A public health reader* (pp. 391–431). San Francisco: Jossey-Bass.

World Health Organization. (2001). *International classification of functioning, disability and health*. Geneva: Author.

World Health Organization. (2010). *A conceptual framework for action on the social determinants of health*. Geneva: Author.

World Health Organization, Commission on Social Determinants of Health. (2008). *Closing the gap in a generation: Health equity through action on the social determinants of health: Commission on Social Determinants of Health final report*. Geneva: Author.

Yerxa, E. J., Clark, F., Frank, G., Jackson, J., Parham, D., Pierce, D., Stein, C., & Zemke, R. (1989). An introduction to occupational science, a foundation for occupational therapy in the 21st century. In J. A. Johnson & E. J. Yerxa (Eds.), *Occupational science: The foundation for new models of practice.* (pp. 1–17). New York: Haworth Press.

Yerxa, E. J., Clark, F., Frank, G., Jackson, J., Parham, D., Pierce, D., . . . & Zemke, R. (1990). Occupational science: The foundation for new models of practice. *Occupational Therapy in Health Care, 6*(4), 1–17.

Young, I. M. (1990). *Justice and the politics of difference.* Princeton, NJ: Princeton University Press.

Young, I. M. (2002). *Inclusion and democracy.* Oxford, England: Oxford University Press.

Zeldenryk, L., & Yalmambirra (2006). Occupational deprivation: A consequence of Australia's policy of assimilation. *Australian Occupational Therapy Journal, 53,* 43–46. http://dx.doi.org/10.1111/j.1440-1630.2005.00530.x

Chapter 4.

THE CHANGING LANGUAGE OF CROSS-CULTURAL PRACTICE

Roxie M. Black, PhD, OTR/L, FAOTA

Chapter Highlights

- Historical Transitions in Language Describing Cross-Cultural Practice
  - Cultural Tolerance
  - Cultural Sensitivity
  - Cultural Competence
- Current and Developing Language and Concepts in Cross-Cultural Practice
  - Cultural Responsiveness
  - Cultural Humility
  - Cultural Intelligence
  - Cultural Safety
  - Cultural Congruence
  - Cultural Proficiency
  - Cultural Effectiveness

Key Terms and Concepts

- ✧ Critical reflection
- ✧ Cultural competence
- ✧ Cultural congruence
- ✧ Cultural effectiveness
- ✧ Cultural humility
- ✧ Cultural intelligence
- ✧ Cultural metacognition

- ✧ Cultural proficiency
- ✧ Cultural safety
- ✧ Cultural sensitivity
- ✧ Cultural skills
- ✧ Cultural tolerance
- ✧ Culturally responsive care

This chapter defines and analyzes the various terms used to describe cross-cultural interactions encountered in health care practice to clarify their meanings and processes. Several of these terms denote constructs that are built on frameworks and characteristics found in the cultural competence literature but indicate a specific focus that helps differentiate them. However, the terms and language used in the cultural effectiveness arena share more similarities than differences.

Historical Transitions in Language Describing Cross-Cultural Practice

This volume uses the term *cultural effectiveness* rather than *cultural competence* in its title, reflecting the most recent change in language describing this practice skill. As the idea of cultural effectiveness evolved, the term *effectiveness* was preceded by such terms as *tolerance, sensitivity,* and *competence.*

Cultural Tolerance

At the beginning of the 20th century, when immigration was at high levels in the United States, the phrase **cultural tolerance** emerged in the literature. Merriam-Webster (2016a) defines *tolerance* as "sympathy or indulgence for beliefs or practices differing from or conflicting with one's own," which sounds like a positive trait, but *tolerate* is defined in another sense as "to allow (something that is bad, unpleasant, etc.) to exist, happen, or be done" (Merriam-Webster, 2016b). Thus, the term *cultural tolerance* is not necessarily positive: "At best, it reflects a neutrality" (Hecht & Baldwin, 1998, p. 67). Goldberg (1997) viewed tolerance as negative "because it always is enacted out of a power position that demeans through condescension and makes prejudice and discrimination acceptable" (as cited in Hecht & Baldwin, p. 67).

Reflection 4.1. Tolerance

- Consider a time when you tolerated a person with whom you had to spend some time. What did that feel like to you?

Cultural Sensitivity

Beginning in the 1950s and 1960s, the social structure of the United States began to shift as a result of the civil rights movements, which promoted the rights of women, African-Americans, and people with disabilities. During this time, the language of diversity changed to include the phrase **cultural sensitivity.** The civil rights movements heightened the awareness and sensitivity of health care professionals to members of minority and disadvantaged groups (Sachdev, 1997).

Chen (1997), in a review of the term *intercultural sensitivity,* stated that "intercultural sensitivity can be conceptualized as an individual's ability to develop a positive emotion towards understanding and appreciating cultural differences" (p. 5). Chen believed that cultural sensitivity was related to the affective recognition and acceptance of others. During and after the 1960s, people learned about those who differed from themselves, and even learned to accept them at some level, but there was no behavioral requirement in the language of cultural sensitivity to act in any particular manner toward people who were different from oneself.

Cultural Competence

Not until the mid-1980s did the term **cultural competence** become prevalent in the health care literature, particularly in nursing, clinical psychology, and social work. Madeline Leininger (1988), a nurse who founded and developed transcultural nursing, was one of the first authors to use the term.

Occupational therapy was slow to follow. Although clients' uniqueness related to sociocultural identity has been discussed in the occupational therapy literature since the first standards were written in 1925 (Black, 2002), only within the past few decades have occupational therapy scholars been writing about cultural competence (Black & Wells, 2007; Bonder, Martin, & Miracle, 2002; Dillard et al., 1992; Suarez-Balcazar et al., 2009).

The difference between *cultural competence* and the preceding terminology is that inherent in its definition is a behavioral aspect or move to action. Cultural competence requires us to not just tolerate or be sensitive to others but also to respond to them in a particular fashion. Many definitions of cultural competence have been put forth in the growing body of literature related to culture and cultural competence, some of which are included in Exhibit 4.1. Each definition indicates that to become culturally competent, health care professionals must actively engage with people who differ from themselves.

Current and Developing Language and Concepts in Cross-Cultural Practice

Although much of the early literature indicated that cultural competence includes particular components

---

Exhibit 4.1. Definitions of *Cultural Competence*

The process of actively developing and practicing appropriate, relevant, and sensitive strategies and skills in interacting with culturally different persons (American Occupational Therapy Association, 2011, p. 2).

A set of congruent behaviors, attitudes, and policies that come together in a system, agency, or among professionals and enable that system, agency, or those professionals to work effectively in cross-cultural situations (Cross, Bazron, Dennis, & Isaacs, 1989, p. iv).

Application of knowledge, skill, attitudes, and personal attributes required . . . to provide appropriate care and services in relation to the cultural characteristics of clients. Cultural competence includes valuing diversity, knowing about the cultural norms and traditions of the populations being served, and being sensitive to these while providing care to individuals (Canadian Nurses Association, 2004, p. 15).

Educational initiatives that aim to teach providers the key tools and skills to deliver quality care to diverse populations (Betancourt, Green, Carrillo, & Ananeh-Firempong, 2003, p. 297).

---

such as cultural self-awareness and attitudes, cultural knowledge, and cultural skill, several scholars, in an effort to further explain the complexities and nuances of intercultural experiences, have since expanded these notions and are conceptualizing, finding, or developing new terminology. Some of the new concepts include *cultural responsiveness, cultural humility, cultural intelligence, cultural safety, cultural congruence,* and *cultural proficiency.* To clarify this often confusing plethora of cultural verbiage, this section defines and analyzes the commonalities and differences between and among the terms and concepts and explains how each of these intersects with the notion of *cultural effectiveness* (see Table 4.1).

Cultural Responsiveness

The term **culturally responsive care** was first used in psychology and mental health publications nearly 20 years ago in the context of the culturally responsive family systems perspective (Turnbull &

Turnbull, 1996) and mental health care to non-majority groups (Baca & Koss-Chioino, 1997; Yurkovich, Clairmont, & Grandbois, 2002). In nursing and the general health care literature, culturally responsive care for specific populations (e.g., Hmong refugees; Parker & Kiatoukaysy, 1999) has been addressed, and components of culturally responsive care have been examined (Goldman, Monroe, & Dube, 1996). In education journals, culturally responsive practices were first described in 1995 (Wlodkowski & Ginsberg, 1995) and have flourished since; a database search for this chapter found more written about cultural responsiveness in education journals than in health care journals.

Muñoz (2007) was one of the first to emphasize culturally responsive care in occupational therapy. After studying occupational therapy practitioners and their conceptualization of culture when working with clients, he developed a model describing culturally responsive care as involving "the

Table 4.1. Characteristics of Approaches to Intercultural Interactions

Term	Self-Awareness	Cultural Knowledge	Cultural Skills	Open, Willing Attitude	Cross-Cultural Experience	Critical Reflection	Consideration of Context
Cultural responsiveness	√	√	√		√		√
Cultural humility	√			√			
Cultural intelligence	√	√			√	√	√
Cultural safety	√	√	√			√	√
Cultural congruence	√	√	√		√		
Cultural proficiency	√	√	√	√	√		
Cultural effectiveness	√	√	√	√	√	√	√

interaction of five interdependent components which comprise processes of providing care and one contextual component [the diversity context] that illuminates environmental factors influencing the provision of culturally responsive caring" (Muñoz, 2007, pp. 265–266). The five components he addressed include

1. Generating cultural knowledge about culturally diverse clients;
2. Building cultural awareness of self, including one's own cultural heritage and biases;
3. Applying cultural skills during assessment and intervention;
4. Engaging with culturally diverse others, including through direct encounters with culturally diverse populations in professional and personal contexts; and
5. Exploring multiculturalism, "a reflective process whereby practitioners demonstrate an intentional drive to continually broaden their cultural understanding and pursue a personal journey of multiculturalism" (Muñoz, 2007, p. 267).

Reflection 4.2. Cultural Heritage

- What is your cultural heritage?
- How has it influenced the occupations you engage in?
- Does your family share any rituals or celebrations related to this heritage?

Muñoz (2007) explained that culturally responsive care results from "the synergistic interaction of [these] five components" (p. 273), several of which complement earlier models of cultural competence. Muñoz argued that the context within which cross-cultural interactions occur can influence these components. The idea of *interactions* is where Muñoz improves on the traditional view of cultural competence, which rarely speaks to the context of interactions but instead focuses solely on self-awareness and attitudes, cultural knowledge, and cultural skills (Campinha-Bacote, 2002; Cross et al., 1989; Saldana, 2001).

Occupational therapy practitioners recognize the influence of context on occupational performance, including social interaction skills, and the inclusion of cross-cultural interactions within the practice

context in Muñoz's (2007) model of culturally responsive care is an important addition to the discourse. Discussing his choice of the term *cultural responsiveness,* Muñoz stated,

> Responsiveness conveys the give and take and the adjustments and reactions that occur when exploring and reacting to cultural aspects of care. Responsiveness also communicates a state of being open to the process of building mutuality with a client and to accepting that the cultural-specific knowledge one has about a group may or may not apply to the person you are treating. (p. 274)

Since Muñoz published his research in 2007, a limited number of occupational therapy authors have written about culturally responsive care within the context of their own practice (e.g., Iwama, Thomson, & MacDonald, 2009).

Cultural Humility

Some authors have issued a "call for cultural humility" as necessary for the teaching of professionalism in health care (Cruess, Cruess, & Steinert, 2010, p. 357). *Cultural humility* is a

> process that requires humility as individuals continually engage in self-reflection and self-critique as lifelong learners and reflective practitioners. It requires humility in how physicians bring into check the power imbalances that exist in the dynamics of physician–patient focused interviewing and care, and it is a process that requires humility to develop and maintain mutually respectful and dynamic partnerships with communities. (Tervalon & Murray-García, 1998, p. 118)

Juarez et al. (2006) discussed cultural humility as an attitude of learning about cultural differences and cultivating self-awareness. They argued that humility allows health care professionals "to consciously be aware of culture and patient uniqueness during each visit" (p. 98). Self-reflection on one's cross-cultural interactions is a hallmark of this approach.

Hook, Davis, Owen, Worthington, and Utsey (2013) suggested that openness to others is closely related to the concept of humility (p. 353) and that humble health professionals are able to maintain an attitude of other orientation:

> For a therapist to develop a strong working relationship and conduct effective [therapy] with a client who is culturally different, the therapist must be able to overcome the natural tendency to view one's own beliefs, values, and worldview as superior, and instead be open to the beliefs, values, and worldview of the diverse client. (p. 354)

Culturally humble therapists approach clients with a sense of naiveté and do not assume that because they have worked with a similar client, the current client will react in the same way (Ridley, Mendoza, Kanitz, Angermeier, & Zenk, 1994).

Some scholars add that to be successful as a culturally humble therapist, one must engage in self-reflection and self-critique as a lifelong learner (Chang, Simon, & Dong, 2012; Juarez et al., 2006; Tervalon & Murray-García, 1998). Hook et al. (2013) viewed cultural humility as a virtue or disposition rather than a competency, such as self-awareness, knowledge, or skill, which are typically expected in cultural competence.

Besides self-reflection and self-critique, Chang et al. (2012) identified three additional elements of cultural humility: (1) learning from clients, (2) partnership building, and (3) maintaining a lifelong process of cultivating humility. Fully engaging in careful listening with clients enables practitioners to address the power inequities found in client–practitioner interactions and helps them avoid cultural stereotyping (Chang et al., 2012, p. 273). Developing mutually respectful partnerships with culturally diverse clients and communities benefits clients through health advocacy. Chang et al. also believed that developing cultural humility is a lifelong process and an active approach to "being in the world and being in relationship with others and self" (p. 273).

Although the literature review for this chapter found nothing published in the occupational therapy literature on cultural humility, it is an important concept that must be considered when discussing the effectiveness of cross-cultural interactions in occupational therapy practice. It isn't as broad a concept as cultural responsiveness or cultural competence because it focuses mainly on the practitioner's attitudes rather than knowledge and skill development. However, becoming culturally humble aids practitioners in learning about clients' cultures and beliefs and provides guidance for practitioner behavior when interacting with culturally diverse clients.

Cultural Intelligence

One of the newest terms used in the management literature is *cultural intelligence,* which "has enormous potential in helping to explain effectiveness in cross cultural interactions" (Thomas et al., 2008, p. 123). To define cultural intelligence, Thomas and colleagues (2008) first agreed on a definition of *intelligence* "as the abilities necessary for adaptation to, as well as selection and shaping of, an environmental context" (p. 124). Addressing context integrates well with occupational therapy philosophy, which always considers the client's context during a therapeutic interaction.

Thomas (2006) had previously defined *cultural intelligence* as "the ability to interact effectively with people who are culturally different," but after considering the complexity of the notion of intelligence, Thomas and colleagues (2008) expanded the concept and the definition of **cultural intelligence** to "a system of interacting knowledge and skills, linked by cultural metacognition, that allows people to adapt to, select, and shape the cultural aspects of their environment" (p. 126). Thomas et al. argued that "knowledge of cultural identities [both the practitioner's and the client's], values, attitudes, and practices makes for greater predictability in social interaction, more accurate attributions, and ultimately more effective intercultural behavior" (p. 128).

Cultural metacognition, or the process of actively examining one's thinking, assumptions, and behavior regarding intercultural interactions (Chua, Morris, & Mor, 2012), is a pivotal construct in Thomas et al.'s (2008) concept of cultural intelligence. It is a reflective process that requires more intentional thought than the self-awareness requirement of cultural competence; it "involves maintaining heightened awareness of, and enhanced attention to, the current cultural experience or present reality, including awareness of the assumptions, emotions, motivations, intentions, behaviors, and skills of oneself and culturally different others" (Thomas et al., 2008, p. 131). Because of the focus on all facets of the cross-cultural interaction, Thomas and colleagues believed that practitioners can have more control over their own responses by recall-ing earlier learned knowledge relevant to the current interaction, thinking about and determining not to react to any negative responses, and choosing posi-tive responses related to previously determined goals. In other words, more intentional thinking about the process, coupled with knowledge and skills, results in effective cross-cultural interactions.

Reflection 4.3. Interactions and Critical Thinking

- Do you think every cross-cultural interaction should require this kind of critical thinking and reflection? Why or why not?
- When would an interaction not require this?

Crowne (2013), citing Ang et al. (2007), stated that cultural intelligence may include "cultural judg-ment, decision-making, cultural adaptation, and task performance" (p. 6). In her study of the effects of length and breadth of varied cultural exposures on cultural intelligence, Crowne found that exposure to various forms of culture significantly influenced cultural intelligence, indicating the importance of cultural travel and other cross-cultural experiences in developing cultural intelligence and cultural skills.

Cultural Safety

Cultural safety, a term coined by Maori nurse Irihapeti Ramsden (1992), is "shared respect, shared meaning, shared knowledge and experience and is learning together with dignity and truly listening" (p. 21). This concept emerged out of the necessity to correct erroneous beliefs regarding the Maori people held by the dominant society in New Zealand by attributing their present-day plight to their culture rather than to the consequences of colonialism and chronic cycles of poverty (Papps & Ramsden, 1996).

Cultural safety concerns the social, economic, and political location of groups in a society that have traditionally been dominated, silenced, and oppressed. By examining the influence of histor-ical and socioeconomic contexts on the health of individuals and health care services, practitioners are able "to unveil often deeply rooted, and largely unconscious and unspoken, assumptions of power held by health educators, students, and providers, and to transfer some of this power to health care

recipients" (Gerlach, 2012, pp. 152–153). These ideas resonate with the espoused beliefs and inclu-sive values of client-centered occupational therapy. The United States, with its history of colonization and slavery—two influential historical legacies whose consequences are reenacted in a myriad ways today—is an appropriate context within which to examine the applicability of cultural safety to occu-pational therapy.

The idea of cultural safety is inherently contro-versial because it challenges the dominant paradigm that systemically perpetuates disadvantages. Cul-tural safety is a "radical, politicized understanding of cultural consideration, effectively rejecting the limited culturally competent approach for one based not on knowledge but on power" (Brascoupé & Waters, 2009, p. 10). Cultural safety goes beyond cultural competence and cultural sensitivity and sit-uates differences encountered in any multicultural context in historical contexts and consequences. It requires health care professionals to reflect on social inequality, power, privilege, and oppression and to dig for the systemic roots of inequities.

Although the construct of cultural safety is yet to be tested and evaluated, it appears to be an applica-ble ethical response in any stratified and diverse so-ciety (Woods, 2010). It has been gaining acceptance in health care education, practice, and research with diverse populations in countries with a history of colonization, such as Canada and Australia.

A study in Israel by Arieli, Friedman, and Hirschfeld (2012) revealed four challenges that Jewish and Arab students experienced in exploring cultural safety: (1) feeling safe to present minority cultures to a majority group, (2) dealing with the tendency of groups to deny the existence of con-flict, (3) discussing the dynamics of oppression, and (4) creating conditions in which people can freely choose their individual and group identi-ties. These findings are similar to those of critical debriefings with students after service-learning experiences in communities they typically would not interact with, putting them outside their com-fort zone (Jyothi Gupta, personal communication, December 2015). Cultural safety provides a "criti-cal and inclusive perspective of culture" that may promote critical discussions and deeper insights into culture, health, and health disparities by giv-ing voice to members of society who are typically silenced and marginalized from mainstream dis-course (Gerlach, 2012, p. 151).

Scholars in occupational therapy have challenged the profession's Eurocentric value-laden assumptions and influences on the therapeutic encounter and processes (Hammell, 2011; Hammell & Iwama, 2012; Jungerson, 2002; Kantartzis & Molineux, 2011; Kirsh, Trentham, & Cole, 2006). To provide authentic client-centered practice in meeting the occupational needs of all members of society, the professional community must examine its discourse and practices through the lens of cultural safety.

Cultural Congruence

Cultural congruence "is a process of effective interaction between the provider and client" facilitated by an understanding of the cultural contexts of both (Schim & Doorenbos, 2010, p. 259). Whereas the concept of *cultural competence* emphasizes the provider's understanding of cultural diversity, cultural awareness, cultural sensitivity, and culturally competent behaviors, Schim and Doorenbos's (2010) model also includes an analysis of client-level dynamics and awareness of cultural confounders.

The client level of Schim and Doorenbos's (2010) model "consists of those patient, family, and community attitudes, beliefs, and behaviors that represent areas of greatest similarity and difference both between and within cultural groups, subgroups, and individuals" (p. 261). In this model, the client can be an individual, his or her family or close friends, or even the community in which the client works and lives.

Cultural confounders, which include racism, sexism, classism, homophobia, and unacknowledged privilege, are barriers to culturally congruent care, and an important task of practitioners is to be sensitive to them. Other cultural confounders are institutional and organizational barriers, and practitioners must recognize and deal with them to provide effective interventions. Such sensitivity enhances the fit between the provider and the client by enabling congruence in thought and action between the two (Quigley, Sperber, & Drossman, 2011; Rashed, 2013). Barrera and Corso (2002) noted that the key to culturally congruent care lies in "the ability to craft respectful, reciprocal, and responsive effective interactions across diverse cultural parameters" (p. 103).

Schim and Doorenbos (2010) believed that the construct of culturally congruent care advances the field by promoting the recognition "that it is in a dynamic interaction between clients and providers that care occurs and that both client, patient, family and provider attitudes, perceptions, and behaviors influence outcomes" (p. 262). Although the role of the provider is similar to that envisioned in cultural competence, addition of the client level and acknowledgment of sociocultural barriers called for in culturally congruent care can help providers enhance and adapt their cross-cultural interactions to provide culturally effective care.

Cultural Proficiency

The concept of *cultural proficiency* is the final step in the cultural competence continuum developed by Cross and colleagues (1989). The other five levels of the continuum are (1) cultural destructiveness, (2) cultural incapacity, (3) cultural blindness, (4) cultural precompetence, and (5) cultural competence (Exhibit 4.2).

Exhibit 4.2. Cultural Competence Continuum

Cultural destructiveness	Purposeful destruction of a culture through attitudes, policies, or actions
Cultural incapacity	Trivialization, blaming, or devaluation of a culture
Cultural blindness	Failure to acknowledge differences between cultures, typified by the belief that culture makes no difference and that all people are the same; disregard for cultural strengths and encouragement of assimilation
Cultural precompetence	Beginning awareness of cultural differences and one's lack of knowledge about work with diverse clients
Cultural competence	Acceptance of and respect for difference; continual work to improve self-awareness, knowledge of cultures and difference, and cross-cultural interactions; continual work to increase effectiveness in practice
Cultural proficiency	High esteem for culture and promotion of cultural competence in others; engagement in lifelong learning to continually increase effectiveness in serving the needs of diverse groups; maintenance of a vision of creating a socially and culturally just environment

Note. Definitions adapted from Lindsey, Robins, Lindsey, & Terrell, 2009; Wittman & Velde, 2002.

Other authors have also identified cultural proficiency as a higher level of cultural competence. Within the nursing literature, Wells (2000) stated that cultural competence does not "achieve the level of cultural development necessary to meet the health care needs of a diverse population" (p. 189) but that cultural proficiency as a philosophical and behavioral approach extends cultural competence in a way that guides and prescribes behaviors toward diverse clients.

Achieving cultural proficiency requires more than just improving one's self-awareness and cultural knowledge and skills, all of which are the characteristics of cultural competence. Cultural proficiency also requires a shift in one's philosophy and worldview regarding effective interactions with diverse populations. Lindsey, Robins, Lindsey, and Terrell (2009) identified the following guiding principles for cultural proficiency:

- Culture is a predominant force in society.
- People are served in varying degrees by the dominant culture.
- People have individual and group identities.
- Diversity within cultures is vast and significant.
- Each cultural group has unique cultural needs.
- The best of both worlds enhances the capacity of all.

These statements speak to a more broadly encompassing view of the underlying assumptions of cross-cultural care. This view assumes a belief in the rightness of and positive results for all in effective cross-cultural interactions, a positive moral stance that has global ramifications. Baron (2007) spoke to this when he described cultural proficiency as a "moral imperative" (p. 52). Within a health care setting, cultural proficiency "endorse[s] the positive role culture can play in a person's health and wellbeing" (Shaya & Gbarayor, 2006, p. 3).

Cultural Effectiveness

The concept of cultural proficiency integrates well with the concept of *cultural effectiveness*, and in some cases the terms are used interchangeably. **Cultural effectiveness** is "the ability to interact with people from different cultures so as to optimise the probability of mutually successful outcomes" (Stone, 2006, p. 338). It is the goal or preferred clinical and therapeutic outcome of many of the concepts discussed in this chapter and the ultimate destination

for best practice in intercultural interactions. Although cross-cultural effectiveness has been discussed in the business and management literature for years (Caligiuri & Tarique, 2012; Fisher & Hartel, 2003; Hopkins, Hopkins, & Gross, 2005), it has received limited attention in the health care literature.

Núñez (2000) found the notion of cultural effectiveness preferable to that of cultural competence because cultural effectiveness "implies that the caregiver is effective in interactions that involve individuals of different cultures and that neither the caregiver's nor the patient's culture offers the preferred view" (p. 1071). Núñez criticized the idea of cultural competence because it "implies a discrete knowledge set that focuses on the culture of the patient only as something 'other' and therefore aberrant from the norm" (p. 1071) and may actually perpetuate stereotypes.

One reason why this text's editors felt it was important to move the focus from cultural competence to cultural effectiveness is because *competence* connotes an end achievement. Gupta (2008) noted that the term *cultural competence* "inadvertently implies that a hypothetical end-point exists that can be reached by acquiring the right knowledge and skills and attitudes needed to work with persons of different cultures" (p. 3). In reality, developing cultural competence is both a lifelong process and an ongoing but attainable goal that can be met during each therapeutic interaction.

Culturally effective care does require the practitioner to develop his or her own cultural self-awareness and a strong knowledge base in several areas, including the client's culture, the practitioner's culture, the health care culture, and the sociopolitical culture of the society within which intervention occurs. It also requires the practitioner to develop **cultural skills,** including effective communication, interpersonal, and attitudinal skills. Many of these skills are developed through both classroom lessons and practice in cross-cultural interactions.

Cultural effectiveness also requires practitioners to engage in **critical reflection** on their practice, consistent with cultural metacognition identified in the cultural intelligence literature (Thomas et al., 2008). Stedman and Thomas (2011) explored how occupational therapy practitioners in Australia modified their practice to ensure clinical effectiveness with Aboriginal clients and found reflection to be an important skill.

Critical reflection is reminiscent of Schon's (1983) discussion of reflection in and reflection on practice, which he developed because of "growing skepticism about professional effectiveness" (p. 13). He argued that it is not enough for health care professionals to be skilled in their practice; to be truly effective, they must make an intentional effort to think about and reflect on what they are doing with a client during the therapeutic session, to use an evaluative thinking process to adapt the intervention as it unfolds, and to consider and reflect on that process after therapy has ended. This careful consideration and deep clinical reasoning are part of culturally effective practice.

Reflection 4.4. Culturally Effective Practitioner–Client Interaction

Reflect on the difference between *cultural competence* and *cultural effectiveness*.

- Which construct speaks clearly of an interaction between a practitioner and a client?
- How would you recognize culturally effective care in practice?

Summary

The language and terminology of cross-cultural practice have evolved and continue to change. Although language shifts and our understanding of culture develops, the terms and approaches described in this chapter highlight the importance of effective cross-cultural practice. Because *diverse* means "anyone who is not you" (Núñez, 2000, p. 1072), the goal of occupational therapy interactions should always be effective care, no matter who the client might be.

References

American Occupational Therapy Association. (2011). *Advisory opinion for the Ethics Commission: Cultural competency and ethical practice.* Bethesda, MD: Author. Retrieved from http://www.aota.org/-/media/corporate/files/practice/ethics/advisory/cultural-competency.pdf

Ang, S., Van Dyne, L., Koh, C., Ng, K. Y., Templer, K. J., Tay, C., & Chandrasekar, N. A. (2007). Cultural intelligence: Its measurement and effects on cultural judgment and decision making, cultural adaptation and task performance. *Management and Organization Review, 3,* 335–371. http://dx.doi.org/10.1111/j.1740-8784.2007.00082.x

Arieli, D., Friedman, V. J., & Hirschfeld, M. J. (2012). Challenges on the path to cultural safety in nursing education. *International Nursing Review, 59,* 187–193. http://dx.doi.org/10.1111/j.1466-7657.2012.00982.x

Baca, L. M., & Koss-Chioino, J. D. (1997). Development of a culturally responsive group counseling model for Mexican American adolescents. *Journal of Multicultural Counseling and Development, 25,* 130–141. http://dx.doi.org/10.1002/j.2161-1912.1997.tb00323.x

Baron, D. (2007). Cultural proficiency: A moral imperative. *Principal Leadership, 8,* 52–54.

Barrera, I., & Corso, R. M. (2002). Cultural competency as skilled dialogue. *Topics in Early Childhood Special Education, 22,* 103–113. http://dx.doi.org/10.1177/02711214020220020501

Betancourt, J. R., Green, A. R., Carrillo, J. E., & Ananeh-Firempong, O. (2003). Defining cultural competence: A practical framework for addressing racial/ethnic disparities in health and health care. *Public Health Reports, 118,* 293–302. http://dx.doi.org/10.1016/S0033-3549(04)50253-4

Black, R. M. (2002). Occupational therapy's dance with diversity. *American Journal of Occupational Therapy, 56,* 140–148. http://dx.doi.org/10.5014/ajot.56.2.140

Black, R. M., & Wells, S. A. (2007). *Culture and occupation: A model of empowerment in occupational therapy.* Bethesda, MD: AOTA Press.

Bonder, B., Martin, L., & Miracle, A. (2002). *Culture in clinical care.* Thorofare, NJ: Slack.

Brascoupé, S., & Waters, C. (2009). Cultural safety: Exploring the applicability of the concept of cultural safety to aboriginal health and community wellness. *Journal of Aboriginal Health, 5*(2), 6–41. Retrieved from http://www.naho.ca/jah/english/jah05_02/V5_I2_Cultural_01.pdf

Caligiuri, P., & Tarique, I. (2012). Dynamic cross-cultural competencies and global leadership effectiveness. *Journal of World Business, 47,* 612–622. http://dx.doi.org/10.1016/j.jwb.2012.01.014

Campinha-Bacote, J. (2002). The process of cultural competence in the delivery of healthcare services: A model of care. *Journal of Transcultural Nursing, 13,* 181–184. http://dx.doi.org/10.1177/10459602013003003

Canadian Nurses Association. (2004). *Promoting culturally competent care.* Ottawa: Author.

Chang, E., Simon, M., & Dong, X. Q. (2012). Integrating cultural humility into health care professional education and training. *Advances in Health Science Education, 17,* 269–278. http://dx.doi.org/10.1007/s10459-010-9264-1

Chen, G.-M. (1997, January). *A review of the concept of intercultural sensitivity.* Paper presented at the meeting of the Pacific and Asian Communication Association, Honolulu.

Chua, R. Y. J., Morris, M. W., & Mor, S. (2012). Collaborating across cultures: Cultural metacognition and affect-based trust in creative collaboration. *Organizational Behavior and Human Decision Processes, 118*, 116–131.

Cross, T., Bazron, B., Dennis, K., & Isaacs, M. (1989). *Towards a culturally competent system of care* (Vol. 1). Washington, DC: CASSP Technical Assistance Center.

Crowne, K. A. (2013). Cultural exposure, emotional intelligence, and cultural intelligence: An exploratory study. *International Journal of Cross Cultural Management, 13*, 5–22. http://dx.doi.org/10.1177/1470595812452633

Cruess, S. R., Cruess, R. L., & Steinert, Y. (2010). Commentary— Linking the teaching of professionalism to the social contract: A call for cultural humility. *Medical Teacher, 32*, 357–359. http://dx.doi.org/10.3109/01421591003692722

Dillard, M., Andonian, L., Flores, O., Lai, L., MacRae, A., & Shakir, M. (1992). Culturally competent occupational therapy in a diversely populated mental health setting. *American Journal of Occupational Therapy, 46*, 721–726. http://dx.doi.org/10.5014/ajot.46.8.721

Fisher, G. B., & Hartel, E. J. (2003). Cross cultural effectiveness of Western expatriate–Thai interactions: Lessons learned for IHRM research and theory. *Cross Cultural Management, 10*(4), 4–28. http://dx.doi.org/10.1108/13527600310797667

Gerlach, A. (2012). A critical reflection on the concept of cultural safety. *Canadian Journal of Occupational Therapy, 79*, 151–158. http://dx.doi.org/10.2182/cjot.2012.79.3.4

Goldberg, D. T. (1997). *Racial subjects: Writing on race in America.* New York: Routledge.

Goldman, R. E., Monroe, A. D., & Dube, C. E. (1996). Cultural self-awareness: A component of culturally responsive patient care. *Annals of Behavioral Science and Medicine, 3*, 37–46.

Guerra, P. L., & Nelson, S. W. (2007). Cultural proficiency. *Journal of Staff Development, 28*(3), 59–60.

Gupta, J. (2008). Reflections of one educator on teaching cultural competence. *Education Special Interest Section Quarterly, 18*(3), 3–4.

Hammell, K. W. (2011). Resisting theoretical imperialism in the disciplines of occupational science and occupational therapy. *British Journal of Occupational Therapy, 74*, 27–33. http://dx.doi.org/10.4276/030802211X12947686093602

Hammell, K. W., & Iwama, M. K. (2012). Wellbeing and occupational rights: An imperative for critical occupational therapy. *Scandinavian Journal of Occupational Therapy, 19*, 385–394. http://dx.doi.org/10.3109/11038128.2011.611821

Hecht, M. L., & Baldwin, J. R. (1998). Layers and holograms: A new look at prejudice. In M. L. Hecht (Ed.), *Communicating prejudice* (pp. 57–84). Thousand Oaks, CA: Sage.

Hook, J. N., Davis, D. E., Owen, J., Worthington, E. L., & Utsey, S. O. (2013). Cultural humility: Measuring openness to culturally diverse clients. *Journal of Counseling Psychology, 60*, 353–366. http://dx.doi.org/10.1037/a0032595.

Hopkins, W. E., Hopkins, S. A., & Gross, M. A. (2005). Cultural diversity recomposition and effectiveness in monoculture work groups. *Journal of Organizational Behavior, 26*, 949–964. http://dx.doi.org/10.1002/job.355

Iwama, M. K., Thomson, N. A., & Macdonald, R. M. (2009). The KAWA model: The power of culturally responsive occupational therapy. *Disability and Rehabilitation, 31*, 1125–1135. http://dx.doi.org/10.1080/09638280902773711

Juarez, J. A., Marvel, K., Brezinski, K. L., Glazner, C., Towbin, M. M., & Lawton, S. (2006). Bridging the gap: A curriculum to teach residents cultural humility. *Family Medicine, 38*, 97–102. Retrieved from http://www.montefiore.org/documents/Bridging-the-Gap-A-Curriculum-to-Teach-Residents-Cultural-Humility.pdf

Jungerson, K. (2002). Cultural safety: Kawa Wakaruruhau— An occupational therapy perspective. *New Zealand Journal of Occupational Therapy, 49*(1), 4–9. Retrieved from http://www.otboard.org.nz/wp-content/uploads/2014/12/Cultural-Safety-_An-Article-2006.pdf

Kantartzis, S., & Molineux, M. (2011). The influence of Western society's construction of a healthy daily life on the conceptualization of occupation. *Journal of Occupational Science, 18*, 62–80. http://dx.doi.org/10.1080/14427591.2011.566917

Kirsh, B., Trentham, B., & Cole, S. (2006). Diversity in occupational therapy: Experiences of consumers who identify themselves as minority group members. *Australian Occupational Therapy Journal, 53*, 302–313. http://dx.doi.org/10.1111/j.1440-1630.2006.00576.x

Leininger, M. M. (1988). Leininger's theory of nursing: Cultural care diversity and universality. *Nursing Science Quarterly, 1*, 152–160. http://dx.doi.org/10.1177/089431848800100408

Lindsey, R. B., Robins, K. N., Lindsey, D. B., & Terrell, R. D. (2009). Cultural proficiency: Changing the conversation. *Leadership, 38*(4), 12–15.

Merriam-Webster. (2016a). *Tolerance.* Retrieved from http://www.merriam-webster.com/dictionary/tolerance

Merriam-Webster. (2016b). *Tolerate.* Retrieved from http://www.merriam-webster.com/dictionary/tolerate

Muñoz, J. P. (2007). Culturally responsive caring in occupational therapy. *Occupational Therapy International, 14*, 256–280. http://dx.doi.org/10.1002/oti.238

Núñez, A. E. (2000). Transforming cultural competence into cross-cultural efficacy in women's health education. *Academic Medicine, 75*, 1071–1080. Retrieved from http://philadelphiaujima.servauntgroup.com/wp-content/uploads/2012/06/culturalcompetenceandCCefficacyinWHed.pdf

Papps, E., & Ramsden, I. (1996). Cultural safety in nursing: A New Zealand experience. *International Journal for Quality in*

Health Care, 8, 491–497. http://dx.doi.org/10.1093/intqhc /8.5.491

Parker, M., & Kiatoukaysy, L. N. (1999). Culturally responsive health care: The example of the Hmong in America. *Journal of the American Academy of Nurse Practitioners, 11*, 511–518. http://dx.doi.org/10.1111/j.1745-7599.1999.tb01220.x

Quigley, E. M. M., Sperber, A. D., & Drossman, D. A. (2011). *Journal of Clinical Gastroenterology, 45*(8), i–ii.

Ramsden, I. (1992). Teaching cultural safety. *New Zealand Nursing Journal, 85*(5), 21–23.

Rashed, M. A. (2013). Culture, salience, and psychiatric diagnosis: Exploring the concept of cultural congruence and its practical application. *Philosophy, Ethics, and Humanities in Medicine, 8*(5). http://dx.doi.org/10.1186/1747-5341-8-5

Ridley, C. R., Mendoza, D. W., Kanitz, B. E., Angermeier, L., & Zenk, R. (1994). Cultural sensitivity in multicultural counseling: A perceptual schema model. *Journal of Counseling Psychology, 41*, 125–136. http://dx.doi.org/10.1037 /0022-0167.41.2.125

Sachdev, P. (1997). Cultural sensitivity training through experiential learning: A participatory demonstration field education project. *International Social Work, 40*, 7–25. http:// dx.doi.org/10.1177/002087289704000102

Saldana, D. (2001). *Cultural competency: A practical guide for mental health service providers.* Austin: University of Texas at Austin, Hogg Foundation for Mental Health.

Schim, S. M., & Doorenbos, A. Z. (2010). A three-dimensional model of cultural congruence: Framework for intervention. *Journal of Social Work in End-of-Life and Palliative Care, 6*, 256–270. http://dx.doi.org/10.1080/15524256.2010.529023

Schon, D. A. (1983). *The reflective practitioner: How professionals think in action.* New York: Basic Books.

Shaya, F. T., & Gbarayor, C. M. (2006). The case for cultural competence in health professions education. *American Journal of Pharmacy Education, 70*(6), 124. http://dx.doi.org /10.5688/aj7006124

Stedman, A., & Thomas, Y. (2011). Reflecting on our effectiveness: Occupational therapy interventions with Indigenous clients. *Australian Occupational Therapy Journal, 58*, 43–49. http://dx.doi.org/10.1111/j.1440-1630.2010.00916.x

Stone, N. (2006). Conceptualising intercultural effectiveness for university teaching. *Journal of Studies in International Education, 10*, 334–356. http://dx.doi.org/10.1177 /1028315306287634

Suarez-Balcazar, Y., Rodawoski, J., Balcazar, F., Taylor-Ritzler, T., Portillo, N., Barwacz, D., & Willis, C. (2009). Perceived levels of cultural competence among occupational therapists. *American Journal of Occupational Therapy, 63*, 498–505. http://dx.doi.org/10.5014/ajot.63.4.498

Tervalon, M., & Murray-García, J. (1998). Cultural humility versus cultural competence: A critical distinction in defining physician training outcomes in multicultural education. *Journal of Health Care for the Poor and Underserved, 9*, 117–125. http://dx.doi.org/10.1353/hpu.2010.0233

Thomas, D. C. (2006). Domain and development of cultural intelligence: The importance of mindfulness. *Group and Organizational Management, 31*(1), 78–99. http://dx.doi .org/10.1177/1059601105275266

Thomas, D. C., Elron, E., Stahl, G., Ekelund, B. Z., Ravlin, E. C., Cerdin, J.-L., . . . Lazarova, M. B. (2008). Cultural intelligence: Domain and assessment. *International Journal of Cross Cultural Management, 8*, 123–143. http://dx.doi .org/10.1177/1470595808091787

Turnbull, A. P., & Turnbull, H. R. (1996). Self determination within a culturally responsive family systems perspective: Balancing the family mobile. In L. E. Powers, G. H. S. Singer, & J. A. Sowers (Eds.), *On the road to autonomy: Promoting self-competence among children and youth with disabilities* (pp. 195–200). Baltimore: Paul H. Brookes.

Wells, M. I. (2000). Beyond cultural competence: A model for individual and institutional cultural development. *Journal of Community Health Nursing, 17*, 189–199. http://dx .doi.org/10.1207/S15327655JCHN1704_1

Wittman, P., & Velde, B. P. (2002). The Issue Is—Attaining cultural competence, critical thinking, and intellectual development: A challenge for occupational therapists. *American Journal of Occupational Therapy, 56*, 454–456. http:// dx.doi.org/10.5014/ajot.56.4.454

Wlodkowski, R. J., & Ginsberg, M. B. (1995). *Diversity and motivation: Culturally responsive teaching.* San Francisco: Jossey-Bass.

Woods, M. (2010). Cultural safety and the socioethical nurse. *Nursing Ethics, 17*, 715–725. http://dx.doi.org/10.1177 /0969733010379296

Yurkovich, E. E., Clairmont, J., & Grandbois, D. (2002). Mental health care providers' perception of giving culturally responsive care to American Indians. *Perspectives in Psychiatric Care, 38*, 147–156. http://dx.doi.org/10.1111/j.1744-6163 .2002.tb01565.x

Section II.

CHARACTERISTICS OF CULTURAL EFFECTIVENESS

Chapter 5.

MODEL FOR CULTURE EFFECTIVENESS

Shirley A. Wells, DrPH, OTR, FAOTA; Roxie M. Black, PhD, OTR/L, FAOTA; and Jyothi Gupta, PhD, OTR/L, FAOTA

> *To be culturally effective doesn't mean you are an authority in the values and beliefs of every culture. What it means is that you hold a deep respect for cultural differences and are eager to learn, and willing to accept, that there are many ways of viewing the world.*
> **Okokon O. Udo (as cited in Clowes, n.d., p. 2)**

Chapter Highlights

- Culture and the Clinical Encounter
- Importance of Cultural Effectiveness for Health Professionals
- Conceptual Framework of the Cultural Effectiveness Model
- The Cultural Effectiveness Model

Key Terms and Concepts

- ✧ Abstract liberalism
- ✧ Awareness
- ✧ Color blindness
- ✧ Color-blind racism
- ✧ Color evasion
- ✧ Communication
- ✧ Conflict Theory
- ✧ Critical analysis
- ✧ Critical reflection
- ✧ Cultural Effectiveness Model
- ✧ Cultural effectiveness
- ✧ Cultural knowledge
- ✧ Cultural pluralism
- ✧ Cultural racism
- ✧ Cultural skill

- ✧ Description
- ✧ Education
- ✧ Evaluation
- ✧ Functional Theory
- ✧ Interactionist Theory
- ✧ Minimization of racism
- ✧ Multicultural education
- ✧ Multiculturalism
- ✧ Naturalization
- ✧ New perspectives
- ✧ Power evasion
- ✧ Reflection
- ✧ Reflection-for-action
- ✧ Reflection-in-action
- ✧ Reflection-on-action

✧ Reflective learning
✧ Self-awareness
✧ Self-exploration

✧ Sociology
✧ Synthesis

Health care providers have a responsibility to develop self-awareness, gain knowledge about other cultures, and cultivate skills to effectively accomplish their clients' health care goals. They must also interact and communicate within multicultural societies and critically reflect on the experiences in which they have effectively responded to client needs and preferences.

The need for culturally effective health care providers comes with the dilemmas of not only quantifying effectiveness in multicultural interaction and integrating culture into health care procedures and teaching approaches but also identifying a model for developing this competency. In this chapter, we introduce the Cultural Effectiveness Model and outline the process for becoming a culturally effective health care provider. Using this model, we explore a framework and process that providers, students, practitioners, and systems can use to increase their ability to effectively adapt, negotiate, collaborate, and function in a multicultural environment.

Culture and the Clinical Encounter

Culture is a part of everyone's life. Every person is influenced by a unique combination of cultural orientations and influences and belongs to various cultural groups that direct and shape his or her multicultural identity. When people interact, culture mediates their interactions (Fitzgerald, 1992; Lott, 2010). As a result, health care consumers and providers approach health care situations with their unique communication characteristics, health beliefs, and customs.

Clients Seeking Health Care

As the American population is multiracial, multicultural, and multilingual, those seeking and providing health care are increasingly diverse. Moreover, the culture of these people is not static but fluid, full of differences within the same ethnic or social groups because of age cohort, gender, political association, class, religion, ethnicity, and even personality (Hasnain et al., 2011; Kleinman & Benson, 2006).

Health Care Providers

The modern health care system is also influenced by differences in the sexual identity, age, educational background, and occupation of health care providers. These different cultural influences affect the provision of effective and quality health care (Black & Wells, 2007). Therefore, every clinical encounter is a cross-cultural interaction.

Cultural influences challenge health care providers to perform assessments and to develop intervention plans with clients who may not share a common language with them; who may have a different understanding of the nature of work, leisure, and self-care; and who may have differing beliefs, values, attitudes, and behaviors. By understanding and accepting the client's values and beliefs, providers can more effectively assess, facilitate, and negotiate better outcomes.

As the United States becomes more racially and ethnically diverse, providers need to respond to consumers' varied perspectives and preserve and protect those cultural traditions that contribute to good health (Institute of Medicine, 2013). Different points of view can complicate health care and make it difficult for both the providers and clients to achieve appropriate and effective care.

Importance of Cultural Effectiveness for Health Professionals

Cultural effectiveness is working successfully with people whose cultural background differs from yours in a manner that embodies respect, sensitivity, and recognition of difference. It refers to an ability to interact effectively with people and systems of different cultures and socioeconomic backgrounds. It is the integration and transformation of knowledge about people and groups of people into specific standards, policies, practices, and attitudes used in settings to increase the quality of services—thereby producing better outcomes (McDaniel, 2014; Watson, 2010). Culturally effective services are respectful of and responsive to the beliefs and practices and cultural and linguistic needs of diverse populations. Clowes (n.d.) suggested five elements of cultural effectiveness:

1. Awareness and acceptance of difference
2. Awareness of own cultural values
3. Understanding the dynamics of difference
4. Development of cultural knowledge
5. Ability to adapt practice to the cultural context of the client.

Clowes (n.d.) argued that cultural effectiveness is not about lists of cultural characteristics, it is about investing open-mindedness and curiosity into communication—developing and expressing genuine warmth, thoughtfulness, and respect for different cultural orientations is needed to enhance the effectiveness of health care delivery.

Practitioners have an obligation to understand and appreciate the differences that exist and to plan for these differences in the delivery of care, because culturally adapted intervention will positively affect service delivery and will overcome cross-cultural bumps (Clowes, n.d.; Hasnain et al., 2011). Cultural beliefs and communication styles affect how we discuss our health problems, influence the way we describe our symptoms, change the way we define reactions to illness, and may affect health outcomes.

Cost of Cultural Ineffectiveness

The consequences of cultural ineffectiveness can be significant. Miscommunication, distrust, and misunderstanding between clients and providers can result. The provider may not understand why the client does not comply with the intervention plan. The client may reject the health care provider even before any one-on-one interaction occurs because of nonverbal cues that do not fit expectations, such as lack of interpreter services, lack of culturally and linguistically appropriate health education material, or stereotyping (Betancourt & Green, 2010; Hasnain et al., 2011). From either perspective, accepting societal stereotypes and beliefs about others who differ in some way from the dominant culture can lead to avoidance, lack of respect, and stigmatization, which, in turn, can influence how people are treated (Waite, Nardi, & Killian, 2014).

Challenges of Culturally Effective Practice

Caring for clients from different cultures presents a variety of challenges. The relationship between culture and health-related behavior is inherently complex. Clients' cultural and ethnic backgrounds shape their views of illness and well-being in the physical, emotional, and spiritual realms and affect their perceptions of health care as well as the outcomes of treatment (Genao, Bussey-Jones, Brady, Branch, & Corbie-Smith, 2003; Kleinman & Benson, 2006; Kundhal, 2003). Health-seeking behaviors, when and to whom we go for care, and the length of time we remain in care are determined, in part, by cultural beliefs about illness.

Sharing Information

Participants of the health care system must share relevant information and coordinate many different activities to effectively accomplish their health care goals. Occupational therapists and occupational therapy assistants depend on receiving information from their clients about health histories and symptoms, lifestyles, and concerns to make appropriate intervention decisions (American Occupational Therapy Association, 2014).

Similarly, clients depend on receiving clear and descriptive information about health care treatment and strategies from their providers. Members of the health care team also depend on sharing pertinent information with each other to provide effective care (Joint Commission, 2010). Yet, the client, provider, and team members are all likely to have very different cultural orientations and understandings regarding the provision of health care on the basis of their personal cultural interaction, influences, experiences, and professional training (Kratzke & Bertolo, 2013).

These different points of view are a positive thing! They can generate a broad base of information that encourages a holistic view of the client's condition, needs, and health care. However, they can also complicate health care if there is lack of respect. Given the need for cultural effectiveness in health care practice, a thorough, systemic, and integrated learning process—which incorporates self-exploration, knowledge, skills, and reflection—is needed to address the issue of acquiring cultural competence.

Reflection 5.1. Attributes of a Culturally Effective Practitioner

- What are the attributes of a culturally effective practitioner?

Conceptual Framework of the Cultural Effectiveness Model

The conceptual framework for the Cultural Effectiveness Model has been developed from two schools of thoughts: (1) sociology and (2) education. *Sociology* is the study of human social relationships and patterns of behavior as social beings. *Education* is the act of acquiring knowledge. Each makes a contribution to becoming culturally effective, and we review both of these perspectives next.

Sociological Perspectives

In sociology, three theoretical perspectives have shaped the study of and have described the interaction between minority and majority groups in a society: Functional Theory, Conflict Theory, and Interactionist Theory. *Functional Theory* examines the theoretical support for maintaining a harmonious society and seeking new and different adjustments to restore equilibrium when dysfunction occurs. Functionalists believe that a stable, cooperative social system is the basis of society. Rapid social changes, such as demographic changes, require compensating adjustments. If these adjustments do not occur, tension and conflicts are created between the groups (Parrillo, 1997).

Conflict Theory emphasizes the tension and conflicts that result when different groups compete for limited resources. Conflict theorists see disequilibrium and change as the norm because of societal inequalities. Group cohesiveness and struggle against oppression are necessary to effect social change (Parrillo, 1997).

Interactionist Theory focuses on the personal interaction patterns in everyday life. Essential to this perspective is the belief that people operate within a socially constructed perception of reality. Interactionists conclude that shared expectation and understanding, or lack of the same, explain intergroup relations. Through better communication and intercultural awareness, minority–majority interaction patterns can improve (Parrillo, 1997). The conceptual framework for the Cultural Effectiveness Model ascribes more to the Interactionist Theory.

Color Blindness

Another sociological assumption that underlies the need for the Cultural Effectiveness Model is the ideology of *color blindness*, which posits that the best way to end discrimination is by treating people as equally as possible without regard to race, culture, or ethnicity. Color blindness deemphasizes the significance of race in shaping social outcomes and individual opportunities (Burke & Banks, 2012; Neville, Awad, Brooks, Flores, & Bluemel, 2013; Williams, 2011).

Neville et al. (2013) described two interrelated domains of color blindness as

1. *Color evasion,* which is the "denial of racial differences by emphasizing sameness" (p. 457), and
2. *Power evasion,* which is the "denial of racism by emphasizing equal opportunities" (p. 457).

"People are just people." "I don't see color." "We're all just human." Pretending not to see race does not make the problems of race go away. Racism—both personal and systemic—is about the social value we assign to people and their actions based on their physical attributes. It is not about what you see but what you perceive and how you're told to behave (Obasogie, 2013). Color blindness maintains these problems because they are not addressed as racial problems. People of color experience subtler social cues that hint at biased tendencies.

Color-blind racism treats individuals as equally as possible, without regard to race, culture, or ethnicity. But we are not equal and never have been. Race does exist, and it does matter for what happens to people. Bonilla-Silva (2006) demonstrated that the central frame of what he termed *color-blind racism* includes

- *Abstract liberalism* (i.e., belief in equal opportunity while justifying racial inequality and opposing affirmative action as preferential treatment),
- *Naturalization* (i.e., allows the U.S. White majority to reject any consideration of racial phenomena because these phenomena are natural and not man-made),
- *Cultural racism* (i.e., relies on culturally based arguments—such as "Mexicans do not put much emphasis on education," or "Blacks have too many babies"—to explain the standing of minorities in society), and
- *Minimization of racism* (i.e., the belief that racial discrimination is lessening or has disappeared and thus is no longer a central factor affecting minorities' life chances).

Color-blind racial ideology (CBRI) favors explanations for continuing racial inequality that are race neutral. It removes racism, past and present, as explanatory factors for disparities. Avoiding race can narrow or skew one's view of the world and lead to disconnection and distrust. Color blindness equates color with something negative or a problem: "I don't see your color; I just see you." For people of color whose race is core to their identities, this causes them to feel invisible. In a color-blind society, negative racial experiences are denied, cultural heritages are rejected, and unique perspectives are invalidated (Greenberg, 2015; Neville et al., 2013; Williams, 2011).

Mounting empirical data suggest that color evasion, evident in ideologies such as color blindness, is ineffective and promotes interracial tension and potential inequality (Bonilla-Silva & Dietrich, 2011; Neville et al., 2013). Williams (2011), the director of the Center for Mental Health Disparities at the University of Louisville, suggested that color blindness alone is not sufficient for healing racial wounds on a national or personal level and could be a form of racism.

Practitioners should not be blind to a person's culture or racial identity. Color blindness ignores the experiences of being stigmatized by society and does not foster equality, respect, or trust. As Williams (2011) emphasized, "It represents an empathetic failure on the part of the therapist; it merely relieves the therapist of his or her obligation to address important racial differences and difficulties" (p. 2).

Cultural Pluralism

The type of interaction between ethnic people and those of the dominant culture promoted by the Cultural Effectiveness Model is based on the views and values expressed in the ideology and theory of cultural pluralism, which is often denoted as multiculturalism. *Cultural pluralism* refers to the presence of many cultures in society that coexist in a supportive and conducive environment (Muchenje, 2012).

According to pluralist theorists, individual ethnic groups have a right to exist on their own terms within the larger society while retaining their unique cultural heritages. *Multiculturalism* recognizes the cultural diversity present in society. It acknowledges, highlights, values, and celebrates cultural differences. It fosters personal friendships and organizational alliances (McCabe, 2011).

Multicultural Education Perspectives

The term *multicultural education* is used to describe a wide variety of programs and practices related to educational equity, women, ethnic groups, language minorities, low-income groups, and people with disabilities (Banks & Banks, 2010). Multicultural education was created during the social protest of the 1960s and 1970s (Banks, 2009).

Characteristics of Multicultural Education

Grounded in the philosophy of cultural pluralism and principles of equality, mutual respect, acceptance, understanding, and moral commitment to social justice, multicultural education stresses the importance, legitimacy, and vitality of ethnic and cultural diversity in shaping the lives of individual people, groups, and nations (Baptiste, 1979). Multicultural education recognizes the diversity of cultural differences that exist in a pluralistic society (Banks, 2009; Sleeter & Grant, 2007).

School as a Social System

Multicultural education views the school as a social system that should be transformed to bring about educational equality; all major components must be substantially changed. "A major goal of multicultural education is to help students to develop the knowledge, attitudes, and skills needed to function within their own microcultures, the U.S. macroculture, other microcultures, and the global community" (Banks & Banks, 2010, p. 25).

Learning Process

Multicultural education offers opportunities to deal directly with cultural diversity and to integrate others' perspectives into the learning process. It encourages learners to view different cultures as sources of learning and enrichment.

Learning is viewed as a tapestry of perspectives. Multicultural education focuses on how to learn rather than learning specific information. It emphasizes the importance of people sharing their stories and learning from the stories of others. It also takes into account the learner, his or her learning style, and the extent to which the learner has changed relative to the material (Banks & Banks, 2004). Multicultural education is a continuing process with the idealized goals of actualizing educational equality and eradicating all forms of discrimination (Banks & Banks, 2010).

Learning Through Reflection

In addition to being framed by sociological and education perspectives, the Cultural Effectiveness Model is based on the idea of learning through reflection. Many health care professionals use their knowledge and past experiences to develop and provide effective care. *Reflection* is the deconstruction of events and interactions (i.e., critical thinking) that allows practitioners to learn, grow, and develop in and through practice (Harrison, 2012).

Learning through reflection must occur throughout the provision of culturally effective care. Practitioners deal with the effects and influence of illness on their clients, which includes their perceptions and the ways they ascribe meanings to signs, symptoms, treatment, and health that may prompt different actions. Critical reflection and thinking encompass investigating and imagining alternative scenarios that are client-centered and acknowledge the complexity of the practice environment (McClure, 2005; Oelofsen, 2012).

Experience

We learn a lot from formal education, but learning research shows that we also learn by doing. Through experience, we learn to

- Absorb (i.e., read, hear, feel),
- Do (i.e., activity), and
- Interact (i.e., socialize; Wertenbroch & Nabeth, 2000).

Occupational therapy practitioners draw on experiences to distinguish relevant information and to assess the risks of different courses of action. Experience allows the professional to analyze instantaneously the factors that could affect the performance or the outcome (Casey, 2014; Hinett, 2002; Schön, 1983).

Critical Reflection

We learn by reflecting on experiences (Leung, Pluye, Grad, & Weston, 2010). Deliberate reflection provides the professional with a process to develop professional judgment and to choose a particular course of action. *Critical reflection* is the "mental process of trying to structure or restructure an experience, a problem, or existing knowledge or insights" (Korthagen, 2001, p. 58). It can be seen as a way to improve the quality and depth of cultural effectiveness.

Schön (1983) suggested that the capacity to reflect on action so as to engage in a process of continuous learning was a defining characteristic of professional practice. The process of critical reflection provides a framework for connections and enables us to distinguish among important cornerstones of learning, prominent features, and background in a way that is meaningful and acceptable (Hinett, 2002).

When we reflect, we deeply consider something about which we might not otherwise have given much thought. We consciously examine our experiences, actions, feelings, and responses and then interpret or analyze them so that we can learn (Atkins & Murphy, 1993; Leung et al., 2010). Typically, we reflect by asking ourselves questions about

- What we did,
- How we did it, and
- What we learned from doing it.

Critical reflecting on experiences encourages insight and complex learning. When done alone, we foster our own growth. When done with others, we enhance our learning (Costa & Kallick, 2008).

Reflective Learning

Reflective learning is "the process of internally examining and exploring an issue of concern, triggered by an experience, which creates and clarifies meaning in terms of self, and which results in a changed conceptual perspective" (Atkins & Murphy, 1993, p. 1189). It enables the person to accept responsibility for his or her personal growth, to link professional development to practical outcomes, to see value in each learning experience, and to see how to use new knowledge and skills in future activities (Davys & Beddoe, 2009).

Atkins and Murphy (1993) identified three stages in the reflective processes:

1. *Awareness*—an awareness of uncomfortable feelings and thoughts, negative or positive; an out-of-the-ordinary experience that causes you to begin reflecting.
2. *Critical analysis*—a critical analysis of the situation that leads to an examination of feelings and knowledge; it may involve the generation of new knowledge requiring the process of critical thinking or talking with colleagues to learn from their experiences.

3. *New perspectives*—the development of a new perspective on the situation; moving from a position of a detached observer to one of becoming involved.

Reflective learning is neatly described by Ruch (2000) as

> a holistic, creative and artistic phenomenon which endeavors to hold theory and practice together in a creative tension. It also allows for uncertainty and mistakes and acknowledges the humanity of practitioners and clients. Reflective learning which acknowledges the complexity, diversity and emotionality of situations offers more scope for student practitioners to reach informed decisions which, by embracing the breadth of knowledge which influence decisions, could help avoid defensive, routinized and ritualistic responses. (p. 108)

Repetition and practice help us to learn, but they do not substitute for the process of actively thinking about how we did, what we did well, and what we did less well. With the aid of a simple prompt question (e.g., "What might I do better next time?" or "What could I do differently?"), we have the potential to draw on the past and present and direct ourselves to a better future. It is this power to effect change that makes reflective practice so fundamental to higher education and to the creation of lifelong learners (Brigden & Purcell, 2004; Hinett, 2002). To provide culturally effective care, practitioners must engage in critical reflection throughout the process of obtaining knowledge, skills, and self-awareness.

The Cultural Effectiveness Model

The *Cultural Effectiveness Model* refers to a process designed to foster understanding, acceptance, knowledge, and constructive relations among people of various cultures and differences (Figure 5.1). The model assumes that

- All people have a variety of multicultural influences.
- Differences exist among and within cultures.
- Everyone has been affected and molded by more than one culture and therefore is a multicultural being.
- Each person has the right to be respected for his or her uniqueness and cultural heritage.
- Becoming culturally competent is a life-long process.
- Cultural effectiveness is a professional and ethical obligation.
- Cultural effectiveness enhances the quality of health care delivery.

The development of the Cultural Effectiveness Model was built on Wells and Black's (2000) Cultural Competency Model, in which three constructs were identified: (1) self-exploration, (2) knowledge,

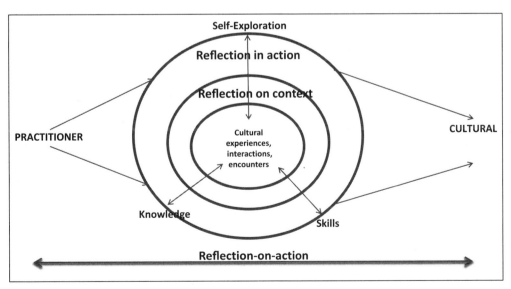

Figure 5.1. The Cultural Effectiveness Model.

and (3) skills. The model needed to be expanded to include new knowledge in the field and to depict the process of delivering culturally effective health care. We have added a fourth construct, *critical reflection,* to emphasize the importance of the thinking process necessary to develop and improve one's self-awareness, knowledge, and skills to provide culturally effective care. Evidence-based and interprofessional collaborative practice necessitates reflection to allow professionals to search for solutions that go beyond their own vision of what is possible. Before a change to practice can occur, clinicians need to reflect on what is being practiced.

The Cultural Effectiveness Model is designed as a tool for developing the knowledge, skills, and reflection that occupational therapy practitioners need to progress toward delivering effective care. It provides a foundation for understanding interaction patterns within environmental, social, and cultural contexts. It can assist the practitioner in adapting, negotiating, and collaborating within our changing society as well as effecting social changes.

The skills of becoming a critically reflective practitioner engaging in reflective practice, whether as a clinician or educator, are vital to delivering culturally effective care. Other personal components necessary to be culturally effective—such as attitudes, behaviors, and perceptions—are not directly addressed but are infused during the learning process.

The Cultural Effectiveness Model aims to assist people in developing the following elements of cultural effectiveness (Clowes, 2014):

- Increase awareness and acceptance of difference
- Increase awareness of own cultural values
- Understand the dynamics of difference
- Develop cultural knowledge and skills
- Adapt practice to the cultural context of the client.

The Cultural Effectiveness Model also aims to assist people in developing:

- Reflective learning and practice skills
- Knowledge of the progression to providing culturally effective care.

The Cultural Effectiveness Model furnishes a clear framework for developing and assessing one's progress toward becoming culturally effective:

To succeed, workers [health care providers] need an awareness and acceptance of cultural differences, an awareness of their own cultural values, an understanding of the dynamics of differences in the helping process, a basic knowledge about the client's culture, knowledge of the client's environment, and the ability to adapt practice skills to fit the client's context. (Cross, Bazron, Dennis, & Isaacs, 1989, p. 32)

With the Cultural Effectiveness Model, the areas in which intervention for change can occur include self-exploration and awareness, cultural knowledge, cultural skills, and critical reflection (see Figure 5.1 and Exhibit 5.1).

Self-Exploration and Awareness

Self-exploration is the process of conducting self-examination of one's own biases toward other cultures and the in-depth exploration of one's cultural and professional background (Campinha-Bacote, 2007). It requires looking inward, learning to recognize when old information no longer applies, and using this knowledge of self. Because bias, stereotyping, prejudice, and clinical uncertainty on the part of health care providers contribute to racial or ethnic disparities in health care (Foege, 2010; Henry J. Kaiser Family Foundation, 2012), self-exploration is essential for cultural effectiveness.

Knowledge of one's self enables the practitioner to be aware of and take responsibility for his or her own emotions and attitudes as they affect his or her professional behaviors. It furnishes the therapist with an understanding of his or her own cultural assumptions about human behavior, values, biases, preconceived notions and personal limitations, as well as the medical culture's biases and of the degree to which he or she is conditioned by these (Gannam, 2014).

Self-exploration is an internal, personal experience, but it is not always a risk-free and pleasant process. It requires the ability to recognize when the judgmental, noncaring self interferes with the ability to reach out, to explore, and to help others. Acknowledging one's own vulnerability in self-introspection can encourage direct communication with others, bolster personal integrity, and assist in determining whether you have any biases or negative feelings toward particular cultures (Erlen, 1998).

Exhibit 5.1. Self-Exploration and Awareness

Goal: To build an awareness of one's own cultural heritage.
Objectives:
- To expand cultural self-awareness.
- To provide the person with an understanding of his or her own culture and of the degree to which he or she is conditioned by it.
- To increase tolerance and acceptance of different values, attitudes, behaviors, and perceptions.

Cultural Knowledge
Goal: To understand that no one culture is intrinsically superior to another; to recognize individual and group differences and similarities.
Objectives:
- To foster the affirmation of all cultures, especially those that, because of minority status, have received a disproportionate amount of negative reinforcement from society.
- To prepare for effective personal adjustment to the stress of intercultural experiences.
- To open avenues of learning and growth that multicultural experiences make accessible.

Cultural Skills
Goal: To develop mastery of appropriate, relevant, and sensitive strategies and skills in communicating and interacting with people from different cultures.
Objectives:
- To develop intercultural communication skills.
- To integrate cognitive, affective, and experiential learning.
- To develop the ability to seek information about the economic, political, and social stresses, and the aspirations of various cultures or ethnic groups within a society.

Critical Reflection
Goal: To facilitate personal growth, professional growth, and meaningful change.
Objectives:
- To foster the habit of reflection as a means of continuing learning.
- To develop critical analysis skills.
- To promote the process of synthesis of new knowledge and experiences.

Awareness of one's own race, ethnicity, and cultural diversity as well as the ability to recognize how these may affect practice is also crucial to the process of becoming a culturally effective practitioner. In actuality, the following culturally appropriate questions need to be answered:

- Who am I in the racial, ethnic, or cultural diversity sense?
- What kind of messages have I received about people from different cultures?
- How accurate is the information I have about people from different cultures?
- How do I usually react to members of other cultures?
- How open am I to learning and interacting with other cultural groups?

A heightened self-awareness and a greater awareness of diversity lead to a realization that, for many people, race, ethnicity, gender, religion, sexual identity, appearance, and disability are forces that shape movement through the life cycle and determine appropriate marriage partners, language, dietary selections, and the various subtleties of daily life. Self-exploration opens avenues of learning and growth. Culturally effective health care providers have beliefs and attitudes that demonstrate

- Awareness of their own ethnic cultural heritage, and how it personally and professional affects their definitions of normality and abnormality and the process of providing services.
- Insight about how oppression, *isms,* (i.e., racism, sexism, classism), discrimination, and stereotyping affect them personally and professionally.
- Awareness of their social impact on others, including an awareness of their communication style differences.
- Ability to seek and integrate experiences that broaden understanding of one's own culture and the culture of others.
- Ability to assess and reflect on the impact of cultural interactions.

Reflection 5.2. Things I Learned as a Child

Much of what we value and feel was learned when we were children. To assist in identifying your myths and biases, recall when and what you learned about each of these groups as a child, then complete the sentences. Be honest with yourself.

- Smart people...
- Asian Americans...
- Rich people...
- Native Americans...
- Hispanics...
- Gays, lesbians, bisexuals, and transgender persons...
- Women...
- Men...
- Lazy people...
- White Americans...
- African Americans...
- Muslims...
- Catholics...

Cultural Knowledge

Cultural knowledge is the process in which the health care provider seeks and obtains a sound educational base about culturally diverse groups (Campinha-Bacote, 2007). It also includes knowledge of health-related beliefs, values, disease incidence and prevalence, and treatment efficacy among diverse groups. Cultural knowledge about other groups promotes understanding and allows occupational therapy practitioners and students to adapt the way in which services are delivered. The greater the shared knowledge, the less likely there are to be misunderstandings.

Many of us have experienced situations in which we are aware of and sensitive to differences, but lacked the specific knowledge of the other cultures or systems involved to avert problems, develop solutions, or acknowledge interplay of cultures. Cultural knowledge allows the therapist to look at an interaction from multiple perspectives, including the culture in which the interaction occurs, cultures of the people involved, and the culture of the society or system.

Gaining cultural knowledge to know *what, who,* and *how* to ask for information should be a desirable goal for a culturally effective practitioner.

Practitioners need to explore the client's culture in terms of family structure and hierarchy, family roles, social attitudes toward seeking help, and the role of spirituality. Kleinman and Benson (2006) proposed the use of what they call *revised cultural formation* to give clients and their family members an opportunity to educate the provider about their culture and views. Using this approach, clinicians can perform a "mini-ethnography" organized by six steps (Kleinman & Benson, 2006, p. 1674):

- *Step 1: Ethnic identity*
  In this step, one affirms and acknowledges a person's racial and ethnic identity and experiences.
- *Step 2: What is at stake?*
  In this step, one assesses all impacts of an illness episode on patients and their loved ones, including close relationships, material resources, religious commitments, and even life itself.
- *Step 3: The illness narrative*
  In this step, one listens to the patient's narrative about the illness and its meaning.
- *Step 4: Psychosocial stressors*
  In this ongoing process, one focuses on the psychosocial problems associated with the illness and its treatment.
- *Step 5: Influence of culture on clinical relationships*
  In this step, one critically self-reflects on the interaction effects of the cultures of the patient, health care system, and provider. One also examines culture in terms of its influence on clinical relationships.
- *Step 6: The problems of a cultural competency approach*
  In this step, one is in danger of overemphasizing cultural differences that could lead to a failure to resolve health problems.

Finding out what matters most to another person is not a technical skill but an elective empathy with the client. The clinicians can then use the information in thinking through treatment decisions and negotiating or collaborating with the client.

The average practitioner cannot achieve comprehensive knowledge about any group, population, or culture. It is more important to know *where* and *how* to obtain the necessary detailed information for use in specific cases. Both formal and informal education coupled with cross-cultural experiences are important avenues for learning. The literature evidence suggests a variety of roads to obtaining cultural knowledge. Providers need to explain to clients that gathering information is one way that the client can bring his or her collaboration into the health care delivery process.

A culturally effective health care provider has cultural knowledge and experience that demonstrate

- Specific efforts to acquire knowledge of the language, values, customs, and beliefs of another culture.
- Understanding about the effects of gender, race, ethnicity, religion, disability, sexual identity, appearance, nationality, geographic location, and lifestyle on human development.
- Basic knowledge about the effects, real or perceived, of institutional and individual discrimination on interaction and use of services.
- Knowledge about the influence of culture on behaviors and needs.
- Knowledge about the worldviews of different cultural and ethnic groups.

Reflection 5.3. Cultural Knowledge

There are many unwritten cultural rules at play when engaging with people.

- What are the rules for eye contact in your community?
- Are they similar or different in another culture?

Cultural Skill

Cultural skill is the ability to use knowledge of self and others to (1) improve cultural interaction and conduct a cultural assessment; (2) collect culturally relevant data during assessments; and (3) practice appropriate, sensitive, and relevant intervention strategies (Campinha-Bacote, 2007; Gannam, 2014). It involves incorporating diverse and multiple perspectives when working with others and having the ability to negotiate and facilitate sharing, acquiring, and mastering strategies, techniques, and approaches for communicating and interacting with people from different cultures. Cultural skill manifests itself in a therapist's ability to accurately interpret and respond to nonverbal or other cultural cues (Agency for Healthcare Research and Quality, 2004).

Shifting One's Own Values

Being a culturally skilled practitioner requires a person to step out of his or her value orientation to identify and interpret what is important in understanding another cultural group (Taylor, 2005). Doing so requires

the practitioner to shift from the role of an authority figure to one of a learner. Such practitioners can improve their effectiveness by using modalities and defining goals that are consistent with their clients' life experiences and cultural values (Gannam, 2014). Such effectiveness can lead to behavioral adaptations and collaboration.

Communication

Cultural skill includes communicating in a manner that is linguistically and culturally appropriate. **Communication** is the flow and exchange of information among those involved in the provision and receipt of care, including interpersonal exchanges and exchanges between people and organizations. Communication encompasses knowledge of the "contextual use of the language; paralanguage variations such as voice, volume, tone, and intonations as well as nonverbal communications such as eye contact, facial expression, touch, body language, spatial distancing practices, and acceptable greetings" (Purnell, 2002, p. 195).

Language and culture are inherently interrelated and interdependent. Cultural and linguistic effectiveness of health professionals can contribute to the health literacy of their clients by improving communication and building trust. Proficiency in cultural communication has been described as skills in communicating with members of diverse cultural groups to achieve desired objectives (Watson, 2010).

Mutual communication (expressive and receptive) conveys a commitment to involvement in an interactive process that involves negotiation until the information is correctly understood by both parties (Joint Commission, 2010). Improved communication skills can lead to increased consumer satisfaction as well as an improved understanding of and compliance with diagnoses and treatment regimens (Agency for Healthcare Research and Quality, 2004).

Competence in cultural skill expedites the ability of providers and clients to collaborate, plan, and deliver mutually beneficial care that will improve rehabilitation outcomes (Hasnain et al., 2011; Joint Commission, 2010). Culturally effective health care providers demonstrate:

- Ability to use, send, and interpret a variety of communication skills, both verbal and nonverbal, to bridge the gap among cultures;

- Ability to negotiate, collaborate, and facilitate a shared understanding with their client and his or her family;
- Ability to generate, modify, and adapt a variety of intervention strategies to accommodate the particular need of the client and his or her family;
- Knowledge to be creative and resourceful in identifying and using cultural value systems on the behalf of the client;
- Skills and knowledge to learn about other cultures; and
- Capability to assess discriminatory intent and discriminatory effect in their interactions and services.

Reflection 5.4. Interpersonal Relationships

- What personal qualities and skills do you have that will help you establish interpersonal relationships with people from other cultural or diverse groups?
- What personal qualities and skills may be detrimental?

Critical Reflection

The encircling construct to cultural effectiveness is critical reflection. As discussed earlier in this chapter, it bridges learning and experiences, allowing people to look back on their interactions and think about what they have experienced. It involves describing, analyzing, and evaluating thoughts, assumptions, beliefs, theory base, and actions (Casey, 2014).

Reflective practice entails a personal commitment to continuous learning and improvement and allows higher level thinking processes (York-Barr, Sommers, Ghere, & Montie, 2001). Schön (1983) distinguished between two types of practice (reflection-in-action and reflection-on-action) in the following way:

- **Reflection-in-action** is concerned with practicing critically. It refers to reflection that takes place during the action (e.g., a therapy student working with a client on an exercise program is making decisions about the suitability of particular exercises, which exercise to do next, and judging the success of each exercise while he or she is conducting the activity).
- **Reflection-on-action** occurs after the activity has taken place when you are thinking about what

you (and others) did, judging how successful you were and whether any changes to what you did could have resulted in different outcomes. This is usually the type of reflection that students are asked to write about as part of their fieldwork experiences.

Killion and Todnem (as cited in Reagan, Case, & Brubacher, 2000) distinguished a third type of reflective practice, **reflection-for-action,** which serves to guide future action.

Fade (n.d.) translated the three types of reflective practice as

1. Looking forward (prospective reflection),
2. Looking at what we are doing now (spective reflection), and
3. Looking back (retrospective reflection).

Therefore, reflective practice involves understanding what the practitioner does before engaging with the client (*looking forward—prospective reflection/ reflection-for-action*) and while working with the client (*looking at what you are doing now—spective reflection/reflection-in-action*), and after engaging with the client (*looking back—retrospective reflection/ reflection-on-action*). For health care providers, critical reflection is about making sense of work-based experiences.

To become a reflective practitioner, according to Brigden and Purcell (2004), the person needs to acquire the following skills:

- **Self-awareness**—the ability to analyze feelings. This skill involves an honest examination of how the situation has affected the person and how the person has affected the situation.
- **Description**—the ability to recognize and recollect salient events. This skill entails recalling similar signs and symptoms and describing a new finding.
- **Critical analysis**—the ability to examine components of a situation. This skill entails examining knowledge, challenging assumptions, as well as imagining and exploring alternatives.
- **Synthesis**—the process of integrating new knowledge or experience. This skill involves the development of new perspective.
- **Evaluation**—the ability to make a judgment about the value of something. This skill comprises judging or assessing the worth of something.

Reflection 5.5. Self-Reflection

Choose someone you remember observing or interacting with at some point today. Write a story about this activity from your perspective.

- What did you learn about your perceptions by writing the story?
- What thoughts or feelings about the activity came out in your writing?
- Would you change your behavior or interaction?
- How would you use this reflection?

Summary

The Cultural Effectiveness Model is a conceptual model that focuses on the process of developing and delivering cultural effectiveness in health care. It can be used to help practitioners answer the question "Is it possible to deliver culturally effective care?" in the affirmative. It can also be used to develop plans for people to practice in a multicultural environment that celebrates and respects cultural differences. The more occupational therapy practitioners examine their practice and articulate effective culturally appropriate interventions, the more health care delivery will improve. Each person will add to his or her knowledge base, through both positive and negative experiences, developing his or her expertise over time.

Reflection 5.6. Being a Culturally Effective Practitioner

- How can you use the Cultural Effectiveness Model to become culturally effective?

References

Agency for Healthcare Research and Quality. (2004, August). *Setting the agenda for research on cultural competence in health care: Introduction and key findings.* Rockville, MD: Author. Retrieved from http://www.ahrq.gov/research/findings/fact sheets/literacy/cultural/index.html

American Occupational Therapy Association. (2014). Occupational therapy practice framework: domain and process (3rd ed.). *American Journal of Occupational Therapy, 68*(Suppl.1), S1–S48. http://dx.doi.org/10.5014/ajot.2014.682006

Atkins, S., & Murphy, K. (1993). Reflection: A review of the literature. *Journal of Advance Nursing, 18,* 118–119. http://dx.doi.org/10.1046/j.1365-2648.1993.18081188.x

Banks, J. A. (Ed.). (2009). *The Routledge international companion to multicultural education.* New York: Routledge.

Banks, J. A., & Banks, C. A. M. (Eds.). (2004). *Handbook of research on multicultural education* (2nd ed.). San Francisco: Jossey-Bass.

Banks, J. A., & Banks, C. A. M. (2010). *Multicultural education issues and perspectives* (7th ed.). New York: Wiley.

Baptiste, H. P. (1979). *Multicultural education: A synopsis.* Washington, DC: University Press of America.

Betancourt, J. R., & Green, A. R. (2010). Commentary: Linking cultural competence training to improved health outcomes: Perspectives from the field. *Academic Medicine Issue, 85,* 583–585. http://dx.doi.org/10.1097/ACM.0b013e3181d2b2f3

Black, R. M., & Wells, S. A. (2007). *Culture and occupation: A model of empowerment in occupational therapy.* Bethesda, MD: AOTA Press.

Bonilla-Silva, E. (2006). *Racism without racists: Color-blind racism and the persistence of racial inequality in the United States* (2nd ed.). Lanham, MD: Rowman & Littlefield.

Bonilla-Silva, E., & Dietrich, D. (2011). The sweet enchantment of color-blind racism in Obamerica. *The ANNALS of the American Academy of Political and Social Science, 634,* 190–206. http://dx.doi.org/10.1177/0002716210389702

Brigden, D., & Purcell, N. (2004, October). *Focus: Becoming a reflective practitioner.* Retrieved from http://iicrd.org/sites/default/files/resources/Becoming_a_reflective_practitioner_0.pdf

Burke, M. A., & Banks, K. H. (2012). Sociology by any other name: Teaching the sociological perspective in campus diversity programs. *Teaching Sociology, 40,* 21–33. http://dx.doi.org/10.1177/0092055X11418686

Campinha-Bacote, J. (2007). *The process of cultural competence in the delivery of healthcare services: The journey continues* (5th ed.). Cincinnati, OH: Transcultural C.A.R.E. Associates.

Casey, T. (2014). Reflective practice in legal education: The stages of reflection. *Clinical Law Review, 20,* 317–354. Retrieved from http://www.law.nyu.edu/sites/default/files/upload_documents/Timothy%20Casey%20-%20Stages%20of%20Reflection_0.pdf

Clowes, L. (n.d.). *Cultural effectiveness* [PowerPoint slides]. Retrieved from http://www.nhcebis.seresc.net/document/filename/388/Cultural_Effectiveness_presentation.pdf

Costa, A. L., & Kallick, B. (2008). Learning through reflection. In A. L. Costa & B. Kallick (Eds.), *Learning and leading with habits of mind: 16 essential characteristics for success* (pp. 221–225). Alexandria, VA: Association for Supervision and Curriculum Development.

Cross, T. L., Bazron, B. J., Dennis, K. W., & Isaacs, M. R. (1989). *Towards a culturally competent system of care* (Vol. 1). Washington, DC: Child and Adolescent Service System Program, Georgetown University Child Development Center, Technical Assistance Center.

Davys, A. M., & Beddoe, L. (2009). The Reflective Learning Model: Supervision of social work students. *Social Work Education, 28,* 919–933. http://dx.doi.org/10.1080/02615470902748662

Erlen, J. A. (1998). Culture, ethics, and respect: The bottom line is understanding. *Orthopedic Nursing, 17*(6), 79–82. http://dx.doi.org/10.1097/00006416-199811000-00012

Fade, S. (n.d.). *Learning and assessing through reflection: A practical guide. Making practice-based learning work.* Retrieved from http://electronicportfolios.org/reflection/RoyalBromptonV3.pdf

Fitzgerald, M. H. (1992). Multicultural clinical interactions. *Journal of Rehabilitation, 58,* 38–42.

Foege, W. (2010). Social determinants of health and health care solutions. *Public Health Reports, 125*(Suppl. 4), 8–10. Retrieved from https://www.ncbi.nlm.nih.gov/pmc/articles/PMC2882969/

Gannam, V. (2014). *Guidelines for developing cross-cultural effectiveness.* Retrieved from https://www.problemgambling.ca/EN/ResourcesForProfessionals/Pages/GuidelinesforDevelopingCrossCulturalEffectiveness.aspx

Genao, I., Bussey-Jones, J., Brady, D., Branch, W. T., & Corbie-Smith, G. (2003). Building the case for cultural competence. *American Journal of Medical Sciences, 326,* 136–140. http://dx.doi.org/10.1097/00000441-200309000-00006

Greenberg, J. (2015). *7 reasons why 'colorblindness' contributes to racism instead of solves it.* Retrieved from http://everydayfeminism.com/2015/02/colorblindness-adds-to-racism/

Harrison, J. (2012). Professional learning and the reflective practitioner. In S. Dymoke (Ed.), *Reflective teaching and learning in the secondary school* (2nd ed., pp. 7–40). Newbury Park, CA: Sage.

Hasnain, R., Kondratowicz, D. M., Borokhovski, E., Nye, C., Balcazar, F., Portillo, N., . . . Gould, R. (2011). Do cultural competency interventions work? A systematic review on improving rehabilitation outcomes for ethnically and linguistically diverse individuals with disabilities [Technical Brief No. 31]. *Focus.* Retrieved from http://ktdrr.org/ktlibrary/articles_pubs/ncddrwork/focus/focus31/Focus31.pdf

Henry J. Kaiser Family Foundation. (2012, November 30). *Disparities in health and health care: Five key questions and answers.* Retrieved from http://kff.org/disparities-policy/issue-brief/disparities-in-health-and-health-care-five-key-questions-and-answers/

Hinett, K. (2002). *Improving learning through reflection—Part one.* York, England: Higher Education Academy. Retrieved from http://www.academia.edu/9174568/Improving_learning_through_reflection_-_part_one

Institute of Medicine. (2013). *Leveraging culture to address health inequities: Examples from native communities: Workshop summary.* Washington, DC: National Academics Press.

Joint Commission. (2010). *Advancing effective communication, cultural competence, and patient- and family-centered care: A roadmap for hospitals.* Oakbrook Terrance, IL: Author.

Kleinman, A., & Benson, P. (2006). Anthropology in the clinic: The problem of cultural competency and how to fix it. *PLoS Medicine, 3,* 1673–1676. http://dx.doi.org/10.1371/journal.pmed.0030294

Korthagen, F. A. (2001). A reflection on reflection. In F. A. Korthagen (Ed.), *Linking practice and theory: The pedagogy of realistic teacher education* (pp. 51–68). Mahwah, NJ: Erlbaum.

Kratzke, C., & Bertolo, M. (2013). Enhancing students' cultural competence using cross-cultural experiential learning, *Journal of Cultural Diversity, 20,* 107–111.

Kundhal, K. K., & Kundhal, P. S. (2003). Cultural diversity: An evolving challenge to physician–patient communication. *JAMA, 289,* 94–96. http://dx.doi.org/10.1001/jama.289.1.94

Leung, K. H., Pluye, P., Grad, R., & Weston, C. (2010). A reflective learning framework to evaluate CME effects on practice reflection. *Journal of Continuing Education in the Health Professions, 30,* 78–88. http://dx.doi.org/10.1002/chp.20063

Lott, B. (2010). *Multiculturalism and diversity: A social psychological perspective.* Malden, MA: Wiley.

McCabe, J. (2011). Doing multiculturalism: An interactionist analysis of the practices of a multicultural sorority. *Journal of Contemporary Ethnography, 40,* 521–549. http://dx.doi.org/10.1177/0891241611403588

McClure, P. (2005). *Reflection on practice.* Retrieved from http://cw.routledge.com/textbooks/9780415537902/data/learning/8_Reflection%20in%20Practice.pdf

McDaniel, G. (2014, January 3). *The business of culturally competent care: Aggressively addressing cultural needs is not only good for society, it's also good for the bottom line of healthcare organizations.* Retrieved from http://nursing.advanceweb.com/Features/Articles/The-Business-of-Culturally-Competent-Care.aspx

Muchenje, F. (2012). Cultural pluralism and quest for nation building in Africa: The rationale for multicultural education. *Journal of Sustainable Development in Africa, 14,* 70–81. Retrieved from http://www.jsd-africa.com/Jsda/Vol14No4-Summer2012B/PDF/Cultural%20Pluralism%20and%20the%20Quest%20for%20Nation%20Building.Francis%20Muchenje.pdf

Neville, H. A., Awad, G. H., Brooks, J. E., Flores, M. P., & Bluemel, J. (2013). Color-blind racial ideology: Theory, training,, and measurement implications in psychology. *American Psychologist, 68,* 455–466. http://dx.doi.org/10.1037/a0033282

Obasogie, O. K. (2013). *Blinded by sight: Seeing race through the eyes of the blind.* Stanford, CA: Stanford University Press.

Oelofsen, N. (2012). Developing practical reflective skills (1/2): Personal learning. *British Journal of Healthcare Assistants, 6,* 294–297. http://dx.doi.org/10.12968/bjha.2012.6.6.294

Parrillo, V. N. (1997). *Strangers to these shores: Race and ethnic relations in the United States* (5th ed.). Boston: Allyn & Bacon.

Purnell, L. (2002). The Purnell Model for cultural competence. *Journal of Transcultural Nursing, 13,* 193–196. http://dx.doi .org/10.1177/10459602013003006

Reagan, T. G., Case, C. W., & Brubacher, J. W. (2000). *Becoming a reflective educator: How to build a culture of inquiry in the schools* (2nd ed.). Thousand Oaks, CA: Corwin.

Ruch, G. (2000). Self and social work: Towards an integrated model of learning. *Journal of Social Work Practice, 14,* 99–112. http://dx.doi.org/10.1080/02650530020020500

Schön, D. (1983). *The reflective practitioner: How professionals think in action.* New York: Basic Books.

Sleeter, C. E., & Grant, C. A. (2007). *Making choices for multicultural education: Five approaches to race, class, and gender* (5th ed.). New York: Wiley.

Taylor, R. (2005). Addressing barriers to cultural competence. *Journal for Nurses in Staff Development, 21,* 135–142. http:// dx.doi.org/10.1097/00124645-200507000-00001

Waite, R., Nardi, D., & Killian, P. (2014). Examination of cultural knowledge and provider sensitivity in nurse managed health centers. *Journal of Cultural Diversity, 21,* 74–79. Retrieved from https://www.researchgate.net/publication/263861568 _Examination_of_cultural_knowledge_and_provider _sensitivity_in_nurse_managed_health_centers

Watson, J. R. (2010, March–April). Language and culture training: Separate paths? *Military Review,* 93–97. Retrieved from http://www.dtic.mil/dtic/tr/fulltext/u2/a518175.pdf

Wells, S. A., & Black, R. (2000). *Cultural competency for health professionals.* Bethesda, MD: American Occupational Therapy Association.

Wertenbroch, A. & Nabeth, T. (2000). *Advanced Learning Approaches & Technologies: The CALT Perspective.* http://www .calt.insead.edu/Publication/CALTReport/calt-perspective .pdf

Williams, M. T. (2011, December 27). Colorblind ideology is a form of racism. *Psychology Today.* Retrieved from https://www .psychologytoday.com/blog/culturally-speaking/201112 /colorblind-ideology-is-form-racism

York-Barr, J., Sommers, W. A., Ghere, G. S., & Montie, J. (2001). *Reflective practice to improve schools: An action guide for educators.* Thousand Oaks, CA: Corwin.

Section II.A.

SELF-AWARENESS, ATTITUDES, AND THE CONCEPT OF POWER

Chapter 6.

CULTURAL SELF-AWARENESS, CRITICAL REFLECTION, AND TRANSFORMING ATTITUDES

Roxie M. Black, PhD, OTR/L, FAOTA

The starting point of any education programme [in cultural effectiveness] should . . . be an exploration of the students' own cultural values, beliefs, and practices, including their own prejudices.
Kate Gerrish & Irina Papadopoulos (1999, p. 1454)

Chapter Highlights

- Understanding Cultural Self-Awareness
- Developing Cultural Self-Awareness
- Cross-Cultural Practice
- Transforming Attitudes

Key Terms and Concepts

✧ Critical reflection
✧ Cross-cultural exchange
✧ Cultural identity
✧ Cultural self-awareness

✧ Enlightened consciousness
✧ Oppression
✧ Self-discovery
✧ Self-reflection

A major characteristic identified in the Cultural Effectiveness Model is cultural self-awareness (or *self-reflection,* a synonymous term used elsewhere in this text), which is developed through a critical self-reflection process. Supported by topical literature, this chapter defines *cultural self-awareness* and explores the reflective process, ending with a discussion of the attitudinal shift that often results from this process. The reflection a person does to

develop cultural self-awareness is intense and personal in nature.

Understanding Cultural Self-Awareness

Cultural self-awareness is the recognition a person has of being a unique person with a specific cultural background that influences his or her beliefs, values, attitudes, and behaviors. Of all the aspects of cultural effectiveness, many scholars agree that cultural self-awareness is the most important (Harry, 1992; Lynch & Hanson, 1998) and is the first step in becoming culturally effective (Black & Wells, 2007; Pedersen, 2001; Weaver, 1999). Emphasizing the importance of cultural self-awareness, Papadopoulos, Tilki, and Lees (2004) stated that it "constitutes an essential first stage in the process of achieving cultural competence; unless one goes through this stage, it is unlikely that s/he can become culturally sensitive, . . . competent[,]" and ultimately effective (p. 9).

Cultural self-awareness has a place in education. Knutson (2006) stated that "one of the most basic and important goals of intercultural education . . . is to lead students to some understanding of the notion of culturally determined behaviour . . . so that they begin to see themselves, not just others, as culturally *marked*" (p. 22). Therefore, "Byram's seminal definition of an inter-cultural speaker includes recognition of self and other as socially constructed" (Knutson, 2006, p. 598).

Social construction of the self is not a new concept. Decades ago, Damen (1987) argued that awareness of the social construction of the self is a corollary to awareness of others:

> Cross-cultural awareness involves uncovering and understanding one's own culturally conditioned behavior and thinking, as well as the patterns of others. Thus, the process involves not only perceiving the similarities and differences in other cultures but also recognizing the givens of the native culture. (p. 141)

Because self-awareness parallels awareness of others, Leonard and Plotnikoff (2000) referred to *cultural self-awareness* as the "heart of cultural competence" (p. 51).

Developing Cultural Self-Awareness

Becoming culturally self-aware is an ongoing process that may be difficult. Occupational therapy students and practitioners are often skilled in identifying their own strengths and weaknesses, which is an aspect of self-awareness. Cultural self-awareness,

however, is more complex and goes beyond those skills. People with cultural self-awareness know and understand themselves at a deeper level.

Self-Reflection

Developing a deep level of self-awareness requires engaging in focused *self-reflection,* which includes recognizing and examining one's culture and subcultures, values and beliefs, as well as biases and prejudices. It also requires reflection on how one values and responds to people who differ in age, gender, class, race, ethnicity, sexual orientation, religion, ability, and political leanings (these groups define a person's social location).

Such self-reflection demands that people challenge their perspectives. Pedersen (2001) stated, "Increased awareness requires challenging our assumptions about ourselves and about other groups and worldviews to discover those basic underlying assumptions which we each assume to be so obviously true that no truth or evidence is required. The tendency is to otherwise assume that others see the world the same way as ourselves" (p. 21). Although few authors have discussed the process of how to achieve self-awareness, López (2008), who referred to *self-awareness* as an affective (i.e., related to emotions) goal in the process of learning about culture and diversity, identified the following steps as part of this process:

- Making it a habit to check one's reactions to the communication with diverse others
- Learning to understand and become aware of one's impact on others
- Understanding and confronting issues of systemic racism, power imbalance, and insensitivity, which is crucial to gaining effective self-awareness
- Breaking habits of obliviousness and making habits of self-reflection
- Reflecting on one's relationship with the client in light of what has been learned about culture. (p. 47)

Cultural Identity and Self-Discovery

Cultural identity refers to being able to associate with and feel like part of a group based on its culture. Although culture often refers to heritage or race, cultural identity can be found in social classes, locality, generation, or other types of groups (www.reference .com, 2016). *Cultural identity* is a narrower term than cultural self-awareness and specifically refers to group membership.

Self-discovery is the personal process one goes through to learn about oneself as a cultural being. Self-discovery helps students and practitioners learn their cultural identity and gives them a deeper sense of self in a diverse world as well as an openness that enhances their empathy with people from different cultural backgrounds (Black, 2002). Because self-discovery and cultural self-awareness contribute so tremendously to how people understand the "nature and construction" of their cultural identity, it's important that they understand how their cultural background shapes their values and beliefs, including health beliefs and practices (Papadopoulos et al., 2004, p. 10).

Reflection 6.1. Social Status

- How does your age, nationality, gender, sexual identity, religion, ethnicity, socioeconomic status, or ability affect your social status?
- Which of these factors can you change?
- Which factors would you want to change? Why?
- How do your unique characteristics benefit you in your society?
- Do any of your characteristics limit you in some way?

Enlightened Consciousness

Culturally self-aware people recognize the characteristics of their own culture and social location and know how these characteristics influence their values, beliefs, behaviors, and choices. In addition, they are mostly comfortable with cultural differences between themselves and others and are sensitive to issues of culture in all interactions (Wells & Black, 2000). McPhatter (1997) referred to this cultural self-awareness as *enlightened consciousness.* She believed that enlightened consciousness is a fundamental transformational process that results in the

> reorienting [of] one's primary worldview . . . . It often requires a radical restructuring of a well-entrenched belief system that perceives oneself and one's culture, including values and ways of behavior, as not only preferred, but clearly superior to another's. The ultimate goal of this shift in mind-set is to create a belief in and acceptance of others on the basis of equality solely because of a sense of shared humanity. (pp. 262–263)

McPhatter (1997) was not talking about simply completing a few self-awareness exercises. Rather, she emphasized the gravity of this work and the need for ongoing and sustained practice. This depth of analysis is not always easy, especially for students and practitioners from the dominant social group. In the United States, that group tends to consist of people who are White, middle or upper class, financially secure, able-bodied, heterosexual, and male. For those whose characteristics fall into this group, self-analysis necessitates recognizing and grappling with one's privilege and reflecting on how it may affect client–practitioner interactions.

Reflection 6.2. Unrealized Benefits

- Does your skin color match that of people who are dominant in your society?
- If it does, do you ever think about what hidden benefits you enjoy because of it? List 3 of those benefits.

Reflection 6.3. Bias and Fear

- Are there groups of people that you are biased against, or in some way fear? Consider where these feelings and attitudes arise from.

Cross-Cultural Practice

In occupational therapy practice, "students must be able to acknowledge their own cultural backgrounds and not feel threatened by their own cultural identifications, especially when they differ with that of the client" (Chau, 1990, as cited in Sowers-Hoag & Sandau-Beckler, 1996, p. 43). The editors of this book believe that the actual practice of cross-cultural experiences, coupled with a metacognitive type of critical reflection, must be present to develop cultural effectiveness within one's practice.

Cross-Cultural Exchanges

A *cross-cultural exchange* is any verbal or nonverbal interaction between two or more people who share similarities and differences. Although many people think cross-cultural exchanges can occur only between people who are ethnically different, almost any interaction is cross-cultural, including the following examples of practitioners and their clients:

- A 30-year-old man working with a geriatric population
- A Protestant White woman working in southern Texas with a mainly Mexican and Catholic population
- A 47-year-old man working in a mental health program with teens
- An African American woman working in Vermont, where there is limited ethnic diversity
- The only person in the occupational therapy department who is not a person of color
- A woman from California working with multiple immigrants and refugees from Asia and Mexico
- An evangelical Christian working with a client who is homosexual.

Each of these examples might be a formula for ineffective interactions, particularly if the practitioner has not yet developed cultural self-awareness, knowledge, and skills. Although many occupational therapy programs incorporate content and goals for the development of cultural awareness, knowledge, and skills, critical reflection and cultural effectiveness in practice can be developed only when opportunities for cross-cultural exchanges are available. There is also significant evidence on the positive impact of cross-cultural experiences on the development of cultural competence (e.g., Hoffmann, Messmer, Hill-Rodriguez, & Vazquez, 2005; Nelson et al., 2011; Pearson et al., 2007; Vaughan, 2005).

Critically Reflective Practice

Critical reflection of cross-cultural experiences is necessary for effective practice. Even novice practitioners can improve practice skills if they have developed critical reflection skills to apply both during and after the intervention. However, these experiences cannot happen without the opportunity for face-to-face interactions with people that are different from oneself.

Critical reflection is "consciously looking and thinking about experiences, actions, emotions, feelings and responses then interpreting them in order to learn from them" (Boud, Keogh, & Walker, 1985, as cited in Paterson & Chapman, 2013, p. 133). Paterson and Chapman (2013) expressed the belief of many health professionals that reflection is "a critical part of learning from experience and is important

in developing and maintaining competency across a practitioner's practice lifetime" (p. 133).

Reflection goes beyond scientific knowledge and thinking in practice. Redmond (2004) stated, *"Reflection,* in the context of learning, is a generic term for those intellectual and affective activities in which individuals engage to explore their experiences in order to lead to new understandings and appreciations" (p. 3; emphasis added). It requires a kind of introspection that is integrative in nature. Reflection is conscious and systematic and "challeng[es] a person's understanding of themselves, their attitudes and behaviors so that any biases are unearthed, thus allowing that individual to become more critical about their views of practice and the world" (Jasper & Rolfe, 2011, p. 235).

Much has been written about critical reflection in health care (Burton, 2000; Hannigan, 2001; Redmond, 2004), but the literature on the effects of critical reflection in cross-cultural interactions is limited. However, Lie, Shapiro, and Najm (2010) examined a clerkship program with diverse clients that intentionally incorporated written reflection followed by reflective discussion. They found that students' discussion of their cross-cultural interactions resulted in "better, more nuanced understanding" of these encounters (p. 119).

In a study of the results of a 4-year program of service learning with a diverse population, the authors distinguished between *reflection,* that is, the commonplace thinking about past events, and *Reflection,* a "more intentional, structured and directed process that facilitates exploration for deeper, contextualized meaning linked to learning outcomes (Eyler, Giles, & Schmiede, 1999, as cited in Rice & Pollack, 2000, p. 124). The latter is the type of reflection needed for cultural effectiveness.

Eyler et al. (1999, as cited in Rice & Pollack, 2000) also pointed out that critical reflection includes examining

- One's experiences, opinions, perspectives, and social positionality;
- One's relation to people (e.g., clients, families, other staff members) at their clinical and service-learning sites; and
- The ways in which oppression is often perpetuated through community service that is insensitive to the needs of others as a result of people who are unaware of the impact of their privileged status in society. (p. 124)

They concluded by stating that the development of critical reflection should be a "central element" in the education for service-learning with a diverse population, and the authors of this book concur.

Critical reflection goes beyond what is expected for cultural competence but must be included in the development of cultural effectiveness, especially for occupational therapy practitioners who recognize the importance of cultural context in their interactions with all clients. See Chapter 8, "Acquiring Cultural Self-Awareness," for examples of how to achieve this level of reflection. Developing cultural self-awareness and practicing critical reflection of cross-cultural experiences transform people, helping to change their attitudes and beliefs about people who are culturally different from themselves.

Reflection 6.4. Critical Reflection

- Have you ever attempted to critically reflect upon your interactions with someone who is different from you?
- What did you learn?

Transforming Attitudes

Transforming attitudes requires understanding oppression. In Chapter 3, "Sociopolitical Dimensions of Participation: Occupational Justice," Gupta describes the sociopolitical determinants that help to maintain the oppression that many nondominant groups of people still experience in the United States. She describes *oppression* as disadvantage and injustice suffered by some people in daily experiences through unquestioned norms and habits, unconscious assumptions, and cultural stereotypes. Bias, stereotypes, and prejudice against disadvantaged groups are the attitudes and behaviors that maintain oppression.

Several decades ago, in recognizing oppression's contribution to health disparities and how it affects health care, many health-related professions (e.g., nursing, clinical psychology, social work, occupational therapy) developed training modules in an effort to educate people and change attitudes and behaviors. This purpose of this undertaking was to make their constituents more culturally competent.

Within the past decade, research has found that health care provider education interventions are finally beginning to change attitudes toward nondominant

groups of people (Beach et al., 2005; Campbell, Sullivan, Sherman, & Magee, 2011). Positive attitudes noted in the evidence include an openness to and acceptance of differences, respect for individual people and their personal beliefs, an interest in the health beliefs of each client, a willingness to collaborate with clients on intervention plans, and an eagerness to learn more about people's cultural backgrounds.

A complete change in attitude will not happen overnight. It takes time, energy, education, deep reflection, and dedication for personal transformation to occur. As difficult as this work might be, it is necessary if occupational therapy practitioners are to provide the most effective care.

Reflection 6.5. Difference

What is your attitude when a stranger whose ethnicity is different from yours—
- Stops you on a busy street and asks for money?
- Stops you on a country road and asks for directions?
- Is accompanied by several noisy young children in a grocery store?
- Is sitting beside you at your child's basketball game?
- Cuts you off to get to an exit when you are driving?

Now consider these same questions if a person of your own ethnicity does the same, and answer these questions:

- Is there a difference in how you feel about the two in comparison?
- If there is a difference, reflect on why this is so, consider what you might want to change about it, and determine what your response might be at a future interaction.

Summary

"Solely addressing the importance of learning about the *other's* culture is not sufficient [to develop cultural effectiveness because] it absolves individuals from learning and understanding the impact of their own sociopolitical and ethnocentric biases on their work with clients who are racially/ethnically or culturally different from themselves" (Negi, Bender, Furman, Fowler, & Prickett, 2010, p. 224). This chapter has emphasized the importance of critical self-reflection in the development of cultural competence and cultural effectiveness in practice. The examination of oneself contributes to attitudinal shifts that encourage the openness to difference and the acceptance of others that are necessary for effective cross-cultural and global interactions required for today's occupational therapy practitioners.

References

Beach, M. C., Price, E. G., Gary, T. L., Robinson, K. A., Gozu, A., Palacio, A., . . . Cooper, L. A. (2005). Cultural competency: A systematic review of health care provider educational interventions. *Medical Care, 43*, 356–373. http://dx.doi.org/10.1097/01.mlr.0000156861.58905.96

Black, R. M. (2002). *The essence of cultural competence: Listening to the voices of occupational therapy students.* Doctoral Dissertation, Lesley University, Cambridge, MA.

Black, R. M., & Wells, S. A. (2007). *Culture and occupation: A model of empowerment in occupational therapy.* Bethesda, MD: AOTA Press.

Boud, D., Keogh, R., & Walker, D. (1985). *Reflection: Turning experience into learning.* London: Kogan Page.

Burton, A. J. (2000). Reflection: Nursing's practice and education panacea? *Journal of Advanced Nursing, 31*, 1009–1017. http://dx.doi.org/10.1046/j.1365-2648.2000.01395.x

Campbell, A., Sullivan, M., Sherman, R., & Magee, W. P. (2011). The medical mission and modern cultural competency training. *American College of Surgeons, 212*, 124–129. http://dx.doi.org/10.1016/j.jamcollsurg.2010.08.019

Damen, L. (1987). *Culture learning: The fifth dimension in the language classroom.* Reading, MA: Addison-Wesley.

Gerrish, K., & Papadopoulos, I. (1999). Transcultural competence: The challenge for nurse education. *British Journal of Nursing, 8*, 1453–1457. http://dx.doi.org/10.12968/bjon.1999.8.21.1453

Hannigan, B. (2001). A discussion of the strengths and weaknesses of "reflection" in nursing practice and education. *Journal of Clinical Nursing, 10*, 278–283. http://dx.doi.org/10.1111/j.1365-2702.2001.00459.x

Harry, B. (1992). Developing cultural self-awareness: The first step in values clarification for early interventionists. *Topics in Early Childhood Special Education, 12*, 333–350.

Hoffmann, R. L., Messmer, P. R., Hill-Rodriguez, D. L., & Vazquez, D. (2005). A collaborative approach to expand clinical experiences and cultural awareness among undergraduate nursing students. *Journal of Professional Nursing, 21*, 240–243. http://dx.doi.org/10.1016/j.profnurs.2005.06.001

Jasper, M., & Rolfe, G. (2011). Critical reflection and emergence of professional knowledge. In G. Rolfe, M. Jasper, &

D. Freshwater, *Critical reflection in practice.* London: Palgrave Macmillan.

Knutson, E. M. (2006). Cross-cultural awareness for second/foreign language learners. *Canadian Modern Language Review, 62*, 591–610. http://dx.doi.org/10.3138/cmlr.62.4.591

Lie, D., Shapiro, J., & Najm, W. (2010). Reflective practice enriches clerkship students' cross-cultural experiences. *Journal of General Internal Medicine, 25*(Suppl. 2), 119–125. http://dx.doi.org/10.1007/s11606-009-1205-4

Leonard, B. J., & Plotnikoff, G. A. (2000). Awareness: The heart of cultural competence. *AACN Clinical Issues, 11*, 51–59.

López, A. S. (2008). Making and breaking habits: Teaching (and learning) cultural context, self-awareness, and intercultural communication through case supervision in a client-service legal clinic. *Washington University Journal of Law and Policy, 28.* Retrieved from http://digitalcommons.law.wustl.edu/wujlp/vol28/iss1/4

Lynch, E. W., & Hanson, M. J. (1998). *Developing cross-cultural competencies: A guide for working with children and their families* (2nd ed.). Baltimore: Paul H. Brookes.

McPhatter, A. R. (1997). Cultural competence and child welfare: What is it? How do we achieve it? What happens without it? *Child Welfare, 76*, 255–278. Retrieved from http://mha.ohio.gov/Portals/0/assets/Learning/CulturalCompetence/Subgroups/Youth/Full%20Articles/CC.Child.Welfare.pdf

Negi, N. J., Bender, K. S., Furman, R., Fowler, D. N., & Prickett, J. S. (2010). Enhancing self-awareness: A practical strategy to train culturally responsive social work students. *Advances in Social Work, 11*, 223–234. Retrieved from https://journals.iupui.edu/index.php/advancesinsocialwork/article/view/482/1787

Nelson, A., Gray, M., Jensen, H., Thomas, Y., McIntosh, K., Oke, L., & Paluch, T. (2011). Closing the gap: Supporting occupational therapists to partner effectively with First Australians. *Australian Occupational Therapy Journal, 58*, 17–24. http://dx.doi.org/10.1111/j.1440-1630.2010.00912.x

Papadopoulos, I., Tilki, M., & Lees, S. (2004). Promoting cultural competence in health care through a research-based intervention in the UK. *Health and Social Care, 1*, 107–116. Retrieved from http://researchonline.lshtm.ac.uk/id/eprint/19364

Paterson, C., & Chapman, J. (2013). Enhancing skills of critical reflection to evidence learning in professional practice. *Physical Therapy in Sport, 14*, 133–138. http://dx.doi.org/10.1016/j.ptsp.2013.03.004

Pearson, A., Srivastava, R., Craig, D., Tucker, D., Grinspun, D., Bajnok, I., . . . Gi, A. A. (2007). Systematic review on embracing cultural diversity for developing and sustaining a healthy work environment in healthcare. *International Journal of Evidence-Based Healthcare, 5*, 54–91. http://dx.doi.org/10.1111/j.1479-6988.2007.00058.x

Pedersen, P. (2001). Multiculturalism and the paradigm shift in counselling: Controversies and alternative futures. *Canadian Journal of Counseling, 35*(1), 15–25. Retrieved from http://cjc-rcc.ucalgary.ca/cjc/index.php/rcc/article/view/178/408

Redmond, B. (2004). *Reflection in action: Developing reflective practice in health and social services.* Aldershot, England: Ashgate.

Rice, K., & Pollack, S. (2000). Developing a pedagogy of service learning: Preparing self-reflective, culturally aware, and responsive community participants. In C. R. O'Grady (Ed.), *Integrating service learning and multicultural education in colleges and universities* (pp. 115–134). Mahwah, NJ: Lawrence Erlbaum.

Sowers-Hoag, K. M., & Sandau-Beckler, P. (1996). Educating for cultural competence in the generalist curriculum. *Journal of Multicultural Social Work, 4*(3), 37–56. http://dx.doi.org/10.1300/J285v04n03_03

Vaughan, W. (2005). Educating for diversity, social responsibility and action: Preservice teachers engage in immersion experiences. *Journal of Cultural Diversity, 12*(1), 26–30. Retrieved from http://search.proquest.com/openview/4217614caa4cdddcef4e1b564c9d57ab/1?pq-origsite=gscholar

Weaver, H. N. (1999). Indigenous people and the social work profession: Defining culturally competent services. *Social Work, 44,* 217–225. http://dx.doi.org/10.1093/sw/44.3.217

Wells, S. A., & Black, R. (2000). *Cultural competency for health professionals.* Bethesda, MD: American Occupational Therapy Association.

www.reference.com. (2016). *What is the definition of cultural identity?* Retrieved from https://www.reference.com/world-view/cultural-identity-mean-d72c87ffe619d385?qo=cdpArticles#

Chapter 7.

PREJUDICE, PRIVILEGE, AND POWER

Roxie M. Black, PhD, OTR/L, FAOTA

The power and lack of power inherent in the roles of clinician and client and in their cultural group status can affect clinical process and outcome. Practitioners need to understand how these two dimensions of power can affect their clients, themselves, and their work together.
Elaine Pinderhughes (1989, p. 109)

Chapter Highlights

• History of Sociocultural Power and Privilege
• Stereotypes, Prejudice, and Discrimination
• Privilege
• Implications of Power

Key Terms and Concepts

✧ Discrimination
✧ Enablement
✧ Individual discrimination
✧ Insiders
✧ Institutional or organizational discrimination
✧ Occupational apartheid
✧ Outsiders
✧ Participatory power
✧ Personal power
✧ Power
✧ Powerlessness

✧ Prejudice
✧ Privilege
✧ Professional power
✧ Self-fulfilling prophecy
✧ Sociocultural power
✧ Stereotype
✧ Stereotyping
✧ Structural discrimination
✧ Unearned privilege
✧ White guilt
✧ White privilege

Health professionals deal with issues of power on a regular, if not daily, basis.

Being aware that this is occurring is an important aspect of self-reflection. Much has been written in occupational therapy about the empowerment of clients (Kielhofner, de las Heras, & Suarez-Balcazar, 2011; Townsend & Whiteford, 2005), and the reality is that as long as one is in a position of authority in the client–practitioner interaction, regardless of whether this situation is wanted, a power differential exists. Power issues also exist in classrooms, both among students and between students and faculty, and they occur among various cultural groups that influence the way people interact with one another.

It is necessary to explore these issues in occupational therapy practice, education, and research for the purpose of increasing the effectiveness of our interactions with whom we interact. This chapter discusses aspects of power, including privilege (e.g., White privilege), prejudice, discrimination, social justice, professional power, and powerlessness.

History of Sociocultural Power and Privilege

Historically, the United States was colonized by White immigrants who brought a sense of entitlement, power, and ownership that devalued the native inhabitants who are now referred to as Native Americans. These colonists arrived with their own ideas, beliefs, and values—in other words, their culture—that quickly became the dominant manner of thinking and acting. They believed in independence, self-control, and mastery, which resulted in control of the land, products, education, commerce, and religion (Tai & Kenyatta, 1999).

Desire for ownership, control, and power resulted in the seizure of lands previously inhabited by native tribes and the large-scale possession of other human beings as slaves to work those lands. A hierarchy evolved that placed prominent White men at the top of the social ladder with others of different culture, ethnicity, gender, and economic status in inferior positions (Ignatiev, 1995).

Although slavery has been legally eradicated in this country, and laws have been enacted to ensure the rights of all, a legacy of oppression—including racism, sexism, classism, heterosexism, ageism, and ableism—remains. Over the past 4 decades, there has been significant positive movement within these social justice issues; yet, many biases remain and are held in place through stereotypes, prejudice, and discrimination.

Stereotypes, Prejudice, and Discrimination

The terms *stereotype, prejudice,* and *discrimination* are often used somewhat interchangeably when discussing **sociocultural power,** which is the status and control given to individuals and groups of people by a society, based on their cultural status within that society. Although these terms do not mean the same thing, they are closely related.

The simplest way to differentiate them is to recognize **prejudice** as preconceived ideas and attitudes—usually negative—about a particular group of people, often without full examination of the facts about this group. A *stereotype* is a belief about a person or members of a group that may or may not have some basis in fact. Finally, **discrimination** is the overt action people take to exclude, avoid, or distance themselves from others (Hecht, 1998).

Stereotype

Stereotyping occurs when one sees a particular characteristic in one or a few members of a group and generalizes that characteristic to all members of the group. Some common stereotypical statements heard in the United States are included in Exhibit 7.1. Such statements may be true for a few members in the identified groups, but by assuming all members of the groups carry these characteristics, one negates the individuality of each member, rendering their true selves invisible and open to misunderstanding.

Exhibit 7.1. Common U.S. Stereotypes

All African Americans can dance.
All Native Americans are alcoholics.
Obese people are morally weak and lazy.
Jewish Americans are good with money management.
White Americans are racist.
Poor people do not want to improve their lot in life.
Women are emotional.
People in wheelchairs are helpless.

Stereotyping is a type of categorization of people. Allport (1974, as cited in Hecht, 1998) believed that categorization is necessary to daily functioning because it enables people to react quickly to new, incoming stimuli. He suggested, however, that categorization done with stereotyping moves to overgeneralization, which actually can impede the process of encoding, storing, and retrieving information. For example, if people expect an Asian woman to be shy and self-effacing, they may then interact with her on the basis of what they expect to be true rather than on what the reality actually is. This misconception often results in what Neuberg (1991) and others have referred to as a *self-fulfilling prophecy,* which occurs when "an originally false social belief leads to its own fulfillment" (Jussim, 2012, p. 50).

Goldstein (1997) warned of the "powerful cognitive, affective, and behavioral impacts of stereotypes on the perceiver as well as the target" (p. 256). People who are targets of stereotyping may alter their behavior in anticipation of being stereotyped, whereas those who stereotype will respond in a particular way because of their belief in the stereotype. If an occupational therapy practitioner is working with an Asian woman in a therapeutic encounter, he or she may overlook vital factors of her condition or belief system during assessment if he or she stereotypes the client and does not probe for important and necessary information. The Asian woman, perceiving the stereotype projected by the practitioner, also may unwittingly respond in a way that supports the stereotype.

Prejudice

Prejudice, a word that stems from the Latin *praejudicium,* meaning to prejudge or form an opinion without sufficient knowledge or experience, represents the (usually negative) affective aspect of attitudes toward an outgroup (Hackney, 2009). Many people do not realize that they carry prejudicial thoughts against others from different sociocultural groups. They may be far more comfortable in social and work contexts with people who are generally like themselves, and they may avoid strangers or outsiders.

Hackney (2009) suggested that people maintain the use of stereotypes and prejudice because they serve important psychological functions of self-affirmation and justification of the status quo. Reporting on current research, Hackney (2009) stated that "when self-image was threatened, individuals discriminated more against a stereotyped target, which led to an increase in self-esteem" (p. 80). Stereotypes and prejudice rationalize and justify the status quo, which corresponds with how "biases of people with power (ingroup members) reinforce social hierarchies and inequality" (p. 80).

Within sociocultural settings, people fall within certain social groups, some of which are more privileged than others, determining insider or outsider status. Those in the more privileged groups are often seen as the *insiders,* and others with less privilege or power are viewed as *outsiders* (see Figure 7.1). Decades ago, Merton (1972) used these terms when discussing the validity of group knowledge, arguing that insiders claim their knowledge of the group is more valid because they have a closer and more accurate understanding of the group's values, perspectives, and culture. Those who function outside the group, however, claim they have a more objective, and thus more valid, understanding.

When occupational therapy practitioners are trying to understand a certain group, both viewpoints are important and provide insight into social reality. "One's understanding of a group remains incomplete when the perspective of either the insider or the outsider is overlooked" (Banks, 1996, p. 8). Prejudice often occurs unconsciously when people do not have clear knowledge about others from a

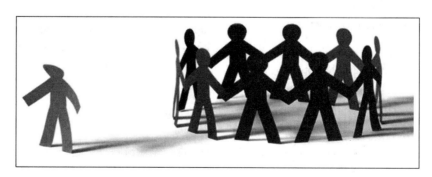

Figure 7.1. Insider–outsider group status.

diverse group and resort to stereotypes as their methods of understanding and judging.

Discrimination

Prejudice (i.e., attitude) and stereotyping (i.e., beliefs about a group) may lead to discrimination (i.e., actions). Lott (1995, as cited in Hecht, 1998) argued that although prejudice and stereotyping are deplorable, discrimination is the social problem. Although people may have prejudicial thoughts, attitudes, and stereotypical beliefs, it is only when they act on these that one sees the evidence of sociopolitical power. Discrimination occurs in many forms—including racism, ageism, heterosexism, classism, and sexism—and at multiple levels. Rothenberg (1998) identified three levels of discrimination: (1) individual, (2) institutional or organizational, (3) and structural.

Individual Discrimination

At an individual level, discrimination may be either intentional or unintentional and may not be motivated by conscious prejudice (Lott, 1995). However, Rothenberg (1998) stated that all discriminatory acts "build on and support prejudicial stereotypes, deny their victim's opportunities provided to others, and perpetuate discrimination regardless of intent" (p. 137). Examples of ***individual discrimination*** include

- Clients and patients who refuse to work with practitioners of color because of their ethnicity
- Teachers who interpret linguistic and cultural differences as indicators of low potential or lack of academic interest on the part of minority students
- Medical office receptionists who make lower income clients wait longer than paying clients, even when the lower income clients made appointments (Rothenberg, 1998).

Reflection 7.1. Discrimination

- Consider a time when you were discriminated against. What was this like for you?

Institutional or Organizational Discrimination

Institutional or organizational discrimination reinforces individual discrimination by instituting rules, policies, and practices that have an adverse effect on nondominant groups, such as people of color, women, older people, people with disabilities, and people with diverse sexual identities. This type of discrimination includes

- Height and weight requirements that are unnecessarily geared to the physical proportions of White men, excluding most women and some people with ethnic backgrounds from certain jobs
- The use of standardized academic tests or criteria geared to the cultural and educational norms of middle-class Whites that are not relevant indicators of successful academic or job performance
- Questions about mental illness on a job application, which then affects the applicant's chance of being hired (Rothenberg, 1998).

Institutional or organizational discrimination often is not an act of conscious prejudice but is considered to be the "normal way" things are done—just part of the organizational climate. People, therefore, are unaware that the practices must be changed despite their discriminatory results, making organizational discrimination more difficult to change than individual discrimination practices.

Structural Discrimination

Structural discrimination is systematic discrimination and occurs among the fields of employment, education, housing, and government. Rothenberg (1998) described a classic style of structural discrimination that reproduces itself this way:

- Discrimination in education denies the credentials to get good jobs, leading to
- Discrimination in employment denies the economic resources to buy good housing, leading to
- Discrimination in housing confines minorities to school districts providing inferior education, closing the cycle in the classic form (p. 140; see Figure 7.2).

All aspects of structural discrimination result in a lack of access for those discriminated against. The complexity of structural discrimination makes change very difficult.

Privilege

Being a member of the dominant sociocultural group affords sociopolitical power and privilege. ***Power*** in is "the capacity to produce desired effects

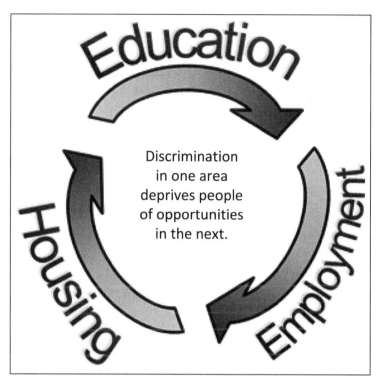

Figure 7.2. Structural discrimination cycle.

on others; it can be perceived in terms of mastery over self as well as over nature and other people" (Pinderhughes, 1989, p. 109). *Privilege* has been defined by Black and Stone (2005) as the entitlements, advantages, and dominance conferred upon groups by society (p. 243). Sociopolitical power gives dominant group members not only mastery over self and others but also the privileges of access to better jobs, education, housing, health care, and material goods. These group members can more easily become decision makers, participants, and policymakers in the dominant discourse than those from outgroups. Power begets privilege and is thoroughly discussed in the "Implications of Power" section.

People who do not share the privileges of the dominant group often are very aware of the differences in power and in access to goods and services. Sometimes these oppressive differences are readily apparent, such as blatant racism that denies people of color access to good education and employment. More often, though, oppression or discrimination is subtle, affecting each person in ways apparent only to those slighted or misused.

For example, several years ago, Shirley Wells (an African American woman) and I were walking in a well-known department store in Maryland, and we passed a cosmetic counter where foundation creams were displayed in various shades of beige. When I recognized none of these creams matched the color of Shirley's skin, I commented on this and asked how she felt about it. She responded that it is frustrating and typical, and that she retaliates by never shopping in this store. Although stores have an increasingly wide array of foundation colors to match the skin tones of almost everyone, this earlier experience exemplifies the subtle yet clear discrimination Shirley faces as an African American woman and the privilege I enjoy as a White woman.

Unearned Privilege

Many scholars have argued that being a member of the dominant group in the United States affords members certain unearned privileges (Frankenberg, 1993; Haney, 1994; McIntosh, 1988). According to Haney (1994), *unearned privilege* includes

freedoms or other benefits given to us simply because we are White, heterosexual, or born into middle-strata economic and social location. Simple examples include names of crayons and bandages as "flesh-colored" actually matching the color of one's skin, while more complex issues relate to lack of access of good schools and jobs to people from lower socio-economic status. Such unearned privilege allows us to generalize from our own experience, to assume that everyone else's is like ours. (p. 5)

White Privilege

White privilege includes the benefits noted above, based on the color of one's skin, with the most privilege given to those with the lightest skin color. McIntosh (1988) compellingly wrote about the privilege of being White:

> I have come to see White privilege as an invisible package of unearned assets which I can count on cashing in each day, but about which I was meant to remain oblivious. White privilege is like an invisible weightless knapsack of special provisions, assurances, tools, maps, guides, codebooks, passports, visa, clothes, compass, emergency gear, and blank checks. (pp. 1–2)

One amazing aspect of being White or male, or possessing other characteristics of power or privilege, is that these characteristics often are invisible to those who have them. People who are White are often taught not to see or be aware of the mantle of privilege within which they are wrapped, reminiscent of the emperor and his new clothes. By not acknowledging these unearned privileges, White people can evade recognizing the power they represent and the responsibility that comes from that awareness (Frankenberg, 1993).

McIntosh (1988) helped increase awareness for White people through her well-known list of 46 ways in which she, as a White woman, benefits from skin color privilege that most people of color cannot count on. The following few items are from that list:

- "I can go shopping alone most of the time, fairly well assured that I will not be followed or harassed."
- "I can do well in a challenging situation without being called a 'credit to my race.'"
- "I am never asked to speak for all people of my racial group."
- "I can be sure that my children will be given curricular materials that testify to the existence of their race."
- "I can be pretty sure that if I ask to talk to the person in charge, I will be facing a person of my race" (McIntosh, pp. 3–4).

Because White people have privileged status, they expect to be responded to in a particular way without even being aware of these expectations or the status associated with them (Lensmire et al., 2013; Solomon & Daniel, 2015). A current example of White privilege in today's world is that the majority of Whites can live in their neighborhoods without the fear that a stray bullet from a gang member could accidently injure or possibly kill them if they go outside.

Challenges of Being White

Although the preceding discussion highlights the privileges and benefits that White Americans are given solely because of their skin color, challenges and problems are inherent within these benefits, especially when one considers becoming culturally aware and culturally effective practitioners. Many Whites have not had to examine or think about what it means to be White. White just is! It is the standard by which others are measured, although its privileges are generally invisible to White members of U.S. society. As Smey (2010) stated, "Being White in a White-dominated society, it is extremely difficult to recognize White privilege" (p. 145).

The invisibility of Whiteness is so complete that people rarely use it as an adjective to describe a specific person or group. One rarely hears phrases such as "the White teacher" or "the White doctor" because being White is the expected standard. However, roles held by other group members are commonly described by their race or ethnicity—for example, "the Jewish banker," "the Chinese lawyer," or "the African professor."

Unexamined Whiteness is maintained partly by the emotion elicited when White Americans begin to evaluate what being White means in the sociopolitical reality of the United States. Examination of privilege and power often results in feelings of guilt, shame, embarrassment, and hopelessness, which often lead to fear, anger, defensiveness, or confusion (Kivel, 1996).

White Guilt

White guilt is often a byproduct of examining what it means to be White (Holzman, 1995). Essayist and culture critic Shelby Steele has written extensively about the concept of White guilt (Steele, 1990, 1998–1999, 2002). Steele (1990) believed that White guilt "springs from a knowledge of ill-gotten advantage. More precisely, it comes from the juxtaposition of this knowledge with the inevitable gratitude one feels for being white rather than black in America" (p. 499).

From his African American perspective, Steele's (1990) contention is that awareness of White people's subjugation of an entire race leads to a sense of guilt and fear, "the fear of what the guilty knowledge says about" Whites (p. 501). In a culture that extols the virtue of strength, guilt and fear generate a sense of vulnerability and discomfiture. It is important, however, to remember Kivel's (1996) words:

There's absolutely nothing wrong with being White or with noticing the difference that color makes. We were born without choice into our families. We did not choose our skin color, native language or culture. We are not responsible for being White or being raised in a White-dominated, racist society in which we have been trained to have particular responses to persons of color. We are responsible to how we respond to racism . . . and we can only do that consciously and effectively if we start by realizing that it makes a crucial difference that we are White. (p. 14)

Kivel has reminded readers that people are responsible for their actions, not their thoughts or what they have been taught.

Reflection 7.2. White Guilt

- If you are White, have you ever experienced White guilt?
- If so, under what conditions?
- Did it or has it become a barrier during cross-cultural interactions?

Considerations for White Practitioners

Although the demographics in the United States are rapidly changing, the majority of the workforce in the major health professions remains White and privileged and will continue to dominate medicine and allied health for the near future (Chapman, Hwang, Both, Thomas, & Deville, 2014; Macura, 2013). Although practices in the United States will

continue to reflect White culture's attitudes, language, values, and beliefs, these practices will also continue to diminish representation for the growing numbers of non-White clients, automatically placing them in vulnerable and unequal power positions.

Occupational therapy practitioners are also in an authoritative position because of their role in the client–practitioner dyad. Because of the multiple vulnerabilities (physical, emotional, and social) of clients, it is the responsibility of the practitioner to try to lessen this power inequity as much as possible within the context of the health care system. They can do this by engaging in the following practices:

- *Develop an accepting attitude.* Understanding that difference does not mean something is better or worse than the White standard.
- *Maintain honesty.* Examining his or her beliefs and values and determining whether he or she harbors biases and prejudices that may affect the care offered to the client.
- *Practicing humility.* Giving up an authoritative stance and humbly admitting the need for additional knowledge about a client's cultural background to develop the most effective intervention plan.
- *Respecting each client.* Providing the foundation for all of the above. Howard (1993) stated, "one of the greatest contributions White Americans can make to cultural understanding is simply to learn the power of respect" (pp. 39–40).

Although it has been noted in some studies that increasing awareness of White privilege has increased awareness of racism and White guilt as well as support for affirmative action (Case, 2007), it is still the privilege and challenge of White practitioners to have an awareness of self and of the inherent power one carries because of his or her dominant status.

Implications of Power

Being aware of and recognizing power is a vital aspect of one's cultural self-awareness, and it must be considered by each practitioner, student, and researcher as one engages in the deep and critical reflection of self before, during, and after cross-cultural interactions.

Personal Power

Everyone is imbued with some level of *personal power*, which Driscoll (1994) labeled as *personal currency* (p. 46) and which Glasser defined as "the need to feel good about ourselves, to believe that we matter and that we have worth and recognition in the eyes of others" (as cited in Litwack, 2004, p. 52). A sense of positive personal power is an awareness of agency, that one can make choices that make a difference in one's life.

Some believe that the pursuit of power is a basic drive and that the "push to exert power is wired in, instinctual" (Person, 2004, p. 64). Most people learn this sense of control and agency very early in life as they discover that a cry, a request, or a pointing finger can result in receiving what they want and need. Watch a young child constantly practice standing and walking, determined after numerous falls and tumbles to successfully walk two steps to his or her parent. A wondrous and satisfied look on the child's face reflects a kind of personal power. It is the look of "I did it! I can do it!" Occupational therapy students experience a similar sense of power and agency when they choose occupational therapy as a profession, enroll in an academic program, and successfully graduate. As Pinderhughes (1989) stated, "A sense of power is critical to one's mental health. Everyone needs it" (p. 110).

Powerlessness

The opposite of personal power is a sense of *powerlessness*, which is the inability to produce an effect, or ineffectiveness. Readers may have felt at some point in their lives that, no matter what they did, their actions did not make a difference. Many people have experienced this feeling but have somehow managed to get through this tough period of their lives, either by their own intrinsic sense of worth or from external support from others.

Moving past difficulty gives people a heightened sense of personal power. However, some people, including some of those with whom occupational therapy practitioners work, rarely have the opportunity to feel powerful. They may have been unloved or abandoned or—because of poverty; racial, ethnic, sexual, or religious oppression; disease; or other sociocultural or health issues—may never have developed a full sense of personal power or lost what they once had. Kronenberg and Pollard (2005) suggested that *occupational apartheid,* the systematized segregation of groups of people from meaningful occupations, also contributes to a sense of meaninglessness and powerlessness.

Professional Power

Occupational therapy practitioners not only experience personal power, but they have earned a certain degree of authority and *professional power,* which is power that comes from a professional's "knowledge and expertise related to the technical, analytical, and interpersonal domains of . . . practice" (Ponte et al., 2007, para. 14). Wilding (1982) believed that professionals are granted power (1) by the members of the public, who accept the "validity and importance" of the activities in which the professional engages (such as occupational therapy assessment and intervention strategies) and (2) by the "unprotesting powerlessness of the groups upon whom . . . professionals practice their ministrations" (p. 60).

Clients depend on practitioners to be knowledgeable and skilled and to provide the best intervention. Most clients come to therapy in a vulnerable and dependent state, with expectations that the therapist will help them return to an active and productive life in which they can continue to participate in the roles and activities that are meaningful to them. Power is an inherent characteristic in this relationship, with the therapist seen as the expert and the client seeking his or her assistance.

Reflection 7.3. Powerfulness

Consider your feelings of powerfulness.

- Are you aware of your personal level of power?
- Are you aware of your level of professional power?

Considering this patient–therapist relationship, professional power is a given for the occupational therapy practitioner and must be acknowledged. If the therapist is part of the dominant social group and his or her client is from a nondominant culture, social power also is an important part of the therapeutic relationship, leaving the client in a type of double jeopardy. Practitioners must be aware of these power relationships and try to diminish them as much as possible. Pinderhughes (1989) warned therapists to be very careful not to use this power as a means of "aggrandizement, to satisfy their own needs for power and esteem not met elsewhere" (p. 10). Pinderhughes interpreted this kind of exploitation as "the most infamous of therapy abuses" (p. 110).

In an examination of the political nature of occupational therapy, Kronenberg and Pollard (2005) contended that one definition of *power* is "as a capacity of actors to determine or change the behaviors or choices of others" (p. 75). In occupational therapy practice, with practitioners having authoritative power over clients, "careful attention is needed to the negotiation of [that] power" (Whiteford & Townsend, 2011, p. 70).

Engaging Clients to Develop Their Own Power

Many ways exist to ameliorate the power differential between the therapist and client. The ability to move from a "power over" model that sometimes occurs in the practitioner–client dyad to a "power with" or *shared power* model takes courage and confidence by the practitioner. It means letting go of some of the authority that identifies occupational therapy practitioners as professionals to share power, but it does not mean diminishing therapists' knowledge and expertise. In fact, therapists' knowledge must be expanded to effectively interact with people within their care in a manner that helps to empower clients within a disempowering health care system.

Although sharing power is an important step in empowering clients, practitioners can make another step as professionals to help clients move to a place of greater agency and control regarding their own health. Borrowing a term found in literature outside of occupational therapy (Buetow, 2013; Norton, 2000), one might consider *participatory power* as a model for interaction with the people and groups with whom one works (see Figure 7.3).

Participatory power is an opportunity for people to become engaged in the decision-making process by listening well, gaining knowledge, and being an active participant in their own health care decisions. Participatory power results in "power from within—the belief in oneself to further develop skills, knowledge and attributes, and to offer them to others" (Norton, 2000, p. 160).

Isn't this what occupational therapy practitioners want for the people with whom they work—the development of a sense of internal power? Shared power happens when one person has a higher power status than another and is willing to share it. There is no clear understanding of how the person who receives the shared power will use it, and there is not a clear expectation.

Participatory power, however, focuses more on equal power, in which each member of the group has a voice and the potential to be a decision maker. It is a true person-centered interactive approach and, if practiced, might potentially result in "communities of health" (Frankford, 1997, p. 210). Using a participatory power approach when interacting with clients is part of the practice of *enablement,* a concept that arose outside the United States more than a decade ago (Polatajko, 2001; Townsend et al., 2007; Townsend & Landry, 2004). Enablement "is distinguished by culturally attuned, participatory, collaborative . . . approaches," and it means that "practitioners employ participatory, empowerment-oriented methods of working in partnership with people and organizations" (Whiteford & Townsend, 2011, p. 68). Enablement is an approach found in client-centered practice.

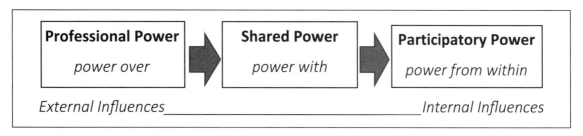

Figure 7.3. Levels of power.

Some may view the model of participatory power as too challenging for clients who may be cultural minorities and who have lived a life filled with discrimination and oppression. However, it is a goal for which practitioners must strive. Whiteford and Townsend (2011) explored participatory occupational justice and the importance of empowerment-oriented approaches to intervention. Providing true opportunities for person-centered voice (i.e., ideas, beliefs, concerns) and decision making, and teaching people to advocate for themselves within regulatory agencies and health care institutions, moves occupational therapy practitioners and clients toward a participatory power model of interaction that strengthens practitioner–client interaction and larger community. Recognizing the power that practitioners hold and moving from shared power to a participatory power relationship is an aspect of self-awareness that moves practitioners toward culturally effective care.

Reflection 7.4. Client Power and Powerlessness

- How will you learn about clients' sense of power or powerlessness?
- What steps will you take to assist your clients to move toward participatory power within their health care settings and experiences?

Summary

Occupational therapy practitioners work in health care settings that are political by nature. An important aspect of cultural self-awareness is the recognition of one's own prejudice and power and how that affects one's relationship with clients, colleagues, and others. In this chapter, I explored the meaning of cultural awareness; stereotypes, prejudice, and discrimination; and power and privilege. I also reviewed how prejudice can affect the practitioner–client relationship.

References

Allport, G. W. (1974). *Six decades of social psychology.* New York: Norton.

Banks, J. A. (1996). *Multicultural education, transformative knowledge, and action.* New York: Teachers College.

Black, L. L., & Stone, D. (2005). Expanding the definition of privilege: The concept of social privilege. *Journal of Multicultural Counseling and Development, 33*(4), 243–255. http://dx.doi.org/10.1002/j.2161-1912.2005.tb00020.x

Buetow, S. (2013). Medical professionalism requires that the best interest of the patient must always come first. *Journal of Primary Health Care, 5,* 76–77. Retrieved from http://www.publish.csiro.au/?act=view_file&file_id=HC13076.pdf

Case, K. A. (2007). Raising White privilege awareness and reducing racial prejudice: Assessing diversity course effectiveness. *Teaching of Psychology, 34,* 231–235. http://dx.doi.org/10.1080/00986280701700250

Chapman, C. H., Hwang, W.-T., Both, S., Thomas, C. R., Jr., & Deville, C. (2014). Current status of diversity by race, Hispanic ethnicity, and sex in diagnostic radiology. *Radiology, 270,* 232–240. http://dx.doi.org/10.1148/radiol.13130101

Driscoll, D. M. (1994). Personal power. *Executive Female, 17*(5), 46–51.

Frankenberg, R. (1993). *White women, race matters: The social construction of Whiteness.* Minneapolis: University of Minnesota Press.

Frankford, D. M. (1997). The normative constitution of professional power. *Journal of Health Politics, Policy, and Law, 22,* 185–221. http://dx.doi.org/10.1215/03616878-22-1-185

Goldstein, S. B. (1997). Methods and techniques. The power of stereotypes: A labeling exercise. *Teaching of Psychology, 24,* 256–258. http://dx.doi.org/10.1207/s15328023top2404_5

Hackney, A. (2009). The diversity monologues: Increasing understanding and empathy, decreasing stereotypes and prejudice. In R. A. R. Gurunge & L. R. Prieto (Eds.), *Getting culture* (pp. 77–89). Sterling, VA: Stylus Publishing.

Haney, E. (1994). *Social location and alliance building.* Unpublished manuscript.

Hecht, M. L. (1998). *Communicating prejudice.* Thousand Oaks, CA: Sage.

Holzman, C. (1995). Rethinking the role of guilt and shame on White women's anti-racism work. In G. M. Enguidanos & J. Adleman (Eds.), *Racism in the lives of women: Testimony, theory, and guides to antiracist practices* (pp. 325–347). New York: Harrington Park.

Howard, G. (1993). Whites in multicultural education: Rethinking our role. *Phi Delta Kappan, 75,* 36–41. Retrieved from http://www.ghequityinstitute.com/gh_articles/whites_in_multicultural_education.pdf

Ignatiev, N. (1995). *How the Irish became White.* New York: Routledge.

Jussim, L. (2012). *Social perception and social reality.* Oxford, England: Oxford University Press.

Kielhofner, G., de las Heras, C. G., & Suarez-Balcazar, Y. (2011). Human occupation as a tool for understanding and promoting social justice. In F. Kronenberg, N. Pollard, & D. Sakellariou (Eds.), *Occupational therapies without borders* (Vol. 2, pp. 269–277). Edinburgh, Scotland: Churchill Livingstone.

Kivel, P. (1996). *Uprooting racism: How White people can work for racial justice.* Philadelphia: New Society.

Kronenberg, F., & Pollard, N. (2005). Overcoming occupational apartheid: A preliminary exploration of the political nature of occupational therapy. In F. Kronenberg, S. S. Algado, & N. Pollard (Eds.), *Occupational therapy without borders: Learning from the spirit of survivors* (pp. 58–86). Edinburgh, Scotland: Churchill Livingstone.

Lensmire, T. J., McManimon, S. K., Tierney, J. D., Lee-Nichols, M. E., Casey, Z. A., Lensmire, A., & Davis, B. M. (2013). McIntosh as synecdoche: How teacher education's focus on White privilege undermines antiracism. *Harvard Educational Review, 83,* 410–431. http://dx.doi.org/10.17763/haer.83.3.35054h14l8230574

Litwack, L. (2004, Spring). Personal power. *Ostomy Quarterly,* 52–53.

Lott, B. (1995). Distance from women: Interpersonal sexist discrimination. In B. Lott & D. Maluso (Eds.), *The social psychology of interpersonal discrimination* (pp. 12–49). New York: Guilford Press.

Macura, K. J. (2013). *Diversity 3.0: Are we there yet?* [Chancellor's Report]. Retrieved from http://www.acr.org/-/media/ACR/Documents/PDF/Pubs/Bulletin%20Archive/2014/Diversity30.pdf

McIntosh, P. (1988). *White privilege and male privilege: A personal account of coming to see correspondences through work in women's studies* (Working Paper No. 189). Wellesley, MA: Wellesley College, Center for Research on Women. Retrieved from http://www.ehcounseling.com/materials/WHITE_PRIVILEGE_MALE_04-02-2003.pdf

Merton, R. K. (1972). Insiders and outsiders: A chapter in the sociology of knowledge. *American Journal of Sociology, 78,* 9–47. Retrieved from http://www.d.umn.edu/cla/faculty/jhamlin/4111/Readings/MertonKnowledge.pdf

Neuberg, S. L. (1991). Expectancy–confirmation processes in stereotype-tinged social encounters: The moderating role of social goals. In M. P. Zanna & J. Olson (Eds.), *Ontario Symposium on Personality and Social Psychology: Vol. 7. The psychology of prejudice* (pp. 103–130). Hillsdale, NJ: Erlbaum.

Norton, M. (2000). Challenges to sharing power in an adult literacy education program. In M. Norton & G. Malicky (Eds.), *Learning about participatory approaches in adult literacy education: Six research in practice studies* (pp. 159–191). Edmonton, AB: Learning at the Centre.

Person, E. S. (2004). Personal power and the cultural unconscious: Implications for psychoanalytic theories of sex and gender. *Journal of the American Academy of Psychoanalysis and Dynamic Psychiatry, 32,* 59–75. http://dx.doi.org/10.1521/jaap.32.1.59.28339

Pinderhughes, E. (1989). *Understanding race, ethnicity, and power: The key to efficacy in clinical practice.* New York: Free Press.

Polatajko, H. J. (2001). National perspective—The evolution of our occupational perspective: The journey from diversion through therapeutic use to enablement. *Canadian Journal of Occupational Therapy, 68,* 203–207. http://dx.doi.org/10.1177/000841740106800401

Ponte, P. R., Glazer, G., Dann, E., McCollum, K., Gross, A., Tyrrell, R., . . . Washington, D. (2007). The power of professional nursing practice—An essential element of patient and family centered care. *Online Journal of Issues in Nursing, 12*(1), 4. http://dx.doi.org/10.3912/OJIN.Vol12No01Man03

Rothenberg, P. S. (1998). *Race, class, and gender in the United States: An integrated study* (4th ed.). New York: St. Martin's Press.

Smey, J. W. (2010). Understanding racism. In R. Leavitt (Ed.), *Cultural competence: A lifelong journey to cultural proficiency* (pp. 137–158). Thorofare, NJ: Slack.

Solomon, R. P., & Daniel, B.-J. M. (2015). Discourses on race and "White privilege" in the next generation of teachers. In D. E. Lund & P. R. Carr (Eds.), *Revising the Great White North?* (pp. 193–204). Rotterdam, the Netherlands: Sense Publishers.

Steele, S. (1990). White guilt. *American Scholar, 59,* 497–506.

Steele, S. (1998–1999). The culture of deference. *Academic Questions, 12,* 54–62. Retrieved from http://www1.udel.edu/educ/gottfredson/color/articles/steele.html

Steele, S. (2002, November). The age of White guilt. *Harper's Magazine,* 33–42. Retrieved from http://harpers.org/archive/2002/11/the-age-of-white-guilt/

Tai, R. H., & Kenyatta, M. (1999). *Critical ethnicity: Countering the waves of identity politics.* Lanham, MD: Rowman & Littlefield.

Townsend, E. A., Beagan, B., Kumas-Tan, Z., Versnel, J., Iwama, M., Landry, J., . . . Brown, J. (2007). Enabling: Occupational therapy's core competency. In E. A. Townsend & H. J. Polatajko (Eds.), *Enabling occupation II: Advancing an occupational therapy vision for health, well-being, and justice through occupation* (pp. 87–133). Ottawa, Ontario: CAOT Publications.

Townsend, E. A., & Landry, J. E. (2004). Enabling participation in occupations. In C. Christiansen & C. Baum (Eds.), *Occupational therapy: Overcoming human performance deficits* (3rd ed., pp. 494–521). Thorofare, NJ: Slack.

Townsend, E., & Whiteford, G. (2005). A Participatory Occupational Justice Framework: Population-based processes of practice. In F. Kronenberg, S. S. Algado, & N. Pollard (Eds.), *Occupational therapy without borders: Learning from the spirit of survivors* (pp. 110–126). Edinburgh, Scotland: Churchill Livingstone.

Whiteford, G., & Townsend, E. (2011). Participatory Occupational Justice Framework (POJF 2010): Enabling occupational participation and inclusion. In F. Kronenberg, N. Pollard, & D. Sakellariou (Eds.), *Occupational therapies without borders: Vol. 2. Towards an ecology of occupation-based practices* (pp. 65–84). Edinburgh, Scotland: Churchill Livingstone.

Wilding, P. (1982). *Professional power and social welfare.* Boston: Routledge & Kegan Paul.

Chapter 8.

ACQUIRING CULTURAL SELF-AWARENESS

Roxie M. Black, PhD, OTR/L, FAOTA

> *Raising of self-awareness crucially contributes towards one's understanding of the nature and construction of their cultural identity.*
> **Irina Papadopoulos, Mary Tilki, & Shelley Lees (2004, p. 10)**

Chapter Highlights

- What Is Cultural Self-Awareness?
- Self-Awareness Activities
- Developing Critical Reflection

Key Terms and Concepts

- ❖ Active and deliberate constructive process
- ❖ Contact theory or hypothesis
- ❖ Critical reflection
- ❖ Cultural Effectiveness Model
- ❖ Cultural self-awareness
- ❖ Examination of practice
- ❖ Gibbs reflective cycle
- ❖ Process of personal transformation
- ❖ Reflexivity
- ❖ Self-awareness activities

Cultural self-awareness may be the most important characteristic of culturally effective practitioners, although it can be difficult to achieve. People often do not know what to do to develop this skill, but many activities are available to facilitate self-reflection, which results in increased cultural self-awareness.

To assist students and practitioners to begin to achieve this skill, this chapter identifies and describes activities that can help develop cultural self-awareness. Many of the activities are focused on working with

students but can be modified to be effective with occupational therapy practitioners, educators, and researchers.

What Is Cultural Self-Awareness?

Cultural self-awareness is the recognition of being a unique individual with a specific cultural background that influences personal beliefs, values, attitudes, and behaviors. Because knowing oneself is critical for occupational therapy practitioners, developing cultural self-awareness is important as one interacts with people who are culturally different from oneself. Without cultural self-awareness, the differences that practitioners face during client interactions have the potential to elicit anger, discomfort, confusion, or unconscious prejudicial responses, which may result in ineffective care.

Self-Awareness Activities

This section provides several *self-awareness activities* to facilitate the development of cultural self-awareness.

Activity 8.1. Cultural Object Exercise

Most occupational therapy students are White, and many may not recognize that they come from any particular culture. This exercise is effective in moving people toward seeing themselves as cultural beings and is best accomplished with a smaller group of 15 or fewer. It is a good beginning activity for self-examination because it is emotionally safe.

Purpose: The purpose of this activity is to explore and celebrate cultural differences and recognize cultural similarities on a personal level. This activity introduces cross-cultural perspectives and how these perspectives influence values, beliefs, and communication patterns and styles.

Task: Have students bring an object to class that exemplifies their cultural heritage or their current cultural experience (e.g., family photograph, a piece of jewelry, a religious object, food, any item of personal cultural significance). Have them share what these objects illustrate about their heritage or experience.

Discussion: While the students introduce their object and talk about the meaning it has for them, the instructor keeps track of similarities and differences in the traditions, occupations, and ethnicities identified as well as the importance of family, religion, and other cultural factors, and then leads the group in a discussion that helps to heighten students' awareness of their own culture and that of their classmates. After completing this exercise, students may engage in Activity 8.2.

Reflection 8.1. Family Background

- Think about what is important to you from your family background and why it has meaning for you. Identify 2 or 3 items you might use for the cultural object exercise.

Activity 8.2. Cultural Identity Paper

This activity was described in Nochajski and Matteliano (2008).

Purpose: The purpose of this activity is to help each student develop a deeper understanding of his or her own culture.

Task: Ask students to write a reflective paper on their cultural identity that addresses the following questions:

- How would you describe your own cultural identity?
- What part of your cultural identity has the greatest influence on your interactions with others? How so?
- Are there any conflicting aspects of your cultural identity?
- Think about someone you know from a different culture than yours and describe the similarities and differences between the two cultures. What conflicts could you see arising between members of these two cultures? What aspects of the cultures could be unifying?

Activity 8.3. Family Elder Interview

Purpose: The purpose of this activity is for students to gather stories about their cultural background from an older family member.

Task: Ask students to arrange an interview with an older family member, preferably one who is known to be a good storyteller. They should record the interview for later assessment. Students should

- Ask the family member to talk about the history of the family, why the story is meaningful, what it says about the values of the family, whether the story is typical for his or her particular cultural group, and how the family has changed.

- Summarize what they learned in a written paper, identifying information that was new to them, what surprised them, and what they learned about themselves during this activity.

Activity 8.4. Interview Someone Culturally Different From You

Purpose: This activity has two purposes: for students to get to know someone from a different culture and to reflect on their responses to the information they gather.

Task: Have each student set up an interview with someone who is culturally different from him or her. Students should

- Ask the interviewee to talk about his or her culture and how it affects the way he or she interacts with family, with friends, and with work colleagues.
- Ask the interviewee whether he or she has experienced any barriers to occupational choice and performance as a result of his or her culture.
- Reflect on what effect this interview has on your awareness of yourself in response to this culture.
- Write a short paper or make a presentation to the class, or both, on the information they gathered from the interviewee and what they learned about themselves during this process.

Activity 8.5. Culture and Diversity Training Game, Role Playing, and Simulation

These activities are designed to stimulate discussion and promote self-reflection and respect for others. Many are available online or through other resources.

BAFA BAFA

BAFA BAFA (see http://bit.ly/1XvPqxc) is a game designed to assist people in learning about the differences in cultures and their effects on behavior. Participants are divided into either the Alpha or Beta cultures. "In both cultures the members learn the rules of their culture (customs, rituals and traditions as specified in the instructions of the game), send observers to learn about the other culture, and exchange groups of visitors to experience

each other's cultural norms" (Kim & Lyons, 2003, p. 404).

Barnga: A Game on Cultural Clashes

Barnga: A Game on Cultural Clashes (see http://bit.ly/1OCiHq3). This is a card game designed to assist participants in recognizing how subtle cultural differences can negatively impact a person's ability to function in a new group. "Participants are led to the realization that, in spite of surface similarities, people from other cultures have differences in the way they do things. A person has to reconcile these differences to function effectively in a cross-cultural group" (Pittenger & Heimann, 1998, p. 253).

Brown Eyes, Blue Eyes

Brown Eyes, Blue Eyes (see http://bit.ly/2aAULUJ) is a simulation in which participants are divided into two groups; one group is assigned tasks related to privilege while the others are not and play this out with each other.

At the end of the simulation and before the debriefing, all participants are asked to write down what they feel. These feelings will be revealed during the debriefing as students talk about what it is like to be discriminated against (Byrnes & Kiger, 1988).

Activity 8.6. Films, Books, and Reflective Journaling

Films and books can offer an "inside perspective into the folklore, history and values of a wide variety of cultures" (Schultz, 1999, p. 63). Critical reflection in journals and discussions about films and books also give people an opportunity to explore and consider their own biases and prejudices. Suggested movies include

- *Eat, Pray, Love* (Gardner & Murphy, 2010). After a divorce, a woman takes an around-the-world journey.
- *Children of a Lesser God* (Palmer & Haines, 1986). This movie explores the relationship between a student and teacher at a school for the deaf.
- *Hotel Rwanda* (Bhembe & George, 2004). A hotel manager in Rwanda takes in more than a thousand Tutsi refugees.

- *Memoirs of a Geisha* (Barber & Marshall, 2005). A woman leaves her small village and becomes a famous geisha.
- *Seven Years in Tibet* (Annaud, 1997). An Austrian befriends the Dalai Lama during China's takeover of Tibet.
- *The Hundred Foot Journey* (Blake & Hallström, 2014). An Indian family moves to France and opens a restaurant across from a renowned eatery, resulting in a culture clash.

Suggested books include

- *Daughters of Copper Woman* (Cameron, 1995). The author recounts native Northwest coast myths.
- *I Know Why the Caged Bird Sings* (Angelou, 1969). The story of Maya is used to examine the experience of Blacks in America, among other themes.
- *The Joy Luck Club* (Tan, 1989). Four Chinese women figure out life in San Francisco.
- *The Spirit Catches You and You Fall Down: A Hmong Child, Her American Doctors, and the Collision of Two Cultures* (Fadiman, 1997). A Laotian refugee family argues with California hospital staff over the care of their daughter, who has been diagnosed with epilepsy.

Reflection 8.2. Movies and Books

- What movies have you seen or books have you read that make you think about differences in cultural beliefs and behaviors? Discuss what you learned with a student peer or colleague.

Personal Interaction With Diverse People and Groups

An effective way to learn how to interact with culturally diverse people is to spend time with them (Nesdale & Todd, 2000; Ward, 2004). Learning about other cultures through some of the activities in the previous section is a good beginning, but interacting with diverse others makes a significant difference in a person's attitude and self-awareness.

Contact theory or hypothesis, developed by social scientists beginning with Allport (1954) and studied more recently by Pettigrew (1998, 2008) and Pettigrew and Tropp (2006), infers that contact with people who are culturally different often reduces prejudice, especially if those who are interacting do not hold deep-seated biases and prejudices against each other. However, research indicates that people with strong biases against another group tend to avoid contact with people from that group (Pettigrew, 1998; Pettigrew & Tropp, 2006), so there is no opportunity to diminish prejudice. Therefore, occupational therapy students and practitioners must be given or seek out opportunities to interact with people who differ from themselves and reflect on their reaction to this experience. Such opportunities may include

- Interviewing a person who is culturally different to "gain insight and knowledge about cultural variation and respect for others" (Lenburg, 1995);
- Attending local cultural activities (i.e., cultural fairs and presentations), dining in ethnic restaurants, and visiting a culturally different colleague or peer in their own home and making a point to speak with people and ask them questions about themselves and their culture;
- Visiting an ethnic neighborhood in your community and observing how people live, communicate, and act; and
- Traveling abroad and immersing yourself in the culture.

During and after any of these activities, students must be led through a critical reflection of the experience.

Developing Critical Reflection

Critical reflection is a vital component of the Cultural Effectiveness Model because it requires people to become more analytical and aware of themselves. Mezirow (1990) cited Boud, Keogh, and Walker (1985), who stated that ***critical reflection*** is "a generic term for those intellectual and affective activities in which individuals engage to explore their experiences in order to lead to new understandings and appreciation" (p. 5). Critical reflection involves thinking about what just happened during a cross-cultural interaction and "should challenge a person's understanding of themselves, their attitudes and behaviors so that any biases are unearthed, thus allowing that [person] to become more critical about their views of practice and the world" (Jasper & Rolfe, 2011, as cited in Paterson & Chapman, 2013, p. 3).

Such reflection deepens one's self-awareness and becomes the foundation for more effective clinical practice. As described in the *Cultural Effectiveness Model* (see Chapters 5, "Model for Cultural Effectiveness," and 6, "Cultural Self-Awareness, Critical Reflection, and Transforming Attitudes"), deep reflection after a cultural encounter often results in a change in attitude and behavior for the practitioner, which he or she can then apply to the next cultural encounter (Schon, 1983). Paterson and Chapman (2013) described this process as "an increased understanding and development of moral growth that improves the society in which the individual works" (p. 134).

Duffy (2007) examined the nursing literature on reflection and found the following four critical attributes that define reflective practice (p. 1403):

1. *Examination of practice,* which is used in a structured way to reflect on a particular practice issue such as performing activities of daily living with a Middle Eastern client;
2. *Reflexivity,* which is the consideration of past experiences on the present;
3. *Active and deliberate constructive process,* in which a practitioner "actively considers the various components of a given task, with a view to learning from and using the lessons learnt to improve practice" (p. 1403); and
4. *Process of personal transformation,* in which through "expanding consciousness, . . . individuals become critically aware of old and new self-views and choose to integrate these views into a new self-definition" (p. 1403).

Educators are obligated to guide students in their thinking and provide opportunities for them to develop these attributes through reflection. Reflection can occur through journaling, engaging in small-group discussions, and writing reflective papers that are guided by provocative questions from the instructor, including

- What went well with this experience?
- Was there anything in your encounter that caused you discomfort? If so, examine why it happened.

- What similarities and differences did you notice between you and the client regarding health beliefs and practices?
- Did you make any cultural mistakes? How might you avoid these in a future encounter?
- Was there a language barrier? How did you interact with each other?
- Did you feel satisfied that this was an effective interaction? What might you do to improve the cross-cultural experience?
- Overall, how do you feel about the experience?

The literature also contains several reflective models (e.g., Gibbs, 1988; Johns, 1995; Mezirow, 1990) that instructors can use to aid students in achieving the four critical attributes. The *Gibbs reflective cycle* (Gibbs, 1988; Figure 8.1) is an exemplar because of its clarity of design and instruction. It consists of the following six stages of reflection to be competed after an experience (Paterson & Chapman, 2013):

1. *Description.* Describe what happened during the encounter.
2. *Feelings.* Examine the thoughts and feelings that occurred during the encounter.
3. *Evaluation.* Identify what was positive and challenging about the encounter.
4. *Analysis.* Try to make sense of the situation, and examine the impact it had on your practice.
5. *Conclusion.* Explore the literature and consult with colleagues to understand the situation better, and determine what else could have been done.
6. *Action plan.* Devise a plan for the future that maps alternative approaches if this situation or a similar situation occurs in the future.

Whether the instructor uses guiding questions as part of his or her teaching strategies for reflective activities or a model such as Gibbs's (1988), he or she must make time in the curriculum for students to examine and reflect on their cross-cultural interactions. Finding time to do so within packed courses is often difficult, yet given the evidence that critical reflection enhances student learning and practice (Mann, Gordon, & MacLeod, 2009; Mezirow, 1990), it is imperative that faculty find a way to make the time for this important educational practice.

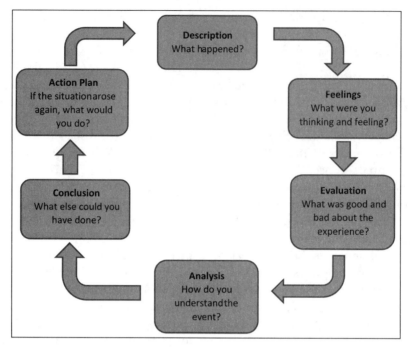

Figure 8.1. Gibbs' reflective cycle.

Reflection 8.3. Meet Someone New

Introduce yourself to a person at work or school who is culturally different from you (in age, ethnicity, sexual orientation, or religion). Spend a little time getting to know each other. As you are communicating with this person, try to be aware of your feelings and think about how the conversation is going. Are you comfortable? Is it an easy or awkward conversation? After the interaction, ask yourself the following questions:

- What were my expectations of this interaction before introducing myself?
- Did the interaction go as planned? Why or why not?
- Did I make any cultural mistakes?
- Did I notice any bias on my part? If so, how would I change my approach during the next cross-cultural interaction?
- How do I feel about meeting the next person who is different? Excited? Anxious? Hesitant?

Summary

Acquiring cultural self-awareness is possible, and numerous suggestions exist in the literature and online to help develop these characteristics. This

chapter identified several ideas that may be effective for occupational therapy students, practitioners, educators, and researchers to help develop the characteristics of self-awareness and critical reflection needed for effective practice.

References

Allport, G. (1954). *The nature of prejudice.* New York: Doubleday.

Angelou, M. (1969). *I know why the caged bird sings.* New York: Random House.

Annaud, J.-J. (Producer & Director). (1997). *Seven years in Tibet* [Motion Picture]. United States: Mandalay Entertainment.

Barber, G. (Producer), & Marshall, R. (Director). (2005). *Memoirs of a geisha* [Motion Picture]. United States: Columbia Pictures.

Bhembe, S. (Producer), & George, T. (Director). (2004). *Hotel Rwanda* [Motion Picture]. United States: United Artists.

Blake, J. (Producer), & Hallström, L. (Director). (2014). *The hundred foot journey* [Motion Picture]. United States: Amblin Entertainment.

Boud, D., Keogh, R., & Walker, D. (1985). *Reflection: Turning experience into learning.* London: Kogan Page.

Byrnes, D. A., & Kiger, G. (1988, October). *Ethical and pedagogical issues in the use of simulation activities in the classroom: Evaluating the "Blue Eyes–Brown Eyes" prejudice simulation.* Paper presented at the Annual Meeting of the Northern Rocky Mountain Educational Research Association, Jackson, WY.

Cameron, A. (1995). *Daughters of copper woman.* Vancouver, BC: Press Gang Publishers.

Duffy, A. (2007). A concept analysis of reflective practice: Determining its value to nurses. *British Journal of Nursing, 16,* 1400–1407. http://dx.doi.org/10.12968/bjon.2007.16.22.27771

Fadiman, A. (1997). *The spirit catches you and you fall down: A Hmong child, her American doctors, and the collision of two cultures.* New York: Farrar, Strauss, & Giroux.

Gardner, D. (Producer), & Murphy, R. (Director). (2010). *Eat, pray, love* [Motion Picture]. United States: Columbia Pictures.

Gibbs, G. (1988). *Learning by doing: A guide to teaching and learning methods.* Oxford, England: Further Education Unit, Oxford Polytechnic.

Johns, C. (1995). Framing learning through reflection within Carper's fundamental ways of knowing in nursing. *Journal of Advanced Nursing, 22,* 226–234. http://dx.doi.org/10.1046/j.1365-2648.1995.22020226.x

Kim, B. S. K., & Lyons, H. Z. (2003). Experiential activities and multicultural counseling competence training. *Journal of Counseling and Development, 81,* 400–408. http://dx.doi.org/10.1002/j.1556-6678.2003.tb00266.x

Lenburg, C. B. (Ed.). (1995). *Promoting cultural competence in and through nursing education: A critical review and comprehensive plan for action.* Washington, DC: American Academy of Nursing.

Mann, K., Gordon, J., & MacLeod, A. (2009). Reflection and reflective practice in health professions education: A systematic review. *Advances in Health Science Education, 14,* 595–621. http://dx.doi.org/10.1007/s10459-007-9090-2

Mezirow, J. (1990). How critical reflection triggers transformative learning. In J. Mezirow (Ed.), *Fostering critical reflection in adulthood* (pp. 1–20). San Francisco: Jossey-Bass. http://dx.doi.org/10.1002/ace.7401

Nesdale, D., & Todd, P. (2000). Effect of contact on intercultural acceptance: A field study. *International Journal of Intercultural Relations, 24,* 341–360. http://dx.doi.org/10.1016/S0147-1767(00)00005-5

Nochajski, S. M., & Matteliano, M. A. (2008). Occupational therapy. In J. Stone & M. A. Matteliano (Series Eds.), *A guide to cultural competence in the curriculum.* Buffalo: NY: Center for International Rehabilitation Research Information and Exchange.

Palmer, P. J. (Producer), & Haines, S. (Director). (1986). *Children of a lesser god* [Motion Picture]. United States: Paramount Pictures.

Papadopoulos, I., Tilki, M., & Lees, S. (2004). Promoting cultural competence in health care through a research-based intervention in the UK. *Diversity in Health and Social Care, 1*(2), 107–115. Retrieved from http://diversityhealthcare.imedpub.com/promoting-cultural-competence-in-healthcare-through-a-research-based-intervention-in-the-uk.pdf

Paterson, C., & Chapman, J. (2013). Enhancing skills of critical reflection to evidence learning in professional practice. *Physical Therapy in Sport, 14,* 133–138. http://dx.doi.org/10.1016/j.ptsp.2013.03.004

Pettigrew, T. F. (1998). Intergroup contact theory. *Annual Review of Psychology, 49,* 65–85. http://dx.doi.org/10.1146/annurev.psych.49.1.65

Pettigrew, T. F. (2008). Future directions for intergroup contact theory and research. *International Journal of Intercultural Relations, 32,* 187–199. http://dx.doi.org/10.1016/j.ijintrel.2007.12.002

Pettigrew, T. F., & Tropp, L. R. (2006). A meta-analytic test of intergroup contact theory. *Journal of Personality and Social Psychology, 90,* 751–783. http://dx.doi.org/10.1037/0022-3514.90.5.751

Pittenger, K. K., & Heimann, B. (1998). Barnga: A game on cultural clashes. *Developments in business simulation and experiential learning, 25,* 253–254. Retrieved from https://journals.tdl.org/absel/index.php/absel/article/viewFile/1059/1028

Schon, D. (1983). *The reflective practitioner: How professionals think in action.* Farnham, England: Ashgate.

Schultz, M. (1999). *Respectful practice: Diversity manual for occupational therapists.* Denver: Author.

Tan, A. (1989). *The Joy Luck Club.* New York: Putnam.

Ward, C. (2004). Psychological theories of culture contact and their implications for intercultural training and interventions. In D. Landis, J. M. Bennett, & M. J. Bennett (Eds.), *Handbook of intercultural training* (3rd ed., pp. 185–210). Thorofare, NJ: Sage.

Section II.B.

CULTURAL KNOWLEDGE

Chapter 9.

HEALTH STATUS AND HEALTH DISPARITIES

Shirley A. Wells, DrPH, OTR, FAOTA

Of all the forms of inequality, injustice in health care is the most shocking and inhumane.
**Dr. Martin Luther King Jr., March 25, 1966, Second National Convention of the Medical Committee
for Human Rights, Chicago (as cited in Munro, 2013, para. 8)**

Chapter Highlights

• Current Efforts to Reduce Health Disparities
• Health Data Sources
• Standards for Data on Race and Ethnicity
• Health Status and Determinants
• Reducing Health Disparities

Key Terms and Concepts

✧ Health behavior
✧ Health care disparity
✧ Health data
✧ Health disparity
✧ Health equity
✧ Health-related behavior

✧ Health status
✧ Health status data
✧ Healthy People initiative
✧ Social determinants
✧ Social determinants of health approach

The United States has made significant progress toward achieving health equity, eliminating health disparities, and improving the health of all residents. People are living longer, healthier, and more productive lives. However, the United States still lags behind dozens of other nations, underperforming in the five dimensions of health (access, quality, efficiency, equity, and healthy lives) and fails to achieve better health outcomes (Davis, Stremikis, Squires, & Schoen, 2014).

Progress has not been similarly experienced by all citizens. Key health outcomes vary greatly by race, sex, socioeconomic status, and geographic location, and there are marked regional differences.

Complex relationships exist among health and biology, genetics, and individual behavior as well as among health and health services, socioeconomic status, the physical environment, discrimination, racism, literacy levels, and legislative policies. Because of these complex relationships, addressing determinants of health must be incorporated into existing approaches to reduce health inequities (Satcher, 2010; U.S. Department of Health and Human Services [DHHS], 2014a).

This chapter explores factors related to health disparities and the sources and difficulties in collecting data and measuring disparities. It also highlights the current statues that contribute to disparities in health and health care.

Current Efforts to Reduce Health Disparities

Health disparities and inequalities are gaps in health and social determinants among segments of the population. Inequities are avoidable, unfair differences in health status seen within and among populations. *Social determinants* of health are the conditions in which people are born, grow, live, work, and age, such as education attainment, access to health food retailers, environmental hazards, and unemployment (Foege, 2010; Mainzer & Moffett, 2011; Sadana & Blas, 2013).

The Centers for Disease Control and Prevention (CDC) and its partners have worked to identify and address the factors that lead to health disparities so that barriers to health equity can be removed (CDC, 2013a). They recognized the need to address health inequities in a systematic way by addressing more than individual factors.

However, eliminating the burden of racial and ethnic health disparities is not easy. The Patient Protection and Affordable Care Act (ACA) of 2010 (Pub. L. 111–148) provides some opportunity to reduce health disparities (DHHS, 2015). States, local communities, and private organizations are engaged in efforts to reduce health disparities through such programs as Racial and Ethnic Approaches to Community Health grants funded by the CDC (DHHS, 2011). These interventions vary in scope and focus on outreach, cultural competency training, and education.

Some private foundations have also developed significant initiatives aimed at reducing disparities, and providers are increasingly undertaking disparity-focused efforts. Achieving health equity requires the hard work of many people and organizations.

Health Data Sources

Reducing health disparities begins with collecting and providing accurate and useful data on causes of disparities. To assess and understand the health of a nation and to develop approaches to sustain it, the U.S. agencies collect and disseminate health data. *Health data* encompass all major areas of health statistics, including population and health status, health resources, health care use, health care expenditures, and program management data.

U.S. Public Health Service

National disease prevention and health promotion initiatives—such as *Healthy People* (i.e., science-based, 10-year national objectives for improving the health of all Americans; https://www.healthypeople .gov/)—have improved the monitoring and reporting of changing health status and emerging risks to health and service delivery. To protect the health of the nation's population, the U.S. Public Health Service (USPHS) gathers a wide variety of timely and reliable data, including epidemiological and statistical information. To meet these needs, USPHS uses various forms of data collection, analysis, and dissemination activities. Health data come from many sources, such as vital records, censuses, birth certificates, industrial records, hospital records, death certificates, registries, and surveys.

National Center for Health Statistics

Health-related statistics and data sources are increasingly available on the Internet. They can be found already neatly packaged or as raw datasets. The most reliable data come from governmental sources or health care professional organizations. The National Center for Health Statistics (NCHS) is one component of the CDC that serves as the federal government's designated agency for general-purpose health statistics. It provides statistical information that guides actions and policies to improve the health of the American people. These health statistics (Health Resources and Services Administration [HRSA], 2013; NCHS, 2014a) permit the government to

- Document the health status of the U.S. population and selected subgroups
- Track the impact of major policy initiative, including the ACA

- Identify disparities in health status and use of health care by race and ethnicity, socioeconomic status, other population characteristics, and geographic region
- Document access to and use of the health care system
- Monitor trends in health indicators
- Support biomedical and health services research
- Provide data to support public policies and programs.

Collaborating with other public and private health partners, NCHS uses a variety of data collection mechanisms to obtain accurate information from multiple sources. This process provides a broad perspective to help us understand the population's health, influences on health, and health outcomes. Sources of data collection include birth and death certificates, patient medical records, personal interviews, standardized physical examinations, lab tests, and facility information. Data are used to compare health indicators over time and across populations and geographic areas.

NCHS supports several data systems that collect information annually or periodically (NCHS, 2014a):

- The National Vital Statistics System collects data on births, deaths, causes of deaths, fetal deaths, marriages, and divorces.
- The National Health and Nutrition Examination Survey, in which adults and children are interviewed about their health and nutritional status, is done on an ongoing basis.
- The National Health Care Surveys monitor the use of medical care (i.e., physicians' offices, ambulatory surgery centers, nursing homes, and home health care agencies), staffing, patient safety, and clinical management of conditions.
- The National Immunization Survey monitors data on childhood immunization coverage.
- The National Survey of Family Growth collects data about family life, marriage and divorce, pregnancy, infertility, use of contraception, and men's and women's health.

In addition to the NCHS, the following centers and agencies collect data from surveys that include items on race and ethnicity: the Center for Chronic Disease and Health Promotion; the Alcohol, Drug Abuse, and Mental Health Administration; the National Institute on Drug Abuse; the National Institute of Mental Health; the Agency for Health Care Policy and Research; the Indian Health Service; the National Institutes of Health (NIH); and the HRSA.

Reflection 9.1. Existing Health Conditions in Your Community

- Analysis of existing conditions relies on available data and, depending on resources and priorities, the collection of new data. Develop an existing health condition profile for your community or state. Collect information from government data sources, public forums, the Internet, individual interviews, and literature.

Standards for Data on Race and Ethnicity

Since 1977, the U.S. government has been collecting aggregated data on race and ethnicity. These data standards stemmed from the responsibilities to enforce civil rights laws and were needed to monitor equal access in housing, education, employment, and other areas for populations that historically had experienced discrimination and differential treatment because of their race or ethnicity. Valid and reliable data are fundamental building blocks for identifying differences in care and developing targeted interventions to improve the quality of care delivered to specific populations. The capacity to measure and monitor quality of care for various racial and ethnic populations rests on the ability both to measure quality of care in general and to conduct similar measurements across different racial, ethnic, and linguistic groups.

Standardized Categories

The Office of Management and Budget (OMB) provides the standardized ethnic categories for collecting these data: Black or African American, White, Asian, American Indian or Alaska Native, and Native Hawaiian or Other Pacific Islander. The only ethnicity choice is one of "yes" or "no" to Hispanic or Latino ethnicity. The OMB's (1997) final guidance allowed people to self-identify their ethnicity and race, and it permitted people to select more than one race or ethnicity. This change authorizes people to more accurately reflect their racial and ethnic background by not limiting responses to only one racial or ethnic category, and it expands reporting options to seven categories (American Indian or Alaska Native, Asian, Black or African American, Hispanic, Native Hawaiian or Other Pacific Islander, White, and Two or More Races; Assistant Secretary for Planning and Evaluation, 2011).

According to the Institute of Medicine ([IOM], 2009), more discrete population data are needed to identify opportunities for quality improvement and outreach. For example, is a Native American child from a Navajo or Choctaw background? Legislation supports the collection of data for disparities reduction, and the data need to continue to be handled properly to maintain the public's trust.

The ACA improves health data collection and analysis strategy on disparities. Section 4302 requires that all health surveys sponsored by the DHHS include standardized information on race, ethnicity, sex, primary language, and disability status. The law also provides the opportunity to collect additional demographic data to improve our understanding of health care disparities. DHHS also plans to collect health data on lesbian, gay, bisexual, and transgender populations (IOM, 2014).

Language Need

Assessing individual language need is an essential first step toward ensuring effective health care communication (IOM, 2009). The Agency for Healthcare Research and Quality (AHRQ, 2010) recommended data collection on the level of English proficiency and preferred spoken language, the language spoken by the person at home, and the language in which he or she prefers to receive written materials. When the person is a child, the language need of the parent or guardian must be determined. Similarly, if an adult has a guardian or conservator, that person's language need must be assessed. Having language-need information facilitates higher quality of services in (1) encounters, (2) analysis of health care disparities, and (3) system-level planning (e.g., determining the need for interpreters and matching patients to language-concordant providers).

Data Availability

Although improvements have been made in data collection, several issues remain on the availability of data on the health status of racial and ethnic-minority populations in the United States. No clearinghouse for statistics lists comprehensive data by race, ethnicity, gender, or socioeconomic status. In terms of race and ethnicity, a wide variety of health data are available for White and African American populations, but considerably fewer national data are available for other ethnic populations. Few tables list any breakdown by ethnicity.

Very limited data are available on the Asian and Pacific Islander populations. National data tend to mask the diversity among Chinese, Japanese, Korean, and recent immigrants from Southeast Asia. Any people of Cuban, Mexican, Puerto Rican, South or Central American, or other Spanish culture or origin, regardless of race, are reported as Hispanics or Latinos. Similarly, national health data on the total Native American population by tribal affiliation are limited (IOM, 2014).

Data Collection Challenges

The data collection process itself can create challenges. First, a clear understanding of why it is important to collect race and ethnicity data is needed. Medical providers may be uncomfortable soliciting this information from patients because they cannot explain why the data are being collected or how the data will be used (AHRQ, 2010). At the same time, patients may be hesitant to provide race and ethnicity data because of concerns around privacy and discrimination. Patients may not understand why health professionals want race and ethnicity data, or they may associate providing race and ethnicity data with discrimination or misuse of the data, such as finding undocumented immigrants (Weissman & Hasnain-Wynia, 2011).

If staff members do not understand the greater accuracy of directly reported data, they may make their own observations of a person's race or ethnicity (AHRQ, 2010). The Health Research and Educational Trust (2013) reported that training on standardized data collection processes can increase compliance, ensure data integrity, and improve patient buy-in. Hospital leadership should assign accountability and monitor data collection efforts to ensure that processes are working as planned. Misperceptions around the legality of data collection and challenges in understanding subpopulations can be addressed by training staff on data collection protocols.

The capacities of varied health information technology systems are another challenge to the data collection processes. Data collection by various entities within the health care system raises the possibility that conflicting data may be assigned to a single person. A person may self-identify in one clinical setting according to a limited set of choices, whereas another setting may offer more detailed options, or the person's race may have been observed rather than requested and then recorded by an intake worker. Not all data systems capture the method through which the data were collected, and some systems do not allow for data overrides (IOM, 2009).

As the nation moves toward national health information technology standards, the interoperability of technology systems has improved to ensure that race, ethnicity, and language data can be collected, stored, and shared. The engagement and support of a hospital's information technology department are important to the success of such efforts (AHRQ, 2010).

Health Status and Determinants

Life expectancy and the overall health of the nation continue to improve for a large number of Americans as a result of an increased focus on preventive medicine, advances in technology, and health education. *Health status* describes the myriad components of the well-being or ill health of the population so that health care professionals can develop interventions for preventing and controlling disease and evaluate the effect of these interventions.

Health status data include various measures, such as the nature and extent of mortality, morbidity, and disability in people and populations, as well as their knowledge, attitudes, and behaviors concerning health and health care (DHHS, 2014a). Americans have taken steps toward better health driven by improvements in more than two-thirds of health measures (United Health Foundation, 2013). Although Americans' life expectancy and health have improved, these gains have lagged behind those in other high-income countries. This health disadvantage prevails even though the United States spends far more per person on health care than any other nation (IOM, 2013).

Life Expectancy

In a recent report, NCHS (2014c) described the health status of the United States as improving. In 2014, life expectancy at birth in the United States for the total population was 78.8 years—76.4 years for men and 81.2 years for women. Life expectancy at birth increased 1.4 years for men and 1.1 years for women. The gap in life expectancy between men and women narrowed from 5.1 years in 2004 to 4.8 years in 2014.

The life expectancy at birth increased more for African American than for the White population. By 2014, the difference had narrowed to 3.4 years, thereby narrowing the gap in life expectancy between these two racial groups. In 2014, the life expectancy for Hispanic persons increased to 81.8 years: 79.2 years for men and 84 years for women.

Between 2004 and 2014, the age-adjusted heart disease death rate decreased 25%. In 2014, 23% of all deaths in the United States were from heart disease and 23% were from cancer, whereas the suicide death rate increased 27%.

Obesity and Smoking

In terms of health risks, the prevalence of obesity among children age 2 to 5 years decreased from 14.0% to 8.9%; moreover, 17.5% of children age 6 to 11 years were obese, and 20.5% of adolescents age 12 to 19 years were obese in 2014. Among adults, those with Grade 1 obesity (i.e., a body mass index [BMI] of 30.0–34.9) increased from 14.8% to 20.6%. Those with Grade 2 obesity (i.e., BMI of 35.0–39.9) rose from 5.2% to 8.8%, and those with Grade 3 or higher obesity (i.e., BMI of 40 or higher) more than doubled from 3.0% to 6.9% (percentages are age-adjusted).

In 2014, 18% of adults were current cigarette smokers, a decline from 2000 (23.2%). Men were more likely than women to be current cigarette smokers (18.8% compared with 14.8%). Nearly one-half (47%) of all adults with hypertension continue to have uncontrolled high blood pressure.

Health Rankings by State

The United Health Foundation (2013), in its America's Health Rankings annual report, listed Hawaii as the healthiest state, followed by Vermont and Minnesota. Mississippi ranked 50th, with Arkansas, Louisiana, Alabama, and West Virginia completing the bottom 5 states. The United Health Foundation also described a decline in ranking for several states: (1) Wisconsin's decline was due to an increase in poor mental health days, a decrease in adolescent immunizations, only marginal improvement in smoking, an increase in obesity, and an increase in violent crime; (2) Maryland's decline was due to increases in child poverty, diabetes, and disparity in health status; and (3) Virginia's decline was due to increases in chlamydia, poor physical health days, and occupational fatalities. Rhode Island experienced increases in drug deaths and infant mortality that affected its decline in rank.

However, large improvements were seen in Wyoming because of a decrease in physical inactivity, an increase in child immunizations, a decline in low-birthweight infants, and a decline in poor physical health days. In Idaho, decreases in children living in poverty, low-birthweight infants, and diabetes contributed to its improvement. In Montana, decreases in smoking, physical inactivity, occupational fatalities, and children living in poverty improved its rank. In New Mexico, decreases in air pollution, cardiovascular deaths, and preventable hospitalizations contributed to its improvement. New York's improvement was due to decreases in smoking, obesity, and the number of people uninsured as well as the increased availability of primary care physicians.

Health Profile for Specific Populations

Of the U.S. population in 2014, racial and ethnic minorities made up 37.9% of the population. Hispanic individuals, 17.4%; multiple-race individuals were 2.0%; American Indians or Alaska Natives were 0.7%; African Americans were 12.4%; Native Hawaiian or other Pacific Islander individuals were 0.2%; and White individuals were 62.1% (NCHS, 2015). According to the Office of Minority Health ([OMH], 2014), the health profiles of the racial and ethnic minority as well as women and men, and older adults are as follows.

African Americans

In 2012, 43.1 million people in the United States were African Americans—alone or in combination. African Americans are the second largest minority population. The death rate for African Americans was generally higher than Whites for heart diseases, stroke, cancer, asthma, influenza, pneumonia, diabetes, HIV or AIDS, and homicide. They are twice as likely to be diagnosed with diabetes as non-Hispanic Whites. In addition, they are more likely to experience complications from diabetes,

such as end-stage renal disease and lower-extremity amputations (OMH, 2014).

Although African Americans have the same or lower rate of high cholesterol as their non-Hispanic White counterparts, they are more likely to have high blood pressure (CDC, 2014). African American women have the highest rates of being overweight or obese compared with other groups in the United States. About 4 out of 5 African American women are overweight or obese. In 2011, African Americans were 1.5 times as likely to be obese as non-Hispanic Whites, and the women were 80% more likely to be obese than non-Hispanic White women (CDC, 2012).

Hispanics and Latino Americans

In 2012, there were almost 53 million Hispanics living in the United States. This group represents 16.9% of the total U.S. population. Among the Hispanic subgroups, Mexicans rank as the largest at 64.3%, followed by Puerto Ricans (9.4%), Central Americans (9.0%), South Americans (5.9%), and Cubans (3.7%). Hispanic health is often shaped by factors such as language and cultural barriers, lack of access to preventive care, and the lack of health insurance (OMH, 2014).

The leading causes of illness and death among Hispanics include heart disease, cancer, unintentional injuries (accidents), stroke, and diabetes. Some other health conditions and risk factors that significantly affect Hispanics are asthma, chronic obstructive pulmonary disease, HIV and AIDS, obesity, suicide, and liver disease. Hispanic adults are 1.7 times more likely than non-Hispanic White adults to have been diagnosed with diabetes by a physician (CDC, 2014).

Among Mexican American women, 78% are overweight or obese, compared with 60.3% of non-Hispanic White women. In 2011, Hispanic Americans were 1.2 times as likely to be obese than non-Hispanic Whites (CDC, 2013d).

American Indians and Alaska Natives

As of 2012, there were an estimated 5.2 million people who were classified as American Indian and Alaska Native alone or American Indian and Alaska Native in combination with one or more other races. This racial group composes 2% of the total U.S. population. Some of the leading diseases and causes of death among American Indians and Alaska Natives are heart disease, cancer, unintentional injuries (accidents), diabetes, and stroke. They also have a high prevalence and risk factors for mental health and suicide, obesity, substance abuse, sudden infant death syndrome (SIDS), teenage pregnancy, liver disease, and hepatitis (OMH, 2014).

American Indians and Alaska Natives have an infant death rate 60% higher than the rate for Whites. The women are 30% more likely than non-Hispanic White women to be obese, and adults are 60% more likely to be obese than non-Hispanic Whites. They are twice as likely to have diabetes as non-Hispanic Whites, and they have disproportionately high death rates from unintentional injuries and suicide. In 2012, the tuberculosis rate for American Indians and Alaska Natives was 6.3, compared with 0.8 for the White population. Data are limited for this population (CDC, 2013b, 2013c).

Asian Americans

According to the 2012 Census Bureau population estimate, 15.5 million Asian Americans live in the United States. Asian American women have the highest life expectancy (85.8 years) of any other ethnic group: Filipino women (81.5 years), Japanese women (84.5 years), and Chinese women (86.1 years). They experience infrequent medical visits because of the fear of deportation, language and cultural barriers, and the lack of health insurance.

Asian Americans are most at risk for cancer, heart disease, stroke, unintentional injuries (accidents), and diabetes. They also have a high prevalence and risk factors for chronic obstructive pulmonary disease, hepatitis B, HIV and AIDS, smoking, tuberculosis, and liver disease. In 2012, tuberculosis was 24 times more common among Asians, with a case rate of 18.9, compared with 0.8 for the non-Hispanic White population (OMH, 2014).

Native Hawaiians and Pacific Islanders

In 2012, there were roughly 1.2 million Native Hawaiians and Pacific Islanders (alone or in combination with one or more races) residing within the United States. This group represents about 0.5% of the U.S. population. Native Hawaiians and Pacific Islanders have higher rates of smoking, alcohol consumption, and obesity. This group also has little access to cancer prevention and control programs.

Some leading causes of death among this population include cancer, heart disease, unintentional injuries (accidents), stroke, and diabetes. Some other health conditions and risk factors that are prevalent among Native Hawaiians and Pacific Islanders are hepatitis B, HIV and AIDS, and tuberculosis. The tuberculosis rate (cases per 100,000) in 2012 was 15 times higher for Native Hawaiians and Pacific Islanders than for the White population (a case rate of 12.3 vs. 0.8; OMH, 2014).

Women and Men

Of the 159.4 million women living in the United States in 2012, 36.4% were considered overweight or obese, 13.7% had fair or poor health, and 32.8% had hypertension. The leading causes of death included heart disease, cancer, and stroke. Moreover, 16% smoked cigarettes, and only 45.7% followed the physical activity guidelines for aerobic activity through leisure-time aerobic activity (OMH, 2014). The percentage of women ages 18 years or older who had 5 or more drinks in 1 day at least once in the past year was 14.2% (DHHS, 2014b).

Of the 154.5 million men, 12.1% reported fair or poor health, 31.4% had 5 or more drinks in 1 day at least once in the past year, and 21.2% currently smoked cigarettes. The leading causes of death were heart disease, cancer, and accidents (unintentional injuries). Moreover, 35% were overweight or obese, and 31.6% had hypertension. Only 53.6% reported meeting the 2008 federal physical activity guidelines for aerobic activity through leisure-time aerobic activity (OMH, 2014).

Older Adults

Of the 43.1 million residents ages 65 years or older in 2012, 22.7% were in fair or poor health, 8.9% smoked cigarettes, and 28.5% had diabetes. The leading causes of death included heart disease, cancer, and chronic lower respiratory disease. The number of nursing home residents ages 65 years or older was 1.3 million.

A large number of this population was obese: men ages 65 to 74 years, 36.4%; men ages 75 years or older, 27.4%; women ages 65 to 74 years, 44.2%; and women ages 75 years or older, 29.8%. Only about 6.45% needed help with personal care from other people (OMH, 2014).

Reflection 9.2. Specific Population's Health Status

- Select a diverse or minority population in your community or state. Develop a health profile for this group.

Health Behaviors and Risk Factors

Health behaviors and risk factors have a significant effect on health outcomes. *Health behavior* refers to a person's beliefs and actions that affect his or her health and well-being. For example, cigarette smoking increases the risk for lung cancer, heart disease, emphysema, and other respiratory diseases. Heavy and chronic use of alcohol and illicit drugs increases the risk for disease and injury. *Health-related behavior* refers to behavior that affects the health and health behaviors of other people, such as risky driving behaviors that endanger vehicle occupants, or parents who shop for groceries, which affects the health of family members (Simons-Morton, McLeroy, & Wendel, 2012).

Motor vehicle–related deaths are a significant cause of preventable death, accounting for 35,332 deaths in the United States in 2010 across all ages. Motor vehicle–related death rates were higher (47%) for young men and women ages 15 to 24 years than for most other age groups.

In 2012, 20.5% of adult men ages 18 years or older and 15.8% of adult women were current cigarette smokers. Nearly one half (47.4%) of adults ages 20 years or older with hypertension continued to have uncontrolled high blood pressure. Excess body weight in children is associated with excess morbidity in childhood and adulthood. In 2012, 17.7% of children ages 6 to 11 years and 20.5% of adolescents ages 12 to 19 years were obese (NCHS, 2014b).

Reflection 9.3. Healthy Living

Living a healthy life requires having adequate housing; a secure and meaningful livelihood; access to schools, parks, and public spaces; safety and freedom from violence; unpolluted air, soil, and water; and a society that promotes not only opportunity and innovation but also cooperation, trust, and equity.

- How would you define *healthy living?*

Reducing Health Disparities

Health disparity refers to a higher burden of illness, injury, disability, or mortality experienced by one population group relative to another group. It is "a particular type of health difference that is closely linked with social, economic, and/or environmental disadvantage" (DHHS, 2014a, para. 5). Health disparities exist when differences in health outcomes or health determinants are observed among populations.

The burden of illness, premature death, and disability disproportionately affect certain populations. Poor health status, disease risk factors, and limited access to health care are often interrelated and have been reported among people with social, economic, and environmental disadvantages. Race or ethnicity, sexual identity, age, disability, socioeconomic status, and geographic location all contribute to a person's ability to achieve good health.

Several factors often working together contribute to these gaps: organization and operation of health care systems; discrimination, bias, and stereotyping among providers; and uncertainty in clinical communication and decision making (IOM, 2013). *Health care disparity* refers to differences among groups in health insurance coverage, access to and use of care, and quality of care.

Over the past 2 decades, the *Healthy People initiative* has focused on disparities. For 2000, its goal was to reduce health disparities among Americans. For 2010, its goal was to eliminate health disparities, and for 2020, its goal is to achieve health equity, eliminate health disparities, and improve the health of all groups (Healthy People, 2016). Healthy People 2020 has defined *health equity* as the "attainment of the highest level of health for all people" (DHHS, 2014a, para. 4), which requires addressing ongoing historical and contemporary injustices, avoidable inequalities, and the elimination of health and health care disparities (DHHS, 2011).

However, eliminating health disparities is challenging and complex. Multiple factors often are associated with health disparities and are difficult to study independently. The sources of disparities are also complex and involve many participants at several levels. Disparities in health and health care limit continued improvement in overall quality of care and population health and result in unnecessary costs.

Areas of Disparities

Even when income, health insurance, and access to care are accounted for, disparities remain (Henry J. Kaiser Family Foundation, 2016). Low performance on a range of health indicators—such as infant mortality, life expectancy, prevalence of chronic disease, and insurance coverage—reveals differences between racial and ethnic-minority populations and their White counterparts.

Health Outcomes

Vulnerable populations have higher rates of health conditions and experience worse health outcomes. According to the American Public Health Association (APHA, n.d.), Americans of diverse racial and ethnic backgrounds experience higher rates of a variety of diseases and health conditions compared with White Americans:

- Twice as many African American, American Indian, and Alaskan Native babies die before age 1 year as compared with White Americans.
- The death rate from HIV and AIDS among African Americans is more than 7 times than that for White Americans.
- Vietnamese American women have a cervical cancer rate nearly 5 times the rate than that for White Americans.

Women may live longer than men, but they also tend to suffer more disease and disability during their lifetime:

- Depression is twice as common among women as compared with men, and it is predicted to be the leading cause of disability by 2020.
- Women are more likely to experience organic brain syndromes and dementias in old age as compared with men.
- Victims of intimate partner violence are 5 times more likely to be women than men.

The CDC's (2013a) Health Disparities and Inequalities Report highlighted key findings on mortality and morbidity:

- The motor vehicle–related death rate for men was approximately 2.5 times that for women. The rate for American Indians and Alaska Natives was 2–5 times that of other races and ethnicities.

- Rates of blood pressure control among adults with hypertension were lowest among Mexican Americans, people without health insurance, those who were never married, and those born outside the United States.
- The infant mortality rate for non-Hispanic Black women was 1.5–3 times that of non-Hispanic White women. American Indian and Alaska Native infants died from SIDS at nearly 2.5 times the rate of White infants.
- Diabetes prevalence was highest among men, people ages 65 years or older, non-Hispanic Blacks, and those of mixed race, Hispanics, people with less than a high school education, those who were poor, and those with a disability.

African American men are more than twice as likely to die from prostate cancer as Whites, and Hispanic women are more than 1.5 times as likely to be diagnosed with cervical cancer. One of the most striking disparities is the disproportionate burden of AIDS cases among Black men. Disparities also occur in life expectancy and mortality. Although the average life expectancy has increased since 1970, these gains have not been evenly distributed. Black males of all ages have the shortest life expectancy compared with all other groups (Henry J. Kaiser Family Foundation, 2016).

Access to Care

Vulnerable populations face increased barriers to accessing care. In its 2011 report on health care quality and disparities, AHRQ (2014) found that low-income people and people of color experienced more barriers to care and received poorer quality care.

Research showed that people with limited English proficiency were less likely than those who were English proficient to seek care even when insured (Kaiser Commission on Medicaid and the Uninsured, 2012). Research also showed differing patient experiences and levels of satisfaction by race, gender, education levels, and language (Henry J. Kaiser Family Foundation, 2016). In 2010, the uninsured rate for adults ages 18 to 34 years was double the rate for adults ages 45 to 64 years. Colorectal screening increased with age, educational level, and household income (CDC, 2013a).

Environment Hazards

Increased exposure to traffic-related air pollution elevated the risk for adverse health outcomes. In

2010, minorities, foreign-born people, and people who spoke Spanish or another non-English language at home were more likely to be living near major highways. The likelihood of working in a high-risk occupation with elevated injury and illness rate was greatest for Hispanics, low-wage earners, those born outside of the United States, those with only a high school education, and men. Work-related death and homicide rates were highest among non-Hispanic Blacks as well as American Indians and Alaska Natives (CDC, 2013a).

Social Determinants of Health

Americans with lower incomes and educational levels report higher rates of disease, disability, and poor health compared with Americans of higher socioeconomic status. Hispanics, Blacks, American Indians, Alaska Natives, and low-income people are much more likely to be uninsured relative to Whites and those with higher incomes. Low-income people also face increased barriers to accessing care, receive poorer quality care, and ultimately experience worse health outcomes (Henry J. Kaiser Family Foundation, 2016).

Lower household income is directly related to an increased risk for chronic conditions in children. The risk for obesity is significantly greater among people with lower income and education, subsequently increasing the risk for diabetes and heart disease. Chronic diseases can actually cause people to fall into poverty when their ability to earn money is compromised by illness (APHA, n.d.).

Where you live when you are poor also determines your health status. Rural Americans are more likely to have chronic illnesses, such as high blood pressure, heart disease, and diabetes. Suicides caused by gun fatalities are disproportionately higher in rural areas. Many rural Americans lack access to treatment because appropriate transportation is either unavailable or too costly or because health care facilities are too far from home. Moreover, they also are less likely to have a health food retailer nearby (CDC, 2013a; National Rural Health Association, 2013).

No single factor can fully explain the U.S. health disadvantage. According to an IOM (2013) panel, four areas are likely:

1. *Health systems.* The United States has a relatively large uninsured population and more limited access to primary care.

2. *Health behaviors.* Americans consume the most calories per person, have higher rates of drug abuse, are less likely to use seat belts, are involved in more traffic accidents that involve alcohol, and are more likely to use firearms in acts of violence.
3. *Social and economic conditions.* The United States has higher levels of poverty and income inequality and lower rates of social mobility. Other countries outpace the United States in the education of young people.
4. *Physical environments.* The environments of U.S. communities are built and designed around automobiles, which discourages physical activity and contributes to obesity.

The U.S. health disadvantage has multiple causes and involves some combination of inadequate health care, unhealthy behaviors, adverse economic and social conditions, and environmental factors, as well as public policies and social values that shape those conditions.

Health disparities are costly, resulting in added health care costs, lost work productivity, and premature death. Recent analysis estimates that 30% of direct medical costs for Blacks, Hispanics, and Asian Americans are excess costs because of health inequities and that, overall, the economy loses an estimated $309 billion per year to the direct and indirect costs of disparities (CDC, 2013a; Henry J. Kaiser Family Foundation, 2016).

Social Determinants of Health Approach

The *social determinants of health approach* involves comprehensive tactics "to improving health, addressing health inequalities, and accelerating health impact" (Dean, Williams, & Fenton, 2013, p. 1) that involve understanding the interaction among behavioral, clinical, policy, systems, occupational, and environmental determinants of health and using cost-effective strategies to achieve sufficient and sustainable population coverage. Addressing heath disparities has primarily focused on diseases, illness, or health care services. However, data have indicated that residents in mostly minority communities continue to have lower socioeconomic status, greater barriers to health care access, and greater risks for (and burden of) disease compared with the general population living in the same county or state (CDC, 2013a; DHHS, 2014a).

Satcher (2010) postulated incorporating a social determinant of health approach with existing approaches to reduce health disparities. Satcher stated that to achieve good health for all, the approach should be broadened to include

> social and structural conditions such as education, housing, employment, living wages, access to health care, access to healthy foods and green spaces, justice, occupational safety, hopefulness and freedom from racism, classism, sexism, and other forms of exclusion, marginalization, and discrimination based on social status. (p. 6)

Health disparities are also related to inequities in education. Good health is associated with academic success. Health risks such as teenage pregnancy, poor dietary choices, inadequate physical activity, physical and emotional abuse, substance abuse, and gang involvement significantly affect how well students perform in school (CDC, 2013a).

School determinants must be considered when working to eliminate child health disparities. Huang, Cheng, and Theise (2013) suggested that focusing attention on the school contexts as social determinants of child health should be a priority. They found that children who attend poor-quality schools with few health resources, more violence, and distressed school climates are more likely to suffer with physical and mental health issues. Because children spend a considerable amount of time in school, it plays a unique role in shaping children's health knowledge, attitudes, behaviors, and health outcomes.

Social Determinants of Health has been added as one of the overarching goals within Healthy People 2020, focusing on ways to address the social and physical environments that promote health for all. The objectives for this goal are designed to reflect five areas: (1) economic stability, (2) education, (3) social and community context, (4) health and health care, and (5) neighborhood and built environment. It is anticipated that more areas and objectives will be added throughout the decade. Healthy People's underlying assumption is

> All Americans deserve an equal opportunity to make the choices that lead to good health. But to ensure that all Americans have that opportunity, advances are needed not only in health care but also in fields such as education,

childcare, housing, business, law media, community planning, transportation, and agriculture. (Office of Disease Prevention and Health Promotion, 2016, para. 4)

Reflection 9.4. Prevention Agenda

- Discuss possible ways to promote a health prevention agenda that includes social conditions for the nation.

Addressing Health Disparities

Addressing health disparities requires multileveled intervention designs that must be locally relevant and integrated into existing systems to function efficiently (Hardy, Bohan, & Trotter, 2013). Sadana and Blas (2013) stated that explicit political commitment, combined with knowledge, is needed to implement policies that reduce health inequities. The ACA aims to reduce health and health care disparities and improve health and health care for vulnerable populations. It increases federal priorities to address disparities by elevating the National Center for Minority Health and Health Care Disparities to an institute within the National Institutes of Health and by creating Offices of Minority Health within key DHHS agencies to coordinate disparity reduction efforts (Henry J. Kaiser Family Foundation, 2016).

The DHHS (2011) has committed to continuously assessing the impact of all policies and programs on racial and ethnic health disparities and promotes integrated approaches, evidence-based programs, and best practices to reduce these disparities. The Health and Human Services Disparities Action Plan (Koh, Graham, & Glied, 2011) to reduce health disparities among racial and ethnic minorities builds on the ACA and is aligned with programs and initiatives such as Healthy People 2020 (DHHS, 2014a).

OMH (2014) has worked to heighten public awareness through programs and initiatives aimed at reducing health and health care disparities and advancing health equity by disseminating targeted information, executing education campaigns, and holding special observances of ethnic and cultural groups. The National Stakeholder Strategy for Achieving Health Equity (OMH, 2011) provides a common set of goals and objectives as well as ideas, suggestions, and comments from thousands of people and organizations across the country for public- and private-sector initiatives and partnerships to help racial and ethnic minorities and other underserved groups reach their full health potential.

Reflection 9.5. Address a Health Disparity

- Develop a simple project to address one health disparity or health care disparity in your community or state that your class, program, or state association could work toward resolving.

Summary

A disparity is an inequality. Health and health care disparities remain a persistent problem in the United States among some population groups in health outcomes, access to health care, adoption of health promoting behaviors, and exposure to health-promoting environments. Some improvements in overall rates and even reductions in some health disparities are noted; however, many gaps persist. Although health and health care disparities are commonly viewed through the lens of race and ethnicity, they occur across a broad range of dimensions and reflect a complex set of individual, social, and environmental factors.

A social determinants of health approach is important for people of all ages; however, it is critical for children whose early development can improve their health throughout the lifespan. Simply collecting data will not ensure that disparities are eliminated. The future health of the nation will be determined by how well we treat populations that continue to experience a disproportionate burden of disease, disability, injury, and death (CDC, 2013a).

References

Agency for Healthcare Research and Quality. (2010). *Race, ethnicity, and language data: Standardization for health care quality improvement: Improving data collection across the health care system.* Retrieved from http://www.ahrq.gov/research/findings /final-reports/iomracereport/reldata5.html

Agency for Healthcare Research and Quality. (2014, May). *2013 national healthcare disparities report* (AHRQ Publication No. 14-0006). Retrieved from http://www.ahrq.gov/sites/default/files /wysiwyg/research/findings/nhqrdr/nhdr13/2013nhdr.pdf

American Public Health Association. (n.d.). *Health disparities: The basics.* Retrieved from http://www.apha.org/~/media /files/pdf/factsheets/hlthdisparty_primer_final.ashx

Assistant Secretary for Planning and Evaluation. (2011). *U.S. Department of Health and Human Services implementation guidance on data collection standards for race, ethnicity, sex, primary language, and disability status.* Retrieved from https:// aspe.hhs.gov/basic-report/hhs-implementation-guidance -data-collection-standards-race-ethnicity-sex-primary-language -and-disability-status

Centers for Disease Control and Prevention. (2012). *Summary health statistics for U.S. adults: National Health Interview Survey, 2011* [Table 31]. Retrieved from http://www.cdc.gov /nchs/data/series/sr_10/sr10_256.pdf

Centers for Disease Control and Prevention. (2013a). *CDC Health Disparities and Inequalities Report—United States, 2013. MMWR, 62*(3). Retrieved from http://www.cdc.gov/mmwr /pdf/other/su6203.pdf

Centers for Disease Control and Prevention. (2013b). Deaths: Final data for 2010. *National Vital Statistics Reports, 61*(4). Retrieved from http://www.cdc.gov/nchs/data/nvsr/nvsr61 /nvsr61_04.pdf

Centers for Disease Control and Prevention. (2013c). *Health behaviors of adults: United States, 2008–2010* [Table 6.1]. Retrieved from http://www.cdc.gov/nchs/data/series/sr_10 /sr10_257.pdf

Centers for Disease Control and Prevention. (2013d). *Health, United States, 2012* [Table 68]. Retrieved from http://www .cdc.gov/nchs/data/hus/hus12.pdf

Centers for Disease Control and Prevention. (2014). *National Diabetes Statistics Report.* Retrieved from http://www.cdc .gov/diabetes/data/statistics/2014statisticsreport.html

Davis, K., Stremikis, K., Squires, D., & Schoen, C. (2014). Mirror, mirror on the wall, 2014 update: How the U.S. health care system compares internationally. *Commonwealth Fund.* Retrieved from http://www.commonwealthfund.org /publications/fund-reports/2014/jun/mirror-mirror

Dean, H. D., Williams, K. M., & Fenton, K. A. (2013). From theory to action: Applying social determinants of health to public health practice. *Public Health Reports, 128*(Suppl. 3), 1–4. Retrieved from http://www.jstor.org /stable/23646711

Foege, W. (2010). Social determinants of health and health care solutions. *Public Health Reports, 125*(Suppl. 4), 8–10. Retrieved from http://www.ncbi.nlm.nih.gov/pmc/articles /PMC2882969/

Hardy, L. J., Bohan, K. D., & Trotter, R. T. (2013). Synthesizing evidence-based strategies and community-engaged research: A model to address social determinants of health. *Public Health Reports, 128,* 68–76. Retrieved from http://www.publichealth reports.org/issueopen.cfm?articleID=3054

Health Research and Educational Trust. (2013). *Reducing health care disparities: Collection and use of race, ethnicity and language data.* Retrieved from http://www.hpoe.org/resources /hpoehretaha-guides/1431

Health Resources and Services Administration. (2013, April). *Compendium of federal data sources to support health workforce analysis.* Retrieved from http://bhpr.hrsa.gov/healthworkforce /data/compendiumfederaldatasources.pdf

Henry J. Kaiser Family Foundation. (2016). *Key facts on health and health care by race and ethnicity.* Retrieved from http://kff .org/disparities-policy/report/key-facts-on-health-and-health -care-by-race-and-ethnicity/

Huang, K. Y., Cheng, S., & Theise, R. (2013). School contexts as social determinants of child health: Current practices and implications for future public health practice. *Public Health Reports, 128*(Suppl. 3), 21–27. Retrieved from http://www .publichealthreports.org/issueopen.cfm?articleID=3044

Institute of Medicine. (2009). *Race, ethnicity, and language data: Standardization for health care quality improvement.* Washington, DC: National Academies Press.

Institute of Medicine. (2013). *U.S. health in international perspective: Shorter lives, poorer health.* Washington, DC: National Academies Press.

Institute of Medicine. (2014). *Capturing social and behavioral domains in electronic health records: Phase 1.* Washington, DC: National Academies Press.

Kaiser Commission on Medicaid and the Uninsured. (2012, August 1). *Overview of health coverage for individuals with limited English proficiency.* Retrieved from http://www.kff .org/uninsured/8343.cfm

Koh, H. K., Graham, G., & Glied, S. A. (2011). Reducing racial and ethnic disparities: The action plan from the Department of Health and Human Services. *Health Affairs, 30,* 1822–1829. http://dx.doi.org/10.1377/hlthaff.2011.0673

Mainzer, H. M., & Moffett, D. B. (2011). Introduction to healthy people in a healthy environment. *Public Health Reports, 126*(Suppl. 1), 1–2. http://dx.doi.org/10.2307/41639258

Munro, D. (2013, August). America's forgotten civil right— Healthcare. *Forbes.* Retrieved from http://www.forbes.com /sites/danmunro/2013/08/28/americas-forgotten-civil-right -healthcare/#6785c0d36ea0

National Center for Health Statistics. (2014a). *Health statistics: How do we know that?* Hyattsville, MD: Author.

National Center for Health Statistics. (2014b). *Health, United States, 2013: In brief.* Hyattsville, MD: Author.

National Center for Health Statistics. (2014c). *Health, United States, 2013: With special feature on prescription drugs.* Hyattsville, MD: Author.

National Center for Health Statistics. (2015). *Health, United States, 2015: In brief.* Hyattsville, MD: Author.

National Rural Health Association. (2013). *Rural health disparities.* Retrieved from http://www.raconline.org/topics/rural -health-disparities/faqs

Office of Disease Prevention and Health Promotion. (2016). *Disparities.* Washington, DC: U.S. Department of Health and Human Services. Retrieved from http://www.healthypeople .gov/2020/about/foundation-health-measures/Disparities

Office of Management and Budget. (1997). *Race and ethnic standards for federal statistics and administrative reporting* (Statistical Policy Directive No. 15, rev.). Washington, DC: Author.

Office of Minority Health. (2011, April). *National partnership for action to end health disparities: National stakeholder strategy for achieving health equity.* Rockville, MD: U.S. Department of Health and Human Services.

Office of Minority Health. (2014). *Minority population profiles.* Retrieved from http://minorityhealth.hhs.gov/omh/browse .aspx?lvl=2&lvlid=26

Patient Protection and Affordable Care Act, Pub. L. 111–148, 42 U.S.C. §§ 18001-18121 (2010).

Sadana, R., & Blas, E. (2013). What can public health programs do to improve health equity? *Public Health Reports, 128*(Suppl. 3), 12–20. Retrieved from http://www.public healthreports.org/issueopen.cfm?articleID=3042

Satcher, D. (2010). Include a social determinants of health approach to reduce health inequities. *Public Health Reports, 125*(Suppl. 4), 6–7. Retrieved from http://www.publichealth reports.org/archives/issueopen.cfm?articleID=2476

Simons-Morton, B., McLeroy, K. R., & Wendel, M. L. (2012). *Behavior theory in health promotion practice and research.* Burlington, MA: Jones & Bartlett.

United Health Foundation. (2013). *America's health rankings: A call to action for individuals and their communities—2013 edition.* Retrieved from http://cdnfiles.americashealthrankings .org/SiteFiles/AnnualDownloads/AnnualReport2013-r.pdf

U.S. Department of Health and Human Services. (2011). *HHS action plan to reduce racial and ethnic disparities: A nation free of disparities in health and health care.* Washington, DC: Author.

U.S. Department of Health and Human Services. (2014a). *Disparities.* Retrieved from http://www.healthypeople.gov/2020 /about/disparitiesAbout.aspx

U.S. Department of Health and Human Services. (2014b). *Women's health and mortality chartbook: 2014 edition.* Washington, DC: Author.

U.S. Department of Health and Human Services. (2015). *About the law.* Retrieved from http://www.hhs.gov/healthcare/rights /index.html

Weissman, J. S., & Hasnain-Wynia, R. (2011). Advancing health care equity through improved data collection. *New England Journal of Medicine, 364,* 2276–2277. http://dx.doi.org /10.1056/NEJMp1103069

Chapter 10.

EXPLORING CULTURAL KNOWLEDGE

Shirley A. Wells, DrPH, OTR, FAOTA

> *Knowledge provides people with materials for reflection and premises for action,*
> *whereas culture also embraces those reflections and those actions.*
> **Fredrik Barth (2002, p. 1)**

Chapter Highlights

- Defining *Knowledge*
- Cultural Knowledge
- Micro- and Macrolevel Knowledge
- Seeking and Acquiring Knowledge

Key Terms and Concepts

✧ Cultural knowledge
✧ Culture general
✧ Culture specific
✧ Deep understanding
✧ Experiential learning
✧ Immersion learning
✧ Knowledge

✧ Macrolevel knowledge
✧ Microlevel knowledge
✧ Middle understanding
✧ Reflection
✧ Reflective writing
✧ Surface understanding

Although cultural sensitivity and awareness are important aspects of providing effective care, cultural knowledge can improve the capacity for culturally effective services. Given the changes in health reform with the Patient Protection and Affordable Care Act (Pub. L. 111–148), combined with the increasing proportion of diversity among the U.S. population, it is critical for health care providers to update their cultural knowledge.

To effectively respond to the needs of the diverse populations they serve, health care providers need to understand and appreciate the cultural differences among different populations and integrate this knowledge into their delivery of patient care. More shared knowledge leads to fewer misunderstandings. In this chapter, I discuss knowledge parameters to foster effectiveness when working with people from different cultures.

Defining *Knowledge*

Knowledge is information, understanding, or skill that you get from experience or education—the awareness of something (Merriam-Webster, n.d.). It provides people with materials for reflection and a premise for action. Knowledge includes feelings, attitudes, information, skills, as well as verbal taxonomies and concepts (Barth, 2002, as cited in Koch, 2009). It encompasses all different ways of understanding that people use to create reality, giving them the capacity to understand the world and give purpose to their actions (Koch, 2009).

Cultural Knowledge

Knowledge varies widely within populations, depending upon spatial, social, and cohort experiences. Knowledge is distributed in population, whereas culture is understood in terms of sharing (Dube & Ngulube, 2012). Culture itself is a shared set of assumptions, values, and norms for a group of people that helps them prioritize what they are going to do and how they are going to get things done. Thus, *cultural knowledge* is sharing information within a population or group of people.

Cultural knowledge is the framework and process in which a health care provider obtains a sound educational base about culturally diverse groups (Campinha-Bacote, 2007). It allows the provider to look at interaction from several perspectives, including the culture in which the interaction occurs, cultures of the people involved, and the culture of the society or system.

Cultural knowledge includes specific knowledge about different cultures and general knowledge about how cultures work (Maznevski, 2008). It involves the core domains of a culture, such as family and kinships, religion and spirituality, time and space, gender, politics, history, language, and economics, all of which are mostly shared and dynamic, changing over time.

Cultural knowledge is a multilevel concept that includes

- *Surface understanding* of culture (i.e., outward behaviors),
- *Middle understanding* (i.e., physical, social, symbolic worlds), and
- *Deep understanding* (i.e., beliefs, values, assumptions; Watson, 2010).

The most comprehensive list of basic cultural knowledge comes from McPhatter (1997), who identified the following as a "grounded knowledge base" necessary for cultural effectiveness:

- Knowledge of the history, culture, traditions and customs, preferred language or primary dialect, value orientation, religious and spiritual orientations, art, music, and folk or other healing beliefs of clients;
- Intimate familiarity with social problems and issues and how they affect a minority group;
- Knowledge of a client's neighborhoods and communities and how they influence their life;
- Strong understanding of the dynamics of oppression, racism, sexism, classism, heterosexism, and other forms of discrimination;
- Knowledge of health and social systems and their effect on disadvantaged groups;
- Awareness of the diversity of family structures; and
- Knowledge of culturally relevant interventions used within the professional structure (pp. 266–270).

Cultural knowledge embodies purposeful practice by facilitating the ability to quickly and accurately comprehend and then appropriately and effectively act.

Reflection 10.1. Unwritten Cultural Rules

People all over the world drink coffee. Some of the unwritten etiquette rules in a coffee shop include (a) stand in line with space between people, (b) use eye contact when ordering, (c) choose a place to sit, and (d) wait for the product.

- Go to a local coffee shop. Observe and uncover the unwritten cultural rules for ordering coffee in your community.
- Are these similar or different from what you have seen in another culture, community, or town?

Micro- and Macrolevel Knowledge

One way to examine cultural knowledge is to organize it into microlevel knowledge and macrolevel knowledge. According to Waite and Calamaro (2010), who completed a study of nursing curriculum on cultural content, *microlevel knowledge* focuses on characteristics, shaped by personal experiences and values, and their training. It is the person's culture, traditions, customs, language, values, beliefs, expectations, preferences, and needs. *Macrolevel knowledge* focuses on information about groups, families, communities, organizations, and the natural environment. It entails understanding the effect that the physical social, economic, and cultural environments have on health care organizations and academic institutions as well as providers delivering care.

In McPhatter's (1997) concentric circles, microlevel knowledge is closest to the person, including his or her culture's characteristics. Moving outward from the client, toward macrolevel knowledge, the awareness of diversity of family structure is found next. The next ring of knowledge incorporates awareness of the client's communities and neighborhoods as well as other external contextual factors (see Figure 10.1).

At the macrolevel, knowledge is more societal than personal, but it involves all people, such as familiarity of social problems and issues that affect minorities, understanding of the dynamics in all forms of oppression, knowledge of health and social systems and their effect on disadvantaged groups, and understanding health disparities.

Having at least a beginning knowledge from these categories leads to knowledge of culturally relevant

interventions. Understanding that there are levels of knowledge may lessen a person's sense of confusion about others and provide some direction in helping plan for cultural effectiveness development. Knowing what one needs to learn, however, does not explain how, where, and when one learns it. The following section explores these options.

Seeking and Acquiring Knowledge

Students already may have gained much of the microlevel and some macrolevel knowledge in undergraduate and graduate coursework. Formal and informal education, coupled with cross-cultural experiences, are important avenues for learning. Current evidence suggests a variety of roads to obtaining cultural knowledge.

Waite and Calamaro (2010) found that knowledge exchange should take place in the classroom setting followed by the clinical setting. The process of knowledge exchange and knowledge development should include interaction between educator and student:

- Preceptor: student → student: patient → *culturally effective outcome*

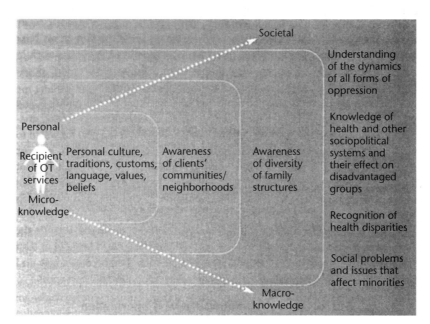

Figure 10.1. Levels of knowledge necessary to deliver culturally relevant occupational therapy (OT) interventions.

- Preceptor: student → preceptor: patient → *culturally effective outcome*
- Preceptor: student → student: practice (Waite & Calamaro, 2010, p. 78).

To achieve culturally effective outcomes, the exchange of knowledge flows from the experienced to the inexperienced and from a structured environment to the clinical setting. Without implementing critical and purposeful teaching strategies, opportunities to develop culturally effective professionals are hindered. In a study among pharmacy students, Okoro, Odedina, Reams, and Smith (2012) found that speaking a language other than English and having exposure to cultural competency instruction with demographic variables were found to be most significantly associated with clinical knowledge of health disparities. Relevant education and training outside the school curriculum potentially improved cultural knowledge of health disparities.

However, the classroom can foster cultural knowledge. In a study exploring the understanding of undergraduate community health students' perceptions of their cultural competencies, Kratzke and Bertolo (2013) found that engaging students firsthand with a new cultural group in a class simulation exercise was essential to enhance their cultural knowledge. An experiential learning exercise was conducted with the cross-cultural BaFá BaFá classroom simulation exercise. The students also received a lecture before the class exercise on topics such as cultural awareness and cultural competencies, reflective writing, and cultural research. The students were assigned to alpha and beta groups with cultural values and expected norms. Each student participated as a visitor to the other group and returned to share his or her observation. The findings showed that having cultural knowledge before interacting with a new group is an essential experience to building skills to work successfully with diverse groups.

According to Waite, Nardi, and Killian (2013), the most beneficial resources for cultural effectiveness ranged from ongoing in-services, online cultural competency workshops, ethnic-specific health educators and consultation, diverse staff, and books. Classroom settings, cultural immersion programs, and provision of in-service to practitioners within the health system setting have also been identified in the literature as effective strategies for developing culturally efficient and effective care (Betancourt & Green, 2010; Larsen & Reif, 2011; Pirkey, Levey, Newberry, Guthman, & Hansen, 2012).

Reflection 10.2. Community Offerings

Learn about your community offerings on culture and diversity. Contact your local library, city hall, museum, church, and so forth to determine what cultural offerings are available.

- Choose one and visit or participate with a friend. Write a journal entry about what this experience was like.
- What did you learn?
- How did you feel?
- With whom did you interact?
- Did it spark your interest?
- Do you want to learn more?

Written Resources

Researching written resources may be the most familiar and, in some ways, easiest approach to learning about other cultures. Many books and resources within the different health care fields describe characteristics of various cultural groups and their effect on health and wellness. Such resources are a good place to begin gaining foundational information, but remember that not all people from the same cultural group share all or any of highlighted characteristics. When written sources alone are used, practitioners must take special care to avoid stereotyping, which would be a disservice to clients (Núñez, 2000).

Other written resources include ethnographies, biographies, or written documentaries. Training manuals, workbooks, and reports from health care organizations provide information about culturally effective approaches for working with diverse groups. Depending on the publishing organization and its focus, these resources may be ***culture general*** (i.e., information that can be used with multiple cultural groups) or ***culture specific*** (i.e., information about one particular group), but all of these resources provide additional, important information about working with diverse populations in a health care arena.

Professional journal articles often contain a plethora of information about cultural groups and competencies from other health professions, such as nursing, social work, and clinical psychology. More information about cultural groups now appears in occupational therapy literature as well. Making time to read some of these resources not only increases cultural knowledge but also establishes a beginning framework of how these concepts are being explored in the profession.

Electronic Resources

Although some Internet sources for cultural knowledge are questionable, online research is a fast and reasonably reliable approach to research. Online research should not be the only approach to learning about different cultures; however, information retrieved through Google Scholar or other online full-text articles and chapters often can be very useful. In addition, both federal and state governments, as well as health organizations and research institutes, offer informative online resources, such as the following websites:

- *U.S. Department of Health and Human Services, Office of Minority Health:* http://minorityhealth .hhs.gov/. This website is a repository of information on health disparity issues specific to African Americans, American Indians and Alaska Natives, Asian Americans, Hispanics, as well as Native Hawaiians and Pacific Islanders.
- *Alaska Native Knowledge Network:* http://ankn.uaf .edu/. This website contains resources related to Native American knowledge systems and ways of knowing and the indigenous languages of the Native people of Alaska.
- *USA.gov:* http://www.usa.gov/. This website provides data about the United States, such as maps and population, demographics, and economic data, as well as resources on other government websites related to cultural and ethnic groups.
- *Centers for Disease Control and Prevention, Office of Minority Health and Health Equity:* http://www .cdc.gov/minorityhealth/. This website monitors and reports on the health status of vulnerable populations and the effectiveness of health programs for these populations.
- *The Henry J. Kaiser Family Foundation (Minority Health):* http://kff.org/state-category/minority -health/. This website contains demographic data on minority populations, medical school graduates, and women's and men's health disparities.
- *U.S. Department of Health and Human Services, Office on Women's Health (Minority Women's Health):* http://www.womenshealth.gov/minority -health/. This website looks at health problems facing specific minority groups and provides links to more in-depth information.

Community Resources and Activities

Many cities and towns celebrate their diversity through art exhibits, festivals, and educational offerings. Taking advantage of these offerings can facilitate learning, often in a personal—and fun—manner. Attending the festivals, smelling delicious foods from various cultures, watching and listening to people interact, enjoying multiple presentations, talking with people, and observing or joining in dancing provides an opportunity to participate in the richness of other cultures in a direct manner.

Eating in ethnic restaurants and conversing with the wait staff is another way to experience different cultures. Local museums highlight various local cultures, as do churches, synagogues, or temples. Although this information may seem commonplace, many people do not take advantage of the resources around them to learn about their culturally different neighbors—visiting these resources can help to develop cultural effectiveness.

Reflection 10.3. Community Makeup

- Describe the makeup and history of your community to provide a context within which to collect data on its current concerns. Describe what matters to people in your community.
- Comment on the types of information that best describe the community (e.g., demographics, history, political climate, civic participation, key leaders, past concerns, geographics, assets).
- Describe the sources of information used (e.g., public records, local people, Internet, maps, phone book, library, newspaper).
- Describe the issues that people in your community care about (e.g., safety, education, housing, health).
- How important are these issues (e.g., perceived importance, consequences for the community)?
- Describe how you collected information and who you listen to in the community.

Conferences and Workshops

Another effective way to gather knowledge is to attend conferences or workshops on culture and diversity. The American Occupational Therapy Association, state occupational therapy associations, other professional organizations, local colleges and universities, places of employment, and local communities all offer such events.

Experiential and Immersion Activities

Experiential learning (i.e., involves actions, movements, and activities) and *immersion learning* (i.e., extensive exposure and involvement) involve activities designed for engagement using experimentation, reflection, thinking, and exercises and represent key nontraditional teaching and learning approaches (Cathcart, Greenspan, & Quin, 2010; Jordi, 2011). The successful use of experiential learning in academic preparation for health professions is supported in the literature (Bonder & Martin, 2013; Kratzke & Bertolo, 2013; Murden et al., 2008; Sharma, LaLinde, & Brosco, 2006). Personal experiences are transformed for learning (Lisko & O'Dell, 2010; Vanlaere, Coucke, & Gastmans, 2010).

Face-to-face interaction with culturally diverse people may be the most exciting and transformative for learners. Waite et al. (2013) suggested that translating simulation experiences and lessons learned into community health settings broadened students' understanding of cultural differences. Such learning may help to develop cross-cultural knowledge and skills needed in the cultural competence learning process.

Reflection

Through the process of *reflection,* a student or practitioner can explore his or her own perspective and integration of cultural knowledge (Núñez, 2000) by examining, comparing, and contrasting (1) his or her culture with the culture of others and (2) his or her assumptions, judgments, and biases about his or her culture and the culture of others. For example, how would you explain finding an apartment to someone trying to orient to U.S. culture? Reflection allows reordering or reworking cultural knowledge, values, and beliefs. The habit of critical reflection is vital for health professionals working with diverse populations.

Reflective writing, which is a written response to new information, can serve to facilitate dialogue with others. It helps people recognize the connections between what they already know and have experienced and what they are in the process of learning. Reflection assists individuals in becoming active and aware of the learning process, focusing not only on what they have learned but also on how they learned it (Branch & Paranjape, 2002). It is an opportunity to gain self-knowledge and to achieve clarity of understanding of the cultural information.

Summary

Cultural knowledge concerns how social groups and identities within a culture relate to and interact with each other. Such knowledge allows practitioners to understand the motivations, social constraints, and traditions of interaction within a culture (Watson, 2010).

Knowledge about the differences in disease presentation by gender, race, ethnicity, and circumstance is essential in providing adequate and effective health care. It can be acquired through formal or informal means. Literature indicates that of the many ways to learn about a person's culture, the most transformative method is through direct contact with people over time. Reflective writing enables a positive impact on cultural intelligence.

References

Barth, F. (2002). An anthropology of knowledge. *Current Anthropology, 43,* 1–18. http://dx.doi.org/10.1086/324131

Betancourt, J. R., & Green, A. R. (2010). Linking cultural competence training to improved health outcomes: Perspectives from the field [Commentary]. *Academic Medicine, 85,* 583–585. http://dx.doi.org/10.1097/ACM.0b013e3181d2b2f3

Bonder, B., & Martin, L. (2013). *Culture in clinical care: Strategies for competence* (2nd ed.). Thorofare, NJ: Slack.

Branch, W. T., & Paranjape, A. (2002). Feedback and reflection: Teaching methods for clinical settings. *Academic Medicine, 77*(12), 1185–1188. Retrieved from http://uthscsa.edu/gme/documents/FeedbackandReflection.pdf

Campinha-Bacote, J. (2007). *The process of cultural competence in the delivery of healthcare services: The journey continues* (5th ed.). Cincinnati: Transcultural C.A.R.E. Associates.

Cathcart, E., Greenspan, M., & Quin, M. (2010). The making of a nurse manager: The role of experiential learning in leadership development. *Journal of Nursing Management, 18,* 440–444. http://dx.doi.org/10.1111/j.1365-2834.2010.01082.x

Dube, L., & Ngulube, P. (2012). Knowledge sharing in a multicultural environment: Challenges and opportunities. *South African Journal of Libraries and Information Science, 78,* 68–77. http://dx.doi.org/10.7553/78-1-48

Jordi, R. (2011). Reframing the concept of reflection: Consciousness, experiential learning, and reflective learning practices. *Adult Education Quarterly, 61,* 181–197. http://dx.doi.org/10.1177/0741713610380439

Merriam-Webster. (n.d.). *Knowledge.* Retrieved from http://www .merriam-webster.com/dictionary/knowledge

Koch, G. (2009). Intercultural communication and competence research through the lens of an anthropology of knowledge. *Forum: Qualitative Social Research, 10*(1), 15. Retrieved from http://nbn-resolving.de/urn:nbn:de:0114-fqs0901153

Kratzke, C., & Bertolo, M. (2013). Enhancing students' cultural competence using cross-cultural experiential learning. *Journal of Cultural Diversity, 20,* 107–111.

Larsen, R., & Reif, L. (2011). Effectiveness of cultural immersion and culture classes for enhancing nursing students' transcultural self-efficacy. *Journal of Nursing Education, 50,* 350–354. http://dx.doi.org/10.3928/01484834-20110214-04

Lisko, S., & O'Dell, V. (2010). Integration of theory and practice: Experiential learning theory and nursing education. *Nursing Education Perspectives, 31,* 106–108.

Maznevski, M. (2008, October). *How cultural intelligence can improve performance: Adapting abroad while being yourself.* Retrieved from http://www.imd.org/research/challenges/TC081 -08.cfm

McPhatter, A. R. (1997). Cultural competence in child welfare: What is it? How do we achieve it? What happens without it? *Child Welfare, 76,* 255–278.

Murden, R., Norman, A., Ross, J., Sturdivant, E., Kedia, M., & Shah, S. (2008). Occupational therapy students' perceptions of their cultural awareness and competency. *Occupational Therapy International, 15,* 191–203. http://dx.doi .org/10.1002/oti.253

Núñez, A. E. (2000). Transforming cultural competence into cross-cultural efficacy in women's health education. *Academic Medicine, 75,* 1071–1079. Retrieved from http://journals.lww .com/academicmedicine/Fulltext/2000/11000/Transforming _Cultural_Competence_into.11.aspx

Okoro, O. N., Odedina, F. T., Reams, R. R., & Smith, W. T. (2012). Clinical cultural competency and knowledge of health disparities among pharmacy students. *American Journal of Pharmaceutical Education, 76*(3), 40. http://dx.doi.org /10.5688/ajpe76340

Patient Protection and Affordable Care Act, Pub. L. 111–148, 42 U.S.C. §§ 18001-18121 (2010).

Pirkey, J. M., Levey, J. A., Newberry, S. M., Guthman, P. L., & Hansen, J. M. (2012). Videoconferencing expands nursing students' cultural realm. *Journal of Nursing Education, 51,* 586–590. http://dx.doi.org/10.3928/01484834-20120823-01

Sharma, N. J., LaLinde, P. S., & Brosco, J. P. (2006). What do residents learn by meeting with families of children with disabilities? A qualitative analysis of an experiential learning module. *Pediatric Rehabilitation, 9*(3), 185–189. http://dx.doi .org/10.1080/13638490600570606

Vanlaere, L., Coucke, T., & Gastmans, C. (2010). Experiential learning of empathy in a care-ethics lab. *Nurse Ethics, 17,* 325–336. http://dx.doi.org/10.1177/0969733010361440

Waite, R., & Calamaro, C. J. (2010). Cultural competence: A systemic challenge to nursing education, knowledge exchange, and the knowledge development process. *Perspectives in Psychiatric Care, 46,* 74–79. http://dx.doi.org/10.1111/j.1744 -6163.2009.00240.x

Waite, R., Nardi, D., & Killian, P. (2013). Examination of cultural knowledge and provider sensitivity in nurse managed health centers. *Journal of Cultural Diversity, 21,* 74–79. Retrieved from https://www.researchgate.net/publication/263861568 _Examination_of_cultural_knowledge_and_provider_sensiti vity_in_nurse_managed_health_centers

Watson, J. R. (2010, March–April). Language and culture training: Separate paths? *Military Review,* 93–97. Retrieved from http://www.dtic.mil/dtic/tr/fulltext/u2/a518175.pdf

Section II.C.

CROSS-CULTURAL SKILLS

Chapter 11.

DEVELOPING CROSS-CULTURAL COMMUNICATION SKILLS

Roxie M. Black, PhD, OTR/L, FAOTA

Health care professionals should understand the effect that different language and non-verbal communication patterns, explanatory models of disease, and contextual factors may have on the expectations of patients and their perceptions of the behavior of [providers]. An appreciation of cultural practices and possible ways to incorporate them into ... treatment can further enhance health care delivery.
Lois M. Nora, Steven R. Daugherty, A. Mattis-Peterson, Linda Stevenson, & L. J. Goodman (1994, pp. 146–147)

Chapter Highlights

- Power of Language
- Communication Skills
- Cross-Cultural Interviewing
- Choosing Effective Cultural Evaluations
- Skillful Attitudes and Active Engagement

Key Terms

- ✧ Attitudes
- ✧ Biased language
- ✧ Cautious willingness
- ✧ Committed willingness
- ✧ Cultural broker
- ✧ Health literacy
- ✧ Inclusive language
- ✧ Interpretation

- ✧ Interviewing
- ✧ Nonverbal communication
- ✧ Personal space
- ✧ Professional jargon
- ✧ Translators
- ✧ Unreflective willingness
- ✧ Volition

One of the main differences between cultural competence and cultural effectiveness compared to cultural sensitivity and cultural tolerance is that the former concepts include the important aspect of skillful action while the latter two pertain only to the affective domain. One must *do* something to be culturally effective: *interact* with people who differ from oneself. In much of the literature on cultural competence, the key characteristic is effective cross-cultural communication skills (Teal & Street, 2008)—being aware of the power of language, having interviewing skills, working with an interpreter (Rosen et al., 2004), offering culturally sensitive and appropriate assessments, and developing the right attitude.

Power of Language

It has been said that whoever does the naming has the power (Wolf, 1982) and that naming links to the exercise of power (King, 1990). Wolf stated that

> Control of communication allows the managers of ideology to lay down the categories through which reality is to be perceived. Conversely, this entails the ability to deny the existence of alternative categories to assign them to the realm of disorder and chaos, to render them socially and symbolically invisible. (p. 386)

Historically in the United States, the "naming" has been done by those who have been dominant and those in powerful positions who have been given the right and "ability to bestow meanings" (Wolf, 1982, p. 386). Nondominant people must abide by the language, discourse, rules, and regulations developed by White western society.

The words one chooses to use hold sociocultural and personal meaning for both the user and the person addressed. Tanno (1997) stated that words and labels convey volumes about assumptions and perceptions. Many words portray bias and prejudicial thoughts, serving to demean and maintain people in oppressed positions. Herbst (1997) identifies more than 850 ethnic and racial terms and expressions that indicate bias in today's U.S. society, all of which "will—in one of their senses, in some ways or context—restrict, misrepresent, or distort how people are known" (p. ix).

Every American grows up knowing, hearing, and sometimes using some of the words identified by Herbst. Although people may not mean to be prejudiced or to show bias toward someone from another group, it is difficult not to make verbal mistakes when raised in a country and society that harbors racism, sexism, homophobia, and other *isms*.

Sometimes slurs are intentionally spoken, but often people use biased language without being aware of the hurt it causes, mainly because much of this language has become part of the accepted vernacular of the dominant discourse. Biased language is that which consciously or unconsciously displays prejudicial views through its words or content. How many of us have referred to older women as "cute little old ladies" without considering that this language diminishes these women and negates the wisdom and experience that are the result of many years of life? Occupational therapy practitioners must be aware of the language they use and how it affect others.

Reflection 11.1. Ethnic Jokes and Slurs

- Have you ever heard an ethnic joke or slur?
- What was your response to it?
- Was the joke or slur against your culture or another's?
- Consider whether this kind of interaction is hurtful. If you believe it is, what can you do to limit or stop this kind of interaction?

Communication Skills

Communication skills incorporate acquiring as well as mastering strategies, techniques, and approaches for communicating and interacting with people from different cultures. These techniques include greetings, asking questions and responding, inclusive language, reducing professional jargon, working effectively with translators and interpreters, being aware of nonverbal communication, and effective cross-cultural interviewing.

Greetings

Learning the appropriate greeting for a person is important in establishing rapport with someone who is culturally different from oneself (see Figure 11.1). For example, a traditional Somali man generally will not shake hands or otherwise touch a female who is not a member of his family. I have learned to ask first whether hand shaking is accepted or not when meeting or being introduced to a man from

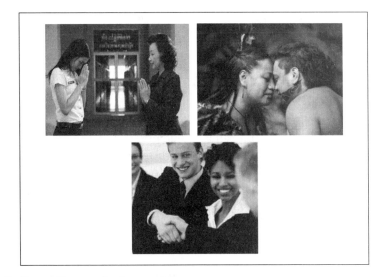

Figure 11.1.   Culturally varied greetings.
Source. Thetaxhaven, ©2007, http://bit.ly/2dSH0Bf. Used with permission via Creative Commons.

Somalia. Because a greeting is often one's first introduction to someone as well as the first impression, using an incorrect, inappropriate, or insensitive approach may negatively affect any interaction that follows with that person.

Reflection 11.2. Greetings

- What ethnic groups live in your community?
- Are you aware of the traditional greetings of these groups?
- Where would you look for that information?
- Once you have the information, plan to practice it by greeting diverse people by their preferred greeting. What kind of response did you get from them?

Asking Questions and Responding

Another communication skill is *learning how to* ask questions of and responding *appropriately to* someone from a different culture (see Figure 11.2). For many people, asking direct questions is perceived as offensive and rude, yet it is expected in the U.S. biomedical approach to patient assessment. Through observation and research, learning the style with which a practitioner can gather information without offending the client or patient is an important skill for effective cross-cultural communication.

For example, during a student trip to China, I experienced the Chinese method of (non)response to a direct question. The Chinese nurses tended to change the subject or generalize about the topic rather than

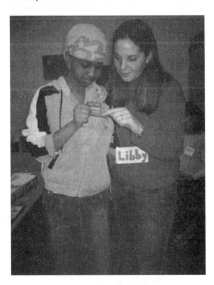

Figure 11.2.   Occupational therapy student responding to a Somali girl's question.
Source. Copyright Roxie M. Black. Used with permission.

answering the question of when the director of the orphanage would be there. Although this kind of response was frustrating to this born-and-bred New Englander who tends to be quite direct, I realized that my frustration or repeated questions were not giving me what I wanted, and finally relaxed and just tried to enjoy the hosts and the setting.

Inclusive Language

Another intentional strategy is to use *inclusive language,* which avoids the use of certain expressions or words that might be considered to exclude particular groups of people. Without reading clients' charts, which may or may not include this information, or having spoken with them earlier, the practitioner will not know the person's sexual or gender orientation. Because we live in a strongly heterosexual society, many practitioners do not consider the sexual identity of the client and will tend to ask about marriage, husbands or wives, or spouses. Getting in the habit of using the terms "partner" or "significant other" will alleviate this cultural mistake, which leaves the homosexual or transgender client feeling alienated or unaccepted.

Professional Jargon

Limiting or omitting professional jargon can facilitate communication with clients. Although the specialized language occupational therapy practitioners, educators, scientists, and researchers use is not intended to diminish or oppress others or to be biased, it separates clients from practitioners and threatens health literacy.

Creating Distance

Some believe that jargon and medical abbreviations not only separate health professionals from their clients but also constitute "an artificial means of defining staff status levels with the profession—from consultant to auxiliary" (Leitch, 1992, p. 50). Hammond (1993) states that the jargon physicians use "transforms common-sense medicine into a cosy, (sic) elite world that is impenetrable to all but the ever-so-clever" (p. 26).

Using the private language of occupational therapy with clients and families may intimidate and silence them, so it is imperative that occupational therapy practitioners communicate with their diverse clients clearly and at the level of language that they understand.

Health Literacy

Many clients, including those who are English speaking, have very poor or limited health literacy skills (Al-Tayyib, Rogers, Gribble, Villarroel, & Turner, 2002; Paasche-Orlow, Parker, Gazmararian, Nielsen, & Rudd, 2005). **Health literacy** is "the degree to which individuals have the capacity to obtain, process, and understand basic health information and services needed to make appropriate health decisions" (Ratzan & Parker, 2004, p. 4).

Research shows correlation between limited health literacy and nondominant groups such as African Americans (Osborn, Paasche-Orlow, Davis, & Wolf, 2007), as well as Hispanic, Native Americans, and adults over the age of 65 (Kutner, Greenberg, Jin, & Paulsen, 2006). Speaking in occupational therapy jargon rarely allows practitioners to communicate well with their clients; rather, it subtly reminds clients that the professionals are part of the dominant group—the authorities, the ones with the knowledge—whereas clients and families are the *other*—the recipients of services and knowledge, the disempowered ones.

Working With Translators and Interpreters

Non-English-speaking persons or people with limited English proficiency with whom occupational therapists work can provide a challenge to effective communication and practice. In a review of Canadian literature, Bowen (2004) concluded that "patients who do not speak an official language often do not receive the same standard of ethical care as other[s]" (as cited in Srivastava, 2007, p. 126).

For example, when I did a site visit with a student who was engaged in a fieldwork experience in a rehabilitation center, an elderly Chinese man who spoke no English and had suffered a cerebrovascular accident was brought into the rehab gym for occupational therapy intervention. No one on staff spoke Mandarin, and he had no English-speaking family with him during that session. Still, this gentleman was warm and friendly, smiling and bobbing his head up and down to signal acquiescence, and it was apparent that the therapists enjoyed working with him while using many gestures and touch to show him what they wanted him to do.

However, I noticed their tone of voice, which often sounded patronizing and infantilizing when speaking with him, and the conversation between the therapists who talked of how "sweet" the patient was and carried out a somewhat inappropriate conversation about him to another staff member in the gym because the patient did not understand what they were saying. The client was not well served by the well-meaning practitioners who inadvertently treated him with limited respect, seemingly due to a lack of understanding of another's language.

If no one on the health care team speaks the client's language, it may be necessary to find a translator, interpreter, or cultural broker to facilitate cross-cultural interactions. Language assistance may include the use of translators, interpreters, or cultural brokers.

Translators, Interpretation, and Cultural Brokers

Translators are generally used to translate a written document, such as an evaluation tool, word for word from one language to another (Su & Parham, 2002), while **interpretation** "involves the spoken word and refers to the process of mediating a verbal interaction between people who speak two different languages" (Srivastava, 2007, p. 128). Interpreters not only translate words but also decode them and "provide the meaning behind the message" (Leavitt, 2010, p. 183).

However, "simply sharing a common language does not necessarily imply sharing of other cultural factors" (Bonder & Martin, 2013, p. 177). It is best if the linguistic expert also understands the health care system and culture. A **cultural broker** is someone who not only speaks both English and the patient's language but also understands the two cultures (including the health care culture) well enough to educate and guide both participants. Bonder and Martin (2013) describe this person as "someone who serves go-between functions for cultural groups that are coming into contact, and they often play peripheral, yet essential roles" (p. 176), including translation services and interacting as a bridge between divergent views of medicine (Bonder & Martin).

Culturally and Linguistically Appropriate Services

The use of linguistic assistants is required by law for health care organizations. The National Standards for Culturally and Linguistically Appropriate Services (CLAS) in Health Care, from the U.S. Department of Health and Human Services (DHHS), Office of Minority Health (2001), address the use of interpreters with patients or consumers with limited English proficiency (Exhibit 11.1).

The standards listed in Exhibit 11.1 (as well as Standard 7) are mandated by law for all recipients of federal funds.

Barriers When Working With Linguist Assistants

Although requirements for linguist assistants are clearly outlined above, skillful use of interpreters or cultural brokers can be problematic. Health care providers may underestimate the need for an interpreter (Srivastava, 2007) because of the following factors:

- Overconfidence in interpretation of nonverbal behavior,
- False fluency, which is the overestimation of one's ability to understand and speak a second language on the part of the provider or client, and
- Perception by the provider that working with interpreters takes too long, is too expensive, or seen as potentially problematic in areas of accuracy and confidentiality (Srivastava, 2007, pp. 129–130).

Another issue with the use of interpreters is the high incidence of medical errors. Flores et al. (2003 as cited in Leavitt, 2010) found an average of 31 errors per clinical encounter, especially with the use of ad hoc interpreters such as family, friends, and community volunteers, who may be helpful in translating factual, nonsensitive data such as name, age, and phone numbers but who may be overwhelmed with the complexity of the health care situation or the interpersonal dynamics with the patient (DHHS, 2001; Leavitt, 2010; Srivastava, 2007). To provide effective care for clients with limited English proficiency, a practitioner who works with culturally diverse clients must be well-versed in the function of linguist assistants and skilled in helping to choose the correct person for each encounter.

Exhibit 11.1. CLAS Standards: Language Access Services

Standard 4. Health care organizations must offer and provide language assistance services, including bilingual staff and interpreter services, at no cost to each patient/consumer with limited English proficiency at all points of contact, in a timely manner during all hours of operation.

Standard 5. Health care organizations must provide to patients/consumers in their preferred language both verbal offers and written notices informing them of their right to receive language assistance services.

Standard 6. Health care organizations must assure the competence of language assistance provided to limited English proficient patients/consumers by interpreters and bilingual staff. Family and friends should not be used to provide interpretation services (except on request by the patient/consumer).

Source. Section from National Standards for Culturally and Linguistically Appropriate Services (CLAS) in Health Care, U.S. Department of Health and Human Services, Office of Minority Health (2001).

Nonverbal Communication

Using nonverbal communication facilitates culturally effective practice (Lynch & Hanson, 1998). Although practitioners may recognize that people from different cultures may gesture differently than they do, not understanding what gestures mean may lead to unintended, rude, or offensive behavior (Black, 2011).

Some cultural groups, such as Arabs or Italians and others from that part of the world, are often more expansive in their gestures than are people from Great Britain and parts of the United States. Various groups of people use different gestures than do those from the United States. For example, to signal "no," Americans shake their heads from side to side, while people from Southern Italy flick their chins, and people from Greece and Turkey signal "no" by jerking their eyebrows and head upward (Black, 2011).

Practitioners should also be sensitive to personal space, or proxemics. **Personal space** is an approximate area around an individual that other people should not physically violate so they feel comfortable and secure. Although this is an individual characteristic, general cultural traits are related to personal space. The British, Canadians, and Americans tend to be low-touch societies, while Mexicans are often more high-touch (Lattanzi & Purnell, 2006). Practitioners should be aware of their own sense of personal space and that of their clients so they will be comfortable and most effective during cross-cultural interactions.

Reflection 11.3. Good Communication

- Generally, do you see yourself as a good communicator? Why or why not?
- Have you had cross-cultural interactions where you felt you communicated well? What made it a positive interaction?
- Have you had a cross-cultural interaction where the communication was not effective? What caused the difficulty?
- What were you feeling during the interaction?
- What do you think the other person was feeling?
- What would you change to improve the communication?

Cross-Cultural Interviewing

Interviewing is one component of a thorough initial evaluation that is "focused on finding out what a client wants and needs to do; determining what a client can do and has done; and identifying supports and barriers to health, well-being, and participation (American Occupational Therapy Association [AOTA], 2014, p. S13).

Interviewing clients is a practice skill in its own right, but it becomes more complex when interviewing someone who is culturally different from the interviewer. Holstein and Gubrium's (2003) fascinating *Inside Interviewing: New Lenses, New Concerns* explains how to deconstruct the process of interviewing with people who are gay, lesbian, transgender, or transsexual, asking if the interview truly represented the thoughts of the interviewee or of the interviewer. Other authors have questioned whether cross-cultural interviewing can be value free and objective (Mullings, 1999) or always biased (Lim, Winter, & Chan, 2006), and some have suggested using narrative interviews to elicit personal stories and points of view of the interviewee (Mattingly & Lawlor, 2000).

Dennis and Giangreco (1996) remind us that "no cookbook approach or checklist will lead professionals to more culturally sensitive family interviews. Instead, cultural sensitivity begins with careful listening and personal reflection" (p. 105), components that have already been discussed in this chapter. Gaining some knowledge of the culture of the client prior to the interview, entering the interview process with an open mind and willing attitude as discussed below, listening to and observing the client with focused attention, and clarifying the meaning of what is being said so that each of person truly understands what the other is saying and what they mean supports an effective cross-cultural interview experience.

Choosing Effective Cultural Evaluations

The *occupational therapy* evaluation should begin with an occupational profile and an analysis of occupational performance, which includes a selection of assessment tools chosen from the hundreds available that evaluate specific skills of the person (AOTA, 2014, p. S13). Most tools used by occupational therapists are designed from a Western point of view and underscored by Western values and may not be appropriate or reliable when used with people from cultures other than the United States. Notable exceptions include the Loewenstein Occupational Therapy Cognitive Assessment (LOTCA) battery (Josman, Abdallah, & Engel-Yager, 2011), the Canadian Occupational Performance Measure (COPM) (Fisher, 2005), and the Assessment of Motor and Process Skills (AMPS), (Buchan, 2002).

Other culturally sensitive tools are available that can be added to the evaluation process that may help build rapport with diverse clients, such as the Sunrise model by Leininger (1988); the ETHNIC tool by Levin, Like, and Gottlieb (2000); and the BELIEF tool by Dobbie, Medrano, Tysinger, and Olney (2003; see Table 11.1). Depending upon the client's needs, the practitioner might choose to include one of these tools as part of the evaluation process or use some of the questions from these tools to add to the occupational profile.

Skillful Attitudes and Active Engagement

Developing an attitude of willingness leads people to engage in the behaviors necessary for effective cross-cultural interactions. Being culturally effective is not a passive position; it takes active engagement and skillful interactions with others. One has to be willing to *do* something to make a difference.

Willingness

Willingness can be defined as a favorable or open disposition toward something. I became aware of the concept of willingness in an earlier study on cultural competence (Black, 2002) and recognized that a positive, respectful attitude is another necessary skill for effective cross-cultural interactions. Although **attitudes** are not skills but dispositions or mental positions people take in relation to something else (Merriam-Webster Dictionary, 1995),

Table 11.1. Culturally Sensitive Assessment Models, Tools, and Questionnaires

Authors	Tool	Reference
Black and Wells	**Cultural Information Questionnaire** Opening statement Questions about meaning of current illness Health beliefs and practices Cultural beliefs and values	Black, R. M., & Wells, S. A. (2007). *Culture and occupation: A model of empowerment in occupational therapy.* Bethesda, MD: AOTA Press.
Leininger	**The Sunrise Model** Cultural values and lifeways Religious, philosophical, and spiritual beliefs Economic factors Educational factors Technological factors Kinship and social ties Political and legal factors	Leininger, M. (1988). Leininger's theory of nursing: Cultural care, diversity, and universality. *Nursing Science Quarterly, 1*(4), 152–160.
Levin, Like, & Gottlieb	**The ETHNIC Tool** **E:** Explanatory (How do you explain your illness?) **T:** Treatment (What treatment have you tried?) **H:** Healers (Have you sought any advice from folk healers?) **N:** Negotiate (Mutually acceptable options) **I:** Intervention (Mutually agreed upon) **C:** Collaboration (With patient, family, and healers)	Levin, S. J., Like, R. C., & Gottlieb, J. E. (2000). ETHNIC: A framework for culturally competent clinical practice. *Patient Care, 9*(Special Issue), 188.
Dobbie, Medrano, Tysinger, & Olney	**The BELIEF Tool** **B:** Health beliefs (What caused your illness/problem?) **E:** Explanation (Why did it happen at this time?) **L:** Learn (Help me understand your belief/opinion) **I:** Impact (How is this illness/problem impacting your life?) **E:** Empathy (This must be very difficult for you.) **F:** Feelings (How are you feeling about it?)	Dobbie, A. E., Medrano, M., Tysinger, J., & Olney, C. (2003). The BELIEF instrument: A preclinical teaching tool to elicit patients' health beliefs. *Family Medicine, 35*(5), 316–319.

attitudes can be learned, like other skills. Therefore, negative attitudes can be unlearned.

People shift their attitudes many times throughout their lifetime, depending on their knowledge and experiences. For example, people might love or hate the Boston Red Sox during one season, depending on the team's standing in the series, or a person may shift attitude about motorcyclists from negative to a more positive viewpoint when a good friend purchases a bike and introduces the joys of riding. In the same way, views of a certain population of people that someone has been taught to fear and hate can also change with increased knowledge and experience. With an attitude of willingness, certain attitudes can be developed and learned.

In Black's 2002 study, participants were asked to identify important characteristics of a culturally competent person, and throughout the interviews, the words *willing* and *willingness* were often spoken. The following are a few of the ways the study participants talked about this concept:

- Willingness to seek out what the differences are
- Willingness to find out what is really going on
- Willingness to accept and experience
- Willingness to listen
- Willingness to understand the situation
- Willingness to let go of assumptions
- Willingness to learn
- Willingness to be open and listen and understand
- Willingness to admit you don't know anything (Black, 2002).

During analysis, it became apparent that the participants were talking about making a conscious choice—a volitional act. Kielhofner (2002) defined *volition* as "a pattern of thoughts and feelings about

oneself as an actor in one's world which occur as one anticipates, chooses, experiences, and interprets what one does" (p. 19). One could infer that a culturally effective person develops and maintains an attitude or disposition that allows him or her not only to be open to certain experiences but also to choose them. Many study participants stated that a person who is culturally competent chooses to have an open mind, chooses to be self-reflective, and chooses to attempt interactions beyond his or her comfort zone. Having the will to do something connotes having and making a choice.

Levels of Willingness

Black's (2002) study showed that not all participants functioned at the same level of willingness or held the same attitude about cross-cultural interactions. Findings suggested three levels of willingness, which include (1) unreflective willingness, (2) cautious willingness, and (3) committed willingness (see Table 11.2).

Unreflective Willingness

Unreflective willingness involves "doing the right thing" because of external societal expectations, not any internal drive. For example, many people now use "politically correct" language by rote, not really thinking about why language has changed to be more respectful, inclusive, and nondisparaging when talking about nondominant groups of people. These people choose to more effectively interact with others because they are expected to and feel that they should.

One study participant told of hearing someone tell ethnic jokes. When questioned about this, she said, "You're supposed to respect other people . . . and part of being a professional is respect for others and their differences, especially when you're a teacher." This

Table 11.2. Levels of Willingness for Cross-Cultural Interactions

Levels	Attitude	Focus	Behavior
Unreflective Willingness	Compliant I'm supposed to act this way	External Societal expectations	"Doing the right thing"
Cautious Willingness	Wants to interact but hesitant Lack of confidence	Internal Fearful of making mistakes	Wants to interact and does but is unsure of skills
Committed Willingness	Excitement "Bring it on!"	Internally motivated	Seeks out opportunities for cross-cultural interactions

Source. Adapted from Black, 2002.

participant recognized that the expected behavior of a professional is to respect others, which means that one does not tell ethnic jokes. She had learned that lesson well, but she did not add anything else to her statement indicating that she had an internal awareness of oppression, injustice, and hurt inherent in such an act. This participant might choose not to tell this kind of joke, but her decision seemed to be grounded in the behavioral expectations for someone in a professional role rather than in a reflective stance regarding the meaning of the act.

Students and practitioners at this level of willingness are moving in a positive direction, but they have much work to do to develop a level of cultural effectiveness that emerges from their own personal values and attitudes. At this level, people may have acquired some cultural knowledge but still need to develop the areas of self- awareness and skill.

Cautious Willingness

At the level of **cautious willingness,** people are willing to learn and behave in more effective interactive patterns but are still hesitant because they either are afraid of making mistakes or they lack confidence in their abilities. The following statement from Black's (2002) study exemplifies this concept.

> I think I am not as culturally competent as I would like to be, because I don't know more about what it means to confront difference . . . .'cause I don't know enough about the difference, the minority, the different cultures. (p. 145)

Although this participant was unsure of her ability and her knowledge, she later indicated that she had a clear understanding of power, inequality, and issues of difference. She had a significant amount of self-awareness and knowledge, but she lacked skill.

People at this level of willingness need more practice with cross-cultural interactions to improve their skill, confidence, and sense of self-efficacy, but they are making good progress toward becoming culturally effective. They have an open and accepting attitude, choosing to interact with others because of an internal drive to connect and an interest in people.

Committed Willingness

Participants exhibiting **committed willingness** were willing to interact with others and sought out

opportunities to do so. They realized that they might make cultural mistakes and that they still had a lot to learn, but they were eager to work with differing cultures and to learn from their mistakes as part of the process. They had a "bring it on" mentality and attitude that was contagious. One participant expressed her committed willingness as follows:

> It's like accomplishing [something]. Look what I've come from! Look what I've learned! This is what it has been preparing you for. Oh, wow! There's a sense of excitement because you realize that there's so much more out there than just . . . backing away. That's the beginning. That's opening a door to a whole new world! (p. 152)

These students' willingness to interact with others came from a strong commitment that clearly embodies Kielhofner's (2002) dynamic interaction among values, interests, and sense of personal causation. Although people showing committed willingness may have much more to learn, their motivation and drive to become culturally effective increases the likelihood that they will succeed.

Reflection 11.4. Willingness

- If you are willing to interact with others who are different from you, what level of willingness best describes you? (1) Unreflective willingness; (2) Cautious willingness; or (3) Committed willingness.
- Would you rather see yourself at another level?
- What steps will you take to move there?

Summary

Skillful and effective communication is a vital part of culturally effective care and is built upon a willingness to learn to interact with people who are different from oneself. This chapter has identified some of the specific ways occupational therapy practitioners communicate with clients, including through the use of translators and interpreters, by using culturally sensitive assessment tools, and through effective interviewing skills. Being an effective communicator is vital for each practitioner, and will serve well when interacting with any client.

References

Al-Tayyib, A. A., Rogers, S. M., Gribble, J. N., Villarroel, M. A., & Turner, C. F. (2002). Effect of low medical literacy on health survey measurements. *American Journal of Public Health, 92*(9), 1478–1480. http://dx.doi.org/10.2105/AJPH.92.9.1478

American Occupational Therapy Association. (2014). Occupational therapy practice framework: Domain & process. (3rd ed.). *American Journal of Occupational Therapy, 68*, (Supplement 1), S1–S51. http://dx.doi.org/10.5014/ajot .2014.682006

Black, R. M. (2002). *The essence of cultural competence: Listening to the voices of occupational therapy students.* Unpublished Doctoral Dissertation. Cambridge, MA: Lesley University.

Black, R. M. (2011). Cultural considerations of hand use. *Journal of Hand Therapy, 24*(2), 104–110. http://dx.doi.org/10.1016 /j.jht.2010.09.067

Black, R. M., & Wells, S. A. (2007). *Culture and occupation: A model of empowerment in occupational therapy.* Bethesda, MD: AOTA Press.

Bonder, B., & Martin, L. (2013). *Culture in clinical care: Strategies for competence.* 2nd ed. Thorofare, NJ: Slack.

Bowen, S. (2004). *Assessing the responsiveness of health care organizations to culturally diverse groups.* Winnipeg: University of Manitoba, Department of Community Health Sciences.

Buchan, T. (2002). The impact of language and culture when administering the Assessment of Motor and Process Skills: A case study. *British Journal of Occupational Therapy, 65*(8), 371–373. http://dx.doi.org/10.1177/030802260206500804

Dennis, R. E., & Giangreco, M. F. (1996). Creating conversation: Reflections on cultural sensitivity in family interviewing. *Exceptional Children, 63*(1), 103–116. http://dx.doi.org /10.1177/001440299606300109

Dobbie, A. E., Medrano, M., Tysinger, J., & Olney, C. (2003). The BELIEF instrument: A preclinical teaching tool to elicit patients' health beliefs. *Family Medicine, 35*(5), 316–319. Retrieved from https://www.stfm.org/fmhub/fm2003/may03 /dobbie.pdf

Fisher, S. (2005). The Canadian Occupational Performance Measure: Does it address the cultural occupations of ethnic minorities? *British Journal of Occupational Therapy, 68*(5), 224–234. http://dx.doi.org/10.1177/030802260506800506

Hammond, P. (1993). Communication breakdown. *Nursing times, 89*(20), 26.

Herbst, P. H. (1997). *The color of words: An encyclopedic dictionary of ethnic bias in the United States.* Yarmouth, ME: Intercultural Press.

Holstein, J. A., & Gubrium, J. F. (2003). *Inside interviewing: New lenses, new concerns.* Thousand Oaks, CA: Sage.

Josman, N., Abdallah, T. M., & Engel-Yeger, B. (2011). Using the LOTCA to measure cultural and sociodemographic effects on cognitive skills in two groups of children. *American Journal of Occupational Therapy, 65*(3), e29–e37. http://dx .doi.org/10.5014/ajot.2011.09037

Kielhofner, G. (2002). *A model of human occupation: Theory and application* (3rd ed.) Baltimore: Lippincott Williams & Wilkins.

King, S. (1990). Naming and power in Zora Neale Hurston's *Their eyes were watching god. Black American Literature Forum, 24*(4), 683–696. http://dx.doi.org/10.2307/3041796

Kutner, M., Greenberg, E., Jin, Y., & Paulsen, C. (2006). *The Health literacy of America's adults: Results from the 2003 national assessment of adult literacy.* Washington, DC: U.S. Department of Education.

Lattanzi, J. B., & Purnell, L. D. (2006). *Developing cultural competence in physical therapy practice.* Philadelphia: F. A. Davis.

Leavitt, R. (2010). *Cultural competence: A lifelong journey to cultural proficiency.* Thorofare, NJ: Slack.

Leininger, M. (1988). Leininger's theory of nursing: Cultural care, diversity, and universality. *Nursing Science Quarterly, 1*(4), 152–160. http://dx.doi.org/10.1177/089431848800100408

Leitch, C. (1992). Understanding sweet nothing. *Nursing Standard, 6*(48), 50–51. Retrieved from http://journals.rcni.com /doi/pdfplus/10.7748/ns.6.48.50.s61

Levin, S. J., Like, R. C., & Gottlieb, J. E. (2000). ETHNIC: A framework for culturally competent clinical practice. *Patient Care, 9*(Special Issue), 188.

Lim, C.-H., Winter, R., & Chan, C. C. A. (2006). Cross-cultural interviewing in the hiring process: Challenges and strategies. *Career Development Quarterly, 54*, 265–268. http://dx.doi.org /10.1002/j.2161-0045.2006.tb00157.x

Lynch, E. W., & Hanson, M. J. (1998). *Developing cross-cultural competencies: A guide for working with children and their families* (2nd ed.). Baltimore: Paul H. Brookes.

Mattingly, C., & Lawlor, M. (2000). Learning from stories: Narrative interviewing in cross-cultural research. *Scandinavian Journal of Occupational Therapy, 7*(1), 4–14. http://dx.doi.org /10.1080/110381200443571

Merriam-Webster Dictionary. (1995). *Attitude.* Springfield, MA: Merriam-Webster.

Mullings, B. (1999). Insider or outsider, both or neither: Some dilemmas of interviewing in a cross-cultural setting. *Geoforum, 30*(4), 337–350.

Nora, L. M., Daugherty, S. R., Mattis-Peterson, A., Stevenson, L., & Goodman, L. J. (1994). Improving cross-cultural skills of medical students through medical school-community partnerships. *Western Journal of Medicine, 161*, 144–147. Retrieved from https://www.researchgate.net/publication/15256770 _Improving_cross-cultural_skills_of_medical_students _through_medical_school-community_partnerships

Osborn, C. Y., Paasche-Orlow, M. K., Davis, T. C., & Wolf, M. S. (2007). Health literacy: An overlooked factor in understanding HIV health disparities. *American Journal of Preventive Medicine, 33*(5), 374–378. http://dx.doi.org/10.1016/j.amepre.2007.07.022

Paasche-Orlow, M. K., Parker, R. M., Gazmararian, J. A., Nielsen, L. T., & Rudd, R. R. (2005). The prevalence of limited health literacy. *Journal of General Internal Medicine, 20*(2), 175–184. http://dx.doi.org/10.1111/j.1525-1497.2005.40245.x

Ratzan, S. C., & Parker, R. M. (2004). Introduction. In C. R. Selden, M. Zorn, S. C., Ratzan, & R. M. Parker, (Eds.). *National Library of Medicine Current Bibliographies in Medicine: Health Literacy.* Vol. NLM, Pub. no. CBM 2000–1. 2000. Bethesda, MD: National Institutes of Health, U.S. Department of Health and Human Services. Retrieved from https://www.nlm.nih.gov/archive//20061214/pubs/cbm/hliteracy.html

Rosen, J., Spatz, E. S., Gaaserud, A. M. J., Abramovitch, H., Weinreb, B.,… Margolis, C. Z. (2004). A new approach to developing cross-cultural communication skills. *Medical Teacher, 26*(2), 126–132. http://dx.doi.org/10.1080/01421590310001653946

Srivastava, R. (2007). Working with interpreters in healthcare settings. In R. Srivastava (Ed.) *The healthcare professional's guide to clinical cultural competence.* (pp. 125–143). Toronto: Elsevier Canada.

Su, C.-T., & Parham, D. (2002). Generating a valid questionnaire translation for cross-cultural use. *American Journal of Occupational Therapy, 56*(5), 581–585. http://dx.doi.org/10.5014/ajot.56.5.581

Tanno, D. V. (1997). Ethical implications in the ethnic "text" in multicultural communication studies. In J. M. Makau & R. C. Arnett (Eds.) *Communication ethics in an age of diversity* (pp. 73–88). Urbana: University of Illinois.

Teal, C. A., & Street, R. I. (2008). Critical elements of culturally competent communication in the medical encounter: A review and model. *Social Science and Medicine, 68*(3), 533–543. http://dx.doi.org/10.1016/j.socscimed.2008.10.015

U.S. Department of Health and Human Services. (2001). *National Standards for Culturally and Linguistically Appropriate Services (CLAS) in Health Care.* Rockville, MD: Office of Minority Health.

Wolf, E. (1982). *Europe and the people without history.* Berkeley: University of California Press.

Chapter 12.

EFFECTIVE PATIENT–PROVIDER COMMUNICATION IN CROSS-CULTURAL ENCOUNTERS

Leanne Yinusa-Nyahkoon, ScD, OTR/L

Communication is the social glue that bonds humans together in relationships, groups, communities, and countries. The strength and quality of those bonds depends on our ability to understand and use communication well.
Bethami A. Dobkin & Roger C. Pace (2003, p. xvii)

Chapter Highlights

- Health Disparities
- Challenges in Clinical Encounters
- National Standards and Initiatives to Improve Patient–Provider Communication
- Traditional and Novel Approaches to Patient–Provider Communication
- Integrating the Standards Into the Clinical Encounter and Beyond the Medical Environment

Key Terms and Concepts

- ✧ Biomedical communication
- ✧ Health beliefs
- ✧ Health literacy
- ✧ Interpretation

- ✧ National Action Plan to Improve Health Literacy
- ✧ National CLAS Standards
- ✧ Translation
- ✧ Virtual patient advocates

Increasingly, diverse patient populations and a demanding health care system have challenged health care professionals' ability to provide high-quality services and to ensure effective patient–provider communication, one of the vital components of such services (Office of Minority Health, 2013a). The Institute of Medicine (2003) reported that complex "historic and contemporary disparities" in access to health care "involve many participants at several levels, including health systems, their administrative and bureaucratic processes, utilization managers, health care professionals, and patients" (p. 1). This chapter focuses on the level of the health care professional and presents recommendations on how to improve patient–provider communication during cross-cultural encounters.

Health Disparities

More than a decade ago, the Institute of Medicine (IOM; 2003) released a report titled *Unequal Treatment: Confronting Racial and Ethnic Disparities in Healthcare.* The report was considered the first comprehensive publication documenting disparities in access to quality health care services among racial and ethnic minorities in the United States (see also IOM, 2012).

More than a decade later, quality health care services are still unevenly distributed to these groups throughout the United States, and low-income populations and residents of the Southern, Middle Atlantic, Pacific, and West North Central census regions have been identified as groups that either tend to have more health disparities or receive suboptimal preventive, acute, and chronic care (Agency for Healthcare Research and Quality [AHRQ], 2015). People of multiple races and those who are lesbian, gay, bisexual, or transgender also experience health disparities; however, the extent of these groups' disparities is not yet well understood.

Providing better patient-centered care to all individuals is an aim of health and health care reform (AHRQ, 2015). Effective patient–provider communication is one area of challenge in efforts to mitigate health disparities and minimize suboptimal health care.

Challenges in Clinical Encounters

Patient–provider communication is influenced by factors inherent in clinical encounters. Common factors that contribute to these challenges include

- Low health literacy among patients,
- Linguistic differences,
- Clinician time constraints,
- Scarcity of diverse and culturally sensitive health care workers,
- Lack of patient centeredness,
- Varied provider listening skills,
- Shortages of health care professionals in certain geographic locations,
- Limited trust in health care practitioners among patients,
- Patients' and providers' health care beliefs, and
- Perceived racism and other perceptions of discrimination (AHRQ, 2003, 2012, 2013, 2015;

Collins, David, Handler, Wall, & Andes, 2004; Debbink & Bader, 2011; Geronimus, 2001; Johnson, Roter, Powe, & Cooper, 2004; Nielsen-Bohlman, Panzer, Hamlin, & Kindig, 2004; Oliver, Goodwin, Gotler, Gregory, & Stange, 2001; Roter et al., 1997).

Provider Emphasis on Biomedical Communication

Effective patient–provider communication is essential "so that patients' needs and wants are understood and addressed and patients understand and participate in their own care" (AHRQ, 2013, Chapter 5, p. 1). However, many clinical interactions consist of provider-dominated *biomedical communication,* in which health care providers direct the conversation, ask closed-ended medical questions, offer clinical information, and limit discussions of psychosocial topics (Roter et al., 1997). This communication pattern interferes with opportunities to elicit patient perspectives and consider patient preferences, which are vital components of evidence-based practice (Carter, Lubinsky, & Domholdt, 2011; Guyatt et al., 2000).

Improving patient–provider communication has been a longstanding priority for researchers and organizations charged with improving health disparities, but communication challenges persist for certain racial groups, low-income patients, and those with limited English proficiency.

When interacting with these clients and their families, health providers have been noted to be less patient centered; to spend fewer minutes planning treatment, answering questions, listening carefully and respectfully, and clearly explaining information; and to be more verbally dominant with biomedical discourse (AHRQ, 2013, 2015; Center for Financing, Access and Cost Trends, 2013a, 2013b, 2013c; Johnson et al., 2004; Office of Minority Health, 2013a; Oliver et al., 2001).

Variations in Health Beliefs

Patients are less likely to comply with health care recommendations they do not understand or that diverge from their health beliefs (Coleman-Miller, 2000; Office of Minority Health, 2013b; Vermeire, Hearnshaw, Van Royen, & Denekens, 2001; Woloshin, Bickell, Schwartz, Gany, & Welch, 1995). Harvard physician and anthropologist Arthur Kleinman defined *health beliefs* as explanatory models of illness and argued that these models differ between clients and providers even when they share similar demographic characteristics. These models diverge further as similarities between the individual client and provider decrease (Cohen, Tripp-Reimer, Smith, Sorofman, & Lively, 1994; Kleinman, 1980; Kleinman, Eisenberg, & Good, 1978; Pachter, 1994; Schouten & Meeuwesen, 2006).

Kleinman et al. (1978) proposed eight questions that health care providers can use to elicit a patient's explanatory model of illness, and others have proposed mnemonic models for eliciting a client's illness experience (Exhibit 12.1; Berlin & Fowkes, 1983; Levin, Like, & Gottlieb, 2000). Clinicians have used Kleinman and colleagues' explanatory model framework to understand the patient's illness perspective, minimize the power differential present during the clinical encounter, and promote effective clinical communication (Arcury, Skelly, Gesler, & Dougherty, 2004; Ashton et al., 2003; Schouten & Meeuwesen, 2006; Simon, 2006; Skelly et al., 2006; Stewart et al., 2000; Suurmond & Seeleman, 2006). However, three decades after Kleinman and colleagues' model was introduced as a staple of clinical communication, health and health care disparities in the United States persist.

Patient–Practitioner Demographic Differences

A comparison of U.S. population and occupational therapy practitioner demographics reveals a challenge particular to occupational therapy clinical encounters. In 2011, 15.0% of Americans lived in poverty and 15.7% had no health insurance (DeNavas-Walt, Proctor, & Smith, 2012); between 2000 and 2010 same-sex partner households

increased 80.4% (Lofquist, Lugaila, O'Connell, & Feliz, 2012). According to the U.S. Census Bureau (2016), 49% of the U.S. population are men, 23% identify themselves as a racial or ethnic minority, 29% hold a bachelor's degree or higher, 13% were born outside of the United States, and 21% speak a language other than English at home. A 2003 study found that only 12% of U.S. adults had proficient health literacy skills, whereas 53% had intermediate health literacy skills, 22% basic health literacy skills, and 14% had below basic health literacy skills (Kutner, Greenberg, Jin, & Paulsen, 2006).

In contrast to U.S. population demographics, 9 of 10 occupational therapy practitioners in the United States are women, and 8 out of 10 self-identify as non-Hispanic White (American Occupational Therapy Association [AOTA], 2015). Some 82% of practitioners are occupational therapists and 98% have a bachelor's degree or higher (AOTA, 2015). It can be assumed that 100% of occupational therapy practitioners have proficient health literacy skills because of their education and training. Because occupational therapy practitioners are likely to provide services to clients who have cultural, educational, health literacy, linguistic, gender, and lifestyle differences, it is important that practitioners understand, become familiar with, and implement evidence-based national recommendations for effective patient–provider communication.

National Standards and Initiatives to Improve Patient–Provider Communication

The U.S. health care system developed national initiatives such as Healthy People 2000, 2010, and most

---

Exhibit 12.1. Eight Questions Health Care Providers Can Use to Elicit a Patient's Explanatory Model of Illness

1. What do you think has caused your problem?
2. Why do you think it started when it did?
3. What do you think your sickness does to you? How does it work?
4. How severe is your sickness? Will it have a short or long course?
5. What kind of treatment do you think you should receive?
6. What are the most important results you hope to receive from this treatment?
7. What are the chief problems your sickness has caused for you?
8. What do you fear most about your sickness?

Source. From "Culture, Illness, and Care: Clinical Lessons From Anthropologic and Cross-Cultural Research," by A. Kleinman, L. Eisenberg, and B. Good, 1978, *Annals of Internal Medicine, 88,* p. 256. Copyright © 1978 by the American College of Physicians. Reprinted with permission.

recently 2020, aimed at achieving health equity, eliminating disparities, and improving the health of all groups in the United States (Centers for Disease Control and Prevention, 2009; Keppel, Pearcy, & Wagener, 2002; U.S. Department of Health and Human Services [DHHS], 2000, 2010).

National CLAS Standards

In 2000, the Office of Minority Health released guidelines for providing culturally sensitive and linguistically appropriate health care—the National Standards for Culturally and Linguistically Appropriate Services in Health Care, known as the ***National CLAS Standards*** (DHHS, 2001). This document was revised and renamed the enhanced National Standards for Culturally and Linguistically Appropriate Services in Health and Healthcare (Office of Minority Health, 2013a) and currently offers 15 best practice recommendations for providing quality health care to an increasingly diverse client population.

Standards 4 through 8 of the National CLAS Standards focus specifically on effective patient–provider communication. These standards read as follows:

- *Standard 4.* Educate and train governance, leadership, and workforce in culturally and linguistically appropriate policies and practices on an ongoing basis.
- *Standard 5.* Offer language assistance to individuals who have limited English proficiency and/or other communication needs, at no cost to them, to facilitate timely access to all health care and services.
- *Standard 6.* Inform all individuals of the availability of language assistance services clearly and in their preferred language, verbally and in writing.
- *Standard 7.* Ensure the competence of individuals providing language assistance, recognizing that the use of untrained individuals and/or minors as interpreters should be avoided.
- *Standard 8.* Provide easy-to-understand print and multimedia materials and signage in the languages commonly used by the populations in the service area.

The National CLAS Standards reflect increased knowledge about patient–provider communication and cultural and linguistic competencies and integrate new national policies and legislation targeting clinical communication (Office of Minority Health, 2013a). For example, the Patient Protection and Affordable Care Act of 2010 (Pub. L. 111–148), described as "the most significant federal effort to reduce disparities in the country's history," encourages providers to participate in trainings about cultural competency and requires that appropriate health care information be made available to patients with low health literacy levels (DHHS, 2011, p. 35).

The National CLAS Standards are consistent with and beneficial to occupational therapy practice. National CLAS Standards 4 through 8 highlight the importance of clear patient–provider communication, especially in interactions with patients who have cultural, health literacy, and linguistic differences. These guidelines are also appropriate when communicating with patients whose socioeconomic status, sexual orientation, or gender identity differ from that of the provider (Office of Minority Health, 2013a).

National CLAS Standard 4 requires ongoing education and training for health care providers to support successful cross-cultural health encounters. Cultural competency curriculum modules based on the initial National CLAS Standards have been developed to ensure cultural and linguistic competencies, and some states have mandated participation for some or all of its licensed health care workers (Office of Minority Health, 2013b).

Reflection 12.1. National CLAS Standards

- Locate the National CLAS Standards online and read them (Office of Minority Health, 2013a). Are they being used in your fieldwork site or workplace?
- Consider how they could be used, and discuss this issue with your classmates or colleagues.

National Action Plan to Improve Health Literacy

Health literacy is the ability to understand, read, and act on health information—for example, following treatment recommendations reviewed during an office visit, determining how much medicine to give a sick child, following the directions on a medical supply box, and interpreting health messages printed on a provider-issued pamphlet (Office of Disease Prevention and Health Promotion, 2010). The ***National Action Plan to Improve Health Literacy*** has offered recommendations to restructure how health information is disseminated in the United States (Office of Disease Prevention and Health Promotion, 2010).

According to the National Action Plan to Improve Health Literacy, health care providers must adopt the universal precautions approach to infectious disease control and ensure that clear communication is the basis for every health information exchange because it is impossible to initially determine a patient's health literacy level (Office of Disease Prevention and Health Promotion, 2010). Providers should assume that all patients have some level of difficulty understanding health information and use clear communication with everyone (Bass, Wilson, Griffith, & Barnett, 2002; Office of Disease Prevention and Health Promotion, 2010; Paasche-Orlow, Schillinger, Greene, & Wagner, 2006; Parker & Kreps, 2005).

Traditional and Novel Approaches to Patient–Provider Communication

The National CLAS Standards and other recommended guidelines suggest that patient–provider communication should always include a balanced discussion of two elements: (1) factual information about the physiological or psychological disease, its related process, and contributing factors based on a patient's race, ethnicity, and culture, and (2) patients' perceptions and attitudes about the illness process (Bobo, Womeodu, & Knox, 1991; Office of Minority Health, 2013a; Scott, 1997). Throughout their professional training, health care providers are taught biomedical communication, so communicating concrete disease information during the clinical encounter is often perceived to be familiar and routine. Consequently, few guidelines for factual communication exist, unlike the numerous models that were developed to facilitate discussion of the patient's illness experience.

The recent focus on culturally and linguistically appropriate health care services and health literacy has launched a reexamination of the traditional means of relaying factual information. The National CLAS Standards, the National Action Plan to Improve Health Literacy, and other publications offer new guidelines when communicating such information to clients (Office of Disease Prevention and Health Promotion, 2010; Office of Minority Health, 2013a).

New models of patient–provider education espouse the concept of universal literacy precautions described in the National Action Plan to Improve Health Literacy, reflect the National CLAS Standards, and embrace the Healthy People 2020 objectives for health communication (DHHS, 2013; Office of Disease Prevention and Health Promotion, 2010; Office of Minority Health, 2013a). For example, Koh and colleagues' (2012) model of effective patient–provider communication incorporates conventional provider actions as well as novel actions that extend beyond the traditional clinical encounter. The model's recommended provider actions include

- Creating reminders about what patients should bring to the next office visit;
- Developing simple medical forms and offering to help patients fill out these required forms;
- Listening to patients' symptoms and concerns;
- Explaining medical information using simple, lay terminology;
- Discussing treatment options and answering related questions;
- Developing a treatment plan collaboratively with patients;
- Asking patients to confirm their comprehension of the treatment plan in their own words;
- Providing simple handouts to reinforce treatment recommendations; and
- Following up with patients and helping schedule future visits.

Reflection 12.2. Model Implementation

- How many of the actions recommended in the model of effective patient–provider communication would you feel comfortable using at your fieldwork site or workplace?
- Are any of these already being implemented?
- Are there any barriers to incorporating these ideas?

Integrating the Standards Into the Clinical Encounter and Beyond the Medical Environment

The recent national focus on culturally and linguistically appropriate services and health literacy has expanded the traditional conceptualization of patient–provider interactions to extend beyond oral communication and include provider actions beyond the clinical encounter. Although many health care decisions and discussions are initiated when patients and their health care providers are together at the clinical encounter, facilitated by language assistance, much of this communication process continues as patients interpret often unfamiliar and complex health information outside of the medical environment through print materials and the use of information technology (Office of Minority Health, 2013a).

Language Assistance

National CLAS Standards 5, 6, and 7 highlight the importance of clear verbal communication during the clinical encounter. Collectively, these standards recommend that language assistance, including qualified interpreters, professional translation services, and trained bilingual staff, are offered to patients, their caregivers, and their health care advocates and proxies who have limited or no English proficiency, low health literacy, or other communication challenges (Joint Commission, 2010; National Health Law Program, 2010; Office of Minority Health, 2013a).

According to these guidelines, language assistance services should be offered at no cost to the patient and are required of all health care institutions and systems receiving federal funding support (Office of Minority Health, 2013a). The standards further highlight that it is important for health care providers to be aware of the language assistance services offered within their health care organization and to notify patients of these services verbally and in writing in the patient's primary language (Office of Minority Health, 2005, 2013a).

Interpretation is assistance with oral communication between people who do not speak the same language, and *translation* provides access to written information in a person's native tongue. Options for interpretation and translation services, including technological approaches and recommendations for how to offer these services at reduced cost, are available (Sperling, 2011).

Interpretation is the language assistance service most frequently needed to facilitate effective patient–provider communication, and according to the National Health Law Program (2010), qualified

interpreters demonstrate specific skill competencies, including dual language proficiency, knowledge of the health care system, cultural competence, and strong interpersonal skills. Although it might be convenient, using family members, friends, and other untrained adults or minors as interpreters during a clinical encounter or unqualified translators of medical information should be avoided (Office of Minority Health, 2013a).

Reflection 12.3. Exercise in Identifying Language Barriers

You accompany your Level I fieldwork educator, Mya, to a home therapy session. Mya tells you that the client, Charles, was recently evaluated and found to be at risk for falls within his home. Some safety concerns with activity of daily living tasks, such as cooking and bathing, were also noted. Charles's home is a one-bedroom apartment in an independent living high-rise building for older adults. On the fourth floor, you ring the doorbell to Charles's apartment, and a little girl age 8 to 10 years opens the door. "Are you here to see my grandfather?" she asks. You and Mya simultaneously respond, "Yes," and enter the apartment. A tall man pushing a rolling walker with a walker basket attached approaches you and says "Hi," but then he quickly looks behind both you and Mya. "Where's the lady . . . the interpreter?" he asks. "No English!"

- According to the National CLAS Standards, what should you do in this situation?
- Would it be appropriate to ask the granddaughter to provide interpretation?
- Whose responsibility is it to provide interpretation services?
- Explore virtual interpretation on the Internet, using computer software and also via smartphone apps. Is it appropriate to use virtual interpretation in this scenario?

Print Materials

Print materials are often provided during the clinical encounter, and some are used to reinforce key clinical messages once patients return home and to their communities. Examples include

- Informed consent forms and other legal documents,

- Prevention and treatment instructions, and
- Health education brochures, pamphlets, and flyers (Office of Minority Health, 2013a).

The National CLAS Standards highlight the importance not only of translation into patients' native language by a qualified translator but also of integrating appropriate pictograms and graphics, simple language, and friendly visual organization and designs into these print materials to effectively convey the information being communicated. Studies have shown that picture-based instructions and graphics promote better understanding of health risks and the need to take medication as prescribed (Ancker, Senathirajah, Kukafka, & Starren, 2006; Katz, Kripalani, & Weiss, 2006; Kripalani et al., 2007; Lipkus, Samsa, & Rimer, 2001; Yin et al., 2008).

Use of Information Technology

In addition to enhancing print communication, the use of information technology is an emerging means of effective health communication. Because of the increasing complexity of health information and the limited time and resources within some health care settings, most clients need additional information, skills, and supportive relationships to meet their health needs that can be provided via the Internet, through multimedia approaches, and in the form of virtual patient advocates (Office of Minority Health, 2013a).

Internet

The Office of the Surgeon General advised clinicians to use credible web-based health information to supplement traditional oral and written health communication, and Healthy People 2020 outlines objectives for using health information technology to connect with culturally diverse populations, promote health, and prevent disease (National Prevention Council, 2011; DHHS, 2013). Existing websites such as healthfinder.gov offer current, evidence-based prevention and wellness information; health care providers are also encouraged to identify and create sites that target the specific needs of their patient population.

The increased prevalence of Internet accessibility has revolutionized the way health information is communicated. In 2012, 81% of adults in the United States reported using the Internet, and of those, 72% reported looking online for health information (Fox & Duggan, 2013a). Internet use is most prevalent among younger Americans; 94% of people ages 18–29 years reported Internet use (Zickuhr & Smith, 2012). Consequently, numerous health websites and online health interventions have been developed to target young adults (Crutzen et al., 2011). Such efforts have proved successful; 75% of adolescents and young adults who searched the Internet for health information later used this information to initiate a health-related conversation with a layperson or medical professional or to change an unhealthy behavior (Rideout, 2001).

Minority groups such as African Americans report less home Internet access and overall online use than White Americans; however, the digital divide appears to be decreasing, making Internet-based health education a viable intervention strategy for many minority groups (Dickerson et al., 2004; Economics and Statistics Administration & National Telecommunications and Information Administration, 2011; Kind, Huang, Farr, & Pomerantz, 2005). Technological advances have also allowed cell phones to be used for health communication. In the United States, 85% of adults own a cell phone, and approximately 31% of cell phone owners use their phone to look up health information, the majority using smartphones (Fox & Duggan, 2012).

Multimedia

Because of widespread Internet use for health information, the National Action Plan to Improve Health Literacy encourages multimedia approaches such as use of video for patient education; computer-based data gathering, tracking, and management; online participatory interventions; and virtual interpreters and other virtual health interactions (Joint Commission, 2010; Office of Disease Prevention and Health Promotion, 2010). Adolescents reportedly prefer computerized risk assessments over traditional paper assessments or in-person interviews because they find the computer less judgmental than a clinician and therefore are willing to disclose more personal health risks (Paperny, 1997).

In addition to being an effective means for assessment, studies show that computer-based interventions are also effective and result in increased knowledge among adolescents and young adults after both single and multiple interactions (Tudor-Locke et al., 2004). The use of health-related technology is also expanding among adults; 27% of adult Internet users report using some form of technology to track a health indicator such as weight, diet, exercise, or health symptoms (Fox & Duggan, 2013b).

Virtual Patient Advocates

Clinicians are also using animated characters with humanlike characteristics called **virtual patient advocates** (VPAs) to deliver evidence-based health interventions. VPAs emulate face-to-face verbal interactions with people, including the use of hand gestures, facial expressions, and body posture, and are particularly effective because they

- Rely minimally on text comprehension;
- Can be accessed as frequently as the patient prefers, enhancing recall of critical information;
- Provide consistent, culturally accepted, individualized health promotion messages;
- Are cost-effective because the VPA interacts with multiple patients without the need for office visits or extensive clinician time;
- Are user friendly and can be designed to resemble the target population; and
- Can assess comprehension and track health behaviors (Bickmore, Gruber, & Picard, 2005; Cassell, Sullivan, Prevost, & Churchill, 2000; McQuiggan & Lester, 2007).

Patients have enjoyed interacting with VPAs in lieu of nursing staff to review hospital discharge recommendations (Bickmore et al., 2010; Project RED, 2014), and in a recent study, 80% of participants felt that it was easy to "talk" to the VPA during an intervention, 73% reported that they trusted the VPA, and 87% felt comfortable telling the VPA everything about their health (Gardiner et al., 2013).

Other Applications

Technological advances have implications for practitioners and the overall U.S. health care system. Healthy People 2020 suggested that state health departments use social marketing methods to prevent disease and promote wellness (DHHS, 2013), and the Health Information Technology for Economic and Clinical Health component of the American Recovery and Reinvestment Act of 2009 (Pub. L. 111–5) encouraged health care organizations to adopt electronic health records (Office of the National Coordinator for Health Information Technology, 2011). Ideally, consumers will someday have meaningful access to and use of their electronic health records including after-visit summaries, discharge instructions, patient reminders, and tailored health education (Koh et al., 2012).

Summary

Improved health communication is one of the primary focus areas of Healthy People 2020, and several national objectives target this component of optimal patient–provider encounters and describe a culturally and linguistically sensitive U.S. health care workforce. Achieving these objectives requires health care providers, including occupational therapy practitioners, to do the following

- Consistently offer patients easy-to-understand health care instructions
- Ensure patient comprehension and ability to follow through with health care recommendations
- Demonstrate satisfactory health communication skills by carefully listening to patients and explaining information in ways they understand
- Offer patients support in completing required medical forms
- Show respect for patients' perspectives and preferences
- Spend adequate time with patients
- Involve patients in health care decisions in accordance with patients' participation preferences
- Offer personalized health information resources to support patient self-management
- Provide the opportunity for patients to manage personal health information (i.e., care received, test results, upcoming appointments) on the Internet
- Communicate with patients online (DHHS, 2013).

These initiatives expand the traditional boundaries of effective patient–provider communication, and occupational therapy practitioners must be aware of, understand, and implement these current recommendations. Collectively, the evidence-based, best-practice approaches described in this chapter provide a framework for health care practitioners striving to improve the health and health care services of all patients and populations throughout the United States.

References

Agency for Healthcare Research and Quality. (2003). *National healthcare disparities report.* Rockville, MD: Agency for Healthcare Research and Quality, U.S. Department of Health and Human Services.

Agency for Healthcare Research and Quality. (2012). *National healthcare disparities report 2011.* Rockville, MD: Agency for Healthcare Research and Quality, U.S. Department of Health and Human Services.

Agency for Healthcare Research and Quality. (2013). *National healthcare disparities report 2012.* Rockville, MD: Agency for Healthcare Research and Quality, U.S. Department of Health and Human Services.

Agency for Healthcare Research and Quality. (2015). *2014 National healthcare quality and disparities report.* Rockville, MD: Agency for Healthcare Research and Quality, U.S. Department of Health and Human Services

American Occupational Therapy Association. (2015). *2015 AOTA salary and workforce study.* Bethesda, MD: AOTA Press.

American Recovery and Reinvestment Act of 2009, Pub. L. 111–5, 123 Stat. 115, 516 (Feb. 19, 2009).

Ancker, J. S., Senathirajah, Y., Kukafka, R., & Starren, J. B. (2006). Design features of graphs in health risk communication: A systematic review. *Journal of the American Medical Informatics Association, 13,* 608–618. http://dx.doi.org/10.1197/jamia.M2115

Arcury, T. A., Skelly, A. H., Gesler, W. M., & Dougherty, M. C. (2004). Diabetes meanings among those without diabetes: Explanatory models of immigrant Latinos in rural North Carolina. *Social Science and Medicine, 59,* 2183–2193. http://dx.doi.org/10.1016/j.socscimed.2004.03.024

Ashton, C. M., Haidet, P., Paterniti, D. A., Collins, T. C., Gordon, H. S., O'Malley, K., . . . Street, R. L. (2003). Racial and ethnic disparities in the use of health services: Bias, preferences, or poor communication? *Journal of General Internal Medicine, 18,* 146–152. http://dx.doi.org/10.1046/j.1525-1497.2003.20532.x

Bass, P. F., Wilson, J. F., Griffith, C. H., & Barnett, D. R. (2002). Residents' ability to identify patients with poor literacy skills. *Academic Medicine, 77,* 1039–1041.

Berlin, E., & Fowkes, W. A. (1983). A teaching framework for cross-cultural health care. *Western Journal of Medicine, 139,* 934–938.

Bickmore, T., Gruber, A., & Picard, R. (2005). Establishing the computer–patient working alliance in automated health behavior change interventions. *Patient Education and Counseling, 59,* 21–30. http://dx.doi.org/10.1016/j.pec.2004.09.008

Bickmore, T. W., Pfeifer, L. M., Byron, D., Forsythe, S., Henault, L., Jack, B., . . . Paasche-Orlow, M. (2010). Usability of conversational agents by patients with inadequate health literacy: Evidence from two clinical trials. *Journal of Health Communication, 15*(Suppl. 2), 197–210. http://dx.doi.org/10.1080/10810730.2010.499991

Bobo, L., Womeodu, R. J., & Knox, A. L., Jr. (1991). Society of General Internal Medicine symposium principles of intercultural medicine in an internal medicine program. *American Journal of the Medical Sciences, 302,* 244–248. http://dx.doi.org/10.1097/00000441-199110000-00010

Carter, R. E., Lubinsky, J., & Domholdt, E. (2011). *Rehabilitation research: Principles and applications* (4th ed.). St. Louis: Elsevier/Saunders.

Cassell, J., Sullivan, J., Prevost, S., & Churchill, E. (2000). *Embodied conversational agents.* Cambridge, MA: MIT Press.

Center for Financing, Access and Cost Trends, Agency for Healthcare Research and Quality. (2013a). *Medical Expenditure Panel Survey, 2013, Table 4.2: Among children under age 18 who had a doctor's office or clinic visit reported in the last 12 months, percent distribution of how often their health providers listened carefully to their parents, United States, 2013.* Generated interactively. Retrieved from http://bit.ly/2ao8Qld

Center for Financing, Access and Cost Trends, Agency for Healthcare Research and Quality. (2013b). *Medical Expenditure Panel Survey, 2013, Table 4.4: Among children under age 18 who had a doctor's office or clinic visit in the last 12 months, percent distribution of how often their health providers explained things clearly, United States, 2013.* Generated interactively. Retrieved from http://bit.ly/2ajFLqd

Center for Financing, Access and Cost Trends, Agency for Healthcare Research and Quality. (2013c). *Medical Expenditure Panel Survey, 2013, Table 4.8: Among children under age 18 who had a doctor's office or clinic visit in the last 12 months, percent distribution of how often their health providers spent enough time with them and their parents, United States, 2013.* Generated interactively. Retrieved from http://bit.ly/2aENQsf

Centers for Disease Control and Prevention. (2009). *Healthy People 2000.* Retrieved from http://www.cdc.gov/nchs/healthy_people/hp2000.htm

Cohen, M. Z., Tripp-Reimer, T., Smith, C., Sorofman, B., & Lively, S. (1994). Explanatory models of diabetes: Patient practitioner variation. *Social Science and Medicine, 38,* 59–66. http://dx.doi.org/10.1016/0277-9536(94)90300-X

Coleman-Miller, B. (2000). A physician's perspective on minority health. *Health Care Financing Review, 21,* 45–56.

Collins, J. W., David, R. J., Handler, A., Wall., S., & Andes, S. (2004). Very low birth weight in African American infants: The role of maternal exposure to interpersonal racial discrimination. *American Journal of Public Health, 94,* 2132–2138.

Crutzen, R., de Nooijer, J., Brouwer, W., Oenema, A., Brug, J., & de Vries, N. K. (2011). Strategies to facilitate exposure to Internet-delivered health behavior change interventions aimed at adolescents or young adults: A systematic review. *Health Education and Behavior, 38,* 49–62. http://dx.doi .org/10.1177/1090198110372878

Debbink, M. P., & Bader, M. D. M. (2011). Racial residential segregation and low birth weight in Michigan's metropolitan areas. *American Journal of Public Health, 101,* 1714–1720. http://dx.doi.org/10.2105/AJPH.2011.300152

DeNavas-Walt, C., Proctor, B. D., & Smith, J. C. (2012). *Income, poverty, and health insurance coverage in the United States: 2011* (Publication No. P60-243). Washington, DC: U.S. Department of Commerce.

Dickerson, S., Reinhart, A. M., Feeley, T. H., Bidani, R., Rich, E., Garg, V. K., & Hershey, C. O. (2004). Patient Internet use for health information at three urban primary care clinics. *JAMA, 11,* 499–504. http://dx.doi.org/10.1197/jamia.M1460

Dobkin, B. A., & Pace, R. C. (2003). *Communication in a changing world.* New York: McGrawHill.

Economics and Statistics Administration, & National Telecommunications and Information Administration. (2011). *Exploring the digital nation computer and Internet use at home.* Washington, DC: U.S. Department of Commerce.

Fox, S., & Duggan, M. (2012). *Mobile health 2012.* Washington, DC: Pew Research Center's Internet & American Life Project.

Fox, S., & Duggan, M. (2013a). *Health online 2013.* Washington, DC: Pew Research Center's Internet & American Life Project.

Fox, S., & Duggan, M. (2013b). *Tracking for health.* Washington, DC: Pew Research Center's Internet & American Life Project.

Gardiner, P., Hempstead, M., Ring, L., Bickmore, T., Yinusa-Nyahkoon, L., Tran, H., . . . Jack, B. (2013). Reaching women through health information technology: The Gabby preconception care system. *American Journal of Health Promotion, 27*(3), S11–S20. http://dx.doi.org/10.4278/ajhp .1200113-QUAN-18

Geronimus, A. T. (2001). Understanding and eliminating racial inequalities in women's health in the United States: The role of the weathering conceptual framework. *Journal of American Medical Women's Association, 56,* 133–150.

Guyatt, G. H., Haynes, R. B., Jaeschke, R., Cook, D. J., Green, L., Naylor, C. D., . . . Richardson, W. S. (2000). Users' guides to the medical literature: XXV. Evidence-based medicine: Principles for applying the Users' Guides to patient care. *JAMA, 284,* 1290–1296. http://dx.doi.org/10.1001 /jama.284.10.1290

Institute of Medicine. (2003). *Unequal treatment: Confronting racial and ethnic disparities in healthcare.* Washington, DC: National Academies Press.

Institute of Medicine. (2012). *How far have we come in reducing health disparities? Progress since 2000: Workshop summary.* Washington, DC: National Academies Press.

Johnson, R. L., Roter, D., Powe, N. R., & Cooper, L. A. (2004). Patient race/ethnicity and quality of patient–physician communication during medical visits. *American Journal of Public Health, 94,* 2084–2090.

Joint Commission. (2010). *Advancing effective communication, cultural competence, and patient- and family-centered care: A roadmap for hospitals.* Retrieved from http://www.jointcommission .org/assets/1/6/ARoadmapforHospitalsfinalversion727.pdf

Katz, M. G., Kripalani, S., & Weiss, B. D. (2006). Use of pictorial aids in medication instructions: A review of the literature. *American Journal of Health-System Pharmacy, 63,* 2391–2397. http://dx.doi.org/10.2146/ajhp060162

Keppel, K. G., Pearcy, J. N., & Wagener, D. K. (2002). *Trends in racial and ethnic-specific rates for the health status indicators: United States, 1990–98* (Healthy People Statistical Notes No. 23). Hyattsville, MD: National Center for Health Statistics.

Kind, T., Huang, Z. J., Farr, D., & Pomerantz, K. L. (2005). Internet and computer access and use for health information in an underserved community. *Ambulatory Pediatrics, 5,* 117–121. http://dx.doi.org/10.1367/A04-107R.1

Kleinman, A. (1980). *Patients and healers in the context of culture: An exploration of the borderland between anthropology, medicine, and psychiatry.* Berkeley: University of California Press.

Kleinman, A., Eisenberg, L., & Good, B. (1978). Culture, illness, and care: Clinical lessons from anthropologic and cross-cultural research. *Annals of Internal Medicine, 88,* 251–258. http://dx.doi.org/10.7326/0003-4819-88-2-251

Koh, H. K., Berwick, D. M., Clancy, C. M., Baur, C., Brach, C., Harris, L. M., & Zerhusen, E. G. (2012). New federal policy initiatives to boost health literacy can help the nation move beyond the cycle of costly "crisis care." *Health Affairs, 31,* 434–443. http://dx.doi.org/10.1377 /hlthaff.2011.1169

Kripalani, S., Robertson, R., Love-Ghaffari, M. H., Henderson, L. E., Praska. J., Strawder, A., . . . Jacobson, T. A. (2007). Development of an illustrated medication schedule as a low-literacy patient education tool. *Patient Education and Counseling, 66,* 368–377. http://dx.doi.org/10.1016/j.pec .2007.01.020

Kutner, M., Greenberg, E., Jin, Y., & Paulsen, C. (2006). *The health literacy of America's adults: Results from the 2003 National Assessment of Adult Literacy* (Publication No. NCES 2006–483). Washington, DC: U.S. Department of Education, National Center for Education Statistics.

Levin, S. J., Like, R. C., & Gottlieb, J. E. (2000). ETHNIC: A framework for culturally competent clinical practice. *Patient Care, 34*(9), 188–189.

Lipkus, I. M., Samsa, G., & Rimer, B. K. (2001). General performance on a numeracy scale among highly educated samples. *Medical Decision Making, 21,* 37–44. http://dx.doi .org/10.1177/0272989X0102100105

Lofquist, D., Lugaila, T., O'Connell, M., & Feliz, S. (2012). *Households and families 2010: 2020 Census briefs*. Washington, DC: U.S. Census Bureau.

McQuiggan, S. W., & Lester, J. C. (2007). Modeling and evaluating empathy in embodied companion agents. *International Journal of Human–Computer Studies, 65*, 348–360. http://dx.doi.org/10.1016/j.ijhcs.2006.11.015

National Health Law Program. (2010). *What's in a word? A guide to understanding interpreting and translation in health care*. Retrieved from http://www.healthlaw.org/images/stories/whats _in_a_word_guide.pdf

National Prevention Council. (2011). *National prevention strategy*. Washington, DC: U.S. Department of Health and Human Services, Office of the Surgeon General.

Nielsen-Bohlman, L. T., Panzer, A. M., Hamlin, B., & Kindig, D. A. (2004). *Health literacy: A prescription to end confusion*. Washington DC: National Academies Press.

Office of Disease Prevention and Health Promotion. (2010). *National action plan to improve health literacy*. Washington, DC: U.S. Department of Health and Human Services.

Office of Minority Health. (2005). *A patient-centered guide to implementing language access services in healthcare organizations*. Washington, DC: U.S. Department of Health and Human Services. Retrieved from http://minorityhealth.hhs .gov/Assets/pdf/Checked/HC-LSIG.pdf

Office of Minority Health. (2013a). *National standards for culturally and linguistically appropriate services (CLAS) in health and health care: A blueprint for advancing and sustaining CLAS policy and practice*. Washington, DC: U.S. Department of Health and Human Services. Retrieved from https://www.thinkcultural health.hhs.gov/pdfs/EnhancedCLASStandardsBlueprint.pdf

Office of Minority Health. (2013b). *A physician's practical guide to culturally competent care* [Online course]. Washington, DC: U.S. Department of Health and Human Services. Retrieved from https://cccm.thinkculturalhealth.hhs.gov/default.asp

Office of the National Coordinator for Health Information Technology. (2011). *Federal health information technology strategic plan 2011–2015*. Washington, DC: U.S. Department of Health and Human Services.

Oliver, M. N., Goodwin, M. A., Gotler, R. S., Gregory, P. M., & Stange, K. C. (2001). Time use in clinical encounters: Are African-American patients treated differently? *Journal of the National Medical Association, 93*, 380–385.

Paasche-Orlow, M. K., Schillinger, D., Greene, S. M., & Wagner, E. H. (2006). How health care systems can begin to address the challenge of limited literacy. *Journal of General Internal Medicine, 21*, 884–887. http://dx.doi.org/10.1111 /j.1525-1497.2006.00544.x

Pachter, L. (1994). Culture and clinical care: Folk illness beliefs and behaviors and their implications for health care delivery. *JAMA, 271*, 690–694. http://dx.doi.org/10.1001/jama.271.9.690

Paperny, D. M. (1997, Summer). Computerized expert health assessment with automated health education. *Permanente Journal, 1*(1), 32–37. Retrieved from http://www.thepermanente journal.org/files/Summer1997/healthed.pdf

Parker, R., & Kreps, G. L. (2005). Library outreach: Overcoming health literacy challenges. *Journal of the Medical Library Association, 93*(4), S81–S85.

Patient Protection and Affordable Care Act, Pub. L. 111–148, 42 U.S.C. §§ 18001–18121 (2010).

Project RED. (2014). *Project RED (Re-Engineered Discharge)*. Retrieved from http://www.bu.edu/fammed/projectred/

Rideout, V. (2001). *Generation Rx.com: How young people use the Internet for health information*. Menlo Park, CA: Kaiser Family Foundation.

Roter, D. L., Stewart, M., Putnam, S. M., Lipkin, M., Stiles, W., & Inui, T. S. (1997). Communication patterns of primary care physicians. *JAMA, 277*, 350–356. http://dx.doi.org/10.1001 /jama.1997.03540280088045

Schouten, B. C., & Meeuwesen, L. (2006). Cultural differences in medical communication: A review of the literature. *Patient Education and Counseling, 64*, 21–34. http://dx.doi .org/10.1016/j.pec.2005.11.014

Scott, C. J. (1997). Enhancing patient outcomes through an understanding of intercultural medicine: Guidelines for the practitioner. *Maryland Medical Journal, 46*, 175–180.

Skelly, A. H., Dougherty, M., Gesler, W. M., Soward, A. C., Burns, D., & Arcury, T. A. (2006). African-American beliefs about diabetes. *Western Journal of Nursing Research, 28*, 9–29.

Simon, C. E. (2006). Breast cancer screening: Cultural beliefs and diverse populations. *Health and Social Work, 31*(1), 36–43. http://dx.doi.org/10.1093/hsw/31.1.36

Sperling, J. (2011). *Communicating more for less: Using translation and interpretation technology to serve limited English proficient individuals*. Washington, DC: Migration Policy Institute.

Stewart, M., Brown, J. B., Donner, A., McWhinney, I. R., Oates, J., Weston, W. W., & Jordan, J. (2000). The impact of patient-centered care on outcomes. *Journal of Family Practice, 49*, 796–804.

Suurmond, J., & Seeleman, C. (2006). Shared decision-making in an intercultural context: Barriers in the interaction between physicians and immigrant patients. *Patient Education and Counseling, 60*, 253–259. http://dx.doi.org/10.1016/j.pec .2005.01.012

Tudor-Locke, C., Bassett, D. R., Swartz, A. M., Strath, S. J., Parr, B. B., Reis, J. P., & Ainsworth, B. E. (2004). A preliminary study of one year of pedometer self-monitoring. *Annals of Behavioral Medicine, 28*, 158–162. http://dx.doi .org/10.1207/s15324796abm2803_3

U.S. Census Bureau. (2016). *QuickFacts: United States*. Retrieved from http://www.census.gov/quickfacts/table/PST045215/00

U.S. Department of Health and Human Services. (2000). *Healthy People 2010: Understanding and improving health* (2nd ed.). Washington, DC: U.S. Government Printing Office.

U.S. Department of Health and Human Services. (2001). *National standards for culturally and linguistically appropriate services in health care: Final report.* Rockville, MD: Author.

U.S. Department of Health and Human Services. (2010). *Healthy People 2020: Disparities.* Retrieved from http://www.healthypeople.gov/2020/about/DisparitiesAbout.aspx

U.S. Department of Health and Human Services. (2011). *HHS action plan to reduce racial and ethnic health disparities: A nation free of disparities in health and healthcare.* Washington, DC: Author.

U.S. Department of Health and Human Services. (2013). *Healthy People 2020: Health communication and health information technology.* Retrieved from http://www.healthypeople.gov/2020/topicsobjectives2020/overview.aspx?topicid=18

Vermeire, E., Hearnshaw, H., Van Royen, P., & Denekens, J. (2001). Patient adherence to treatment: Three decades of research. A comprehensive review. *Journal of Clinical Pharmacology and Therapeutics, 26,* 331–342. http://dx.doi.org/10.1046/j.1365-2710.2001.00363.x

Woloshin, S., Bickell, N. A., Schwartz, L. M., Gany, F., & Welch, H. G. (1995). Language barriers in medicine in the United States. *JAMA, 273,* 724–728. http://dx.doi.org/10.1001/jama.1995.03520330054037

Yin, H. S., Dreyer, B. P., van Schaick, L., Foltin, G. L., Dinglas, C., & Mendelsohn, A. L. (2008). Randomized controlled trial of a pictogram-based intervention to reduce liquid medication dosing errors and improve adherence among caregivers of young children. *Archives of Pediatric Adolescent Medicine, 162,* 814–822. http://dx.doi.org/10.1001/archpedi.162.9.814

Zickuhr, K., & Smith, A. (2012). *Digital differences.* Washington, DC: Pew Research Center. Retrieved from http://www.pewinternet.org/2012/04/13/digital-differences

Section II.D.

PLAN FOR EFFECTIVENESS AND REFLECTION

Chapter 13.

CONSTRUCTING A PERSONAL PLAN TO DEVELOP CULTURAL EFFECTIVENESS

Roxie M. Black, PhD, OTR/L, FAOTA

To prepare students to be effective practitioners, we must design curricula that enable them to lessen or eradicate the disparities of care for populations who come from divergent backgrounds, to effectively partner with them in health care decisions, and to function as their health care advocates.
Ana E. Núñez (2000, p. 1071)

Chapter Highlights

- Strategic Planning for Change
- Determine Your Level of Willingness to Engage
- Establish Goals and Action Steps
- Engage in Self-Awareness Activities
- Develop Support Systems
- Develop Resources to Improve Your Cultural Knowledge
- Seek Knowledge Through Intercultural Experiences
- Critically Reflect on Your Interactions
- Periodically Reevaluate Your Goals and Progress

Key Terms and Concepts

✧ Cautious willingness
✧ Committed willingness
✧ Critical reflection

✧ Support systems
✧ Unreflective willingness

Culturally effective care has the potential to reduce health disparities. Evidence "indicates that culturally effective services may improve health outcomes, increase the efficiency of clinical and support staff, and result in greater client satisfaction with services" (Anderson, Scrimshaw, Fullilove, Fielding, & Normand, 2003, p. 68).

Earlier chapters of this text outlined the characteristics needed for effective cross-cultural interactions, which include cultural self-awareness, a willing attitude of openness and engagement, knowledge of diverse others, cross-cultural skills, and critical reflection. Acquiring such skills and knowledge can be a complex and lifelong process, but using a strategic approach such as the one discussed in this chapter simplifies and guides the process. This chapter describes a strategic approach to constructing a personal plan to develop cultural effectiveness that anyone can follow on his or her own, inside and outside of the classroom. Parts of the process, such as learning about a specific cultural group, may be relatively brief, but the entire process can continue throughout one's lifetime.

Strategic Planning for Change

Although each cross-cultural interaction has the potential to change the participants in myriad ways, the type of change (e.g., positive or negative, superficial or substantive) cannot be predicted, and practitioners cannot control the results of this interplay. However, those who wish to be more prepared and effective in communicating with people who are different from themselves can intentionally and strategically develop a plan for change.

Formal education for culturally effective care may be obtained by multiple means, as evidenced in Section IV, "Culture and Education," of this text. However you approach developing a plan to advance your cultural effectiveness, you'll need training to address your developmental needs. Such training can involve a variety of methods, including minilectures, group discussions, interactive exercises, role-playing, selected readings, videos, and videotaping clients and colleagues followed by discussion of issues noted. Community tours and visits, discussion with community members, and home visits all can be part of your personal plan. Because learning about others and reflecting on your own beliefs and biases can evoke strong emotions, training and learning may be most effective when you set aside time for critical reflection on the emotions that are elicited and examination of the desired responses.

The following steps are recommended in constructing your personal plan; take these steps in the order that works best for you:

- Determine your level of willingness to engage.
- Establish goals and action steps.
- Engage in self-awareness activities.

- Develop support systems.
- Develop resources to improve your cultural knowledge.
- Seek knowledge through intercultural experiences.
- Critically reflect on your interactions.
- Periodically reevaluate your goals and progress.

Table 13.1 provides an outline for constructing a personal plan to achieve cultural effectiveness, and Table 13.2 shows an example of a specific plan.

Determine Your Level of Willingness to Engage

Research indicates that people engaged in cross-cultural interactions do so with varying levels of motivation or willingness (Black, 2002). When planning to improve your cross-cultural interaction skills, it helps if you first determine whether your willingness level is

1. Unreflective willingness,
2. Cautious willingness, or
3. Committed willingness.

People who demonstrate *unreflective willingness* choose to interact with diverse others because they are expected to and feel that they should. *Cautious willingness* can be observed in people who demonstrate a willingness to learn and behave in a more effective manner but are hesitant because of a lack of confidence in their abilities or fear of making mistakes. *Committed willingness* is seen in those who are not only willing to interact with others but also seek out opportunities to do so. More information about these levels can be found in Chapter 11, "Developing Cross-Cultural Communication Skills." Once you have identified where you are starting from in your personal plan for change, you can engage in other activities to develop your cultural self-awareness.

Establish Goals and Action Steps

Your level of willingness will determine the goals you choose. Identify 3 to 5 clear, achievable goals that will guide your progress. Determine specific, measureable action steps for each goal and a reasonable timeline for achieving these steps. The dates on the timeline should be no longer than a year's time, and

Table 13.1. Constructing a Personal Plan to Develop Cultural Effectiveness

Step	Activities to Promote Change
Determine your level of willingness to do this work.	Review the three levels of willingness found in Chapter 11 of this book. Determine the level that best describes you.
Establish goals and action steps.	Develop concrete action steps and a timeline. (See Table 13.2 for a sample plan.) Action steps addressing the basic components of self-awareness, knowledge, skills, and critical reflection must be part of the plan.
Engage in self-awareness activities that help you assess your personal context.	Seek out activities that facilitate self-reflection. Examine your values, beliefs, behaviors, roles, biases, perceptions, knowledge, work and personal ethics, health beliefs, family roles and relationships, and communication style. Being honest about yourself is necessary for understanding who you are and how you view the world. Admitting to both the negative and positive aspects of your personality is essential for making changes and acquiring new knowledge and skills. From this assessment, determine what areas you need to work on.
Develop support systems.	Developing support systems is difficult and ongoing. Seek out allies, colleagues, advocates, and role models to help you through this process. You'll need a safe environment to discuss issues and concerns openly, freely, and without fear of being judged. Support systems will help you deal with the discomfort that occurs when your views and beliefs are challenged.
Develop resources to improve your cultural knowledge.	Find and examine sources of information, tools, and people who will increase your knowledge base. Locating and securing training materials, advisers, courses, consultants, and mentors are vital to developing cultural effectiveness.
Seek knowledge through intercultural experiences.	Attend cultural celebrations and ceremonies in your area, including faith-based rituals that are open to the public. Visit restaurants, museums, and the homes of peers who are culturally different from you.
Critically reflect on your interactions.	During and after intercultural interactions and experiences, make the time to consider your reactions and feelings. Ask yourself the following questions: • Did I experience any bias or stereotyping? • Was I comfortable during the interaction? • Was I satisfied with my responses during the interaction? • Might I have responded in a more effective manner? • What did I learn during this interaction about myself? • About the other person or group? • How will I improve on my actions during the next interaction?
Periodically reevaluate your goals and progress.	Review your goals and action steps and determine whether you have met your goals and made progress on your action steps. Revise unmet goals and develop new goals.

Table 13.2. Example of a Personal Plan

Goal	Action Step	Date	Measure
I will learn more about Somali culture.	I will read 2 books written about the culture.	Complete by December 15	First book completed by November 15, 2nd by December 15
I will attend events where I can interact with Somalis.	I will attend 2 Somali cultural celebrations.	Complete by February 28	First celebration attended December 31st, 2nd by February 28
I will get to know my Somali classmates.	I will introduce myself and spend time with them between classes and during lunch.	Complete by Thanksgiving	Met with them at least once per week through Thanksgiving
I will monitor and reflect on my own reactions during and after interactions with Somali peers.	I will keep a weekly journal of personal reflections and discuss it with a trusted friend.	Meet at least 2 times between September and late November	Completed reflective journal and met with friend on September 12 and November 20

some activities may be completed within a shorter time frame. Identify the measurement you will use to determine the successful completion of your activities.

Engage in Self-Awareness Activities

During the process of improving self-awareness, one asks, Who am I? The purpose is to determine the need for change to be a more effective practitioner. The process includes an honest examination of your values, beliefs, behaviors, roles, biases, perceptions, knowledge, personal ethics, and health beliefs, among others. It is important to identify, recognize, and admit to both negative and positive characteristics in your personality and beliefs so you can determine which attributes you might choose to change. Recognizing how these attributes and attitudes shape your interactions with others is an important first step toward changing your practice to respect differences in others. Such differences are not limited to race and ethnicity but also extend to socioeconomic status, gender identity, religion, age, and ability, among others.

Although self-awareness is probably the most difficult characteristic to attain, there are many resources to help you honestly review your own values, beliefs, and behaviors. Numerous self-awareness activities can be found in the literature, in Chapters 8, "Acquiring Cultural Self-Awareness," and 11, "Developing Cross-Cultural Communication Skills," in this book, and on diversity training sites online. Exhibit 13.1 provides a self-awareness activity I have successfully used with students.

Develop Support Systems

Many people and organizations can be your *support systems* during this process. Support systems may include your student peers, your program faculty, your family and friends, and organizations such as your local library, a clinic that supports refugees and immigrants in your area, or local senior organizations. These supports are "safe places" where you can discuss your concerns, doubts, and progress without fear of criticism or reprisal.

As you seek out these settings and people, remember to look for people and places where you know that you can talk and ask questions freely and safely about intercultural interactions.

Reflection 13.1. Self-Assessment

- Some people have a difficult time examining themselves in an honest manner. Do you?

Develop Resources to Improve Your Cultural Knowledge

While working toward increased cultural self-awareness, you can begin gathering information about diverse groups of people and the sociopolitical issues they face. Guidance on working with diverse people and populations can be found in the following documents:

- National Standards for Culturally and Linguistically Appropriate Services (CLAS) in Health and Health Care (Office of Minority Health, 2013)
- Accreditation standards for occupational therapy education (Accreditation Council for Occupational Therapy Education, 2012)
- *Occupational Therapy Code of Ethics (2015)* (American Occupational Therapy Association 2015; see also Slater, 2016).

You also can seek knowledge through scholarly books, novels, and videos and documentaries about various cultures that identify their beliefs about health, wellness, and illness. For example, understanding a culture's folk medicine can help you see benefits and appropriate uses of traditional health beliefs and behaviors in the treatment process. Understanding the sociocultural climate, the socially dominant forces and hierarchies, and the oppression of those who belong to nondominant groups is necessary to understanding the lives of members of those groups.

Reflection 13.2. Personal Traditional Beliefs

- Does your family have any traditional approaches to illnesses that are similar to folk medicine?
- What are they? Share with a colleague or peer.

Seek Knowledge Through Intercultural Experiences

Some of the best cultural knowledge comes from interactions with people from diverse backgrounds.

Exhibit 13.1. Assessing How You Relate to Various Groups of People

The following are different levels of response you might have toward a person or a cultural group:

- *Greet:* I feel I can greet this person warmly and sincerely welcome him or her.
- *Accept:* I feel I can honestly accept this person as he or she is and be comfortable enough to listen to his or her problems.
- *Help:* I feel I would genuinely try to help this person with his or her problems as they might relate to or arise from the label or stereotype given to him or her.
- *Background:* I feel I have the background of knowledge or experience to be able to help this person.
- *Advocate:* I feel I could honestly be an advocate for this person.

Below is a list of types of people. Read the list, and place a check mark by anyone you would not hesitate to greet, accept, help, and so forth. Try to respond honestly, not as you think might be socially or professionally desirable. Your answers are only for your personal use in clarifying your initial reactions to different people.

Type of Person	Greet	Accept	Help	Have Background On	Advocate
Haitian					
Child abuser					
Muslim					
Neo-Nazi					
Mexican American					
Catholic					
Elderly person with dementia					
IV drug user					
Native American					
Prostitute					
Jehovah's Witness					
Convict					
Somali					
Gay man or lesbian					
Person with AIDS					
African American					
Atheist					
Member of the Ku Klux Klan					
Alcoholic					
White American					
Amish					
Unmarried pregnant teen					
Transgender person					

Source. Adapted from *Strategies for Working With Culturally Diverse Communities and Clients,* by E. Randall-David, 1989, Washington, DC: Association for the Care of Children's Health. Copyright © 1989 by The Association for the Care of Children's Health. Adapted with permission.

In my experience, showing respect and interest and politely asking questions about someone's culture and beliefs are usually met with acceptance and positive interactions.

Structured opportunities to work with people from other cultures and ethnicities provide valuable, practical, and specific knowledge and might include

- Visiting a community you would like to learn more about and performing a community assessment, which involves walking or driving around and taking note of the community's places of worship, grocery stores, parks, recreational facilities, and neighborhood restaurants;
- Engaging with culturally or ethnically organized student groups, medical groups, or community

groups and asking about specific health issues important to their community; and

- Arranging a panel of traditional healers (e.g., *curanderos,* herbalists, shamans, medicine men and women) or practitioners of alternative medicine to discuss their methods and cultural beliefs.

The result of such exploration is increased cultural knowledge and the beginning of cultural skill development.

Critically Reflect on Your Interactions

Assessing your own performance and behavior during and after any cross-cultural interaction or intercultural experience is a vital and unique component of developing cultural effectiveness. This self-assessment can be done through the application of ***critical reflection:*** "The purpose of reflection is to work out what is already known and add new information with the result of drawing out knowledge, new meaning and a higher level of understanding" (Moon, as quoted in Paterson & Chapman, 2013, p. 134).

Several strategies are used in critical reflection. You may choose to write in your personal plan that you will keep a journal in which you reflect on your cross-cultural interactions. Or you may set time aside for thoughtful consideration after an interaction, perhaps using a list of pertinent questions to facilitate your thinking. These questions might include the following:

- Did I experience any bias or stereotyping?
- Was I comfortable during the interaction?
- Am I satisfied with my responses during the interaction?
- Might I have responded in a more effective manner?
- What did I learn during this interaction
  - About myself?
  - About the other person or group?
- How will I improve on my actions during the next opportunity to do so?

Another effective strategy is to have someone observe the cross-cultural interaction between you and a client and then give a critical evaluation of your

performance. This information can be considered during your self-reflection. Exhibit 13.1 provides an activity that can further aid your self-assessment.

Reflection 13.3. Assessing How You Relate

Ask each member of a class or a group of friends to complete the activity in Exhibit 13.1. When completed, compare your results with the others in the group. Consider the following questions during your discussion:

- Were you surprised at any of your responses? What other feelings (e.g., anger, embarrassment) did you experience?
- If there were types of people that you would not want to address, talk about what your options might be if you confronted them in your occupational therapy practice.
- If you needed to work with people from a population that you have negative feelings about, could you provide them with effective care? Why or why not?
- What does the *Occupational Therapy Code of Ethics* (AOTA, 2015) say about this kind of practice dilemma?

Periodically Reevaluate Your Goals and Progress

The final step in constructing a personal plan to develop cultural effectiveness is to regularly evaluate your progress. Evaluation is the time to review your goals and action steps and determine whether you have met your goals and made progress on your action steps. If you have, what goals would you like to achieve next? Questions to ask include the following:

- Am I more open to others who are different from me?
- Have I increased my knowledge of the diverse groups with whom I work?
- Am I more comfortable and skilled in interacting with diverse others?
- If I have not yet met all the goals in my personal plan, are they the most appropriate goals, or should I consider others?
- What should be my next steps?

Summary

This chapter outlined a way to develop a personal plan that will help you become a more culturally effective practitioner. Providing culturally effective care to your clients is mandated in many occupational therapy documents. Becoming a culturally effective occupational therapy practitioner takes time, motivation, and a willingness to critically evaluate and consider your performance as you interact with diverse persons and groups.

References

Accreditation Council for Occupational Therapy Education. (2012). 2011 Accreditation Council for Occupational Therapy Education (ACOTE') standards. *American Journal of Occupational Therapy, 66*(Suppl.), S6–S74. http://dx.doi.org/10.5014/ajot.2012.66S6

American Occupational Therapy Association. (2015). Occupational therapy code of ethics (2015). *American Journal of Occupational Therapy, 69*(Suppl. 3), 6913410030. http://dx.doi.org/10.5014/ajot.2015.696S03

Anderson, L. M., Scrimshaw, S. C., Fullilove, M. T., Fielding, J. E., & Normand, J., Task Force on Community Preventive Services. (2003). Culturally competent healthcare systems: A systematic review. *American Journal of Preventive Medicine, 24*(3 Suppl.), 68–79. Retrieved from https://www.thecommunityguide.org/social/soc-AJPM-evrev-healthcare-systems.pdf

Black, R. M. (2002). *The essence of cultural competence: Listening to the voices of occupational therapy students.* Unpublished doctoral dissertation. Lesley University, Cambridge, MA.

Núñez, A. E. (2000). Transforming cultural competence into cross-cultural efficacy in women's health education. *Academic Medicine, 75*(11), 1071–1080. Retrieved from http://journals.lww.com/academicmedicine/Fulltext/2000/11000/Transforming_Cultural_Competence_into.11.aspx

Office of Minority Health. (2013). *National standards for culturally and linguistically appropriate services (CLAS) in health and health care: A blueprint for advancing and sustaining CLAS policy and practice.* Washington, DC: U.S. Department of Health and Human Services. Retrieved from https://www.thinkculturalhealth.hhs.gov/pdfs/EnhancedCLASStandardsBlueprint.pdf

Paterson, C., & Chapman, J. (2013). Enhancing skills of critical reflection to evidence learning in professional practice. *Physical Therapy in Sport, 14,* 133–138. http://dx.doi.org/10.1016/j.ptsp.2013.03.004

Randall-David, E. (1989). *Strategies for working with culturally diverse communities and clients.* Washington, DC: Association for the Care of Children's Health.

Slater, D. Y. (Ed.). (2016). *Reference guide to the Occupational Therapy Code of Ethics (2015 ed.).* Bethesda, MD: AOTA Press.

Section III.

CULTURE AND CLINICAL PRACTICE

Chapter 14.

CULTURE AND CLINICAL PRACTICE

Shirley A. Wells, DrPH, OTR, FAOTA

We ain't what we want to be; we ain't what we gonna be; but thank God, we ain't what we was.
African American folk saying (Johnson, 1995, p. 14)

Chapter Highlights

- Culture and Clinical Interaction
- Culture and Clinical Reasoning
- Culture and Clinical Practice
- Culture and Evaluation
- Cultural Knowledge in Practice
- Culture and the Occupational Therapy Process
- Cultural Approach to Health Service Delivery

Key Terms and Concepts

✧ Clinical reasoning
✧ Conditional reasoning
✧ Critical reflection
✧ Cultural brokering
✧ Cultural clinical interaction
✧ Cultural humility
✧ Cultural knowledge
✧ Cultural safety
✧ Culturally effective care
✧ Diagnostic reasoning
✧ Ethnocentrism

✧ Ethnorelativism
✧ Interactive reasoning
✧ Interprofessional collaborative practice
✧ Logical reasoning
✧ Narrative reasoning
✧ Outcomes
✧ Pragmatic reasoning
✧ Procedural reasoning
✧ Professional reasoning
✧ Scientific reasoning

Understanding the meaning of culture, cultural effectiveness, and health disparities and incorporating these meanings into practice constitute a mission many occupational therapy practitioners and students have embraced. Much has been published in the area of diversity and cultural sensitivity that educates practitioners and students about different cultural values and norms and describes the health beliefs and practices of various racial, ethnic, and cultural groups (Balcazar, Suarez-Balcazar, Taylor-Ritzler, &

Keys, 2009; Bonder & Martin, 2013; Office of Minority Health, 2014). The medical literature supports the assertion that an understanding of the health beliefs and behaviors of particular cultural groups can lead to a better understanding of how individual clients perceive and take action to address illness and can improve practitioners' clinical judgment (Andrés-Hyman, Ortiz, Anez, Paris, & Davidson, 2006; Hickling, 2012; Institute of Medicine [IOM], 2013; Kleinman & Benson, 2006).

Many practitioners and students lack a clear understanding of how to integrate culture into their daily practice of decision making, assessment, and intervention. It is one of the least developed aspects of occupational therapy knowledge on a practical level. Poor integration of cultural knowledge into clinical practice can result in a sense of dissatisfaction and disharmony for both clients and providers. Practitioners may feel inadequate in their intervention choices, leading to inappropriate treatment models. This chapter presents practical ways to integrate culture into the daily clinical process, including incorporating culture into clinical assessments and evaluations, using cultural knowledge and skills to design intervention strategies, and reflecting on the outcomes.

Culture and Clinical Interaction

A plethora of literature focuses on the influence of culture on health and health care, the therapeutic relationship, and treatment outcomes, as well as the need for provider training and education. Health care professionals are challenged to understand the cultural needs of their clients, to collaborate with their clients, and to integrate awareness of multiple cultures to provide culturally effective client-centered care.

An essential step in establishing a satisfying and productive therapeutic relationship is acknowledging that multiple cultures are involved in the relationship and that every clinical encounter is a *cultural clinical interaction.* The multiple cultures involved in any given clinical encounter include, at a minimum,

- The personal or familial culture of the provider,
- The personal or familial culture of the client and his or her family,
- The traditional medical culture, and
- The culture of the primary medical system (Fitzgerald, 1992; see Figure 14.1).

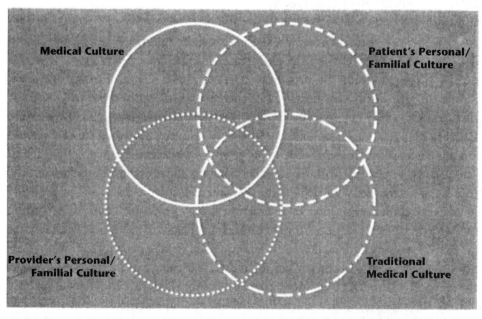

Figure 14.1. The four overlapping cultures present in clinical interactions.
Note. From "Multicultural Clinical Interactions," by M. H. Fitzgerald, 1992, *Journal of Rehabilitation, 58,* p. 39 Copyright © 1992 by the National Rehabilitation Association. Adapted with permission.

Awareness of these multiple cultures is fairly easy to maintain when the participants in the interaction come from obviously different cultural backgrounds, but it is more difficult when the participants have similar backgrounds and appearances (American Evaluation Association [AEA], 2011).

Skills Required in Cultural Clinical Interactions

Cultural diversity is a fact in the United States. Every person is a product of multiple cultures and interprets reality through his or her cultural filters. In a multicultural health care environment, practitioners must engage in cultural brokering, cultural safety, and cultural humility to provide client-centered care and improve the health outcomes of ethnic and racial minority populations (see Exhibit 14.1).

Cultural brokering is a health care intervention through which the professional uses his or her cultural and health science knowledge and skills to negotiate with the client and the health care system for an effective, beneficial health care plan (Wenger, 1995, as cited in National Center for Cultural Competence, 2004). The strength of cultural brokering is in its emphasis on respect, caring, understanding, and patience in health care encounters (Warda, 2000).

Adopting a culturally safe approach to client care can benefit individuals, providers, institutions, and health care systems. *Cultural safety* is achieved when the services provided are based in the culture of the individual seeking the services (IOM, 2013). Culturally safe care is delivered in the client's language and is consistent with the client's traditional practices.

Cultural humility is the recognition by service providers of the common disconnect between clients and providers. It integrates a lifelong commitment to engaging in self-evaluation and critique, to addressing the power imbalances in the provider–client relationship, and to developing mutually beneficial partnerships (Tervalon & Murray-García, 1998). The process of developing cultural humility helps providers acknowledge and address the imbalance of power that naturally exists in the client–provider interaction. Through the use of client- and

---

Exhibit 14.1. Guidelines for Creating a Multicultural Approach and Environment

- Expect every client, family, colleague, or person to be different. (A "client" is not "just a client.") Each individual has his or her own identity, culture, ethnicity, background, experiences, and lifestyle.
- The culture and lifestyle of people matter. Being aware of and respecting differences are not enough: Knowledge about the impact of these differences must be integrated into all your interactions.
- Take into account the client's culture and how it affects and shapes the individual.
- Acknowledge that some health beliefs and practices are derived from basic needs and may have little basis in reality. Also be aware that some practices you consider to be "primitive" do serve a purpose for the person within the culture and must be respected.
- Be cognizant of gender and age. These characteristics influence the approach the practitioner uses and the perceptions held by the client, family, or caregiver about the practitioner.
- Use good basic health care practices, such as completing a thorough assessment with the client and family, checking diet restrictions before planning or initiating a cooking activity, involving the client and family in the program, and doing an assessment of the home environment.
- Look for cues, both verbal and nonverbal, that will help you involve the client in the treatment session.
- Be flexible and adaptable in your treatment of the client, and avoid a cookbook approach.
- Be aware of your personal biases and how they may affect the therapeutic relationship.
- Don't misjudge people because of their accent or grammar.
- Avoid being patronizing or condescending. Use language that fosters trust and alliance.
- Use an interpreter if you are not fluent in the client's preferred language. If an interpreter is unavailable, learn basic words, phrases, or sentences in that language to show that you're making an effort to identify with the client.
- Be aware of discriminatory intent vs. discriminatory effect; that is, a policy, test, or standard that is applied equally to all has the effect of excluding minorities vs. someone receiving different treatment than others because of his or her race, age, sex, national origin, religion, or disability. Be an agent of change.
- Listening to the client and being responsive to his or her needs is a demonstration of cultural competence. It is important to understand the world from the perspective of the client, family, and caregiver.

Source. American Occupational Therapy Association (1996).

family-focused interviewing and care, practitioners can develop humility, and a mutually respectful partnership between the provider and client can be maintained (IOM, 2013).

Reflection 14.1. Mrs. Garcia: Cultural Food Beliefs

During an inpatient treatment session, Mrs. Garcia, a 32-year-old woman recovering from a spinal fusion, tells you that she is hungry. You ask her why. She states, "I did not eat breakfast this morning; the food was cold, and I can't eat cold food."

- What cultural health belief system does this client subscribe to?

- What questions might you ask to clarify this situation?

- What cultural knowledge do you need to gather? Where will you find the needed information?

Need for Interprofessional Collaborative Practice

As interprofessional practice takes hold in the delivery of health care, it can serve to maximize accessibility to health care and to facilitate effective cross-cultural caregiving by health care professionals who are not members of minority groups (Bridges, Davidson, Odegard, Maki, & Tomkowiak, 2011; Minore & Boone, 2002). *Interprofessional collaborative practice* occurs when health care workers from different professional backgrounds work together with clients, families, and communities to deliver the highest quality client- and family-centered care (World Health Organization, 2010).

From a literature review of cultural competence and interprofessional practice, Purden (2005) concluded the following:

- Interprofessional collaboration should include local paraprofessionals and key community workers and professionals.
- Professional and community leaders should facilitate opportunities for professionals and paraprofessional community members to collaborate on actual client care situations.

- The sustainability and relevance of interprofessional community health programs and services require the support and participation of the community.

Successful collaboration is likely to result in services that are a blend of ideas and perspectives from traditional healing practice and conventional Western health care. The principles of interprofessional collaborative practice, such as openness, mutual respect, inclusiveness, responsiveness, and understanding of one another's roles, are fundamental to the delivery of culturally competent services to racial and ethnic-minority communities and to communities at large (Interprofessional Education Collaborative Expert Panel, 2011).

Culture and Clinical Reasoning

Occupational therapy practitioners use professional reasoning and critical thinking to plan, direct, develop, and reflect on interventions that are acceptable, meaningful, and satisfying to clients (Schell, 2014). Clinical reasoning helps practitioners establish a framework for intervention and care that preserves or maintains the client's cultural perspective, accommodates and negotiates change to promote the client's health, and repatterns and restructures cultural beliefs and behaviors as necessary (Kleinman & Benson, 2006).

Occupational therapy practitioners already use clinical reasoning as a guide to organize and articulate their thinking in clinical practice to individualize treatment, facilitate functional performance, and create positive outcomes for their clients. Thus, clinical reasoning is the perfect process for infusing culture into daily practice (American Occupational Therapy Association [AOTA], 2014; Bass, 2014; Mu, Coppard, Bracciano, Doll, & Matthews, 2010).

Aspects of Clinical Reasoning

Reasoning is the metacognitive analysis health care providers engage in when they "actually think about thinking" (Schell, 2014, p. 384). *Clinical reasoning* is an umbrella term to include all the complex reasoning processes that health care providers use when thinking about their client, the disability, the situation, and the personal and cultural meanings that the client gives to the disability, the situation, and the self (Fleming, 1991; Schell, 2014). The term *professional reasoning* is sometimes used and is a broader term for the reasoning process all professionals engage in regardless of setting (e.g., medical, educational, community; AOTA, 2014; Schell & Schell, 2007).

Occupational therapy practitioners use theoretical principles and models, knowledge about the effects of conditions on participation, and available evidence on the effectiveness of intervention to guide their thinking. In clinical practice, experienced practitioners engage in multiple clinical reasoning episodes for each client. Practitioners use cognitive and scientific reasoning to integrate the client's history, evaluation information, and cultural context into an individualized intervention plan (Schell, 2014). Clinical reasoning is challenging and requires determination and active engagement in deliberate practice and continued learning; it also requires reflection on activities designed to improve performance (Ericsson, Whyte, & Ward, 2007).

Occupational therapy practitioners reconstruct the client's ability to function and perform daily life tasks within his or her cultural context. Practitioners and clients work on rebuilding clients' sense of self, ways of accomplishing tasks and engaging in activities, and ways of viewing themselves and their lives (AOTA, 2014). The practitioner, to accomplish this, uses a variety of reasoning strategies. Fleming and Mattingly (1994) described the reasoning of occupational therapy practitioners as not one, but several forms of thinking, including narrative, interactive, pragmatic, conditional, and procedural reasoning, all of which provide practitioners with ways to understand a person's illness experience:

- *Narrative reasoning* focuses on the client's occupational story, life history, cultural background, activities, and roles the client values.
- *Interactive reasoning* is used in looking for the meaning of the disease or disability to the client. It also encompasses the interpersonal interaction between the practitioner and the client.
- *Pragmatic reasoning* is used in considering the treatment environment and possibilities for treatment within the given environment. The practitioner's values, knowledge, abilities, and

experience, as well as the client's social and financial resources, also are considered.
- *Conditional reasoning* is used to continuously modify treatment as necessary to enable the person to function in the future.
- *Procedural reasoning* is used in identifying problems and interventions on the basis of the client's disease or impairment and may reflect the habits and culture of the setting. Procedural reasoning involves the evaluative process of obtaining data necessary to select an intervention, including interview, observation, and formal evaluation using standardized measures.

Schell (2014) described the *scientific reasoning* that practitioners engage in when providing care as comprising scientific inquiry methods such as hypothesis testing, theory-based decision making, and application of statistical evidence to clinical decisions. Scientific reasoning is based on an understanding of heath conditions that affect clients and is used to decide on interventions. It involves the use of applied *logical reasoning,* which is the ability to think through problems and apply strategies to solve them, and *diagnostic reasoning,* which involves investigation and analysis of the cause or etiology of conditions. Diagnostic reasoning is based on the science and evidence of practice.

Occupational therapy practitioners use clinical reasoning to understand clients from the clients' own point of view—in other words, to see clients as the clients see themselves. Using narrative and interactive reasoning, practitioners attempt to understand the meanings people make of themselves and their lives, families, environment, and culture. Failure to assess cultural considerations in the clinical reasoning process can prevent practitioners from establishing a therapeutic relationship based on equality and mutual respect and may create reluctance in the client to participate in the treatment program (Black & Wells, 2007).

Critical Reflection

The encircling construct for clinical reasoning and cultural effectiveness is *critical reflection.* During the clinical process, the practitioner seeks to understand what worked, what did not work, why changes occurred, and what the changes mean for the client's future (Schell, 2014; Schon, 1983). Reflective practitioners participate in critical reflection before engaging with the client to become aware of their thinking processes, to track how their thinking developed over time, and to become more confident and competent as practitioners (Leung, Pluye, Grad, & Weston, 2010; Oelofsen, 2012).

Practitioners who are able to think critically rely on reflection, induction, deduction, analysis, challenge of assumptions, and evaluation of data and information to guide decision making. Critical reflection skills are essential to assist practitioners in rethinking outmoded approaches to health care, health promotion, and prevention of illness and complications, especially when cultural views are involved. Therefore, learning and reflection improve the quality and effectiveness of the interaction.

Culture and Clinical Practice

Success in clinical practice depends on the awareness that people have reasons for their decisions and behaviors, regardless of whether they can articulate those reasons or whether the health care worker recognizes what they are (AOTA, 2014; Kleinman & Benson, 2006). Culture plays a significant role in the decisions and behaviors of not only clients but also of providers. Using a set of behavioral standards developed according to the norms of the practitioner or medical system to assess a client from another culture is a cultural imposition.

In a review of cultural competence in nursing education, Waite and Calamaro (2010) concluded that

students and practicing nurses must be prepared to easily understand the influence of

---

Reflection 14.2. Culturally Different Client: Clinical Reasoning

Using the aspects of clinical reasoning (narrative, interactive, pragmatic, conditional, procedural, and scientific reasoning), how would you solicit and integrate cultural information for the following client?

Yesenia, a 48-year-old Mexican American woman, was found by her daughter at home with a broken hip. This is her third bone fracture—following bretaks to her right wrist and left humerus—in the past 12 months. She was diagnosed with osteoporosis and has a family history of diabetes and high blood pressure. Examination revealed limited active range of motion (ROM) of the right hip in all planes and increased pain with all movement, decreased right lower-extremity weight bearing, and difficulty walking. She also has decreased muscle strength of both upper extremities and limited ROM of the right wrists. She has been placed on a calcium-enriched diet and supplement.

Yesenia is the daughter of migrant farm workers. She has been married for 30 years and is the mother of 4 daughters and 2 sons, ranging in age from 16 to 25. She has worked as a laborer and store clerk and is currently not working. She lives with her husband and 4 children in a one-level three-bedroom house.

Finish the chart:

Reasoning	Client Information	Questions to Solicit Cultural Information
Narrative	A 48-year-old Mexican American woman Fracture of right wrists and left humerus in the past 12 months; diagnosed with osteoporosis.	What cultural group do you identify with? How would you describe your family structure? Describe your spirituality or religious practice or belief? In what language do you prefer to discuss your health and treatment: English or Spanish?
Interactive	Examination revealed limited active ROM of the right hip in all planes and increased pain with all movement, decreased right lower-extremity weight bearing, and difficulty walking. She also has decreased muscle strength of both upper extremities and limited ROM of the right wrists; currently not working.	What do you think caused your problem(s)? Have you tried any home remedies, medicines, folk or traditional treatment for your problem/illness? How would you describe a state of wellness or good health? A state of poor health? Are there any cultural, religious, or spiritual beliefs or practices that may influence your care?
Pragmatic		
Conditional		
Procedural		
Scientific		

culture in individuals' perceptions of their health needs and in their responses to the healthcare services they receive. Clinicians must also understand that the degree of clients' compliance with and their response to treatment will be significantly affected by the degree of congruence between their expectations and the care they receive. It is, therefore, essential that nurses be prepared to provide care that is culturally competent. We can no longer ask if nurses are ready to meet this challenge; it is an expected mandate for those who are practicing from an ethical perspective. (pp. 78–79)

According to the *Occupational Therapy Practice Framework: Domain and Process* (AOTA, 2014), engagement and participation in occupation take place within contexts, which include culture: "Cultural context includes customs, beliefs, activity patterns, behavior standards, and expectations accepted by the society of which a client is a member. It influences the client's identity and activity choices, and practitioners must be aware of these norms" (p. S9). The practitioner's understanding that all people are products of their own culture; have knowledge of other cultures; and are able to bridge cultures can lead to positive, rewarding, and effective clinical interactions.

Awareness of the relationships among culture, clinical reasoning, and practice enables a culturally effective approach to health care, which leads to adaptation, negotiation, collaboration, and appropriate intervention strategies (Andrés-Hyman et al., 2006). Gathering explicit details and in-depth information about the client's background and cultural beliefs provides a realistic clinical image of clients and paints a picture of an individual with unique interests, values, goals, abilities, and priorities. Clinical reasoning and reflection help practitioners center on the particulars of the client rather than on their general condition or limiting factors (Fleming, 1991), moving the clinical intervention from a diagnostic to a client- and family-centered approach.

Culture and Evaluation

Many assessment tools used in health care settings have overwhelmingly incorporated Western values, ethics, theories, and standards. Many are based on the sociocultural norms of the White, middle-class population and the social expectations and values of the majority cultural group (Brown & Bourke-Taylor, 2014). Such assessment tools are not always appropriate for use with members of ethnic and culturally diverse populations because the interpretation of the results may lead to nonoptimal treatment approaches (Hinkle, 1994). Although many tools have been adapted or validated for cross-cultural use, the increasing cultural and ethnic diversity in the United States makes the elimination of overt or subtle biases an important issue (Sousa & Rojjanasrirat, 2010).

Cultural Bias in Evaluation

According to the American Evaluation Association (AEA, 2011), evaluations cannot be culture free. Those who engage in evaluation do so from perspectives that reflect their values, their ways of viewing the world, and their culture. Cultural differences and behaviors between the evaluator and the person being evaluated may influence performance on an assessment. For example, clients evaluated in an unfamiliar system or by a provider who is culturally different often exhibit adjustment behavior (AEA, 2011). In stressful environments, adjusting cultural responses makes survival possible. Clients will alter their behavior to reach a harmonious relationship with their environment. They search for some level of balance or acceptance with the environment, others, or themselves.

Culture shapes the ways in which evaluation questions are conceptualized, which in turn influence what data are collected, how the data will be collected and analyzed, and how data are interpreted. Culture not only influences the client but also the patterns of interaction within the evaluation setting and process.

Cultural factors such as language, education level, generation, literacy level, and comfort in test-taking situations might influence and restrict testing (Brown & Bourke-Taylor, 2014; Muñoz, 2010). Behaviors such as eye contact, tone of voice, and greetings are culturally dependent and varied. Evaluators run the risk of making an incorrect assessment if they interpret clients' behaviors according to what they mean in the majority culture (AEA, 2011; Andrews & Boyle, 2003; Muñoz, 2010). For example, an evaluator who is not aware of values placed on different modes of communication within Deaf and hard-of-hearing communities (e.g., use of sign language, lip reading, or personal assistive listening devices) can miss important individual differences regarding ways of interacting. Evaluator bias can be both conscious and unconscious.

Reflection 14.3. Culturally Different Client: Evaluator Bias

Evaluators run the risk of making an incorrect assessment if they interpret clients' behaviors according to what they mean in the mainstream culture.

- How would you assess a client who views time differently from you?

Selecting Appropriate Assessment Tools

Assessment tools should be used as an aid to understanding the client. Providers choosing to use a standardized tool with members of a different population need to look at the purpose of the assessment, the needs of the individuals being assessed, and the types of modification or accommodation to be used (Bass, 2014; Brown & Bourke-Taylor, 2014). Performance on standardized assessments by diverse clients may not provide accurate information about the clients (Miller, Linn, & Gronlund, 2009). If standardized tests and assessments are used, they need to be interpreted in the context of the client's culture. Accurate evaluation is the first step in effective and culturally appropriate treatment provision.

Reflection 14.4. Assessment Tools and Cultural Diversity

Select an occupational therapy assessment tool and evaluate its usefulness with culturally diverse clients.

- Has the test been standardized on a variety of racial and ethnic populations?
- How would you interpret its results for members of culturally diverse groups?

Cultural Knowledge in Practice

Cultural knowledge—that is, specific knowledge about other cultures—is as necessary to the reasoning process as medical knowledge. Cultural knowledge promotes understanding, awareness of self, reflection, and empathy. It enables practitioners to recognize individual differences and similarities, affirm the culture of the client, and open avenues to learning and

growth. Such information, however, should never be used as part of a cookbook approach to treatment of clients. Culturally effective evaluators work to avoid reinforcing cultural stereotypes and prejudice (AEA, 2011). Rather, cultural knowledge provides a starting point for gathering information, asking questions, and establishing rapport with the client.

Lack of knowledge about other cultures, as well as lack of awareness of one's own biases and values, can lead to misinterpretation of evaluation results. Avoiding *ethnocentrism,* or the tendency to evaluate other groups according to the values and standards of one's own ethnic group (*American Heritage Stedman's Medical Dictionary,* 2002), and developing *ethnorelativism,* or acceptance of other groups, societies, and cultures without judgment (Bennett, 2004), help practitioners become effective evaluators (Muñoz, 2010). Culturally effective evaluators recognize and are responsive to differences between and within cultures and subcultures.

Culture and the Occupational Therapy Process

Practitioners can easily incorporate cultural queries into the occupational therapy process of evaluating, intervening, and targeting outcomes (AOTA, 2014). Experienced practitioners can immediately observe significant data, draw conclusions, and initiate appropriate care because of their knowledge, skill, and experiences. Expert practitioners appear to perform these processes in a way that seems automatic or instinctive (Bass, 2014), but the inclusion of culture in the process is a learned skill (AEA, 2011). For students to learn to manage complex cultural scenarios effectively, it is essential that they understand the process of and steps in clinical reasoning in the evaluation process.

Phase 1: Occupational Profile

In the initial assessment phase, data are gathered, hypotheses are formulated, and decisions are made for further action. The *occupational profile* is the "summary of a client's occupational history and experiences, patterns of daily living, interests, values, and needs" (AOTA, 2014, p. S13).

The information gathered during this phase provides an understanding of the client's cultural background and ethnic identity. It helps the practitioner determine at the outset whether standard treatment approaches should be modified. As part of this inquiry, it is important to

- Ask the client whether he or she has cultural, religious, or spiritual beliefs or practice that may influence care;
- Acknowledge and affirm the client's cultural or ethnic experiences and illness;
- Determine whether the client uses any complementary or alternative practices;
- Demonstrate sensitivity to the client's needs and preferences such as language, title, eye contact, and ways of addressing family members;
- Support the client's ability to understand and act on health information (e.g., ask how he or she prefers to receive information, such as by reading, hearing, or viewing it); and
- Identify dietary needs or restrictions that may affect care (e.g., ask whether religious or spiritual beliefs or customs require or forbid eating certain foods and how traditional foods are eaten).

How the practitioner approaches the individual client sets the stage for all further therapeutic interactions between them and influences the client's ability to trust the provider and health system. Knowledge of specific cultural and ethnic groups and an awareness of their own values and biases enable practitioners to create a wide range of appropriate responses to the client's needs (see Exhibit 14.2).

During the data-gathering phase, the provider can determine whether a cultural conflict may exist between himself or herself and the client, including whether or not the provider is the best individual to serve the client. Culturally effective providers are aware of and comfortable with differences between themselves and their clients and are sensitive to circumstances that may prompt them to refer clients to others for provision of services. For example, a practitioner asked to provide occupational therapy services to someone who is gay but feels uncomfortable interacting with this person because of religious or spiritual beliefs should refer the client

---

Exhibit 14.2. Eliciting Cultural Information in Clinical Interaction

Questions regarding the current illness:
- What is your general understanding about your illness?
- What do you think caused your problem?
- Why do you think it started?
- How severe is your illness? How long do you think it will last?
- What are the main problems your illness has caused for you?
- Have you tried any home remedies, medicines, or folk or traditional treatments for your illness? Did they help? Are you still using them?
- What type of treatment do you think you should receive?
- What results do you hope to receive from the treatment?
- Is there any other information that would be helpful in designing a workable treatment plan?

Questions regarding health beliefs and practices:
- Do you adhere to a religious healing system (e.g., Seventh Day Adventist, West African voodoo, fundamentalist sect, Pentecostal beliefs)?
- Do you adhere to a cultural healing system (e.g., Asian healing system, Raza or Latino *curanderismo*)?
- How is illness explained in your culture (e.g., germ theory, presence of evil spirits, imbalance between hot and cold, yin and yang, disequilibrium between nature and people)?
- Do you rely on cultural healers (e.g., medicine man or woman, shaman, *curandero*, Chinese herbalist, spiritualist, minister, *hougan* [voodoo priest])?
- What types of cultural healing practices and remedies do you and your family use (e.g., massage to cure *empacho*, coining, wearing of talismans or charms for protection against illness)?
- How would you describe a state of "wellness" or "good health"? A state of "poor health" or "illness"?

Questions regarding cultural beliefs and values:
- Are there any taboos or restrictions on who can see a woman's or man's body?
- Are there any taboos or other beliefs connected with mental illness?
- Describe your spirituality or religious practices and beliefs.
- What cultural, racial, or ethnic groups do you identify with?
- How would you describe your family structure?
- What type of support system or network is available to you?
- Who is the primary decision maker in your family?

Source. Black & Wells (2007), p. 258.

to another practitioner to ensure that the client receives quality care.

Constructing a narrative and life history of the client, whether formally or informally, allows the provider to frame problems and limitations in a cultural context. This process also gives practitioners a way to share with colleagues their ideas about what is going on with a particular client; discuss with the client and his or her family specific client-centered issues; and plan culturally appropriate strategies with the client, treatment team members, and other professionals.

Phase 2: Analysis of Occupational Performance

During the second phase of the evaluation process, the *analysis of occupational performance,* practitioners explore clients' occupational problems using assessment tools and instruments, cultural knowledge, and professional and technical knowledge. Analysis of occupational performance entails evaluating the selected occupation result from the "dynamic transaction among the client, the context and environment, and the activity or occupation" (AOTA, 2014, p. S14), along with the culture of the client.

Culturally effective practitioners not only look for physical causes of complaints but also encourage clients to talk about why they are ill. This step is particularly relevant to some cultural groups. For example, some Hispanic clients do not differentiate between physical and emotional illness and may present with physical complaints when in fact the cause is an emotional problem.

When selecting an assessment strategy, practitioners should understand the validity, reliability, and test construction process of any instruments or tools they consider. Many assessment tools have not been standardized for ethnic populations, so caution should be used when interpreting test results. Unless cultural differences are accounted for, inappropriate treatment strategies may be selected (Bass, 2014; Brown & Bourke-Taylor, 2014).

For example, a 6-year-old child raised on a Native American reservation is labeled a slow learner because he is shy and quiet in class, responds only when called on or when spoken to, avoids eye contact and looks down at the floor, and does not engage in conversations with the other children. Within the Native American culture, children are taught to respect and honor their elders; a bowed head is a sign of respect. Also, looking at people directly in the eye is considered a sign of hostility or impoliteness, and children are expected to be seen but not heard (Wells, 1994). If health care institutions and providers are not attuned to the culture of their clients, outcomes can be negative (IOM, 2013).

Phase 3: Intervention

Occupational therapy intervention includes "skilled services provided by therapists in collaboration with clients to facilitate engagement in occupations related to health, well-being, and participation" (AOTA, 2014, p. S14). Practitioners examine what they know about clients, consider their cultural knowledge, and apply professional and technical data to develop goals and intervention strategies. During intervention, practitioners articulate their understanding of clients' problems from a contextual and cultural perspective and apply theoretical reasoning.

The intervention process consists of development of the intervention plan, implementation of the plan, and intervention review. This process ensures that treatment matches clients' expectations, which are grounded in their cultural values and behaviors, and the health care provider's responsibilities, which are grounded in his or her professional orientation.

The intervention process allows practitioners to integrate effective communication, cultural skills, and client- and family-centered care into discussion about treatment options, risks, and alternatives (Joint Commission, 2010). Before engaging a client in intervention planning, practitioners must address the client's communication needs and health literacy; clients must be able to understand presented information and fully participate in the conversation so that practitioners can obtain informed consent, provide client education, and meet any accommodation needs.

During intervention implementation, practitioners implement, monitor, reassess, and modify intervention strategies. They continually and systematically collect specific information not only about performance changes but also about cultural values, beliefs, and behaviors. If the intervention is not beneficial or in line with clients' cultural expectations, practitioners can alter or terminate the therapy. Practitioners should

- Monitor changes in the client to determine whether new or more severe impairments develop during the course of treatment;
- Notify the client and family of ongoing opportunities to ask questions;
- Adapt existing procedures to better involve the client and family; and
- Support the client's ability to understand the health information being given by speaking in plain language, avoiding professional jargon, using the teach-back method to assess understanding, and using trained interpreters.

Practitioners should accommodate the client's cultural, religious, or spiritual beliefs and practice whenever possible by doing the following:

- Respect the client's needs or preferences for modesty. Uncover only parts of the body necessary for examination and treatment; use full gowns,

robes, or clothing for walking and transporting; and provide privacy in dressing, bathing, and toileting training.
- Respect culture and religious restrictions on touching, distance, and modesty when the provider is of the opposite sex or younger or older than the client.
- Ask whether there are specific times of the day to avoid scheduling treatment to respect religious or spiritual practices.
- Inform the client of any changes in dietary needs or feeding behaviors that may arise because of the medical condition or impairment.

The client should be involved in the therapy delivery model. Cultural traditions and preferences should shape the delivery of care, not the other way around. Incorporating cultural traditions and preferences during interventions requires cultural humility to recognize any disconnects between client and provider, provision of cultural safety during care, and use of cultural knowledge in conjunction with Western medicine (IOM, see Exhibit 14.3).

Exhibit 14.3. Culturally Sensitive Intervention Strategies

- Become aware of the cultural group's inclinations on issues of privacy, self-disclosure, familial power and distribution, discussion of intimate matters with a person outside the family, use of formally organized helping institutions, and context in which help is or should be offered.
- During assessments, consider the socioenvironmental impacts as well as individual psychological reactions.
- Become familiar with non-Western medical beliefs and practices.
- Take advantage of opportunities to learn about people and their cultures. Listening and showing a willingness to learn and share experiences can be invaluable.
- During discharge or termination planning, make an effort to connect the client to the positive elements of support in their community.
- Avoid recommending and training clients in the use of equipment that is financially impractical, culturally inappropriate, or culturally unacceptable to the client and his or her family.
- Avoid patronizing or condescending approaches.
- Understand the communication style of the group. Observe for clues—verbal or nonverbal—that may indicate preferences.
- Develop a wide variety of verbal and nonverbal responses that will facilitate involvement of the client.
- Become familiar with special terminology used by the client.
- Use an interpreter if you are not fluent or effective in the preferred language of the client. Learn basic words, phrases, and sentences in the target language.
- If an interpreter is used, meet with him or her to discuss information to be given and received from the client, the interpreter's style and approach to the client, and cultural practices and beliefs of the client's cultural group.
- Involve the client and family members in goal setting.
- Discuss with the client and family how potential treatment goals and outcomes may alter typical cultural roles and practices. Let the client and family decide how and to what extent they wish to engage in the new behavior.
- Be flexible and adaptable in your approach. Take into account the client's culture, environment, age, gender, religion, life history, principal stressors, geographic location, sexual orientation, educational level, appearance, nationality, ethnicity, communication style, and abilities.

Source. From "Clinical Consideration in Treating Minority Women Who Are Disabled," by S. A. Wells, 1991, *OT Practice, 2*(4), pp. 13–22. Copyright © 1991 by S. A. Wells. Used with permission.

Phase 4: Targeting Outcomes

According to the *Framework,* **outcomes** "are the end result of the occupational therapy process; they describe what clients can achieve through intervention" (AOTA, 2014, p. S16). Outcomes are used to measure progress, adjust goals, and prepare for discharge, and are woven throughout the occupational therapy process.

Cultural misunderstanding can affect practitioners' ability to assist their clients in achieving optimal outcomes. Outcomes should be developed within the cultural and environmental context of the client. Practitioners should incorporate cultural needs during discharge and follow-up, providing discharge instructions that include the client's cultural and literacy needs and identifying follow-up providers and facilities that can meet the client's cultural needs. When culturally effective care is provided, clients' response to care is improved, compliance increases, and engagement with the health system is more likely (IOM, 2013).

Cultural Approach to Health Service Delivery

The demographic changes in the United States over past decades have significantly altered the clinical milieu. Practitioners must strive to provide high-quality clinical services. A growing body of research documents that client experiences, including poor health outcomes and lower quality of care, are related to race, ethnicity, language, disability, and sexual orientation, compromising health care delivery and services (Agency for Healthcare Research and Quality, 2014; Hickling, 2012). The IOM (2000) noted that the cultural approach is client centered, effective, efficient, timely, safe, and equitable. The cultural approach to health care involves providing care that does not vary in quality because of personal characteristics such as gender, race, ethnicity, geographic location, and socioeconomic status. Within this quality framework, health care providers need to be equipped to deliver health care services to increasingly diverse individuals and families.

Studies have shown that incorporating concepts of cultural competence and client- and family-centeredness into the care process can increase client satisfaction with and adherence to treatment

(Bartlett, Blais, Tamblyn, Clermont, & MacGibbon, 2008; Wolf, Lehman, Quinlin, Zullo, & Hoffman, 2008). The American Academy of Pediatrics (2011) defined **culturally effective care** as "the delivery of care within the context of appropriate physician knowledge, understanding, and appreciation of cultural distinctions leading to optimal health outcomes" (para. 1) and established guiding principles for a multicultural approach to the delivery of care:

- Communicate, by attitude and behavior, openness to different cultures.
- Be willing to adapt, if possible, clinical practice to acknowledge clients,' families,' and caregivers' culture.
- Demonstrate a commitment to professional development aimed at acquiring new cultural knowledge and skills.
- Consider that often the variability within cultures (e.g., between affluent and poor African-Americans) may be more pronounced than that between cultures.

Bazaldua and Sias (2004) described the interaction between a provider and a client as a cross-cultural exchange of attitudes that require the use of the R.E.S.P.E.C.T. Model of Cross-Cultural Communication (Welch, 1998):

- *Rapport.* Develop it by understanding the client's point of view and avoid assumptions.
- *Empathy.* Remember that clients are seeking advice and acknowledgment of their feelings and concerns.
- *Support.* Assist clients by understanding their social context and involving their family.
- *Partnership.* Work with clients regarding the intervention plan and negotiate if necessary.
- *Explanations.* Teach concepts and verify that clients understand them.
- *Cultural Competence.* Your responsibility is to be knowledgeable about your own biases and preconceptions and to respect the client's beliefs and culture.
- *Trust.* Assuring reliance is essential and requires patience.

The AEA (2011) described a starting point for developing and implementing a culturally competent evaluation. Essential practices for culture competence are as follows:

- *"Acknowledge the complexity of cultural identity."* Evaluators recognize, respond to, and work to reconcile differences between and within cultures and subcultures.
- *"Recognize the dynamics of power."* Evaluators work to avoid reinforcing cultural stereotypes and prejudice in their work.
- *"Recognize and eliminate bias in social relations."* Evaluators are thoughtful and deliberate in their use of language and other social relations to reduce bias when conducting evaluations.
- Use *"culturally congruent epistemologies, theories, and methods."* Evaluators seek to understand how the constructs are defined by cultures and are aware of the many ways epistemologies and theories can be used; the ways data can be collected, analyzed, and interpreted; and the diversity of contexts in which findings can be disseminated.
- *"Continue self-assessments."* Monitor the extent to which you can serve as an open, responsive instrument given relevant attributes of an evaluation context."

Summary

Because cultural differences are always present in health care encounters, occupational therapy practitioners must serve as cultural brokers among the many cultures with which they interact. Integrating culture into the daily clinical reasoning and occupational therapy process enables practitioners to bridge cultures and use a holistic approach to care, allowing each client to be seen as an individual with his or her own identity, culture, experiences, background, and lifestyle. Interacting in this manner moves the clinical intervention from a diagnostic approach to a client- and family-centered approach.

Commitment to acquiring the awareness, knowledge, and skills and engaging in the critical reflection needed to provide culturally effective and safe care can benefit practitioners through increased confidence in their ability to address the needs of various groups. This commitment can help practitioners skillfully and respectfully negotiate the implications of diversity in the clinical setting, thereby improving the health of diverse clients through true partnership at the client-centered and community levels.

Reflection 14.5. Judy: Schizophrenia

Judy, a 25-year-old woman, was admitted to the psychiatric unit after being arrested for arson when she set fire to the local soup kitchen. She was diagnosed with schizophrenia. Her chart reveals that she is of biracial heritage; her mother is White and her father is Haitian. She has lived with her parents off and on in a small Midwestern town. She was often picked up by the police for loitering, panhandling, and creating a public disturbance.

Judy's mother reported that Judy had been a happy, caring, and studious person who wanted to be a teacher. She attended the local college until 5 years ago, when she began exhibiting behaviors such as talking to herself, hearing voices, and being fascinated with fire. She had occasional outbursts about her White half abusing her Haitian half. On admission to the unit, she exhibited a flat affect, immobility, and difficulty organizing her thoughts.

Her parents commented that they had failed her and that being biracial caused stress for her. They thought that evil spirits possessed their daughter and that their only hope was an intervention by a voodoo priest.

- How does this situation challenge or fit with your values and belief system?
- What cultural biases might interfere with your interaction with the parents? Why or why not?
- How would you advise this family? How would you support the client?
- Whose cultural value system would you use to evaluate the client? Whose system would you promote to the client?
- Would you be willing to work with a voodoo priest? Why or why not?

References

Agency for Healthcare Research and Quality. (2014). *2013 national healthcare disparities report* (Publication No. 14-0006). Rockville, MD: Author.

American Academy of Pediatrics. (2011). *Culturally effective care toolkit.* Retrieved from https://www.aap.org/en-us/professional-resources/practice-support/Patient-Management/Pages/Culturally-Effective-Care-Toolkit.aspx?nfstatus=401&nftoken=00000000-0000-0000-0000-000000000000&nfstatusdescription=ERROR:+No+local+token

American Evaluation Association. (2011). *American Evaluation Association statement on cultural competence in evaluation.* Fairhaven, MA: Author. Retrieved from http://www.eval.org/p/cm/ld/fid=92

American Heritage Stedman's Medical Dictionary. (2002). *Ethnocentrism.* Boston: Houghton Mifflin.

American Occupational Therapy Association. (1996). *Creating a multicultural approach and environment* [Video]. Bethesda, MD: Author.

American Occupational Therapy Association. (2014). Occupational therapy practice framework: Domain and process (3rd ed.). *American Journal of Occupational Therapy, 68*(Suppl.1), S1–S48. http://dx.doi.org/10.5014/ajot.2014.682006

Andrés-Hyman, R. C., & Ortiz, J., Anez, L. M., Paris, M., & Davidson, L., (2006). Culture and clinical practice: Recommendations for working with Puerto Ricans and other Latinas(os) in the United States. *Professional Psychology: Research and Practice, 37,* 694–701. http://dx.doi.org/10.1037/0735-7028.37.6.694

Andrews, M. A., & Boyle, J. S. (2003). *Transcultural concepts in nursing care* (4th ed.). Philadelphia: Lippincott Williams & Wilkins.

Balcazar, F. F., Suarez-Balcazar, Y., Taylor-Ritzler, T., & Keys, C. B. (2009). *Race, culture, and disability: Rehabilitation science and practice.* Boston: Jones & Bartlett.

Bartlett, G., Blais, R., Tamblyn, R., Clermont, R. J., & MacGibbon, B. (2008). Impact of patient communication problems on the risk of preventable adverse events in acute care settings. *Canadian Medical Association Journal, 178,* 1555–1562. http://dx.doi.org/10.1503/cmaj.070690

Bass, J. D. (2014). Assessment identification and selection. In J. Hinojosa & P. Kramer (Eds.), *Evaluation in occupational therapy: Obtaining and interpreting data* (4th ed., pp. 35–45). Bethesda, MD: AOTA Press.

Bazaldua, O. V., & Sias, J. (2004). Cultural competence: A pharmacy perspective. *Journal of Pharmacy Practice, 17,* 160–166. http://dx.doi.org/10.1177/0897190004264812

Bennett, M. J. (2004). Becoming interculturally competent. In J. Wurzel (Ed.), *Toward multiculturalism: A reader in multicultural education* (2nd ed., pp. 62–77). Newton, MA: Intercultural Resource Corporation.

Black, R., & Wells, S. (2007). *Culture and occupation: A model of empowerment in occupational therapy.* Bethesda, MD: AOTA Press.

Bonder, B., & Martin, L. (2013). *Culture in clinical care: Strategies for competence* (2nd ed.). Thorofare, NJ: Slack.

Bridges, D. R., Davidson, D. A., Odegard, P. S., Maki, I. V., & Tomkowiak, J. (2011). Interprofessional collaboration: Three best practice models of interprofessional education. *Medical Education Online, 16,* http://dx.doi.org/10.3402/meo.v16i0.6035

Brown, T., & Bourke-Taylor, H. (2014). Accommodating diversity issues in assessment and evaluation. In J. Hinojosa & P. Kramer (Eds.), *Evaluation in occupational therapy: Obtaining and interpreting data* (4th ed., pp. 221–240). Bethesda, MD: AOTA Press.

Ericsson, K., Whyte, A., & Ward, J. (2007). Expert performance in nursing: Reviewing research on expertise in nursing within the framework of the expert-performance approach. *Advances in Nursing Science, 30,* 58–71. Retrieved from https://www.researchgate.net/publication/6506676_Expert_Performance_in_Nursing_Reviewing_Research_on_Expertise_in_Nursing_Within_the_Framework_of_the_Expert-Performance_Approach

Fitzgerald, M. H. (1992). Multicultural clinical interactions. *Journal of Rehabilitation, 58,* 38–42.

Fleming, M. H. (1991). Clinical reasoning in medicine compared to clinical reasoning in occupational therapy. *American Journal of Occupational Therapy, 45,* 988–996. http://dx.doi.org/10.5014/ajot.45.11.988

Fleming, M. H., & Mattingly, C. (1994). Giving language to practice. In C. Mattingly & M. H. Fleming (Eds.), *Clinical reasoning: Forms of inquiry in therapeutic practice* (pp. 3–21). Philadelphia: F. A. Davis.

Hickling, F. W. (2012). Understanding patients in multicultural settings: A personal reflection on ethnicity and culture in clinical practice. *Ethnicity and Health, 17,* 203–216. http://dx.doi.org/10.1080/13557858.2012.655266

Hinkle, J. (1994). Practitioners and cross-cultural assessment: A practical guide to information and training. *Measurement and Evaluation in Counseling and Development, 27,* 103–115.

Institute of Medicine. (2000). *Crossing the quality chasm: A new health system for the 21st century.* Washington, DC: National Academies Press.

Institute of Medicine. (2013). *Leveraging culture to address health inequalities: Examples from Native communities: Workshop summary.* Washington, DC: National Academies Press.

Interprofessional Education Collaborative Expert Panel. (2011). *Core competencies for interprofessional collaborative practice: Report of an expert panel.* Washington, DC: Interprofessional Education Collaborative.

Johnson, V. (1995). *Heart full of grace: A thousand years of Black wisdom.* New York: Simon & Schuster.

Joint Commission. (2010). *Advancing effective communication, cultural competence, and patient- and family-centered care: A roadmap for hospitals.* Oakbrook Terrace, IL: Author.

Kleinman, A., & Benson, P. (2006). Anthropology in the clinic: The problem of cultural competency and how to fix it. *PLoS Medicine, 3*(10), e294. http://dx.doi.org/10.1371/journal .pmed.0030294

Leung, K. H., Pluye, P., Grad, R., & Weston, C. (2010). A reflective learning framework to evaluate CME effects on practice reflection. *Journal of Continuing Education in the Health Professions, 30*(2), 78–88. http://dx.doi.org/10.1002/chp.20063

Miller, M. D., Linn, R. L., & Gronlund, N. E. (2009). *Measurement and assessment in teaching* (10th ed.). Upper Saddle River, NJ: Pearson Education.

Minore, B., & Boone, M. (2002). Realizing potential: Improving interdisciplinary professional/paraprofessional health care teams in Canada's northern Aboriginal communities through education. *Journal of Interprofessional Care, 16,* 139–147. http://dx.doi.org/10.1080/13561820220124157

Mu, K., Coppard, B. M., Bracciano, A., Doll, J., & Matthews, A. (2010). Fostering cultural competency, clinical reasoning, and leadership through international outreach. *Occupational Therapy in Health Care, 24,* 74–85. http://dx.doi .org/10.3109/07380570903329628

Muñoz, J. P. (2010). Evaluating special populations. In J. Hinojosa, P. Kramer, & P. Crist (Eds.), *Evaluation: Obtaining and interpreting data* (3rd ed., pp. 275–293). Bethesda, MD: AOTA Press.

National Center for Cultural Competence. (2004). *Bridging the cultural divide in health care settings: The essential role of cultural broker programs.* Washington, DC: National Center for Cultural Competence, Georgetown University Center for Child and Human Development, Georgetown University Medical Center.

Oelofsen, N. (2012, June). Developing practical reflective skills (1/2): Personal learning. *British Journal of Healthcare Assistants, 6,* 294–297. http://dx.doi.org/10.12968/bjha.2012.6.6.294

Office of Minority Health. (2014). *Minority population profiles.* Retrieved from http://minorityhealth.hhs.gov/omh/browse .aspx?lvl=2&lvlid=26

Purden, M. (2005). Cultural considerations in interprofessional education and practice. *Journal of Interprofessional Care, 19*(Suppl. 1), 224–234. http://dx.doi.org/10.1080 /13561820500083238

Schell, B. A. B. (2014). Professional reasoning in practice. In B. A. B. Schell, G. Gillen, & E. S. Cohn (Eds.), *Willard and Spackman's occupational therapy* (12th ed., pp. 384–397). Baltimore: Lippincott Williams & Wilkins.

Schell, B. A. B., & Schell, J. W. (2007). *Clinical and professional reasoning in occupational therapy.* Baltimore: Lippincott Williams & Wilkins.

Schon, D. A. (1983). *The reflective practitioner: How professionals think in action.* New York: Basic Books.

Sousa, V. D., & Rojjanasrirat, W. (2010). Translation, adaptation and validation of instruments or scales for use in cross-cultural health care research: A clear and user-friendly guideline. *Journal of Evaluation in Clinical Practice, 17,* 268–274. http://dx .doi.org/10.1111/j.1365-2753.2010.01434.x

Tervalon, M., & Murray-García, J. (1998). Cultural humility versus cultural competence: A critical distinction in defining physician training outcomes in multicultural education. *Journal of Health Care for the Poor and Underserved, 9,* 117–125. http:// dx.doi.org/10.1353/hpu.2010.0233

Waite, R., & Calamaro, C. J. (2010). Cultural competence: A systemic challenge to nursing education, knowledge exchange, and the knowledge development process. *Perspectives in Psychiatric Care, 46,* 74–80. http://dx.doi.org/10.1111/j.1744 -6163.2009.00240.x

Warda, M. R. (2000). Mexican Americans' perceptions of culturally competent care. *Western Journal of Nursing Research, 22,* 203–224. http://dx.doi.org/10.1177/01939450022044368

Welch, M. (1998). *Enhancing awareness and improving cultural competence in health care. A partnership guide for teaching diversity and cross-cultural concepts in health professional training.* San Francisco: University of California at San Francisco. Available at http://cirrie.buffalo.edu/culture/curriculum/resources /models.php

Wells, S. A. (1991). Clinical consideration in treating minority women who are disabled. *OT Practice, 2*(4), 13–22.

Wells, S. A. (1994). *A multicultural education and resource guide for occupational therapy educators and practitioners.* Bethesda, MD: American Occupational Therapy Association.

Wenger, A. F. (1995). Cultural context, health and health care decision making. *Journal of Transcultural Nursing, 7*(1), 3–14.

Wolf, D. M., Lehman, L., Quinlin, R., Zullo, T., & Hoffman, L. (2008). Effect of patient-centered care on patient satisfaction and quality of care. *Journal of Nursing Care Quality, 23,* 316–321. http://dx.doi.org/10.1097/01.NCQ.0000336672 .02725.a5

World Health Organization. (2010). *Framework for action on interprofessional education and collaborative practice.* Geneva: Author. Retrieved from http://apps.who.int/iris/bitstream /10665/70185/1/WHO_HRH_HPN_10.3_eng.pdf

Chapter 15.

CULTURE AND ETHICAL PRACTICE

Shirley A. Wells, DrPH, OTR, FAOTA

> *It not the color of the skin that makes the man, but the principles formed within the soul.*
> **Maria W. Stewart (quoted in Johnson, 1995, p. 102)**

Chapter Highlights

- Types of Ethics
- Moral Principles
- Ethical Decision Making
- Bioethics
- Culture and Ethics
- Ethics in Clinical Practice

Key Terms and Concepts

- ✧ Advance directive
- ✧ Applied ethics
- ✧ Autonomy
- ✧ Beneficence
- ✧ Bioethics
- ✧ Clinical ethics
- ✧ Code of ethics
- ✧ Compensatory justice
- ✧ Conflict
- ✧ Cultural bioethics
- ✧ Deontological approach
- ✧ Descriptive ethics
- ✧ Dilemma
- ✧ Distributive justice
- ✧ Environmental ethics
- ✧ Ethical decision making
- ✧ Ethical dilemmas

- ✧ Ethic of diversity framework
- ✧ Ethics
- ✧ Health care ethics
- ✧ Informed consent
- ✧ Justice
- ✧ Metaethics
- ✧ Moral principles
- ✧ Morals
- ✧ Neuroethics
- ✧ Nonmaleficence
- ✧ Normative ethics
- ✧ *Occupational Therapy Code of Ethics*
- ✧ Particularist ethics
- ✧ Public health ethics
- ✧ Regulatory and policy bioethics
- ✧ Social ethics
- ✧ Social justice

❖ Standards of care
❖ Theoretical ethics
❖ Universalist ethics

❖ Utilitarian approach
❖ Veracity
❖ Virtue ethics

Ethical choices have assumed major importance in health care as advances in medical technology and rising costs have forced many practitioners to deal with difficult choices surrounding life and death issues, allocation of resources, and practitioner–client relationships (Pozgar, 2014). The multicultural composition of the U.S. population has added an additional layer of complexity to ethical choices in current practice. Clients and their families, as well as occupational therapy practitioners, bring cultural, religious, and ideological beliefs with them to the health care interaction; for example, clients' cultural beliefs may challenge or conflict with American culture's emphasis on self-reliance and individualism (Ludwick & Silva, 2000). Different cultures hold different values, making it hard to always make the right ethical choice when confronted with differing values. **Ethical dilemmas** in health care occur when clients, family members and caregivers, and practitioners hold differing values (Pozgar, 2014).

In the presence of cultural differences, health care practitioners frequently confront choices that depend more on moral and ethical values than on medical knowledge. The moral consequences of not respecting differences within a multicultural society are raising difficult questions for ethicists, policymakers, researchers, and clinicians. This chapter examines how culture influences the ethics of health care decision making and policy. It also examines the ethical responsibilities of practitioners and the rights of the client and family.

Types of Ethics

The term *ethics* comes from the Greek word *ethos,* meaning "cultural custom or habit." **Ethics** is "a systematic view of rules of conduct that is grounded in philosophical principles and theory; character and customs of societal values and norms that are assumed in a given cultural, professional, or institutional setting as ways of determining right and wrong" (Slater, 2016, p. 291). Ethics are external standards that are provided by the institutions, groups, or culture to which an individual belongs.

For example, occupational therapy practitioners are required to follow the *Occupational Therapy Code of Ethics* (American Occupational Therapy Association [AOTA], 2015) regardless of their own feelings or preferences. The field of ethics involves systematizing, defending, and recommending concepts of right and wrong and acceptable behavior (Fieser, 2014). Purtilo and Doherty (2011) described ethics as "a study of and reflection on everyday morality" (p. 17).

The term **morals,** which is often used interchangeably with the term *ethics,* refers to "personal beliefs regarding values, rules, and principles of what is right or wrong" that "may be culture based or culture driven" (Slater, 2011, p. 226). Morals are ideas about what is right and what is wrong that are deeply ingrained in culture and religion (Pozgar, 2014). *Morals* refers to an individual's own principles regarding right and wrong that can change if an individual's beliefs change (Purtilo & Doherty, 2011). Ethics and morals encompass the principles of conduct that help govern the behaviors of individuals and groups, values and guidelines by which people live, and the justification of these values and guidelines.

In this chapter, *ethics* pertains to professional behaviors and rules provided by an external source, e.g., codes of conduct, whereas *morals* are the basis for personal behavior and rules related to right and wrong. Morals are more abstract, subjective, and often personal or religion-based, while ethics are more practical, shared principles promoting fairness in social, business, and professional interactions. Both ethics and morals may have a part in clinical ethical dilemmas and decision making. For example, in the United States, a doctor may not euthanize a patient, even at the patient's request, according to the ethical standards for health professionals. However, the same doctor may personally believe in a patient's right to die, according to the doctor's own morality (Diffen, n.d.).

Metaethics

The various ethical approaches relevant to everyday decision making are addressed by a field of study called *metaethics.* **Metaethics** is a branch of analytical philosophy that explores the status, foundations, and scope of moral values, properties, and words (DeLapp, 2015). It investigates where our ethical principles come from and what they mean (Fieser, 2014) and explores the nature of goodness and badness, or what it is to be morally right or wrong. Metaethics tries to answers such questions as

- What are people doing when they use the moral words *good* and *right?*
- Where do moral values come from?
- Are things morally right or wrong for all people at all times?
- Does morality vary from person to person, context to context, or culture to culture?

Normative Ethics

Normative ethics gives us practical guidelines or norms that form a societal perspective on ethical behavior. It involves articulating the good habits we should acquire, the duties we should follow, and the consequences of our behavior for others. It is concerned with how people ought to act, what kind of person one ought to be, or what sorts of policies ought to be implemented (Duignan, 2011; Slater, 2016). Normative ethics attempts to answer specific moral questions concerning what people should do or believe. It sets the specific norms and standards for right and wrong action and behavior.

Applied Ethics

Applied ethics is the application and evaluation of the principles and norms that guide practice in particular domains. It involves examining controversial issues that people face in their lives, such as abortion, gun control, gay and lesbian marriage, euthanasia, and capital punishment (Fieser, 2014). It deals with moral problems, such as the obligations (if any) we have toward the world's poor. It addresses the moral permissibility of specific actions and practices (Dittmer, 2014; Gordon, 2012; Petrini, 2007). Subsets of applied ethics include medical ethics, bioethics (discussed in a later section), business ethics, legal ethics, and others.

Descriptive Ethics

Descriptive ethics is concerned with how people actually behave. It focuses on behavior patterns among people in different cultures. It explains moral behavior

and phenomena such as what people believe is primarily important and how societies regulate behavior (e.g., through punishment for certain actions), which are based on the culture they live in (Glannon, 2005). It is also referred to as *behavioral ethics.*

Reflection 15.1. Using Theories of Ethics

Health care practitioners use a combination of theories to determine the correct action to take.

A 41-year-old woman with a diagnosis of multiple sclerosis has been referred to an occupational therapist for an evaluation. During the assessment she informs the therapist that she is being physically abused by her live-in boyfriend. The client asks the therapist to keep the revelation confidential. What action should the therapist take for each of the following type of ethics?

- *Descriptive ethics:* What do you think is right?
- *Normative ethics:* How should you act?
- *Metaethics:* What does *right* even mean?

Virtue Ethics

Virtue ethics concentrates on a person's moral character and his or her motivation for action and personal integrity (Slater, 2016). A virtuous person is one who focuses on doing the good and right thing in relationship to other people by habit rather than according to a set of rules or consequences of conduct. The concept of moral character involves doing the right thing to answer the question, How should I live?

Virtues are those characteristics or traits ascribed to a person who habitually acts in a manner that will be praised by others (Purtilo & Doherty, 2011). Certain character traits such as courage, honesty, and justice are considered virtue principles or characters. "The character of a virtuous person is good as exhibited by his or her unswerving good behavior and actions" (Pozgar, 2014, p. 28). For example, a young man stops his car and helps a woman change her flat tire, refusing money, or a man in a store does not quite have enough money for his purchase, and the person behind him makes up the difference. According to virtue ethics, a person ought to act in ways that exhibit virtue, even if that means doing what might generally be seen as bad or bringing about undesirable consequences such as not qualifying a patient for therapy knowing this is a requirement for the patient's skilled nursing placement (Baranzke, 2012).

Social Ethics

Social ethics focuses on policies that affect the wider community, the protection of the community, and the treatment of each member of the community (O'Sullivan, 2014). It promotes adherence to moral norms in relationships with others and the community as a whole (Slater, 2011). Social ethics varies among different societies and cultures because what is considered right or wrong by a society is influenced by such factors as religious beliefs, economic conditions, and social and cultural factors (Innovateus, 2015). Social ethics thus involves acceptance and tolerance of differences.

Issues such as abortion, euthanasia, the death penalty, animal cruelty, gene manipulation, and cloning have given rise to ethical questions that disturb the equilibrium of society. Opponents of social ethics argue that the rights and interests of individuals should not be sacrificed in favor of the interests of the larger society (Glannon, 2005).

Environmental Ethics

Environmental ethics involves one's moral obligation toward the environment (Davy, 2005). This approach studies the moral relationship of human beings with the environment and its nonhuman contents. For example, concerns about pollution and the depletion of natural resources, dwindling plant and animal biodiversity, the loss of wilderness, the degradation of ecosystems, and climate change are all environmental ethics issues that have entered public consciousness and policy in recent years (Cochrane, 2014).

Theoretical Ethics

Theoretical ethics operates at a more fundamental level and is the systematic effort to understand moral concepts and justify moral principles and theories (Fieser, 2014; Petrini, 2007). It seeks to answer the questions, How do we justify our judgments about the right and the good? What makes a certain action good? What features are relevant when evaluating the moral worth of an action? It is the philosophical study of the main concepts and methods of ethics

and is concerned with the nature of ethical language, the objectivity of ethical beliefs, and the nature of ethical reasoning.

Universalist and Particularist Ethics

Morality, like culture, is different for different people. It can vary from time to time and from person to person. Behavioral standards and moral values accepted by virtually all societies or that can apply to all humans—for example, human rights—may be referred to as *universalist ethics. Particularist ethics,* or culture-specific ethics, involves moral norms adhered to by a given cultural community but not by others (e.g., ancestor worship).

Ethics come into play in situations when a shared universal or cultural standard does not automatically apply to a situation and decisions are a function of particular circumstances. Particularists insist that moral problems are solved one by one and that no single principle can be used to guide moral actions. Because moral problems are contextual and complex, all moral judgments must be made in reaction to individual cases by keeping in view all significant aspects of each case (Kihlbom, 2000).

Clinical and Public Health Ethics

Clinical and public health ethics are practical examples of applied ethics. *Clinical ethics* refers to the day-to-day principles used in decision making by practitioners caring for clients (McCullough, 2014). Ethical issues are embedded in every clinical encounter between clients and practitioners because the care of clients always involves both technical and moral considerations. Because clinical practice is characterized by a personal client–practitioner relationship, the practitioners engaged in making difficult ethical decisions are the focus of clinical ethics (Jonsen, Siegler, & Winslade, 2010; McCullough, 2014). According to McClimans, Dunn, and Slowther (2011), clinical ethics help provide a theoretical justification for client-centered care, and client-centered clinical ethical practices can be furthered through ethics consultation, education, and policy development and review.

Because public health actions are often undertaken by governments and are directed at the population level, *public health ethics* involves a systematic process to clarify, prioritize, and justify possible courses of actions (Centers for Disease Control and Prevention,

2014). It is characterized by global attention to whole populations. It seeks to understand and clarify principles and values that guide public health actions as they relate to health conditions; prevention; and the social, economic, and demographic determinants of health and disease (Petrini, 2007).

Moral Principles

Moral principles are used by society to appraise the behavior of individuals and groups. Although these principles are informal rules, not codified laws (Robinson, 2008), they are universally binding and fundamentally transcultural (Boss, 1998), affecting all people regardless of their personal desires, culture, or religion. Moral principles are abstract criteria for evaluating human behavior in its entirety (see Table 15.1).

Moral principles protect members of society against harm and highlight the good in people. Moral principles are grounded in broad theories of ethics. Historically, two theories of justification of conduct have dominated: (1) the utilitarian approach and (2) the deontological approach.

Utilitarian Approach

The *utilitarian approach* to moral conduct assesses an action in terms of its consequences or outcomes. It asks which choice, action, or policy would promote the best possible outcome (Pozgar, 2014; Slater, 2016). The ethical action is seen as the one that produces the greatest good and does the least harm for all stakeholders. This approach tries to

increase the good and reduce the harm done: "The moral worth of an action is determined by its outcome, and thus, the ends justify the means" (Pozgar, 2014, p. 10). Such an approach to health care rationing, for instance, would look for the collective social benefit rather than advantages to individuals. It holds that every entity's interests should be considered equally when making the decision.

Deontological Approach

The *deontological approach* holds that moral conduct must be evaluated in terms of standards alone and that the consequences of conduct are not germane to the evaluation of that conduct. It focuses on one's duties to others and others' rights. It is also referred to as *duty-based ethics* (Pozgar, 2014). The deontological approach to moral conduct involves analyzing people's ability to follow moral codes, laws, and rules (Slater, 2016). For example, according to this approach, it would be wrong to subject a human being to dangerous medical research without the person's consent, even if the consequences of doing so might be to save the lives of many others.

Ethical Decision Making

Good intentions alone are insufficient to guide moral decision making: Consequences matter when applying moral principles and making a judgment. *Ethical decision making* is the mode of reasoning used to recognize, analyze, and clarify ethical problems and decide the right thing to do in a particular case (Pozgar, 2014; Purtilo & Doherty, 2011). It requires

Table 15.1. Principles for Evaluating Moral Choices

Moral Principle	Duty Involved
Consistency	To choose consistently or logically
Self-improvement	To improve one's own knowledge and virtue
Equality	To treat all humans as equal
Justice	To give each person equal and fair consideration
Beneficence	To do good acts and promote happiness
Autonomy	To respect the individual's right to self-determination
Veracity	To tell the truth
Fidelity	To keep promises (e.g., confidentiality); to be loyal
Nonmaleficence	To do no harm
Axiology	To make consistent, harmonious, and coherent choices
Consequences	To consider the foreseeable consequences of actions
Altruism	To respect all people and cooperate with others in the production and enjoyment of shared values

Sources. Boss, 1998; Buford, 1984; Callahan, 1995; Veatch & Flack, 1997.

reflection and logical judgment and involves gathering relevant information, correctly applying ethical knowledge and skills (Purtilo & Doherty, 2011), and reflecting on one's actions from the perspective of moral theories.

According to Callahan (1995), good individual moral decision making encompasses three elements: (1) self-knowledge, (2) knowledge of moral theories and principles, and (3) cultural perception. Self-knowledge is fundamental to ethical decision making because one's feelings, motives, inclinations, and interests both enlighten and obscure moral understanding. Knowledge of moral theories and principles supports one's ability to make good decisions when dealing with people who hold different values. Understanding general ethical principles can help one foster dialogue and facilitate a resolution (Morris, 2003). Cultural perception can challenge and influence ethical decision making. Stereotyping, bias, and ethnocentricity all involve cultural perceptions that can lead one to prejudge people, apply negative generalities about a group unfairly to members of an entire population, or prevent one from making an impartial judgment (Fremgen, 2012).

People are cultural and social beings, reflecting a particular culture at a particular time that shapes how they understand themselves, how they perceive moral problems, and what they view as plausible and feasible responses to moral problems. Recognizing that one's own behaviors are shaped and defined by one's specific culture can lead to collaboration and cooperation in making sound ethical decisions (Wells, 2016). Ethical decision making involves choice and balance. It is not easy when there are multiple routes to take (Chmielewski, 2004; Pozgar, 2014).

Ethical Decision Making in the Health Care Context

What are health care practitioners' duties and obligations to the people whose lives and well-being may be affected by their actions? What do practitioners owe to the common good or the public interest? An ethical decision in health care is different from general ethical decisions because the domain of medicine is different from other areas of human life and because medicine has its own moral approaches and traditions (Pellegrino & Thomasma, 1981). All health care practitioners have written **standards of care** that detail what is minimally required of them,

and standards of care typically address ethical decision making.

Proponents of differences between general and health care ethical decision making argue that making a decision in a medical context requires a detailed and sensitive appreciation of the characteristics of health care practice and of the unique features of sick, injured, and dying people. The medical ethical literature emphasizes the imperative that health care practitioners keep a focus on the well-being of the whole person. Bishop and Scudder (2001) described the core of the health care practitioner as a "caring presence"—that is, a personal presence that assures the other of the practitioner's concern for his or her well-being. Therefore, practitioners must bring trustworthiness to the relationship. It is not that the ethical principles and virtues of medicine are different from the more general principles of ethics; it is the combination of general ethical principles and the context of health care that give health care ethics special consideration.

Ethical Dilemmas in Health Care

An ethical dilemma arises when ethical principles and values are in conflict (Pozgar, 2014). **Conflict** occurs when competing interests create a problem; the *dilemma* occurs after the problem has been created. A **dilemma** arises when a person's concepts of what is right and wrong conflict with what he or she is supposed to do (Allen, 2013). It involves both ethical conflict and conduct; as Purtilo and Doherty (2011) described it, "An ethical dilemma occurs when a moral agent is faced with two or more conflicting courses of action but only one can be chosen as the agent attempts to bring about an outcome consistent with the professional goal of a caring response" (p. 60).

There is no set formula for determining which action to take in an ethical dilemma or conflict. One must carefully weigh the moral principles, select those most compelling in a particular situation, and try to honor as many principles as possible. One must use creativity and reason to make a judgment. More important, ethical decision making requires that one personally enter into the decision-making process. Then, whatever decision is made, one must act on it (Morris, 2003). A decision of conscience blends moral judgment with the will to act on that judgment (Pozgar, 2014).

On the basis of cultural context and beliefs, when two values present themselves and one chooses one value rather than the other, one says that value is more important than the other. For example, a respect for client autonomy that stresses the right of competent clients to make their own choices on the basis of their cultural context can conflict with the principle of beneficence if a client's choice may be harmful.

Use of Codes and Other Ethical Directives

When confronted with an ethical conflict, choice, or decision, health care practitioners may turn to their professional code of ethics or other ethical directives, which may include oaths, prayers, and bills of rights. A *code of ethics* articulates the basis and minimal standards for character and conduct and the basic ethical principles relevant to professional practice. As guidelines for acceptable behaviors by members of a particular group, association, or profession, health care codes of ethics often relate general moral values, duties, and virtues to the unique situations encountered in health care practice. Codes of ethics also prescribe standards to guide professional conduct, principles expressing responsibilities and duties, and rules of specific conducts (Pozgar, 2014).

Professional codes of ethics serve a dual purpose: (1) to promote the integrity and reputation of the profession by maintaining specific standards of practice and (2) to serve society's well-being by protecting clients from incompetent practice. Professional ethics documents provide a moral framework for professional practice and define an ideal standard of practice at which to aim.

At the center of professional ethics codes and other ethical directives lie the values held by the profession. The moral duties articulated in ethics documents may be broad, such as respecting the dignity and self-determination of individuals, or specific, such as maintaining client confidentiality or not engaging in sexual relations with a client. The more general duties permit a certain amount of interpretation in their implementation by the individual practitioner, whereas the more specific ones establish minimum standards for professional behavior. Many groups also provide accompanying guides for professional conduct that attempt to elaborate behaviors consistent with their selected principles and virtues.

Professional ethics documents cannot make a practitioner ethical; they can only inform and guide. Moral guidelines may focus on the character of the individual, with the assumption that moral behavior will flow naturally from a moral person. Professional codes of ethics and other ethical directives ideally serve as something to aspire to. The ethical principles of the *Occupational Therapy Code of Ethics* (AOTA, 2015) that are most relevant to cultural effectiveness are as follows:

- *Principle 1.* Occupational therapy personnel shall demonstrate a concern for the well-being and safety of the recipients of their services. (Beneficence; p. 2)
- *Principle 4.* Occupational therapy personnel shall promote fairness and objectivity in the provision of occupational therapy services. (Justice; p. 5)
- *Principle 6.* Occupational therapy personnel shall treat client, colleagues, and other professionals with respect, fairness, discretion, and integrity. (Fidelity; p. 7)

Wells (2006) recognized that culture may influence how people cope with problems and interact with each other. The ways in which occupational therapy services are planned and implemented need to be culturally sensitive to be culturally effective, so occupational therapy practitioners have an ethical responsibility to be culturally effective practitioners.

Bioethics

Bioethics is the philosophical study of the ethical controversies brought about by advances in biology, research, and medicine (Glannon, 2005). A multidisciplinary field, bioethics blends philosophy, theology, history, and law with medicine, nursing, health policy, and the medical humanities (Center for Practical Bioethics, 2014) and applies ethical principles in health care delivery, medical treatment, and research (Slater, 2016).

The purview of bioethics ranges from the private and individual dilemmas health care workers face (e.g., What should I do here and now?) to the societal choices citizens and legislators face as they try to devise equitable health or environmental policies (e.g., What should we do together as citizens and fellow human beings?) Rather than provide specific answers, bioethics asks relevant questions, such as

- What is the most just way to distribute scarce resources such as health care technology?
- What obligation do health care practitioners have to treat clients in ethically acceptable ways?
- What is society's and individual practitioners' obligation in providing health care to disadvantaged people?
- What is the obligation of health care practitioners to treat clients?

Bioethicists ask these questions in the context of modern medicine and health care to foster public knowledge and comprehension of both moral philosophy and scientific advances. They note how medical technology can change the way we experience the meaning of health and illness and, ultimately, the way we live and die (Center for Practical Bioethics, 2014). Bioethics has brought about significant changes in standards for the treatment of the sick and for the conduct of research.

As the field of bioethics developed, four general areas of inquiry emerged that in practice often overlap: (1) health care ethics, (2) regulatory and policy bioethics, (3) cultural bioethics, and (4) neuroethics (Callahan, 2008; Center for Ethics and Humanities in the Life Sciences, 2014; Post, 2004).

Health Care Ethics

Health care ethics focuses on the ethics of the delivery and provision of health care. It involves questioning the ways human beings are treated in medicine, rehabilitation, and other related fields in light of personal and universal moral principles, rights, and values. Because of its context, health care ethics focuses on individual cases, seeking to determine what has to be done here and now with each client (Gordon, 2014).

Regulatory and Policy Bioethics

Regulatory and policy bioethics involves the development of legal or clinical rules and procedures applied to medical cases or general practices. Examples include the use of fetal tissue in research; the definition of death; and guidelines for do-not-resuscitate orders, euthanasia, cloning, and the rationing of health resources. This area of bioethics seeks to provide legal

and policy solutions to pressing societal problems that are ethically defensible and clinically sensible and feasible (Encyclopedia of Bioethics, 2004).

Cultural Bioethics

Cultural bioethics refers to ethical questions in relation to the historical, ideological, cultural, and social context in which bioethical principles are expressed. Culture has become important in bioethics because of divergent viewpoints and judgments from various cultures regarding many bioethical problems (Beck, 2014). Which practice among the many different practices in many cultures is the right one? Health care practitioners are obligated to fulfill their duties by respecting clients' attitudes and behaviors, but they should also observe common ethical standards with a special interpretation for different backgrounds and various cultures (Zahedi & Larijani, 2009).

Neuroethics

Neuroethics, now a formally recognized discipline, is a field of inquiry closely related to both cognitive neuroscience and bioethics that deals with the ethical implications of neuroscientific knowledge and technology. It involves consideration of the benefits and dangers of brain research, such as the use and effect of psychotropic or brain-altering drugs that change thought, mood, or behavior. Neuroethics can shed new light on the way humans make their decisions and their underlying motivations to act in certain ways (Tieu, 2007).

Culture and Ethics

Ethical dilemmas and conflicts arise frequently in culturally pluralistic settings. Health care dilemmas often occur when there are alternative choices, limited resources, and differing values among clients, family members, and caregivers (Pozgar, 2014). Most questions center on whether health care practitioners are obligated to act in accordance with contemporary medical ethics in the United States or with respect for the cultural differences of their clients and their families' wishes (Ho, 2006; Jotkowitz, Glick, & Gezundheit, 2006; Paasche-Orlow, 2004). Problems arise when participants in the health care setting have different interpretations of illness and treatment, hold disparate values in relation to death and dying, and use language or decision-making frameworks differently (Kleinman & Benson, 2006).

According to Beauchamp and Childress (2013), several general principles form the core of a cross-cultural common morality, including

- *Autonomy:* Respect for the decision-making capacity of the individual;
- *Nonmaleficence:* Avoidance of causing harm;
- *Beneficence:* Provision of benefits and balancing of benefits, burdens, and risks; and
- *Justice:* Fairness in the distribution of benefits and risks.

Although these principles can take different forms in different cultural contexts, they can be useful to consider in judging rightness and wrongness of beliefs and behaviors (Ebbesen, 2011; Zahedi & Larijani, 2009).

Autonomy

The U.S. Constitution and public laws recognize and uphold a person's right to make his or her own decisions about health care. People also have the right to know the risks and benefits of and alternatives to recommended procedures (Pozgar, 2014).

The principle of autonomy and individual rights can be at odds with the values of some cultures and religions, and a focus on individuality can overshadow the interconnectedness of social relationships. Autonomy is relational and situated rather than a matter of individual choice (Zahedi, 2011). Much of the world embraces a value system that places the family, the community, or society as a whole above the individual. In some cases, the good or primacy of the community may take precedence over the individual's autonomy (Crow, Matheson, & Steed, 2000; Zahedi, 2011).

Clients from all cultures want and need the support of their families. Recognizing the culturally prescribed role that families play when a loved one is ill demonstrates respect for individual values and wishes and supports the principle of autonomy (Jotkowitz et al., 2006; Kleinman & Benson, 2006; Zahedi, 2011).

To respect cultural differences encountered in clinical medicine, health care practitioners need to develop a level of comfort with client autonomy. Clinicians can accept a range of views and refrain

---

Case Example 15.1. Autonomy

A **52-year-old Nigerian immigrant** with an abiding fear of cancer visited his doctor because of a small growth on his lip. The pair had a long-standing patient–physician relationship, and the doctor was aware of the patient's fear of cancer. The patient and family were from a culture in which health care practitioners normally inform the family rather than the patient of a diagnosis.

When the biopsy was completed, the patient's son and daughter were informed of the patient's diagnosis and terminal prognosis. They asked that all information be withheld from the patient and one daughter. They reported a strong cultural prohibition against the telling of bad news, explaining that disclosure would discourage hope and might hasten the patient's death. They also expressed the fear that if their sister learned of the prognosis, it would place her unborn child at risk.

- Did this physician have an obligation to inform the patient of the diagnosis, placing autonomy above all other values?
- Or was the physician obligated to follow the family's wish, thereby respecting their cultural custom?

---

from assuming that their clients share their own perspectives (Paasche-Orlow, 2004). Individual beliefs and reactions to illness cannot be ascertained or presumed on the basis of the client's language, education, class, or ethnicity. Issues of autonomy and individual rights, ethical and cultural value systems, and family processes are important in influencing the position and assumptions that clients and health care practitioners carry into and throughout the delivery of health care. Autonomy is at the center of medical decision making regarding truth telling, advance directives, and informed consent (Glannon, 2005; Pozgar, 2014; Zahedi, 2011).

Truth Telling (Veracity)

The ethical principle of **veracity** (i.e., the duty to tell the truth) is central to the practitioner–client relationship. It binds the practitioner to honesty (Purtilo & Doherty, 2011). Veracity is not about disclosing a unilateral truth to the client; it is about an ongoing process of communication with the client (Jotkowitz et al., 2006; Surbone & Zwitter, 2000). The ethical justification for truth telling exists in the legal requirement for complete disclosure and the necessity of avoiding malpractice (Pozgar, 2014).

Cross-cultural differences in truth-telling attitudes and practices have become a major source of debate. The application of truth telling can become a quagmire when multiple cultural views, values, beliefs, and practices are operative. The predominant practice in the United States of disclosing a diagnosis of serious illness to the patient is not considered appropriate by individuals of some ethnic and religious cultures (Fallowfield & Jenkins, 2004). Many Mexican Americans, for example, endorse the view that doctors should not discuss death and dying with their patients because doing so could be harmful to the patient, and this population also tends to place emphasis on family-centered decision-making styles (Candib, 2002). Similarly, Eastern cultures place more emphasis on the collective role of the family in decision making and disclosure.

Lai (2006) argued that truth telling is influenced by four major social–cultural and ethical factors:

1. Family as a key player in medical-related decision making
2. Harmony as an essential value for both the individual and family
3. Taboos about discussing death and related issues
4. Ethical concerns in truth telling (e.g., the predominant value of nonmaleficence [i.e., to do no harm] may lead to not telling the truth).

Surbone (2006) suggested that imposing the truth on unprepared patients whose cultural expectation is to be shielded from painful medical information is culturally disrespectful or ineffective.

Advocates of truth telling believe that sharing information strengthens a trusting client–practitioner relationship (Zahedi, 2011). It is the duty of health care practitioners to ask clients if they wish to receive information and make decisions or if they prefer that their families handle such matters. In recent years, U.S. health care practitioners have learned to use listening skills and to let clients communicate what and how much they want to learn about their disease or condition. It is obligatory for health care practitioners to know how to provide information in a kind and considerate manner (Jotkowitz et al., 2006; Kleinman & Benson, 2006; Paasche-Orlow, 2004).

Informed Consent

Informed consent is a legal and ethical concept that consists of two components: (1) the disclosure of all medical information to the patient and (2) the right of competent patients to decide whether to accept or forgo treatment on the basis of the information given (Glannon, 2005). Although informed consent provides clients with the right to know the potential risks, benefits, and alternatives of a proposed treatment (Pozgar, 2014), it may be inapplicable to members of ethnic groups that traditionally make collective decisions among the family or tribal group (Ho, 2006).

Disclosing risks during an informed consent discussion and offering clients the opportunity to make advance directives can pose problems for adherents to traditional cultural beliefs. The structure of the language in advance directives is not culturally sensitive. For example, the traditional Navajo belief is that health is maintained and restored through positive ritual language. When health care practitioners disclose the risks of treatment in an informed consent discussion, they speak in a negative way, thereby violating the Navajo value of thinking and speaking in a positive way. The Navajo traditionally have believed that thought and language have the power to shape and control events (Jotkowitz et al., 2006; Sico, 2013). A Navajo Indian client would not be likely to prepare an advance directive. The realities of death and attempts to make plans for end-of-life scenarios cause some ethnic groups, such as Mexican Americans and Korean Americans, to shy away from planning because they do not feel that preparing advance directives will bring them or their family any benefit in a situation they believe is out of their hands (Sico, 2013).

Given the increasing diversity of the patient population, waiving informed consent or refusing family requests to withhold information from the patient cannot be taken lightly. It is important to open the channels of communication rather than impose an individualist approach to informed consent that could exacerbate the patient's and family's vulnerability and disharmony (Ho, 2006). Before sharing health information, health care practitioners need to assess the wishes of the patient, including whether the patient wants others present when information is provided (Crow et al., 2000).

Advance Directives

An ***advance directive*** allows people to make their wishes known regarding health decisions that must be made when they are legally incompetent, especially in the case of illness that will end in death (Purtilo & Doherty, 2011). Advance directives include legal documents such as the following (Purtilo & Doherty, 2011; Scott, 2013):

- *Living wills* enable patients to specify the types of treatment they would want to have and, more important, not have.
- *Durable power of attorney* enables patients to specify a surrogate or proxy decision maker to make treatment decisions when the patient is no longer able to (also called *health care proxy*).
- *Medical directives* enable patients to provide legal instructions regarding their preferences for medical care.
- *Do not resuscitate* and *do not intubate orders* are written by a physician and put in the medical record to enable patients to prevent unwanted resuscitative measures.
- *Out-of-facility do not resuscitate order* is a state-approved document designed to enable competent patients with a terminal medical condition to prevent unwanted resuscitative measures by others outside a medical treatment facility.
- *Declaration for mental health treatment* enables competent individuals to declare their wishes concerning future mental health treatment options.

Advance directives are processes accompanied by forms to help reassure clients that their wishes will be honored as much as possible. A key concept underlying advance directives is respect for a patient's right to give informed consent to health-related examination and intervention (Scott, 2013). These directives guide choices for practitioners and caregivers if the patient is terminally ill, seriously injured, in a coma, in the late stages of dementia, or near the end of life.

Reflection 15.2. Advance Directives

- How are occupational therapy practitioners in your setting made aware of existing client advance directives?

Nonmaleficence

The principle of *nonmaleficence* requires health care practitioners to not intentionally harm or injure the client, either through commission or omission, in the performance of their job (McCormick, 2013). The obligation to avoid or minimize the risk of harm is supported not only by commonly held moral convictions but also by the laws of society.

Western societies place greater importance on harmful acts done with deliberate intent than out of neglect or ignorance (Purtilo & Doherty, 2011). Harm can extend beyond physical or psychological harm and may include harm to one's reputation, liberty, or property. What constitutes harm may differ among clients as well as among health care practitioners (Garrett, Braillie, & Garrett, 2010).

This principle affirms the need for medical competence. Medical mistakes may occur; however, this principle articulates a fundamental commitment to protect clients from harm.

Beneficence

The meaning of the principle of *beneficence* is "doing good for others or bringing about good for them" (Slater, 2016, p. 291). It involves actions used to help other people. Health care practitioners have a duty to "prevent harm, remove harm when it is being inflicted and bring about positive good" (Purtilo & Doherty, 2011, p. 83). Health care practitioners must make an active decision to act with compassion, communicate with clients about what is going to happen, and consider the client's needs and feelings. Clients assume that practitioners are there for their benefit and will act with charity and kindness toward them (Purtilo & Doherty, 2011); yet what a clinician may think is good for the client may not be what the client wants or thinks is good for him or her (Kornblau & Burkhardt, 2012).

The goal of providing benefit is at the very heart of population health care: to promote the welfare of people. Should all members of society receive all the medical care they need? Should immunization be mandatory for children regardless of personal or religious belief? Beneficence entails an awareness of the inequality in some social structures (Allen, 2013). Doctors Without Borders, which provides medical care to the less fortunate around the world, is an example of an organization with beneficence as its foundation.

All health care practitioners must strive to improve their clients' health, to do the most good for all clients in every situation. But what is good for one client may not be good for another, so practitioners must consider each situation individually, taking into account cultural values that might conflict with the principle of beneficence.

Case Example 15.2. Ethical Principles

It is the end of the day. You have been treating clients since the 7:30 a.m. dressing program. You even had lunch at your desk while completing paperwork. You can't wait to go home and just relax and rest. But a local physician calls as you are walking out the door and asks you to conduct an evaluation of a male client age 45 years with a multiple sclerosis who is Muslim. Following the principles of nonmaleficence and beneficence, what actions would you take?

Justice

The principle of justice demands that health care practitioners be as fair as possible when offering treatments and allocating scarce medical resources. It is a form of fairness, giving to each that which is his or her due. If a patient arrives at the emergency room with a broken arm before another patient with a broken arm, the one who arrives first would expect to be seen first. However, if the patient who arrives second is bleeding profusely, the first patient would expect that person to be seen first. Practitioners should be able to justify their actions in every situation. The caring response is achieved when individuals or groups are treated fairly and equitably (McCormick, 2013; Purtilo & Doherty, 2011; Slater, 2016; Zahedi & Larijani, 2009).

Distributive justice is concerned with the distribution of health care goods and services. It hinges on the fact that some goods and services are in short supply; when there is not enough to go around, some fair means of allocating resources must be determined. Is everyone entitled to receive health care benefits, and if so, is everyone entitled to the same amount? The principle of distributive justice is the strong motivation behind health care reform to address the needs of the entire population. The principle of distributive justice is based on the use of medical conditions to justify the allocation of resources (e.g., as in Medicare; McCormick, 2013; Purtilo & Doherty, 2011).

Compensatory justice assumes that the allocation of resources should be based on more than medical need alone. The individual's position in society is also a relevant factor (e.g., workers' compensation). *Social justice* focuses on disparities in health and health care allocations (e.g., differences between racial and ethnic groups in health insurance coverage, access to and use of care, and quality of care; Purtilo & Doherty, 2011).

Approaches to the principle of justice foster the societal goals of providing care in the face of limited resources. The principle of justice is applied at the bedside of individual patients but also addressed systemically in laws and policies that govern the access of populations to health care.

Reflection 15.3. Ethics and Health Care Reform

- Identify and discuss ethical challenges that affect occupational therapy practitioners in the era of health care reform.

Ethics in Clinical Practice

The challenge in providing ethical and culturally competent care is in the diversity of meanings that can be applied to similar concepts and principles (Iwama, 2003). The meanings people assign to ideas and concepts are culturally based and culturally driven. Culture shapes people's views of illness and well-being in both the physical and spiritual realms and affects their perceptions of health care and the outcome of treatment. Practitioners may be comfortable with the idea of respecting cultural difference when the client is a competent adult, but when children are involved they may be unwilling to tolerate decisions that result in what they perceive to be compromised care or harm, even when these decisions make sense in the context of a particular culture (Jotkowitz et al., 2006). Cultural effectiveness is key to making sound, ethical, culturally appropriate decisions in clinical practice.

Practitioners and clients may not agree on a common set of cultural values. What may be regarded as morally wrong in one culture may be morally praiseworthy in another (Ho, 2006). For example, the sick role in occupational therapy is viewed as an active role, one in which clients achieve their optimal level of functioning through active participation. In other societies, however, the sick role is a passive role. In Chinese society, for example, it is sometimes believed that a person is chronically ill because of sins committed by family members. Thus, family members may try to do everything for the sick person, encouraging maximum dependence (Zahedi, 2011).

Beliefs and values serve as a basis for moral decision making and vary by culture. Ethics are greatly influenced by the cultural framework in which an interpersonal encounter takes place. Practitioners must be aware of the value assumptions embodied in biomedical approaches and in the culture, power, and ethics of medicine to identify how these assumptions play out in clinical practice (Coward & Hartrick, 2000; Paasche-Orlow, 2004). Clients and their families, as well as health care practitioners, bring many different cultural models of morality and moral reasoning to the clinical setting. Constantly overlapping and interacting cultures can create daily conflicts and dilemmas when providing health care services.

Because present bioethical concepts of moral deliberation offer little insight into how to develop meaningful responses to cultural pluralism, religious diversity, and normal conflicts, Wells (2005) proposed an *ethic of diversity framework* with moral principles and rules of human conduct for finding resolutions in a pluralistic environment (see Exhibit 15.1).

This framework, which includes the principles of understanding, tolerance, standing up to evil, fallibility, respect, cultural competence, justice, and care, can be used to guide decisions when conflicts arise in a multicultural setting. It can help health care practitioners and students engage in moral reasoning and test their moral opinions against those of others. It supports the expectation of differences in all clinical interactions.

The values of ethical relativism and pluralism hold that practitioners respect the moral choices clients make in light of their culture or religious beliefs (Haddad, 2001; Paasche-Orlow, 2004; Zahedi & Larijani, 2009). Embracing these values increases learning opportunities and facilitates cultural effectiveness. Using the ethic of diversity framework as a guideline offers practitioners an opportunity to extend human knowledge by finding wisdom in dissimilar cultural practices. It allows them to teach clients what, from a medical point of view, may

---

Exhibit 15.1. Ethic of Diversity Framework

The following principles can be used to protect clients against harm and to help identify the good of people. These principles collectively assist occupational therapy practitioners in acknowledging differences as "norms."

- *Principle of Understanding:* We seek to understand other cultures before we pass judgment on them.
- *Principle of Tolerance:* We recognize that there are important areas in which intelligent people of good will in fact differ.
- *Principle of Standing Up to Evil:* We recognize that at some point we must stand up against evil, even when it is outside of our own bodies.
- *Principle of Fallibility:* We recognize that, even with the best of intentions, our judgment may be flawed and mistaken.
- *Principle of Respect:* We recognize that all human beings are worthy of respect simply because they are human.
- *Principle of Cultural Competence:* We seek self-exploration, knowledge, and skills to interact effectively and humanely with people different from ourselves.
- *Principle of Justice:* We seek to deal with everyone fairly and equitably in the distribution of goods and services.
- *Principle of Care:* We recognize that the needs of others play a part in all ethical decision making.

Source. From "An Ethic of Diversity," by S. A. Wells, in *Educating for Moral Action: A Sourcebook in Health and Rehabilitation Ethics* (pp. 36–37), by R. B. Purtilo, G. M. Jensen, & C. B. Royeen (Eds.), 2005, Philadelphia: F. A. Davis. Copyright © 2005 by F. A. Davis. Adapted with permission.

damage health and to learn more about the rationale for and techniques of many traditional practices. It assists practitioners in discovering ways to give care to people who have different values and lifestyles in the clinical setting.

A cross-cultural ethical conflict may not have a single, ethically correct resolution but rather many possible resolutions, each with ethical costs and advantages (Pozgar, 2014; Purtilo & Doherty, 2011). Which resolution is ultimately chosen depends on which voices are included in the dialogue. Paasch-Orlow (2004) stated that culturally effective ethical decisions involve learning about culture, embracing pluralism, and minimizing the negative consequences of difference. A sound moral decision requires practitioners to reflect on their own values and biases, interpret the cultures involved, and acknowledge the contributions and principles of moral reasoning.

Reflection 15.4. Personal Code of Ethics

- Write a personal code of ethics, including principles to guide your interactions with culturally diverse individuals.

Summary

Clients bring cultural, religious, and ideological beliefs to every client–practitioner relationship. If health care practitioners' views on the ethical principles that govern decision making conflict with the values held by clients, their families, or their communities, disagreement over cultural values may lead to confrontation. Respecting the beliefs and values of the client is important in establishing an effective therapeutic relationship. Adults have a moral and legal right to make decisions about their own health care and to include their family in making such decisions. Conflicts based on cultural difference can be mediated using strategies that allow both the client and the practitioner the opportunity to clarify their values.

Each health care practitioner must embody an ethic of caring and respect for all groups, a responsibility to condemn unjust medical practices, and a humility and an empathy regarding human suffering. We must discover how to see each person as a cultural being; take the time to learn how the client and family define

ethical values; and give weight to alternative values, social systems, and decision-making styles. As we face the ethical challenges of today—health care reform, widening health disparities, chronic disease management, and electronic medical records (Lachman, 2012)—let's not forget to be ethical and culturally effective practitioners.

Reflection 15.5. Ethic of Diversity

- Is it unethical to deny treatments that are clearly unacceptable by the standards of Western culture but clearly acceptable by the standards of other culture of origin?

References

Allen, J. F. (2013). *Health law and medical ethics for healthcare professionals.* Boston: Pearson.

American Occupational Therapy Association. (2015). *Occupational therapy code of ethics (2015). American Journal of Occupational Therapy, 69*(Suppl. 3), S1–S48. http://dx.doi.org/10.5014/ajot.2015.696S03

Baranzke, H. (2012). "Sanctity-of-life"—A bioethical principle for a right to life? *Ethical Theory and Moral Practice, 15,* 295–308. http://dx.doi.org/10.1007/s10677-012-9369-0

Beauchamp, T. L., & Childress, J. F. (2013). *Principles of Biomedical Ethics* (7th ed.). New York: Oxford University Press.

Beck, D. (2014). Between relativism and imperialism: Navigating moral diversity in cross-cultural bioethics. *Developing World Bioethics, 15,* 162–171. http://dx.doi.org/10.1111/dewb.12059

Bishop, A., & Scudder, J. (2001). Caring presence. In *Nursing ethics: Holistic caring practice* (2nd ed., pp. 41–65). Sudbury, MA: Jones & Bartlett.

Boss, J. A. (1998). *Ethics for life: An interdisciplinary and multicultural introduction.* Mountain View, CA: Mayfield.

Buford, T. O. (1984). *Personal philosophy: The art of living.* New York: CBS College.

Callahan, D. (1995). History of bioethics. In W. T. Reich (Ed.), *Encyclopedia of bioethics* (2nd ed., rev.; Vol. 1, pp. 248–256). New York: Macmillan Reference.

Callahan, D. (2008). Bioethics and policy—A history. In M. Crowley (Ed.), *From birth to death and bench to clinic: The Hastings Center bioethics briefing book for journalists, policymakers, and campaigns* (pp. ix–x). New York: Hastings Center.

Candib, L. M. (2002). Truth telling and advance planning at the end of life: Problems with autonomy in a multicultural world. *Families, Systems, and Health, 20,* 213–228. http://dx.doi.org/10.1037/h0089471

Center for Ethics and Humanities in the Life Sciences. (2014). *What is bioethics?* Retrieved from http://www.bioethics.msu .edu/what-is-bioethics

Center for Practical Bioethics. (2014). *What is bioethics?* Retrieved from http://www.practicalbioethics.org/what-is-bioethics

Centers for Disease Control and Prevention. (2014). *Public health ethics.* Retrieved from http://www.cdc.gov/od/science/integrity /phethics

Chmielewski, C. (2004). *Values and cultures in ethical decision-making.* Retrieved from http://www.nacada.ksu.edu/Resources /Clearinghouse/View-Articles/Values-and-culture-in-ethical -decision-making.aspx

Cochrane, A. (2014). Environmental ethics. In *Internet ency-clopedia of philosophy.* Retrieved from http://www.iep.utm .edu/envi-eth/

Coward, H., & Hartrick, G. (2000). Perspectives on health and cultural pluralism: Ethics in medical education. *Clinical and Investigative Medicine, 23,* 261–266. Retrieved from http:// www.nlc-bnc.ca/eppp-archive/100/201/300/cdn_medical _association/cim/vol-23/issue-4/pdf/pg261.pdf

Crow, K., Matheson, L., & Steed, A. (2000). Informed consent and truth-telling: Cultural directions for healthcare providers. *Journal of Nursing Administration, 30,* 148–152. http://dx.doi .org/10.1097/00005110-200003000-00007

Davy, B. J. (2005). Being at home in nature: A Levinasian ap-proach to pagan environmental ethics. *Pomegranate, 7,* 157–172. http://dx.doi.org/10.1558/pome.2005.7.2.157

DeLapp, K. M. (2015). Metaethics. In *The Internet Encyclope-dia of Philosophy.* Retrieved from http://www.iep.utm.edu /metaethi/

Diffen. (n.d.). *Ethics vs. morals.* Retrieved from http://www.diffen .com/difference/Ethics_vs_Morals

Dittmer, J. (2014). Applied ethics. In *Internet encyclopedia of philosophy.* Retrieved from http://www.iep.utm.edu /ethics/

Duignan, B. (Ed.). (2011). *The Britannica guide to ethics: Think-ers and theories in ethics.* New York: Britannica Educational.

Ebbesen, M. (2011). Cross cultural principles for bioethics. In G. D. Gargiulo (Ed.), *Advanced biomedical engineering.* Rijeka, Croatia: InTech. http://www.intechopen.com/books/advanced -biomedical-engineering/cross-cultural-principles-for-bioethics

Fallowfield, L., & Jenkins, V. (2004). Communicating sad, bad, and difficult news in medicine. *Lancet, 363,* 312–319. http://dx.doi.org/10.1016/S0140-6736(03)15392-5

Fieser, J. (2014). Ethics. In *Internet Encyclopedia of Philosophy.* Retrieved from http://www.iep.utm.edu/ethics/

Fremgen, B. F. (Ed.) (2012). *Medical law and ethics* (4th ed.). Boston: Pearson.

Garrett, T. M., Braillie, H. W., & Garrett, R. M. (2010). *Health care ethics: Principles and problems* (5th ed.). Upper Saddle River, NJ: Pearson Prentice Hall.

Glannon, W. (2005). *Biomedical ethics.* New York: Oxford Uni-versity Press.

Gordon, J. S. (2012). Human rights in bioethics—Theoretical and applied. *Ethical Theory and Moral Practice, 15,* 283–294. http://dx.doi.org/10.1007/s10677-012-9365-4

Gordon, J. S. (2014). Bioethics. In *Internet Encyclopedia of Phi-losophy.* Retrieved from http://www.iep.utm.edu/bioethic/

Haddad, A. (2001). Acute care decisions: Ethics in action. *RN, 64*(3), 21–24. Retrieved from https://dspace.creighton.edu /xmlui/handle/10504/65342

Ho, A. (2006). Family and informed consent in multicultural setting. *American Journal of Bioethics, 6,* 6–28. http://dx.doi .org/10.1080/15265160500394531

Innovateus. (2015). *What influences social ethics?* Retrieved from www.innovateus.net/innopedia/what-influences-social-ethics

Iwama, M. (2003). Toward culturally relevant epistemologies in occupational therapy. *American Journal of Occupational Ther-apy, 57,* 582–588. http://dx.doi.org/10.5014/ajot.57.5.582

Johnson, V. (1995). *Heart full of grace: A thousand years of Black wisdom.* New York: Simon & Schuster.

Jonsen, A. R., Siegler, M., & Winslade, W. J. (2010). *Clinical ethics: A practical approach to ethical decisions in clinical med-icine* (7th ed.). New York: McGraw-Hill.

Jotkowitz, A., Glick, S., & Gezundheit, B. (2006). Truth-telling in a culturally diverse world. *Cancer Investigation, 24,* 786–789. http://dx.doi.org/10.1080/07357900601063972

Kihlbom, U. (2000). Guidance and justification in particularistic ethics. *Bioethics, 4,* 287–309. http://dx.doi.org/10.1111/1467 -8519.00199

Kleinman, A., & Benson, P. (2006). Anthropology in the clinic: The problem of cultural competency and how to fix it. *PLoS Medicine, 3,* 1673–1676. http://dx.doi.org/10.1371/journal .pmed.0030294

Kornblau, B. L., & Burkhardt, A. (2012). *Ethics in rehabilita-tion: A clinical perspective* (2nd ed.). Thorofare, NJ: Slack.

Lachman, V. D. (2012). Ethical challenges in the era of health care reform. *Medsurg Nursing, 21,* 248–250, 245. Retrieved from http://www.nursingworld.org/MainMenuCategories/Ethics Standards/Resources/Ethical-Challenges-in-the-Era-of-Health -Care-Reform.pdf

Lai, Y. (2006, July). *Views from Asia: Truth telling in cancer di-agnosis and progress in Taiwan.* Paper presented at the World Cancer Congress of the Union for International Cancer Control, Washington, DC. Retrieved from https://2006. confex.com/uicc/uicc/techprogram/P10430.HTM

Ludwick, R., & Silva, M. C. (2000). Ethics: Nursing around the world: Cultural values and ethical conflicts. *Online Journal of Issues in Nursing, 5*(3). Retrieved from www.nursingworld.org /MainMenuCategories/ANAMarketplace/ANAPeriodicals /OJIN/Columns/Ethics/CulturalValuesandEthicalConflicts .aspx

McClimans, L. M., Dunn, M., & Slowther, A. M. (2011). Health policy, patient-centred care and clinical ethics. *Journal of Evaluation in Clinical Practice, 17,* 913–919. http://dx.doi.org/10.1111/j.1365-2753.2011.01726.x

McCormick, T. R. (2013). *Principles of bioethics.* Retrieved from https://depts.washington.edu/bioethx/tools/princpl.html#prin2.

McCullough, L. B. (2014). Deliberative clinical ethics: Getting back to basics in the work of clinical ethics and clinical ethicists. *Journal of Medicine and Philosophy, 39,* 1–7. http://dx.doi.org/10.1093/jmp/jht054

Morris, J. F. (2003, February 24). Is it possible to ethical? *OT Practice,* pp. 18–23.

O'Sullivan, J. P. (2014). Josef Fuchs' revised natural law: Possibilities for social ethics. *New Blackfriars, 95,* 379–396. http://dx.doi.org/10.1111/nbfr.12077

Paasche-Orlow, M. (2004). The ethics of cultural competence. *Academic Medicine, 79,* 347–350. http://dx.doi.org/10.1097/00001888-200404000-00012

Pellegrino, E. D., & Thomasma, D. C. (1981). *A philosophical basis of medical practice: Toward a philosophy and ethic of the healing professions.* New York: Oxford University Press.

Petrini, C. (2007). Theoretical models and operational frameworks in public health ethics. *International Journal of Environmental Research and Public Health, 7,* 189–202. http://dx.doi.org/10.3390/ijerph7010189

Post, S. G. (Ed.). (2004). *Encyclopedia of bioethics.* New York : Macmillan Reference.

Pozgar, G. D. (2014). *Legal and ethical issues for health professionals* (4th ed.). Boston: Jones & Bartlett.

Purtilo, R. B., & Doherty, R. F. (2011). *Ethical dimensions in the health professions* (5th ed.). St. Louis, MO: Elsevier/Saunders.

Purtilo, R. B., Jensen, G. M., & Royeen, C. B. (Eds.). (2005). *Educating for moral action: A sourcebook in health and rehabilitation ethics.* Philadelphia: F. A. Davis.

Robinson, L. (2008). Moral principles are not moral laws. *Journal of Ethics and Social Philosophy, 2*(3), 1–22. Retrieved from http://www.jesp.org/PDF/MoralPrinciplesAreNotMoralLaws.pdf

Scott, R. W. (2013). *Legal, ethical, and practical aspects of patient care documentation: A guide for rehabilitation professionals* (4th ed.). Burlington, MA: Jones & Bartlett.

Sico, R. (2013). End-of-life care: The legal, cultural, and interdisciplinary barriers hindering the effective use of advance directives *Annals of Health Law, 22,* 44–63. Retrieved from http://www.luc.edu/media/lucedu/law/centers/healthlaw/pdfs/advancedirective/pdfs/issue10/sico.pdf

Slater, D. Y. (2011). Glossary of ethics terms. In D. Y. Slater (Ed.), *Reference guide to the Occupational Therapy Code of Ethics and Ethics Standards* (pp. 223–228). Bethesda, MD: AOTA Press.

Slater, D. Y. (2016). Appendix A: Glossary of ethics terms. In D. Y. Slater (Ed.), *Reference guide to the Occupational Therapy Code of Ethics* (2015 ed., pp. 291–292). Bethesda, MD: AOTA Press.

Surbone, A. (2006). Telling the truth to patients with cancer: What is the truth? *Lancet Oncology, 7,* 944–950. http://dx.doi.org/10.1016/S1470-2045(06)70941-X

Surbone, A., & Zwitter, M. (2000). Communication with the cancer patient: Information and truth. In *Annals of the New York Academy of Sciences* (2nd ed., pp. 109–118). New York: Johns Hopkins University.

Tieu, M. (2007). Neuroethics: The law and the person. *Bioethics Research Notes, 19*(3). Retrieved from http://www.bioethics.org.au/Resources/Online%20Articles/Opinion%20Pieces/1903%20Neuroethics%20The%20Law%20and%20The%20Person%20MT.pdf

Veatch, R. M., & Flack, H. E. (1997). *Case studies in allied health ethics.* Upper Saddle River, NJ: Prentice-Hall.

Wells, S. A. (2005). An ethic of diversity. In R. B. Purtilo, G. M. Jensen, & C. B. Royeen (Eds.), *Educating for moral action: A sourcebook in health and rehabilitation ethics* (pp. 31–41). Philadelphia: F. A. Davis.

Wells, S. A. (2016). Cultural competency and ethical practice. In D. Y. Slater (Ed.), *Reference guide to the Occupational Therapy Code of Ethics* (2015 ed., pp. 155–160). Bethesda, MD: AOTA Press.

Zahedi, F. (2011). The challenge of truth telling across cultures: A case study. *Journal of Medical Ethics and History of Medicine, 4,* 11.

Zahedi, F., & Larijani, B. (2009). Common principles and multiculturalism. *Journal of Medical Ethics and History of Medicine, 2,* 6. Retrieved from http://www.ncbi.nlm.nih.gov/pmc/articles/PMC3713936/

Chapter 16.

CLIENT-CENTERED, CULTURALLY EFFECTIVE OCCUPATIONAL THERAPY: A PHENOMENOLOGICAL STUDY

Peggy M. Martin, PhD, OTR/L

It is essential that occupational therapists question, listen, and respond to all of their clients, but especially those clients who are the most different from themselves.
Peggy M. Martin (2008, p. 146)

Chapter Highlights

- Background on Culturally Effective Practice
- Method
- Findings
- Discussion
- Implications for Occupational Therapy Practice

Key Terms and Concepts

- ✧ Altruism
- ✧ Being greeted
- ✧ Biomedical communication
- ✧ Coming to therapy
- ✧ Culture
- ✧ Patient-centered communication

- ✧ Phenomenology
- ✧ Put Yourself in My Shoes
- ✧ See Me Like Anybody Else
- ✧ Understand My Culture
- ✧ Worry and Concern

Occupational therapy aims to help people participate in everyday life through the therapeutic use of life activities (Moyers & Dale, 2007). Treatment goals commonly reflect Western cultural values of individualism, independence, materialism, mobility, and productivity (Kondo, 2004; Pierce, 2003). Tension may exist when these professional values are not congruent with those of the client receiving services (Kondo, 2004). Misunderstandings may occur when practitioners do not understand cultural beliefs or cannot adequately communicate using easily understood language.

This chapter reports a study designed to add understanding about the client experience when the client and practitioner differ in ethnic or racial background.

Background on Culturally Effective Practice

Little research has examined culturally effective practice in occupational therapy. Case studies have explored aspects of cultural effectiveness through narratives of therapy episodes. Blanche (1996) analyzed the therapy experience when the client and therapist shared an ethnic and linguistic background, recommending more culturally competent occupational therapy practice. Kondo (2004) described a case in which the assumptions of a Western-based occupational therapist led to misunderstanding about discharge goals. Odawara (2005) analyzed critical incidents in two different therapy episodes with therapists and clients who both identified themselves as part of Japanese communities, adding to an understanding of how cultural values emerge within the therapy relationship.

The study (Martin, 2008) described in this chapter examined the client experience in racially different client–occupational therapist dyads in hopes of uncovering a structure of culturally effective practice. In occupational therapy practice, "all aspects of the domain, including occupations, client factors, performance skills, performance patterns, and context and environment, are of equal value, and together they interact to affect the client's occupational identity, health, well-being, and participation in life" (American Occupational Therapy Association [AOTA], 2014, p. S4). If background similarity between therapist and client leads to a shared understanding of occupations, performance patterns, and context and environment, then how do clients who self-identify as being different from their therapist experience the occupational therapy process?

Practitioner and Client Diversity

The occupational therapy process often occurs with practitioners and clients who differ racially or ethnically. According to the 2015 AOTA Salary and Workforce Study, 90.9% of occupational therapists were women, and 85.3% were White (AOTA, 2015a); in contrast, 2010 Census data indicate that the U.S. general population was 50.8% women (U.S. Census Bureau, 2011a) and 72.4% White (U.S. Census Bureau, 2011b). As a result, occupational therapy practitioners often interact with people who differ in gender and race or ethnicity from themselves. *Culture* refers to beliefs, values, and attitudes shared by members of a social group (Geetz, 1973), so it is likely that occupational therapy practitioners frequently differ culturally from their clients when practicing occupational therapy.

Reflection 16.1. Practitioner vs. U.S. Demographics

Describe a time when you interacted with people who differed from yourself.

- How did you feel?
- What words best describe these feelings (e.g., *inquisitive, uncertain, fearful, comfortable*)?
- Describe a time when your health care provider differed in background from yourself.
- How important is it for rehabilitation practitioners to be members of ethnic communities that they serve?

One element of client–practitioner interaction affected by cultural differences is communication. After reviewing 14 articles published between 1974 and 2004, Schouten and Meeuwesen (2006) concluded that doctors interacting with patients who differed in cultural and ethnic backgrounds had more communication difficulties, behaved less affectively, and provided less health instruction. Patients who differed ethnically from the physician were less verbally expressive and less assertive in medical interactions than were White patients with White physicians.

Research results support the value of focusing on communication in models of culturally competent practice. For example, Burch (2008) concluded that rehabilitation professionals need to develop intercultural skills when working with people of diverse sexual orientations; in their study, occupational therapists, physical therapists, speech therapists, nurses, and physicians reported low levels of knowledge and mastery in interactions with spinal cord–injured clients of diverse sexual orientations.

As a whole, the evidence suggests that practitioner communication skill is linked to client satisfaction; thus, increased practitioner skill in intercultural communication is an important outcome aligning with the Triple Aim of improving the client experience, improving health, and reducing costs (Berwick, Nolan, & Whittington, 2008).

Disparity in Health Outcomes

People have different health outcomes on the basis of their race and ethnicity. Some of this difference is attributed to biological factors, but greater difference is attributed to social or procedural differences in health care practice. White people have better outcomes after stroke (Cruz-Flores et al., 2011), spinal cord injury (Myaskovsky et al., 2011), joint replacement (Freburger et al., 2011), trauma (Englum et al., 2011), and pain (Meghani et al., 2012). Health disparities involving other groups, such as lesbian, gay, and bisexual people (Fredriksen-Goldsen, Kim, Barkan, Muraco, & Hoy-Ellis, 2013) and people with disabilities (Drum, McClain, Horner-Johnson, & Taitano, 2011), also exist.

Hypothesized causes of these disparities include social, economic, geographic, access, health system, and genetic factors. Researchers most often evaluate health outcomes of rehabilitation by post-hospital place of discharge (Englum et al., 2011; Freburger et al., 2011; Meghani et al., 2012), results on national outcome measures such as the FIM™ (Granger, Hamilton, Keith, Zielezny, & Sherwin, 1986; Putnam et al., 2010), or self-perceived health satisfaction scales (Myaskovsky et al., 2011). People of color (non-Hispanic Black and Hispanic individuals) receiving Medicare have higher 30-day readmission rates after postacute inpatient rehabilitation (Ottenbacher et al., 2014). Although researchers acknowledge the complexity of factors influencing this metric, the use of benchmarks such as hospital readmission rates to determine payment has helped uncover disparate health outcomes experienced by people who are racial and ethnic minorities.

The aim of my research was to uncover strategies to improve the quality of occupational therapy for culturally diverse clients. I sought to answer the research question, What is the experience of people discharged from occupational therapy who differ racially or ethnically from their occupational therapist?

Reflection 16.2. Client's Perspective

Culturally effective therapy is client centered; it requires that practitioners understand the presenting problem from the client's perspective.

- What stance, arousal level, or state of mind enables a practitioner to understand the client's perspective?
- Can a practitioner's behavior prevent a client from sharing their perspective?
- How does a practitioner ensure that his or her understanding of the client's concerns aligns with that of the client?

Method

A qualitative phenomenological approach was used to describe the experiences of 5 recipients of occupational therapy who differed from their therapist by race or ethnicity. *Phenomenology* is an approach to research that is based on the premise that knowledge is subjective and experienced. Phenomenology can be used to describe and deepen our understanding of an individual's subjective experiences through his or her expressions of time and relationships (Davidson, 2003). Phenomenology explains a phenomenon (Heidegger, 1962) by analyzing the meanings people hold about the phenomenon and by describing the structure of the phenomenon (Giorgi, 1997).

I sought to describe the structure experienced by people receiving occupational therapy from a therapist different from them in race or ethnicity. I conducted interviews with the 5 participants and transcribed, analyzed, and thematically interpreted the narratives spoken within the interviews with the aim of uncovering the tacit (unexpressed) structure of the phenomena the participants experienced within their intercultural occupational therapy relationships.

All participants had received at least 2 weeks of individual occupational therapy following a framework of intervention determined by their occupational therapist. Specific therapy settings and general intervention approaches were recounted by the participants at the time of interview and are reported within the descriptions of each participant.

Participants

Participants were included in the study if they had been discharged from occupational therapy service within the 3 years preceding the study (2003–2006) and if they identified as being racially or ethnically different from their primary occupational therapist. Participants were excluded if the occupational therapy service did not include intervention or if an interpreter was used during the therapy sessions.

Participants were recruited by flyers posted in public locations near occupational therapy clinics in a large Midwestern health care facility and through purposeful sampling whereby agencies serving people with disabilities included the recruitment text in newsletters. One clinic specializing in the rehabilitation of chronic conditions purposefully contacted discharged clients who might meet the inclusion and exclusion criteria.

After extensive recruitment efforts, 5 individuals who self-identified as racially or ethnically different from their therapist volunteered to give voice to their experience receiving occupational therapy. In 4 of the 5 cases, the therapist was a White woman, and in one case the therapist was a White man. Three participants had most recently been discharged from the same outpatient clinic specializing in the treatment of chronic pain; 1 had received occupational therapy in a school and work setting, and 1 had been discharged from an outpatient rehabilitation clinic. All but 1 participant spoke English as their primary language.

Each participant was asked to select his or her own pseudonym. The following are brief biographies of the participants:

- **Amina** was a wife, mother, worker, and immigrant from Somalia. She was mother to 6 children, all under age 10 years. Amina entered therapy because of a back injury and arm pain and received therapy from an outpatient clinic that specialized in serving people with chronic pain. She spoke English as a second language without the use of an interpreter during therapy sessions.
- **Eagle Cloud** was a 30-something man who described himself as a full-blooded Native American and a person with a disability. He was diagnosed as a young child with fetal alcohol spectrum disorder and received occupational therapy intermittently throughout his childhood. Eagle Cloud had recently been discharged from occupational therapy after being treated for a balance and mobility disorder.

- **Missy** was an African American woman in her mid-40s. She cared for her grandchild while parenting a remaining child at home. Missy had had a strong work history until she was injured at work. Missy had been discharged from occupational therapy and was seeking new career options.
- **Smiley** was an African American man in his early 30s. After surviving a full tour of active wartime duty as a Marine, he returned home and was injured at work. Smiley had recently completed occupational therapy in an outpatient clinic specializing in the management of chronic pain.
- **Suzy,** an African American woman in her mid-40s, had received occupational therapy intermittently throughout her life as a result of living with cerebral palsy. Suzy worked part-time as a disability consultant in a large university. She was recently discharged from occupational therapy to treat an exacerbated fine motor impairment affecting her arm and hand function.

Data Collection: Phenomenological Interviews

I interviewed each participant twice using open-ended questions to gather descriptive information about their experience receiving occupational therapy. The first interview was designed to elicit an experiential narrative to describe receiving occupational therapy from a racially or ethnically different therapist.

Each interview opened with the question, "What is it like to receive occupational therapy when your therapist is racially or ethnically different from yourself?" Additional probing questions were asked to clarify, redirect, or further explore something stated by the participant using questions such as "Can you tell me more about that?" or "How did your body experience that?" When the conversation became more factually than meaningfully descriptive, I asked the question, "Can you tell me of a time when you received health care that was not culturally competent?"

The second interview occurred after I analyzed the first interview and provided the opportunity to clarify statements from the first interview. This interview again began with the question, "What is it like to receive occupational therapy when your therapist is racially or ethnically different from yourself?" After providing an opportunity to answer, I gave each participant a copy of the themes derived from his or her first interview to prompt further description. All interviews occurred at a time and place selected by the participant and were approximately 1 hour in length.

Data Analysis: Phenomenological Text Analysis

All interviews were recorded and transcribed as text. After first reading the text for overall meaning, I divided each text into central units of meaning, adding description to the experience of receiving occupational therapy (van Manen, 1990). Each meaning unit was labeled with words the participant had used, which I later translated into the language of occupational therapy practice (Giorgi, 1997). This process was important in enabling me to more fully understand the experience of the client unencumbered by my previous understandings. For example, one participant described how he "trained" his therapist, saying,

> If you are patient around me, I know what it means to be patient. But if you're all fidgety with me, trying to hurry up and get things done, then I channel, I tend to, people's energy are like super glue to me. If somebody's really fast and not focused, then I'm not going to be focused.

I labeled the meaning unit from the natural attitude as "people's energy are like super glue to me and affect me." Using professional terminology, I translated the label of this meaning unit to "client

performance is affected by therapist arousal level." I then grouped meaning units into themes, each theme describing an essential component of the description of the experience (Giorgi, 1997).

Findings

The following themes emerged from the phenomenological text analysis (see Figure 16.1):

- *Coming to Therapy:* When participants became clients, they felt tensions because their health no longer supported their existing social roles.
- *Worry and Concern:* Participants were filled with uncertainty and worried anticipation.
- *Being Greeted:* The greeting, both personal and physical, helped alleviate participants' anxiety and was perceived as an important invitation.
- *Understand My Culture:* Participants sought understanding, acceptance, and permission to retain their culture within the therapy experience. They experienced feeling cared for when the therapy was at their level—that is, when it was paced appropriately for their rate of work and adapted to their learning style.
- *See Me Like Anybody Else:* Participants spoke of noticing others and watching how others were treated to ascertain whether all clients were treated equally.
- *Put Yourself in My Shoes:* Participants felt cared for when the intervention was "at their level" and "relaxed."

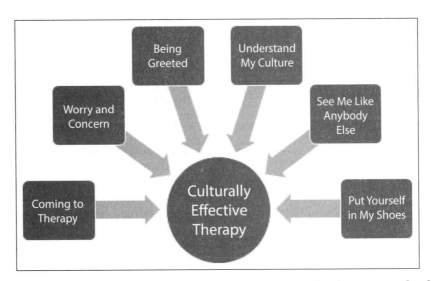

Figure 16.1. Themes uncovered in the phenomenological text analysis.

Themes are discussed in this order to reflect their interdependent nature and the sequence used by the participants to describe their therapy experience.

Coming to Therapy

Participants entered an unknown experience when they came to occupational therapy. An important event preceded each therapy episode; for most, it was when they realized they required help to fill valued social roles. Three of the participants were unable to continue working, either outside or within the home, and expressed this theme as follows:

- *Smiley:* "When I first found out I had to go through therapy, I really didn't want to be bothered with it. I felt, you know, I'll be able to get better. I'll try to stretch and do things my way, but I knew it wasn't working."
- *Amina:* "I was very deficit and I cannot hold my baby long enough, you know? Our body, it work together, what we don't feel when we are healthy."
- *Missy:* "One time, one minute, you can just about do anything you want to do, and then the next minute, you can't barely do anything—you can't even wash clothes and stuff like that." In her second interview, Missy extended her description: "It's ugly. At the point when I first got injured, I was just a waste, 'cause I couldn't do nothin.' What can I do? I can't. I could barely lift up anything, couldn't sweep, vacuum, none of that stuff."

Thus, the Coming to Therapy theme describes the tensions participants felt when their health no longer supported their existing social roles and they became occupational therapy clients.

Reflection 16.3. Welcome

Imagine you are a client at the setting where you work.

- What degree of welcome do you feel when you are scheduled for or learning about your therapy appointment?
- When walking into your setting?
- Identify at least 3 items or actions that could add to the friendly, welcoming atmosphere of your setting.

Worry and Concern

Although each participant's story was different, each used words such as *worry, scary,* and *distress* or described unfilled expectations to characterize their experience of coming to therapy. The participants described their wariness of the new health encounter. Smiley used words, including *nervous, worried,* and, later, *relief.* Smiley recalled his first meeting with the occupational therapist, who quickly made him feel comfortable:

He really relaxed me, [and said] that it's not anything painful or anything that you have to really worry about. Like if I did feel pain, to let him know down the road. But the thing that sticks out in my head most of all was that they were very quick to make you feel comfortable about just joking around and making a comfortable atmosphere for me to deal with. I felt this was real nice because I never had therapy before.

Missy described her own early worry: "When I first went in, I was nervous and everything. Like, are they going to torture me, and all this and that, and get mad if I can't do it, and stuff like that?"

Participants also worried about access to and payment of therapy by their health insurance company, some having already waited a long time for insurance approval. Eagle Cloud said,

The stress was always there because bills was still coming in. My significant other, she was stressed out even though she never pointed a finger, but yet she still gave me support. Basically all the bills were on her, and then still I'm waking up certain days and I'm in a lot of pain, but I still have to try to keep going through with everything. It was difficult.

Stress accompanying the beginning of therapy was compounded by reduced English fluency for Amina, who spoke English with a strong accent:

It's not easy, you know? To be shunned when you are, it's just very limit, you might have a lot of stress, you know? More you know the language, the more you get help or you know you can say your problem: "I have this, and I need [to get] healthy." If your language is very limit, you're pretty much a disabled person. You need to say something to body you cannot express. And even sometime it is interpreter, they didn't help you 'cause you have your *own* feeling, you have your *own* worries, and you say something they are, you know, they didn't say it the way you want.

Therapy was seen as the unknown place to "get healthy" or to regain lost functions. Participants were concerned about whether they would be asked to do things they had never before done, about whether they would get better and return to healthy living, about insurance and financial stability, and about how they would be treated and engaged in occupational therapy. Experiences in the Worry and Concern theme were conveyed in tones of uncertainty and worried anticipation.

Reflection 16.4. Minimizing Stress

Reflect on a past experience you have had with a health care system.

- What prompted your visit?
- What feelings did you experience within the health care encounter?
- List 5 things about this health care visit that positively contributed to your experience.
- Now list 5 things that negatively influenced your experience.
- What themes do you see?

Being Greeted

Friendliness of the staff and therapists helped alleviate participants' worries and concerns. Being greeted was seen as a sign of respect. Smiley described its importance as follows:

> The greeting is respectful. I mean, when I was raised up as a child, my mom always told me, you say, "Hey, how you doin' today?" Or "good morning," "good afternoon," or somethin' like that. Respect was there in that aspect also, not prying into my business. That's respectful to me.

Missy, who disclosed that she had not returned to two different previous therapy clinics, described being greeted at her most recent therapy location:

> They was so nice and sympathetic with me. First I thought of, like, is it just me, or is it everybody who walks through that door, they treatin' the same way? Everybody with a smile

or "hello" and everything else, so it's real nice. If you want coffee or whatever, cappuccino, they got a little bit of some. It was just nice. I liked it. Like I said, I would go back just to be going!

Sometimes the receptionist, as the frontline greeter, greeted participants the most enthusiastically and was a significant reason for participants' return to the clinic. Amina described one receptionist this way:

> She just, you know, accepts you. She knows you. I don't know how I explain her because my English is limited. She so friendly. She looks like she made a lot of effort to make happy the patients. I don't know, she African-American lady, though. I watch her most of time. . . . What I mean is that she has a lot energy to welcome her patients.

Sometimes the physical environment of the clinic contributed to participants' sense of being greeted. Some participants mentioned the presence of a wide variety of magazines, some intended for non-White audiences, as a physical greeting. Others mentioned the types of pictures on the walls and the presence of coffee kiosks as being inviting. The theme of Being Greeted, both personally and physically, communicated how the people and environment of the clinic alleviated participants' anxiety and served as an important invitation to participate in therapy.

Reflection 16.5. Invitation to Participate

Clients feel satisfied when they are greeted and feel welcomed. The initial interview is a critical time for occupational therapy practitioners to learn the presenting story from the client's perspective.

- What specific questions can you use in the initial interview with clients to help them feel greeted and invited to participate?

Understand My Culture

Culture is core to each individual and a vantage point for understanding the cross-cultural therapy encounter. Participants talked of culture using phrases such as *my people, culture people, I was taught, my culture, my background,* and *cultural standards* to voice a connection to an entity bigger than themselves.

Eagle Cloud stated, "[Culture] helps me—not that I ever forget who I am, where I come from and stuff—but it helps me remember who I am." Participants shared stories about being Black in a White world, of being raised by a grandmother who understood the Native American culture, and of being asked to do things in the United States that were against the ways they were taught in their birth country. Amina's story about a therapy intervention held in a therapeutic pool was particularly revealing:

> I don't feel comfortable going man with the pool. I know it is clinic, and I don't feel that I can do something to staring at my body. I don't feel that way. But at the same time, it's not the way I grew up and it's against my culture, you know? Go swimming with the other man if, you know, which is not my husband or someone, you know? And I never do it.

Although Amina discussed her concerns with the therapist, a suitable solution was not found within the therapy episode.

Clients perceived themselves as being different from their therapists. Suzy stated, "When you look around you, you see that most people who have done that and who have gotten somewhere near the top, if not at the top, don't look like you." Later in the same interview, Suzy continued,

> When I came here [place of work], I knew that I was going to be the only person of color. It is the same with getting therapy. I never, I have never in my life seen . . . I take that back. Once, in high school, I had physical therapy at home, and I had an African-American physical therapist, and her name was Suzy. Yes. But I had her for a very limited period of time. I guess I was about 17. She was the only person of color I ever seen in that particular field. Yeah! We had lots of fun!

Eagle Cloud also talked about the benefits of sharing ethnicity with a psychologist who provided care:

> That's the one thing I like about having a Native American psychologist: It's not a power trip or a power struggle about whose beliefs are more real. And that's real easy for people who don't understand the Native American culture and

don't have any sensitivity training—it's easy for them to push their beliefs. And that's the one thing that's not healthy.

The Understand My Culture theme described something to which participants belonged, from which they came, a filter of affordances for opportunity, and a lens for shared understanding when client and therapist shared a culture.

See Me Like Anybody Else

The theme of See Me Like Anybody Else was about the similarity of all individuals. People noticed how they fit with others receiving services and compared their treatment to that of others around them. Smiley said,

> They were watching me, and I was watching them, because I was looking at them do their exercises in therapy, and everyone seemed to have a big amount of contentment in their heart. As far as the treatment that they were receiving and how the therapists were toward them, I felt that everyone did feel they were treated in a humane manner—respectfully, and not stereotyped against or whatever. I just remember a lot of smiling from the other people who were from different countries and some other Afro-Americans that were there. They seemed pretty nice toward me and towards the staff. . . . I noticed that everyone was treated the same, equally. That made me feel more at home, too, to see other people from different countries be treated the same way as I was.

Amina said,

> I can say I don't feel any different. Even outside, with other people who are Cambodi and different culture, different, you know, colonists, American, and I was very comfortable. I don't feel different. I don't feel, you know, dismissed by appointment. I don't feel hate, any, you know, disrespect towards. I just feel respect.

Missy felt similarly, saying, "Wasn't any differences, just like there was no colors or racial things when she was on the job—just treating me like I was a regular person, from the bottom on." The theme of See Me Like Anybody Else described participants noticing others, watching how others were treated, and seeing that all clients were treated equally.

Put Yourself in My Shoes

The theme of Put Yourself in My Shoes describes the empathy that participants wanted to see from their therapists. Caring requires that practitioners pay attention to the individuality of their clients. Put Yourself in My Shoes included the subthemes of Feeling Cared For and Letting Me Be Me. Participants felt cared for when their therapists were compassionate, focused on client performance, expressed overall concern about the client's health, and asked questions and listened to answers.

Participants also felt cared for when the intervention was "at their level" and "relaxed," which Missy explained as follows: "They took their time and asked me my concerns and asked me what it is that I be able to do." For Eagle Cloud, it was feeling that his "inner self has to trust for the outer self to do its work." Therapists, he said, ought to "coddle the inside, work on the outside."

It was important for participants to understand how the therapy activities contributed to getting better and to feel that they were paced for each individual. Smiley said,

> They [therapists] were never pushy. I mean, they was just more or less make it as though it was a suggestion. "Well, Smiley, this is your workout, and this is—your big muscles are strong, but your weak muscles, your small muscles are weak. And this is what we suggest you do. You can do it at home, and . . ." et cetera. When someone suggests somethin' to me rather than tellin' me what to do, it's a whole different world. And suggestions make things or break things.

Eagle Cloud liked being able to be himself, something he linked to cultural sensitivity:

> I think being culturally sensitive means being able to adapt to the learning style. . . . It's sort of like, they're [clients] being flexible with you [therapist], you being flexible with them. So I mean they'll learn your way, but you'll also learn their way. And it will eventually come together. I think that's what culturally competent, what cultural sensitivity means to me. It just means that people are willing to learn my

way as I'm willing to learn theirs. So I think, it's all about flexibility and patience.

Feeling cared for felt like being at home. All but one participant actually used the words "like I was at home" in their descriptions of receiving occupational therapy. Smiley said,

> That's why that individual [client] feels at home. Because he has some attention on him or her, and he feels like they took the time to want to know how I feel. They took the time to make me comfortable. They took the time to make me feel at home, so now I feel like I'm at home.

Amina felt very comfortable with her therapist, saying, "The girl [therapist], I used to make with words, was a nice girl, helping me out, friendly, and talked to me. . . . It helped me a lot to welcome, or I kind of feel, when I graduate from the program, I feel [like] family or close friend." Like Smiley, Missy likened therapy to home: "I felt like I was at home, [as if I] had a personal therapist come to my house taking care of me. Boy, it was nice. It was nice."

Subthemes of Put Yourself in My Shoes

The subtheme Feeling Cared For describes participant experiences in occupational therapy when they felt "coddled," "at home," or "like family." Participants experienced feeling cared for when the therapy was at their level—that is, when it was paced appropriately for their rate of work and adapted to their learning style. Participants wanted to feel tended to as an individual and engaged in a direct relationship with the therapist.

The subtheme Let Me Be Me describes the participant expectation to be viewed as an individual, unique in their abilities and reasons for therapy and distinct in their identity. Eagle Cloud talked of training the therapist to look beyond her formal education to see him as an individual:

> [Training the therapist] can be challenging. It can be rewarding. You know, it just depends on who you're working with, and how willing they are to be trained. That's always hard—to train a therapist who goes by what they were taught before they met me as a person. "Well, that's not what my book says." Well, I'm not that book; I'm one person.

Suzy, a lifelong recipient of occupational therapy, valued being treated as an adult:

I'm not saying that maybe somebody doesn't have their own individual biases; what I am saying is that my overall impression is that you are just treated like an adult who is capable of speaking up for yourself. I think that, in my opinion, that overrides whatever they [therapists] might think of whatever color you are.

Eagle Cloud emphasized autonomy in selecting interventions:

I think the thing that people forget is, each individual lives inside his own body, so he knows his body better than anybody. It's like when somebody, just 'cause they work with me, that's like assuming that they just stepped inside my body every day and said, "Oh, he's got a broken arm. Oh, his leg is bruised. Oh, his clothes are . . . ." It's like, when you get into any profession, you can't ever go into every situation knowing everything.

Participants did not feel permission to be themselves when they perceived care as if they were a "peg on a wall"; this phrase was used to describe therapy experiences when the participant felt "left to the wolves" or unattended and therapy felt too routine and lacking in individualized attention. Participants felt cared for when they felt valued as an individual and engaged in a direct relationship with the therapist.

Reflection 16.6. Empathy

Describe a time when you felt as if someone put himself or herself in your shoes.

- How did this feel?
- What actions did the other person do to contribute to your feeling?

Discussion

Findings within the themes support research conducted elsewhere regarding short-term clinical encounters. Swenson, Zettler, and Lo (2005) investigated patient responses to videotaped doctor–patient vignettes to determine whether patients preferred patient-centered or biomedical communication in a typical office visit (less than 20 minutes in length). *Patient-centered communication* was characterized by responses to patient questions, ideas, and emotions regarding their illness to reach a common ground about the illness, its treatment, and patient and doctor roles. *Biomedical communication* was characterized by a disease-oriented approach to patient problems and a doctor-centered approach to decision making. Swenson and colleagues found that more than twice as many patients preferred the patient-centered approach to communication. Furthermore, they found that patients frequently wanted to feel respected by their doctors, including having permission to partake in the decision-making aspects of the care. Health care professionals, including occupational therapists, should practice client-centered communication to foster culturally sensitive practice.

Recipients of occupational therapy first Come to Therapy, with all the Worry and Concern that clients experience when occupational therapy is indicated. People come to therapy because of a precipitating event in their lives, a time when what they expected of their body did not align with their present experience. Satisfaction with the initial therapy session seemed to be linked to the degree to which their initial expectation of therapy was met. Being Greeted is the invitation to therapy; these participants were drawn into therapy by a friendly tone and a welcoming message.

Understand My Culture speaks to the central role played by culture in the everyday lives of people in need of therapy services. People seek understanding, acceptance, and permission to retain their culture within the therapy experience. Put Yourself in My Shoes describes the nature of therapy encounters over time. Participants wanted the level of empathy from therapists that could be explained as sharing a body that has lived or having a high level of mutuality across the relationship. Three participants reported past therapy experiences in which they did not experience collaborative and client-centered occupational therapy. In these cases, they either transferred to a different therapist or setting or stopped attending therapy and waited until another precipitating event occurred before reattempting therapy at a different location. It is likely that the previous therapists were unaware of how these participants perceived their actions, losing an opportunity to learn more collaborative practice.

Subthemes of Put Yourself in My Shoes include Feeling Cared For and Let Me Be Me. Feeling Cared For described the mutual relationship of the client and therapist. Participants described therapists as caring when they experienced openness to a personal relationship, a result supported by other researchers (le Roux, 2002; Rosa & Hasselkus, 2005; Wilson, 2000), and the trust described by Schwartzberg (2002) that is core to caring. Let Me Be Me represents the autonomy sought by participants within the therapy process. Participants experienced respect for autonomy when the therapist adjusted the pace of therapy, when challenges were presented at a level of possibility, and when the therapist informed or offered suggestions but did not control next steps in therapy. When participants felt permission to be themselves, they voiced a sense of being at home.

Reflection 16.7. Culturally Effective Therapy

Culturally effective, client-centered therapy requires that occupational therapy practitioners value the traditions and rituals of their clients' everyday lives while focusing the assessment and intervention on solving the problem as presented by the client.

- How do you know when a health provider values your everyday traditions?
- Can the therapist focus too much on problem solving in a therapy encounter?

Implications for Occupational Therapy Practice

The purpose of this study was to better understand the therapy experience from the perspective of clients of a different race or ethnicity from their therapist. An understanding of the client experience fosters practical knowledge, skills, and attitudes that help practitioners provide culturally effective service enabling recipients to actively engage in their everyday lives. Implications for occupational therapy practice based on the themes that emerged from this research are offered at both the individual and system levels.

Individual Level

Occupational therapy practitioners need to recognize that culture is embedded within and influences each therapy encounter. Clients who differ from their therapist in race or ethnicity are aware of the dominant White and Western culture of the health care setting. Clients notice when therapists and staff look different from themselves, and they notice when other clients of color receive different service. Although each therapy visit is an opportunity for culturally effective practice, the opportunity may be greatest when clients are first introduced to therapy.

Understand the Problem

Clients have a presenting problem that brings them to therapy. The problem generally affects several occupations within at least one of their meaningful life roles. It is important that therapists quickly learn and understand how the impairment affects their clients' daily lives. Generally, the initial therapy visit begins with an interview, and it is this interview that provides the base for a respectful and culturally effective relationship.

Gently Interview

During the initial therapy visit, clients are often worried, filled with concern, and feeling vulnerable. It is important that therapists be skilled interviewers, asking clients about their reasons for seeking occupational therapy while using gentle probing questions to understand the client's story leading to the therapy appointment. The interview may include questions about strategies the client has already used to solve the presenting problem. Practitioners need to probe for further information using neutral, non-biased questions such as "What happened next?" and "Tell me more about that" to fully understand the presenting problem.

Development of a shared understanding of a client's everyday life may reduce faulty assumptions made by the practitioner based on his or her cultural background. The initial interview provides a tremendous opportunity for the practitioner to understand affected life roles and occupations and the values and beliefs associated with successful performance of these occupations.

It is also important that the interviewing practitioner be in a personal state of openness and willingness to be surprised by the client, much like a phenomenologist strives to be open for the participant interview. This research suggests that culturally effective practice begins with a focused and intentional emphasis by the practitioner on fully understanding the client's problem and its impact on the client's everyday life.

Be Welcoming

Clients feel welcomed when receptionists exude friendliness and when others greet them consistently and respectfully. The greeting received by clients is important. Participants spoke both of the welcoming quality of the physical space and of the friendly greeting they received on entering the therapy area by receptionists and other office staff. Waiting space, pictures on walls, and wait room magazines were all identified as important welcoming messages to the stressed and concerned people who entered.

Empathize and Collaborate

Participants wanted a level of empathy from their therapists that indicated that they had put themselves in the client's shoes. Establishing empathy requires a great deal of collaboration so that the client feels cared for in a way that still supports client autonomy. This collaboration requires mutually establishing treatment goals and determining appropriately challenging intervention plans.

Practitioners should approach each treatment plan as an opportunity to collaborate by finding common goals and mutually determined ways to achieve these goals. Frequent progress checks and questions about the impact of the intervention on the client's everyday life allow practitioners to make ongoing individualized adjustments to therapy, thereby respecting individual preferences and demonstrating openness to different ways of performing.

Reflection 16.8. Interviewing

Practice interviewing an individual about a pivotal experience of his or her past, asking open-ended questions with probing follow-up questions.

- How long does the interview last until the conversation shifts away from the experience?
- Who caused the change in conversation topic?
- How comfortable were you in letting the other person control the content of the conversation?
- Were you satisfied with your level of understanding of the other's experience?

System Level

Expanding outcome measures to include client interviews, deploying resources to support welcoming first-day experiences, and maintaining a focus on client satisfaction constitute infrastructure that supports culturally effective practice. When evaluating client satisfaction, administrators can conduct interviews with past therapy recipients to gather important information about client experiences and quality of care that surveys or questionnaires may miss. Qualitative research practices can contribute valuable information to existing quality improvement outcome metrics for data collection, analysis, and interpretation.

Greet and Welcome

Health care systems should pay particular attention to the initial greeting and ways clients are made comfortable. Procedures used to make appointments, the spaces through which clients enter the health care setting, and the friendliness of a receptionist's greeting are all important to the success of the therapy episode. Settings that encourage feelings of respect and welcome may experience greater client satisfaction, resulting in higher retention and better overall health outcomes.

Communicate Respectfully

Clearly stated organizational values about respectful communication may promote culturally effective practice. It is equally important that therapists embrace these policies in their own interactions and in interactions they observe (e.g., among health care workers or between clients). Practitioners promote culturally effective practice when they correct other health care employees, clients, or family members who use a disrespectful phrase or a biased word.

Participants in this study vigilantly watched and listened to interactions in client–client dyads and client–therapist dyads. One study participant decided not to return to a follow-up appointment after overhearing a racially derogatory word used in a conversation between another client and a therapist. It is important that therapists use neutral, inclusive language at all times and that the health care setting highly values respectful communication.

Reflection 16.9. Communication

Find your institution's written policy about communication.

- Does the policy firmly state a value of respectful communication for all people?
- Is it easily seen by clients in your setting?
- If not, how could this policy be more visible to the public?
- What impact do you think this statement has on clients and staff?

Engage in Altruism

Occupational therapy practice is more than healing bodies, minds, and emotions. Occupational therapy practitioners are grounded in the value of **altruism,** or placing another's needs before their own (AOTA, 2015b). Altruism extends to the very nature of the relationship between the therapist and client. Being altruistic requires a willingness to share the lived experience of the client and to intentionally open oneself to the pain of another's life. One way to do this is to position the client at the center of the experience. *Centering the client* means that health care systems vigilantly monitor health disparities across groups of people, that access to therapy is just and fair, that program outcome evaluations include information from all recipients of service, and that practitioners are aware of their own stereotypes and biases that might impair their ability to listen closely to each client.

Summary

This research describes the experience of recipients of occupational therapy who self-identified as racially or ethnically different from their therapist. The results suggest that when clients feel the intimacy of home, they feel a level of comfort that is desired in therapy. In addition, the results suggest that being in therapy is an interactive relational experience dependent on therapists' understanding clients' distinct cultures and treating each client as they would treat anybody else. Clients feel cared for when therapists are compassionate, are centered on client performance, express concern about the client's health, and ask questions and listen to answers.

Acknowledgment

This research was completed to meet partial requirements for the PhD degree at the University of Minnesota under the expert advisement of Rosemarie Park, PhD, College of Education and Human Development, Department of Work, Community, and Family Education. Dr. Park encouraged recognition of and reflection on the tacit influences affecting the health, well-being, and participation of all people.

References

American Occupational Therapy Association. (2014). Occupational therapy practice framework: Domain and process (3rd ed). *American Journal of Occupational Therapy, 68*(Suppl. 1), S1–S48. http://dx.doi.org/10.5014/ajot.2014.682006

American Occupational Therapy Association. (2015a). *2015 AOTA salary and workforce study.* Bethesda, MD: AOTA Press.

American Occupational Therapy Association. (2015b). Occupational therapy code of ethics (2015). *American Journal of Occupational Therapy, 69*(Suppl. 3), 6913410030. http://dx.doi.org/10.5014/ajot.2015.696S03

Berwick, D. M., Nolan, T. W., & Whittington, J. (2008). The triple aim: Care, health, and cost. *Health Affairs, 27,* 759–769. http://dx.doi.org/10.1377/hlthaff.27.3.759

Blanche, E. I. (1996). Alma: Coping with culture, poverty and disability. *American Journal of Occupational Therapy, 50,* 265–276. http://dx.doi.org/10.5014/ajot.50.4.265

Burch, A. (2008). Health care providers' knowledge, attitudes, and self-efficacy for working with patients with spinal cord injury who have diverse sexual orientations. *Physical Therapy, 88,* 191–198. http://dx.doi.org/10.2522/ptj.20060188

Cruz-Flores, S., Rabinstein, A., Biller, J., Elkind, M. S. V., Griffith, P., Gorelick, P. B., . . . Valderrama, A. L. (2011). Racial–ethnic disparities in stroke care: The American experience: A statement for healthcare professionals from the American Heart Association/American Stroke Association. *Stroke, 42,* 2091–2116. http://dx.doi.org/10.1161/STR.0b013e3182213e24

Davidson, L. (2003). *Living outside mental illness: Qualitative studies of recovery in schizophrenia.* New York: New York University Press.

Drum, C., McLain, M. R., Horner-Johnson, W., & Taitano, G. (2011). *Health disparities chart book on disability and racial and ethnic status in the United States.* Retrieved from http://www.iod.unh.edu/pdf/Health%20Disparities%20Chart%20Book_080411.pdf

Englum, B. R., Villegas, C., Bolorunduro, O., Haut, E. R., Cornwell, E. E., Efron, D. T., & Haider, A. H. (2011). Racial, ethnic, and insurance status disparities in use of post-hospitalization care after trauma. *Journal of American College of Surgeons, 213,* 699–708. http://dx.doi.org/10.1016/j.jamcollsurg.2011.08.017

Freburger, J. K., Holmes, G. M., Ku, L. E., Cutchin, M., Heatwolf-Shank, K., & Edwards, L. J. (2011). Disparities in post-acute rehabilitation care for joint replacement. *Arthritis Care and Research, 63,* 1020–1030. http://dx.doi.org/10.1002/acr.20477

Fredriksen-Goldsen, K. I., Kim, H., Barkan, S. E., Muraco, A., & Hoy-Ellis, C. P. (2013). Health disparities among lesbian, gay, and bisexual older adults: Results from a population-based study. *American Journal of Public Health, 103,* 1802–1809. http://dx.doi.org/10.2105/AJPH.2012.301110

Geetz, C. (1973). *The interpretation of cultures.* New York: Basic Books.

Giorgi, A. (1997). The theory, practice, and evaluation of the phenomenological method as a qualitative research procedure. *Journal of Phenomenological Psychology, 28,* 235–260. http://dx.doi.org/10.1163/156916297X00103

Granger, C. V., Hamilton, B. B., Keith, R. A., Zielezny, M., & Sherwin, F. S. (1986). Advances in functional assessment in medical rehabilitation. *Topics in Geriatric Rehabilitation, 1*(3), 59–74. http://dx.doi.org/10.1097/00013614-198604000-00007

Heidegger, M. (1962). *Being and time* (J. Macquamie & E. Robinson, Trans.). New York: Harper & Row.

Kondo, T. (2004). Cultural tensions in occupational therapy practice: Considerations from a Japanese vantage point. *American Journal of Occupational Therapy, 58,* 174–184. http://dx.doi.org/10.5014/ajot.58.2.174

le Roux, J. (2002). Effective educators are culturally competent communicators. *Intercultural Education, 13,* 37–48. http://dx.doi.org/10.1080/14675980120112922

Martin, P. M. (2008). *Cultural competence in occupational therapy: The client experience* (Doctoral dissertation). Retrieved from ProQuest. (Order No. 3295693)

Meghani, S. H., Potomano, R. C., Tait, R. C., Vallerand, A. H., Anderson, K. O., & Gallagher, R. M. (2012). Advancing a national agenda to eliminate disparities in pain care: Directions for health policy, education, practice, and research. *Pain Medicine, 13,* 5–28. http://dx.doi.org/10.1111/j.1526-4637.2011.01289.x

Moyers, P. A., & Dale, L. M. (2007). *The guide to occupational therapy practice* (2nd ed.). Bethesda, MD: AOTA Press.

Myaskovsky, L., Burkitt, K. H., Lichy, A. M., Ljungberg, I. H., Fyffe, D. C., Ozawa, H., . . . Boninger, M. L. (2011). The association of race, cultural factors, and health-related quality of life in persons with spinal cord injury. *Archives of Physical Medicine and Rehabilitation, 92,* 441–448. http://dx.doi.org/10.1016/j.apmr.2010.10.007

Odawara, E. (2005). Cultural competency in occupational therapy: Beyond a cross-cultural view of practice. *American Journal of Occupational Therapy, 59,* 325–334. http://dx.doi.org/10.5014/ajot.59.3.325

Ottenbacher, K. J., Karmarkar, A., Graham, J. E., Kuo, Y. F., Deutsch A., Reistetter, T. A., . . . Granger, C. V. (2014). Thirty-day hospital readmission following discharge from postacute rehabilitation in fee-for-service Medicare patients. *JAMA, 311,* 604–614. http://dx.doi.org/10.1001/jama.2014.8

Pierce, D. (2003). *Occupation by design: Building therapeutic power.* Philadelphia: F. A. Davis.

Putnam, K., Horn, S., Smout, R., Dejono, G., Deutscher, D., Tian, W., & Hsieh, C. (2010). Racial disparities in stroke functional outcomes upon discharge from inpatient rehabilitation facilities. *Disability and Rehabilitation, 32,* 1604–1611. http://dx.doi.org/10.3109/09638281003611078

Rosa, S. A., & Hasselkus, B. R. (2005). Finding common ground with patients: The centrality of compatibility. *American Journal of Occupational Therapy, 59,* 198–208. http://dx.doi.org/10.5014/ajot.59.2.198

Schouten, B. C., & Meeuwesen, L. (2006). Cultural differences in medical communication: A review of the literature. *Patient Education and Counseling, 64,* 21–34. http://dx.doi.org/10.1016/j.pec.2005.11.014

Schwartzberg, S. (2002). *Interactive reasoning in the practice of occupational therapy.* Upper Saddle River, NJ: Pearson Education.

Swenson, L. L., Zettler, P., & Lo, B. (2005). "She gave it her best shot right away": Patient experiences of biomedical and patient-centered communication. *Patient Education and Counseling, 61,* 200–211. http://dx.doi.org/10.1016/j.pec.2005.02.019

U.S. Census Bureau. (2011a). *Age and sex composition: 2010.* Retrieved from http://www.census.gov/prod/cen2010/briefs/c2010br-03.pdf

U.S. Census Bureau. (2011b). *Overview of race and Hispanic origin: 2010.* Retrieved from http://www.census.gov/prod/cen2010/briefs/c2010br-02.pdf

van Manen, M. (1990). *Researching lived experience: Human science for an action sensitive pedagogy.* London, ON: University of Western Ontario.

Wilson, M. C. (2000). Cross-cultural communication between African American parents and teachers: The role of culture, language and voice. *Digital Abstracts International, 61*(07) (UMI No. 9981798).

Chapter 17.

ADDRESSING CULTURE IN PATIENT ENCOUNTERS

Dianna Michelle Medina, OTD, MOT, OTR/L

Understanding a patient's sociocultural background is extremely important as the occupational therapist helps patients identify and engage in culturally meaningful occupational experiences.
Etsuko Odawara (2005, p. 325)

Chapter Highlights

- Culture and Patient–Provider Relationships
- Case Example of Mohammed Ahmad
- Case Example of Arnaldo Gómez
- Implications for Occupational Therapy Practice

Key Terms and Concepts

✧ Case-based training
✧ Conversational script
✧ Cultural broker
✧ Culture

✧ Patient encounter
✧ Patient–provider relationship
✧ Scripted cards
✧ Therapist–interpreter relationship

Seeking to understand a patient's culture is essential to establishing an effective therapeutic encounter. *Culture* includes traditional beliefs, health practices, values, group norms, and means of self-expression. Black and Wells (2007) discussed the complex ways culture affects health status and outcomes.

Working with multicultural populations provides occupational therapy practitioners with challenges and opportunities to develop trusting patient–provider relationships. Practitioners have a responsibility to include culture in their clinical reasoning. This chapter provides two case examples to highlight barriers related to cultural differences and strategies for resolving challenges. The cases of Mohammed Ahmad and Arnaldo Gómez exemplify how cultural differences between patients and providers can affect participation in therapy and how the use of proactive, culturally considerate strategies can improve the therapeutic relationship, patient and practitioner understanding, and patient participation.

Case Example of Mohammed Ahmad

Mohammed Ahmad, a 55-year-old Saudi Arabian man, experienced a brain injury in his home country. He received medical care in Saudi Arabia and temporarily returned to his home. His family obtained resources for him to come to the United States for rehabilitation because of persistent cognitive and physical deficits. He participated in acute brain injury rehabilitation, after which he was referred to a postacute brain injury rehabilitation program.

Hiring an Interpreter and Cultural Broker

The first task for the program was to hire an interpreter to assist in completing evaluations and treatment; use of trained professional interpreters improves outcomes and accuracy of communication (Flores, 2007). Diamond and Jacobs (2009) indicated that in addition to providing language assistance, an interpreter can also be a *cultural broker* by providing information about the client's cultural beliefs and practices. The program hired an interpreter and asked him to share information about Arabic culture in addition to interpreting for the therapy team. With the interpreter's help, Mohammed could give basic information about himself and his goals in Arabic, his native language. His family provided additional information about his history, injury, and goals.

Mohammed's physical and cognitive impairments affected his performance in many areas of occupation. The occupational therapy services available to him through the program included personal management, housekeeping, money management, meal planning and preparation, and mobility training. After the occupational therapist discussed the available services, Mohammed indicated that his wife and daughter were responsible for cooking and doing laundry at home. Goals were then modified according to Mohammed's cultural and personal preferences, and his treatment plan was tailored to focus on his goals in self-care and leisure.

Working with the interpreter was critical to establishing rapport and building mutual understanding with Mohammed. Diamond and Jacobs (2009) encouraged practitioners to seek help from interpreters to learn patients' names, a simple yet profound approach for building rapport. Through the interpreter, the therapist discovered that the patient preferred to use his family name, Ahmad, over Mohammed, information that was not included in the medical chart. Despite being in a different country, being called Ahmad encouraged him to feel more at ease.

Modifying Treatment

In addition to calling the patient Ahmad, the occupational therapist worked with the interpreter to develop a *conversational script,* a document containing phrases that is used to interact with another individual. The therapist identified commonly used phrases, and the interpreter wrote out the Arabic translations phonetically using the English alphabet so that the therapist could read them aloud. The therapy script included commonly used phrases such as "good morning" and "try again." Using the script, Ahmad's therapist was able to greet, encourage, and dismiss him from every therapy session in Arabic. Diamond and Jacobs (2009) advocated the use of nonfluent language skills to develop rapport with patients. Learning a greeting in the patient's language is a way for a therapist who is nonfluent to interact more dynamically with the patient.

Another way treatment was modified was by having the therapist and Ahmad perform activities simultaneously. The interpreter explained that Ahmad perceived treatment as unfair when he was asked to perform or repeat an activity alone, that family structure in the Arab culture is patriarchal, and that Ahmad did not feel comfortable being directed to do a task. He was more accepting of treatment when he was one of several people doing an activity. Therefore, family members were frequently invited to participate in therapy activities to help him feel comfortable. Ahmad could participate in his rehabilitation program with positive patient–therapist interactions as he pursued goals that were meaningful to him and his family.

(Continued)

Case Example of Mohammed Ahmad *(Cont.)*

Building a Positive Therapist–Interpreter Relationship

The *therapist–interpreter relationship* was critical to establishing a connection with Ahmad and his family. Interpreters can help the therapist build a positive therapeutic relationship with the patient and family by providing a bridge between languages and cultures. Therapists working with interpreters should request assistance with understanding cultural issues, learning names, and learning words in the patient's language to enable them to deliver effective therapy services. Facilities should seek out interpreters who

- Are able and willing to provide cultural information as well as interpretation,
- Are open to working with treatment teams and families, and
- Demonstrate respect as they relay information.

Reflection 17.1. Clinical Reasoning

Practitioner collaboration with treatment team members is valuable to the team and patient.

- What role did the interpreter play in helping the therapist understand Ahmad's culture?

Culture and Patient–Provider Relationships

Culture profoundly influences patient encounters and the patient–provider relationship. A *patient encounter* is the interaction or exchange that occurs between the occupational therapy practitioner and the patient throughout the therapy process. A *patient–provider relationship* is a partnership between the practitioner and the patient established to help the patient meet his or her occupational therapy goals.

Effective patient–provider relationships require occupational therapy practitioners to be aware of their own culture and to seek to understand the culture of the patient. This meeting of cultures is the essence of the patient encounter. Culture is the foundation of the encounter and a necessary tool for establishing and maintaining rapport with a patient. By understanding the patient's customs, expectations, and preferences, the practitioner can begin to create a positive relationship. An effective patient–provider relationship fosters the exchange of ideas and expertise between occupational therapy practitioners and patients.

A good patient–provider relationship can mitigate culture-related challenges during patient encounters, facilitating better communication, more accurate evaluation, and more effective intervention. For example, Medina, Haltiwanger, and Funk (2011) reported that Hispanic men with chronic conditions withheld health-related information from family members and health care providers and that understanding their reasons for withholding information, such as a desire not to burden the family, helped providers adjust their strategies for delivering occupational therapy services. By maintaining culture at the forefront of patient encounters, practitioners build trusting relationships with an evolving understanding of patient preferences.

Reflection 17.2. Your Perspective

- Occupational therapy practitioners have a role in recognizing, promoting, and valuing diversity. Identify a personal cultural value that you hold, and discuss it with a peer. Encourage the peer to identify and share one of his or her cultural values with you.

Implications for Occupational Therapy Practice

Culture can become a building block instead of an obstacle to treatment. The following are recommendations for working with patients from diverse backgrounds:

- Suspend personal judgment when gathering information about a patient.
- When immigration is a concern, inform clients about confidentiality and what it means for their care.

Case Example of Arnaldo Gómez

Arnaldo Gómez was a 30-year-old Hispanic man who sustained a traumatic brain injury during a construction worksite accident. He underwent a craniotomy, the surgical removal of a portion of the skull due to brain swelling and other medical interventions to stabilize his condition (Stedman, 2005). Arnaldo was hospitalized for approximately 3 months from initial hospitalization to completion of inpatient rehabilitation. He received funding for care through workers' compensation, which covered the cost of his medical expenses. After completing inpatient rehabilitation, he was transferred to a postacute residential brain injury rehabilitation program. Members of the treatment team included a physician, nurses, occupational therapists, physical therapists, neuropsychologists, and speech–language therapists. Arnaldo's case was especially complex because of cultural, social, and contextual factors related to his situation.

Arnaldo's primary language was Spanish, and he spoke very limited English. His limited English language proficiency was a barrier to his participation in therapy. Limited English proficiency has been shown to negatively affect the health status and health outcomes of Hispanic people (Diamond & Jacobs, 2009; Timmins, 2002).

Arnaldo also lacked family and community support. He had lived and worked in the United States for less than 2 years at the time of his injury. He had one relative in the United States and infrequent contact with his family in Mexico. In fact, he had not informed his ex-wife or daughter of his accident, even though it had occurred several months previously. Lack of family support and distance from relatives added to the emotional strain he experienced.

Arnaldo, an undocumented immigrant, was also concerned that his immigration status would affect his eligibility to receive workers' compensation. He was assigned a case manager who was able to coordinate care and help him gain access to rehabilitation. However, Arnaldo hesitated to disclose personal information or facts about his previous work situation and the accident. He was suspicious of the therapists when asked questions and held back information that may have been helpful to the treatment team.

Arnaldo completed evaluations for the various therapies and began his comprehensive rehabilitation program to address cognitive, social, physical, and functional deficits. Bilingual support staff interpreted for Arnaldo throughout the evaluation and treatment process. The support staff was residential aides who had no formal training in medical terminology. He perceived that they did not always understand or convey what he was expressing, which left him feeling confused and isolated. Arnaldo attempted to leave and also yelled at his roommate within the first week at the facility. The treatment team perceived Arnaldo's behavioral issues as poor adherence to the rules and recommendations.

Reflection 17.3. Patient Understanding

Patient understanding is critical to promoting active participation in treatment.

- What strategies can you use to make sure your patients have understood your instructions?

Improving Communication

A challenge for the treatment team was to understand how to help Arnaldo stay and benefit from the rehabilitation program. Specifically, it was necessary to understand how his culture influenced his beliefs and behavior. The team sought ways to improve communication with Arnaldo, understand his perspective, and motivate him to participate in rehabilitation.

A bilingual occupational therapist was added to the treatment team to help them understand the difficulties that Arnaldo was having in rehabilitation. This therapist worked to establish a trusting patient–provider relationship with Arnaldo. Building rapport was especially important in this case because of Arnaldo's lack of understanding of the medical system and fear of deportation. The

(Continued)

Case Example of Arnaldo Gómez *(Cont.)*

therapist listened to his story, his concerns, and his hopes for the future. She gained insight about his strengths, weaknesses, and perceptions about health care. Once Arnaldo understood that his care providers could not share his information because they were legally required to treat it as confidential, he was more willing to express his desires and concerns. He had been worried that he was going to be forced to stay at the facility permanently and desperately wanted to go back home.

Arnaldo had a poor understanding of his brain injury and the expectations for him at the rehabilitation center. He felt trapped, having been transferred from one facility to the next since the time of his accident. Furthermore, he resented being taken to an out-of-state rehabilitation center for postacute brain injury treatment. Despite consenting to participate, Arnaldo did not understand that the next phase of rehabilitation would require him to be away from home for several more months. The new therapist communicated to him that this stage of rehabilitation was intended to give him opportunities to demonstrate his independence while being in a supportive environment.

Fostering Self-Advocacy

The team also learned that poor carryover of strategies was actually attributable to Arnaldo's hesitancy to make mistakes. He often refused to participate if he felt that he could not perform a task well. He had difficulty accepting that he was not able to perform tasks such as counting change with the same accuracy or speed as before his injury. Therefore, rather than demonstrate his weakness, he preferred to avoid difficult tasks. What had been seen as a refusal to follow instructions was actually poor understanding of instructions. The therapist focused on fostering Arnaldo's self-advocacy skills in the clinic and in the community, encouraging Arnaldo to ask for clarification when interacting with others. He was also encouraged to use tools to help him be successful, such as using a calculator to stay within his budget when shopping.

One strategy that was implemented was the use of *scripted cards* that had basic requests in Spanish and English. Cards included short phrases in English spelled using Spanish phonetics that he could sound out. He used this strategy with success to make requests such as "next stop" when riding the bus.

Providing Case-Based Training

On a facility level, bilingual residential aides were asked to participate in case-based training to improve the communication between Arnaldo and treatment team. Bilingual support staff may not always have the correct terminology needed to convey complex medical information, but case-based training can help them develop skills needed for basic interpretation (McCabe, Gohdes, Morgan, Eakin, & Schmitt, 2006). *Case-based training* uses patient narratives to teach skills in basic interpretation, relevant terminology, and explanation of approaches to care used in the specified setting. For example, participants in the case-based training learn to interpret word for word instead of summarizing as a means to improve accuracy. Still, it is recommended that trained professional interpreters or bilingual health care providers interpret for patients because they improve communication and patient satisfaction and decrease errors (Flores, 2007).

Reflection 17.4. Patient–Provider Relationship

- How can culturally considerate strategies improve the therapeutic relationship between patient and provider?

Incorporating Culturally Meaningful Occupations

The bilingual occupational therapist incorporated culturally meaningful occupations into treatment to help Arnaldo understand and participate in therapy. During his cooking evaluation, Arnaldo

(Continued)

Case Example of Arnaldo Gómez *(Cont.)*

said, "I haven't had a tortilla in 2 months. I'm sick of eating bread." The therapist modified the evaluation to give the patient the opportunity to prepare a quesadilla (grilled tortillas with cheese) instead of a peanut butter and jelly sandwich. Arnaldo was motivated to regain independence in meal planning and preparation so that he could determine his own menu. Buying and preparing Mexican foods helped Arnaldo feel connected to his roots, thereby bringing a little piece of home to the clinic. An outing to a *carnicería* (butcher shop; see Figure 17.1) focused on developing Arnaldo's skills in independently navigating and interacting with others in the community. In addition, this experience gave Arnaldo the opportunity to speak with others in his native language.

Familiar activities such as *lotería* (Mexican bingo) provided motivation for Arnaldo to work on memory, fine motor skills, and positive social interactions. Letter writing was used to target attention and problem solving but also as a way to promote social ties and open communication with his daughter. Photos and storytelling were used to help Arnaldo recount his injury and draw meaning from his story. He added photos to a notebook as he took on new challenges and reached his therapy goals.

Arnaldo took an active role in his therapy when he understood the reasons for participating in rehabilitation and was able to engage in occupations that were personally meaningful. He reached his therapy goals, including living in an apartment at the rehabilitation facility, shopping, cooking, and navigating the community using the public bus system. He completed the program and demonstrated his independence in

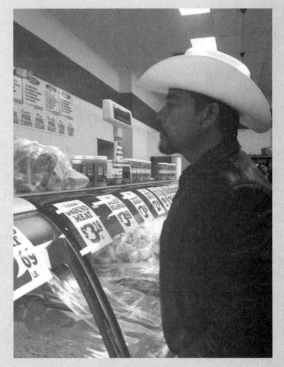

Figure 17.1. Arnaldo shopping at a *carnicería* (butcher shop).
Source. D. Medina. Used with permission.

basic and instrumental activities of daily living. He returned to his home with hopes of becoming a resident and returning to work.

Reflection 17.5. Understanding Patients' Cultural Background

• What resources can you use to better understand the cultural background of your patients?

• Build rapport by asking about the patient's preferred name.
• Ask clients to explain meaningful occupations with which you are not familiar.
• Incorporate culturally meaningful occupations and personal preferences into treatment.
• Modify treatment using pictures or simplified instructions to increase patient understanding of the task.
• Give patients frequent opportunities to ask questions and give feedback.

• Seek out interpreters who are skilled at interpreting the language and sharing the culture of patients being served.
• Check that patients' nonverbal communication matches the content of the words being interpreted.
• Develop a script with simple, commonly used therapy phrases.
• Ask for help from an interpreter or bilingual team member if you feel that your message has not been transmitted accurately.

Summary

Occupational therapy practitioners have a role in recognizing, promoting, and valuing diversity. By integrating culture into the clinical reasoning process, occupational therapy treatment can be more effective. Whether by greeting patients in their language or helping them plan and prepare a traditional meal, practitioners have many opportunities to create cultural connections. Honing in on the cultural essence of patient encounters leads to positive patient encounters and fruitful patient–provider relationships.

References

Black, R. M., & Wells, S. A. (2007). *Culture and occupation: A model of empowerment in occupational therapy.* Bethesda, MD: AOTA Press.

Diamond, L. C., & Jacobs, E. A. (2009). Let's not contribute to disparities: The best methods for teaching clinicians how to overcome language barriers to health care. *Journal of General Internal Medicine, 25,* 189–193. http://dx.doi.org/10.1007/s11606-009-1201-8

Flores, G. (2007). The impact of medical interpreter services on the quality of health care: A systematic review. *Health Services Research, 42,* 727–754. http://dx.doi.org/10.1177/1077558705275416

McCabe, M., Gohdes, D., Morgan, F., Eakin, J., & Schmitt, C. (2006). Training effective interpreters for diabetes care and education: A new challenge. *Diabetes Education, 32,* 714–720. http://dx.doi.org/10.1177/0145721706292101

Medina, D. M. V., Haltiwanger, E. P., & Funk, K. P. (2011). The experience of chronically ill elderly Mexican-American men with spouses as caregivers. *Physical and Occupational Therapy in Geriatrics, 29,* 189–201. http://dx.doi.org/10.3109/02703181.2011.587636

Odawara, E. (2005). Cultural competency in occupational therapy: Beyond a cross-cultural view of practice. *American Journal of Occupational Therapy, 59,* 325–334. http://dx.doi.org/10.5014/ajot.59.3.325

Stedman, T. L. (2005). *Stedman's medical dictionary for the health professions and nursing.* Philadelphia: Lippincott Williams & Wilkins.

Timmins, C. L. (2002). The impact of language barriers on the health care of Latinos in the United States: A review of the literature and guidelines for practice. *Journal of Midwifery and Women's Health, 47*(2), 80–96. http://dx.doi.org/10.1016/S1526-9523(02)00218-0

Chapter 18.

POVERTY, CULTURAL VALUES, AND LIFESTYLES

Anne Cronin, PhD, OTR/L, FAOTA

> *To understand the heart and mind of a person, look not at what he has already achieved, but at what he aspires to.*
> **Khalil Gibran (1918, p. 10)**

Chapter Highlights

- Culture of Poverty
- Occupational Need and Poverty
- Patterns in Poverty: Regional Values
- Patterns in Poverty: Racial Segregation
- Patterns in Poverty: Non-Western Belief Systems
- Patterns in Poverty: Homelessness
- Poverty and Values: Discussion of the Cases
- Implications for Occupational Therapy Practice

Key Terms and Concepts

- ✧ Affordable housing
- ✧ Appalachia
- ✧ Aspiration trap
- ✧ Cultural safety
- ✧ Cultural values
- ✧ Culture of poverty
- ✧ Health literacy
- ✧ Lifestyle
- ✧ Motivational interviewing
- ✧ Occupational justice
- ✧ Occupational need
- ✧ Poverty
- ✧ Poverty traps

Cultural contexts influence lifestyle options for any individual, and lifestyle options equally influence cultural contexts. This chapter describes lifestyles and performance patterns in a way that reflects the multidimensional nature of cultural contexts and cultural values. The chapter proposes that poverty is not a cultural choice but rather a lack of resources that limits lifestyle choices. Consistent with the World Health Organization's (2015) acknowledgment that the conditions in which people are born, grow, work, live, and age shape the conditions of daily life, the focus of this chapter is the impact of poverty on human occupations and the interaction between the lack of resources associated with poverty and the cultural values of the individual.

Consideration of cultural context in health requires a discussion of poverty. Because poverty is undesirable in any cultural context, people living in poverty may themselves be viewed as undesirable and may be devalued or stigmatized by the majority culture. This bias against people living in poverty offers a special challenge to occupational therapy practitioners, regardless of their area of practice or the cultural contexts within which they practice.

Through case examples and reflections, this chapter describes how the lifestyles that emerge when people are born, grow, work, live, and age in conditions of poverty shape their occupational behaviors and their interactions with health care providers.

Culture of Poverty

Poverty is generally understood as a lack of resources, most typically a lack of money, goods, or means of support. Anthropologist Oscar Lewis first used the term *culture of poverty* in 1959 (Lewis, 1959; see also Rosemblatt, 2009). Lewis suggested that poverty was a social phenomenon that resulted in a distinct culture, a culture that was as entrenched as the cultures of race and class. When one thinks of poverty, one usually thinks of tangible things that people should have or should be able to do. Lewis, however, described the culture of poverty as

> a subculture of Western society with its own structure and rationale, a way of life handed on from generation to generation along family lines. . . . It is a culture in the traditional anthropological sense in that it provides human beings with a design for living, with a

ready-made set of solutions for human problems, and so serves a significant adaptive function. (Lewis, 1966, p. 19)

Lewis (1966) viewed the culture of poverty as a social theory that expands on the cycle of poverty and offers a way to explain why people make choices that result in sustaining the cycle of poverty rather than in breaking the cycle and moving toward the economic and social mainstream. Lewis's view was unique in that, in addition to considering lack of resources, he also considered the lifestyle expectations of people living with a chronic lack of resources.

Lewis's (1966) ideas were expanded and began to lose scientific credibility when they were applied, contrary to his original intent, to politics. The "culture of poverty" became a cornerstone of conservative ideology that presumed that bad attitudes and faulty lifestyles caused poverty, not low wages or lack of jobs. Policies based on the culture of poverty ideas reflected the assumption that people might cease to be poor if they simply changed their culture (Small, Harding, & Lamont, 2010). Contemporary scholars (O'Connor, 2001; Small et al., 2010) have rejected this assumption as simplistic and essentially as blaming the victim.

Recent studies have shown culture to be multidimensional and individualist (Copestake & Camfield, 2010; Demetry, Thurk, & Fine, 2015; Mills, 2015; Shavitt, Torelli, & Riemer, 2011). It is no longer believed that members of a societal group always share a culture, or that a group's culture is consistent across individuals or subgroups. However, evidence does show that living in chronic poverty results in changes in aspirations, coping strategies, and lifestyle choices (Copestake & Camfield, 2010). Living in poverty also leads to a pattern of occupational need.

Occupational Need and Poverty

Occupational need occurs when a person encounters difficulties engaging in occupations of daily living. Being able to engage in occupations is influenced by contextual factors, including opportunity, education, and resources. Occupational need is a useful consideration in developing occupational therapy interventions that support prevention and lifestyle change. Chronic poverty and the ways it affects performance of everyday occupations are important to occupational therapy practice and theory.

Poverty has a pervasive impact on occupation, affecting all aspects of the occupational therapy domain including client factors, performance patterns, and performance skills. Figure 18.1 illustrates occupational therapy's domain, which provides a framework for examining the many ways poverty can affect a person. The following examples demonstrate how poverty affects cultural lifestyle and values:

- Parents living in poverty have less access to transportation and more challenging schedules and thus are less able to be active participants in their child's schooling, such as by volunteering at the school, joining the parent–teacher association, or attending parent–teacher meetings.

- Many parents living in poverty have limited education and do not have the resources to support their child through an extended educational process. In addition, they may not value educational achievement and thus may not insist that their child complete school assignments or comply with school expectations.
- Adults living in poverty may become fatalistic, not believing that their actions will have any positive impact on their life choices or on those of their children.
- People living in poverty have few opportunities for playful or gratifying leisure activities.

Because of the sense of helplessness and lack of control over their lives, people living in poverty may

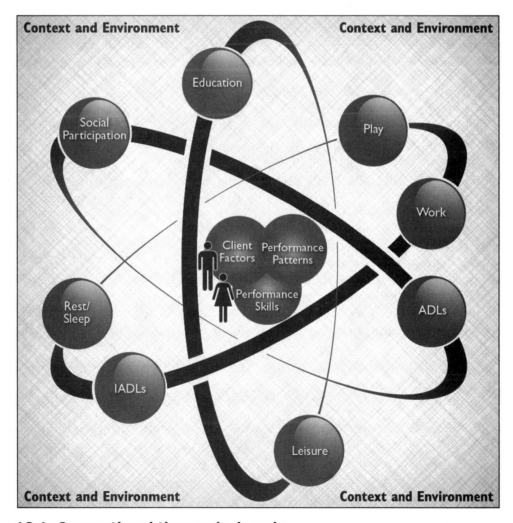

Figure 18.1. Occupational therapy's domain.
Source. From Occupational Therapy Practice Framework: Domain and Process, by American Occupational Therapy Association, *American Journal of Occupational Therapy, 68*(Suppl. 1), p. S5. Copyright © 2014 by the American Occupational Therapy Association. Reprinted with permission.
Note. ADLs = activities of daily living; IADLs = instrumental activities of daily living.

choose to live in the moment, not planning ahead, and not deferring gratification. This view may lead to participation in unhealthy lifestyles, including unprotected sexual activity, substance abuse, and criminal activity. Additional lifestyle patterns that may be influenced by occupational need include food choices, type and frequency of exercise, coping strategies, expectations, perceived self-efficacy, risk-taking behaviors, and adherence to regimens (medical or education) recommended by outsiders.

The *Occupational Therapy Practice Framework: Domain and Process* (3rd ed.; American Occupational Therapy Association, 2014) states that "achieving health, well-being, and participation in life through engagement in occupation is the overarching statement that describes the domain and process of occupational therapy in its fullest sense" (p. S4). For the purposes of this chapter, *lifestyle* is defined as the habits, attitudes, tastes, and moral standards that together constitute the mode of living of an individual or group. Lifestyle may be a choice, but it may also be a response to social, economic, or physical constraints.

The case examples presented in this chapter are intended to illustrate lifestyles that are not typical in North America. Occupational therapy practitioners may find it less easy to address engagement in occupation when the client's lifestyle is unfamiliar and less valued, but they need to consider lifestyles outside their experience with respect and sensitivity. Foundational considerations for occupational therapy practitioners, such as helping clients find appropriate balance in their ability to engage in work, play, leisure, and self-care, may be difficult to assert for clients whose lifestyles are shaped by poverty and deprivation. This chapter considers chronic poverty, homelessness, alienation, and cultural values that are in conflict with mainstream norms.

Reflection 18.1. Considering Occupational Needs

Divide a piece of paper into two columns. In the first column, with as much detail as possible, write down your usual morning routine in preparation for going to work or class. In the second column, list what you might change or omit if you lived in a shelter with others and shared bathroom and kitchen facilities.

- Do you think this potential change in routine would change your outlook on the day to come?

Patterns in Poverty: Regional Values

In the United States, people living in poverty tend to be clustered in certain regions, counties, and neighborhoods (Farrigan & Parker, 2012). One such region is the mid-Atlantic, mountainous region of the United States known as Appalachia.

Although modern ***Appalachia*** is economically diverse, historically people from this region have been associated with chronic poverty. People with this heritage typically relate to a rural farming lifestyle, a strong kinship network, and a distrust of outsiders (Marcum, 2008). In much of modern-day Appalachia, lack of economic opportunities and high unemployment continue (Daniels, 2014; Demetry et al., 2015).

Related to economic problems is what is considered a characteristic of Appalachian culture: an acceptance of subsistence lifestyles and high levels of poverty as normal (Lohmann, 1990). Behringer and Friedell (2006) described the intersection of cultural beliefs and health behaviors as follows: "Appalachians are characterized as proud, private, wanting to 'take care of their own,' and not accepting of charity" (p. 3). The case example of Angel demonstrates how these values can affect the provision of occupational therapy services.

Patterns in Poverty: Racial Segregation

Contemporary studies of poverty have demonstrated that cultural values do not predict poverty and that the values a person expresses are often distinct from his or her behavioral choices (Small et al., 2010). ***Cultural values*** are the commonly held standards for what is good or bad, important or unimportant, right or wrong, and fair or unjust. For example, in the United States, the predominant work ethic does not ensure participation in the workforce. Similarly, a person's ability to articulate the link between obesity and Type 2 diabetes does not always result in efforts toward weight loss and healthy eating.

This distinction between cultural values and behavioral choices is consistent with Thomas's (2011) findings in a review of public health studies that although health literacy provides a foundation for

Case Example: Angel

Angel, age 7 years, was referred to the regional feeding and swallowing clinic by the school occupational therapist working with her. Angel had cerebral palsy and profound cognitive impairment. She was the youngest of four children and lived with her father on a small farm that was 20 miles from the school.

Angel was thin and difficult to feed. Her resistance to eating had caused the school to send letters home to Angel's father. Angel's father told the school, "I take care of my baby; she eats fine." The school staff assumed that Angel's father was detached and disinterested and pursued a referral for a specialist feeding evaluation. The father was told that if he did not take Angel to the clinic appointment, the school would contact child protective services.

Families coming to the clinic for feeding evaluation were instructed to bring the foods and devices (e.g., spoons, bottles) that they typically used and, when possible, to delay the child's breakfast so that he or she would be hungry for the evaluation. At the clinic, Angel and her father were settled behind an observation mirror. The father prepared Angel's breakfast. He opened his bag and brought out a box of instant oatmeal, a thermos, and a large mixing bowl. He proceeded to make 2 quarts of instant oatmeal and added 2 cups of applesauce and 1 cup of dried milk powder. After mixing all of the ingredients, he sat next to Angel and offered her a spoonful. To the amazement of the observers, Angel greedily and contentedly ate a volume of close to 3 quarts of oatmeal with no problems. Angel's father was an attentive caregiver, talking to her and giving her the time she needed to manage each bite.

In the follow-up interview, it was learned that Angel's mother had died giving birth to her and that her father had been her only caregiver since infancy. Because Angel could not speak or defend herself, her father had been reluctant to send her to school. Angel's father distrusted strangers in general and especially distrusted their commitment to the care of his daughter. He had allowed Angel to attend school only when legal action was threatened. At present, he and Angel got up at 5:00 a.m. to prepare her for school. He fed her the big breakfast because "she cannot tell them when she is hungry, and I need to be sure she has enough."

Angel was picked up by the school bus at 6:30 a.m. and had a 90-minute bus ride to school. With the long ride, she was away from home for 9 hours every school day. Angel's father's strategy was to feed her enough to tide her over for the 9 hours and then feed her again as soon as she got home.

With the school's assurance that Angel would be offered food at least three times during her stay at school, Angel's father agreed to cut the size of her breakfast in half. Within a year, Angel was participating in meals and snacks at school with no problems. The feeding difficulty resulted from Angel's feeling overfull rather than to a skill deficit. Angel's father was deeply committed to providing for and protecting her; his approach to this task was what was unexpected. In considering Angel's behavior in school and her father's lack of concern about their queries, the school staff had assumed that Angel's father was detached and disinterested. In this case, the availability of nonjudgmental communication that focused on Angel and her diet at home and at school made the source of the problem clear.

The challenges to the school occupational therapist were caused not by poverty but by a lack of insight into the Appalachian values guiding the actions of Angel's father. The father's focus on self-reliance and the assumption that outsiders (in this case, school staff) could not be trusted to care for his daughter led him to engage in a feeding behavior that was unusual and unexpected. He was not disinterested, but he did not see feeding his daughter as an issue that should be discussed with school personnel. When the topic was introduced, both parties were able to work together and help Angel participate more fully in school activities.

To be effective, occupational therapy practitioners need to understand the unique cultural and economic factors that may influence the help-seeking and health behaviors of cultural groups. It is important to understand that people who have had negative experiences with authority groups may feel alienated and be reluctant to trust or disclose information about their daily occupations and life choices. It is the responsibility of the practitioner to be respectful and responsive to the client, taking the time to build trust and rapport in the therapeutic partnership.

healthy behavior, personal factors such as perceived health status, identity, and fears also influence health behaviors. *Health literacy* is the degree to which a person has the capacity to obtain, communicate, process, and understand health information and services on which to base appropriate health decisions (Patient Protection and Affordable Care Act of 2010, Pub. L. 111–148). Prevention and health literacy efforts result in greater voluntary behavioral change in people at higher socioeconomic levels (Nettle, 2010).

Smith, Curtis, Wardle, von Wagner, and Wolf (2013) noted that health literacy, as typically measured, is a skills-based construct that has not included motivational elements and thus does not correlate strongly with health behaviors or health outcomes. Because of this dynamic, the people in society who face the greatest adversity and health risks are also potentially the ones least motivated to behave in ways that improve their health situation.

Discussions of urban poverty often focus on poverty in racial-minority groups. In spite of policies to increase opportunities for members of minority groups, people of African American and Hispanic cultural backgrounds in urban areas are more likely than non-Hispanic White people to live in racially segregated areas and chronic poverty (Logan & Stults, 2011). Sampson (2008) described these segregated urban neighborhoods as *poverty traps,* arguing that people living in segregated, economically disadvantaged communities are influenced by the beliefs and social behaviors that are common in their community.

For example, when people see graffiti and garbage, do they find it acceptable or see serious disorder? Do they respect the legal system or have a high level of "moral cynicism"? Do they see health care workers as people who have respect and understanding for the challenges they face? If they have limited access to health care, are they likely to limit their contacts with the health care system to medical emergencies only and fail to consider healthy lifestyle changes? Similarly, are people in segregated areas more likely to rely on nontraditional or folk remedies that reflect their cultural heritage rather than look outside their culture to the medical mainstream? The case of Ruby, an African American woman living in an economically disadvantaged (census tract where more than 20% of residents have household incomes below the U.S. poverty level) urban neighborhood, illustrates the implications of living in a poverty trap.

Patterns in Poverty: Non-Western Belief Systems

People living in poverty often struggle to assert their own values in the face of social pressures linking conformity with government aid and to fight against a loss of cultural identity. Rose (2013) described this dilemma in an article titled "People Can't Protect Their Culture When They're on Welfare." Rose quoted Chief Clarence Louie of the Osoyoos Indian band in British Columbia's South Okanagan as saying "You're going to lose your language and culture faster in poverty than you will in economic development" (p. 36).

Cultural safety is defined as an environment that is

> spiritually, socially and emotionally safe, as well as physically safe for people; where there is no assault, challenge or denial of their identity, of who they are and what they need. It is about shared respect, shared meaning, shared knowledge and experience of learning together. (Williams, 1999, p. 213)

The concept of *cultural safety* expands ideas of basic cultural sensitivity to include a consideration of power imbalances in social exchanges, institutional discrimination, and respect for cultural values and practices (Williams, 1999).

For health care providers, fostering cultural safety means providing care that offers health support even when the client has differing health beliefs and values than their own. Distrust and conflicting beliefs can lead people to avoid or refuse health care services. Benedek (1998), through her description of Bessie, a Navajo, illustrated how cultural beliefs can interfere with participation in health care settings: "Bessie . . . bears a lasting distrust. She won't even go to the Indian Health Service Hospital in Tuba City, where the Navajos get free health care. She thinks the doctors make you sicker" (p. 69).

For occupational therapy practitioners working with people who have strong cultural ties that differ from the mainstream, a community-based wellness approach that incorporates the values of the cultural group may be a good way to help bridge the gap. For these people, their cultural identity needs to be supported and reinforced for any intervention strategy to work. Jull and Giles (2012) argued that occupational therapy practitioners need to understand

Case Example: Ruby

Ruby, an African American woman age 58 years, was referred to occupational therapy by her primary care physician at the local free health clinic. Ruby had multiple medical problems, including morbid obesity, hypertension, and Type 2 diabetes. Ruby's health was very fragile, and she did not have private health insurance. At a recent visit to the free clinic, Ruby's blood sugar was so high that they kept her in the office for 6 hours while they titrated insulin into her system to prevent a coma. She was sent home with strict instructions about healthy eating, weight loss strategies, and a new medication regimen that included twice-daily insulin shots.

Ruby had worked as a custodian at the local hospital for most of her adult life. Although her family income routinely fell near the poverty level, through this job she had supported herself and her two daughters. Ruby's recent health problems made it hard for her to manage the physical demands of her job, and when the hospital faced budget cuts, Ruby lost this employment. Since losing her job, Ruby's health had steadily declined.

Ruby lived with her youngest daughter and grandson in a small apartment. Both Ruby and her daughter were unemployed and received a small amount of federal support because of Ruby's medical disability, as well as her daughter's child support. In Ruby's neighborhood, there was an abundance of fast-food chain restaurants and a high-priced convenience store but no true grocery store that carried fresh fruits and vegetables. Ruby's occupational therapist focused on analyzing her daily routines.

Ruby reported that she began each day with her insulin shot and breakfast (usually coffee and a toaster pastry), after which she went out. Twice a week she rode the bus to the local senior center, where she met friends and played board games. At the senior center, Ruby was offered a second breakfast. She commented that she usually ate what was offered because "it's just sociable." On days she did not go to the senior center, Ruby stayed at home to clean and cook, went shopping, or went to medical appointments. She had to take a bus to do real grocery shopping, and so most of the time she bought her food at the corner convenience store, which had only processed and prepackaged foods.

In the late morning, Ruby caught the bus and went to her church. She had been a leader at the church for years and said that the only good thing about being out of work was that she could "offer my hands to God." At the church, Ruby volunteered in the kitchen making sandwiches and wrapping other food items for the sack lunches offered to homeless people. As a volunteer, she earned a free lunch, which typically included a sandwich, potato chips, cookies, and fruit juice.

After the sack lunches were distributed, Ruby helped with cleanup and then walked to the church day care center. She was paid to work as a child care assistant for 15 hours a week to help with the children who came for after-school care. Her grandson was able to attend the program for free as long as she worked there. At the day care center, Ruby had after-school snacks with the children. In the evening, Ruby returned to her apartment, cooked an evening meal, took another insulin shot, and enjoyed her meal in front of the television. After this meal Ruby had time for herself. She stated that she enjoyed watching television, helping her grandson with his homework, baking for friends, talking on the phone, and cleaning the house. She rarely left the house in the evening because she did not have a car and did not feel safe on the bus. Ruby's daughter wanted to become a beautician and sometimes had people come by to do braids and weaves. When her daughter was working, Ruby provided child care and sometimes helped.

When Ruby and the occupational therapist reviewed her routines, Ruby was startled to notice that sometimes she was eating 6 times a day. Although Ruby appreciated saving money by eating free meals when they were available, she realized that in doing this she did not always have control over what she ate and seldom had access to low-calorie food options. Additionally, many of Ruby's routine activities were sedentary.

With the occupational therapist's guidance, Ruby was able to set 3 achievable self-management goals that did not interfere with the activities she valued. The first goal was to limit herself to 3 moderate

(Continued)

Case Example: Ruby *(Cont.)*

meals a day. Ruby agreed that rather than having breakfast at the senior center, she would limit herself to a cup of coffee while she visited with friends. She continued to have lunch at church and agreed to choose a piece of fresh fruit rather than the potato chips. She no longer ate during snack time at the day care center and limited her snacking in the evenings.

A second goal was to increase her activity level. The senior center offered some exercise groups in addition to the games. Ruby had never tried group exercise before but agreed to try with her friends at least twice a week. In addition, Ruby chose to work distributing lunches on the cafeteria line rather than packing the lunches; doing so required her to stand and walk and kept her away from the temptation of the food in the kitchen. Ruby also agreed to take the stairs at home and at church rather than the elevator whenever possible.

A final goal was to stick to a routine every day for monitoring her blood sugar. The clinic gave Ruby a glucose meter to use daily in the morning before eating. The occupational therapist helped her organize a diary to record her glucose level and to note anything new or different that happened during the day that might affect her blood sugar. She agreed to attend a morning lifestyle support group for diabetics at the clinic run by the occupational therapist and to bring her diary to the group meeting. The group goals included use of the glucose monitors, healthy meal preparation, fun ideas for exercise, blood pressure monitoring, and oral and foot care. Ruby enjoyed the group meetings, even recruiting a friend from the senior center to join the group. With the group to look forward to and someone to regularly look at her diary, Ruby paid more attention to her medication and activity level and over time was able to stabilize her diabetes and regain her energy and ability to exercise more.

Ruby benefited from the support of group interventions and was more willing to change her health behaviors when she got support and feedback on a regular basis. For practitioners interested in community change, initiatives to provide fresh food options or exercise activities in Ruby's neighborhood could benefit the community at large. In Ruby's case, her awareness of her limited finances led her to accept free meals whenever they were available; these free meals may have saved her money but were deleterious to her health. Ruby needed help finding ways to meet the challenges imposed by her health condition while still achieving her personal and economic goals. In this case, an intervention focused on lifestyle coaching was a very effective way to improve Ruby's adherence to her health routines.

and develop cultural effectiveness skills to offer culturally safe health care.

The case of Dulakshi describes a young child in an immigrant family with an Eastern belief system profoundly different from the American mainstream. This family, although well educated, lived in poverty and did not understand the American health care system.

Patterns in Poverty: Homelessness

In 2012, the estimated odds of experiencing homelessness in the United States was 1 in 29 for people living in poverty. Figure 18.2 shows the estimated number of homeless people by state in 2013. This figure gives an idea of the prevalence of homelessness in the United States.

The groups at greatest risk for homelessness are poor veterans and people discharged from prisons or jails (National Alliance to End Homelessness [NAEH], 2012). Homelessness is caused by the inability of households to pay for housing; many homeless adults are employed but do not make enough money to manage the costs of housing. "The State of Homelessness in America 2014" (NAEH, 2015) reported that the majority of the homeless population was composed of individual adults, with about 36% of the homeless being family groups. Veterans accounted for 9.5% of the homeless population and 8% were unaccompanied homeless youth (NAEH, 2015). Additionally, 29% of homeless adults were severely mentally ill, 22% were physically disabled, 18% were employed, 17% were victims of domestic violence, 12% were veterans, and 4% were HIV positive (U.S. Conference of Mayors, 2015).

Case Example: Dulakshi

Dulakshi was a 3-year-old girl diagnosed with microcephaly, epilepsy, and global developmental delays. Her family had recently emigrated from Sri Lanka and was seeking services for their daughter. Dulakshi's parents had strong beliefs in the importance of Vedic astrology and horoscope influences. Within this belief system, astrological readings guide many areas of life, such as making decisions about marriage, opening a new business, and moving into a new home.

The family reported that Dulakshi was having difficulty with development because of a particularly bad alignment of her astral influences. A trusted astrologer in Sri Lanka had assured them that the astral problem would resolve and that at the age of 7 years, Dulakshi would become normal and walk. Since her birth, Dulakshi's parents had actively pursued rituals that were recommended to minimize their daughter's "bad time," reflecting a god's anger, and they had chosen these rituals over the traditional therapies (including occupational therapy) that were recommended by physicians in both Sri Lanka and the United States.

During the occupational therapy assessment, the therapist noted that the family had no interest in the child becoming independent or achieving specific goals. They saw her as their karma and their responsibility. The family also did not take her out in public and were resistant to the idea of her attending a preschool program for children with special needs outside of the home. In spite of what seemed like very narrow expectations, when asked what their goals were for Dulakshi, the family said that they wanted her to function like a normal child.

The occupational therapist chose to focus on the family's strengths, which included a strong social and family support network and their good intentions for their daughter. The therapist chose to focus intervention on the parents using the strategy of motivational interviewing, which offered a culturally safe approach to open a dialogue to educate the family and develop a therapy plan for the child that was respectful of the parent's beliefs.

Motivational interviewing is nonjudgmental, nonconfrontational, and nonadversarial (Brobeck, Bergh, Odencrants, & Hildingh, 2011). The interviews were designed to be culturally safe and avoid a direct challenge to the family's beliefs. The therapist focused on understanding the parents' values and helping them understand the potential supports available to them through the public schools and the public health system.

Over time, the parents gained awareness of the potential problems caused by Dulakshi's condition and agreed to participate in occupational therapy and attendance at school. Following this process, the family agreed to send Dulakshi to school with her mother two mornings a week. When the mother saw that Dulakshi seemed to enjoy the activities and the other children, she became an advocate for increasing Dulakshi's school participation. The family came to value school participation as a positive event that helped minimize the impact of Dulakshi's "bad time." They did not change their views about her condition, but they did allow therapeutic interventions to support her development and prepare her for school.

In this case, a compromise was achieved that all parties felt was beneficial for the child. It was likely that Dulakshi's family would continue to be challenged by American educational and health care expectations for their child, but the initial positive experience may have encouraged them to be more open to future dialogue about strategies to best serve their daughter.

This case offers an example of a belief system that is challenging to U.S.-trained occupational therapists. Rather than correcting a family that has such a belief system or directly challenging their values, the occupational therapist should focus on building understanding and mutual respect. As the family gains confidence that the occupational therapist will include them in goal setting and respect their concerns, the therapist may be able to serve as a cultural broker for the family as they address the challenges of life in a new country.

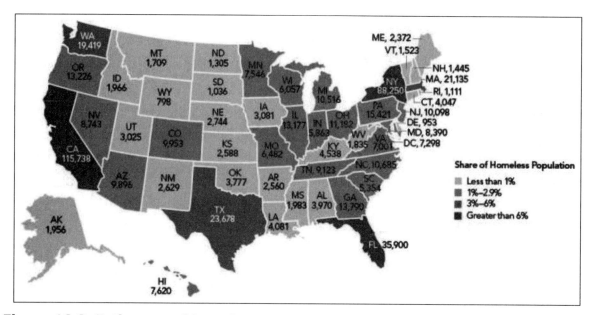

Figure 18.2. Estimates of homeless people by state, 2015.
Source. Reprinted from *The 2015 Annual Homeless Assessment Report* (AHAR) to Congress, by the U.S. Department of Housing and Urban Development, 2015, p. 12.

A survey conducted by the U.S. Conference of Mayors (2015) identified lack of affordable housing as the leading cause of homelessness among families with children. This illustrates that homelessness is as much about access to ***affordable housing*** as it is about employment. Access to affordable housing is affected by national and regional economic trends. For example, the National Alliance to End Homelessness (2014) reported that during the economic recession of 2008 to 2011, more than 6.5 million households were spending more than 50% of their income for housing expenses. Similarly, the NAEH (2009) reported a 32% jump in the number of home foreclosures between April 2008 and April 2009, paralleling the economic recession.

Fair market rent is the amount of money a given property would command if it were open for leasing at the moment. According to the National Low Income Housing Coalition (2013), a renter in 2012 needed an estimated annual income of $39,080 for a two-bedroom rental unit at the fair market rent rate. The Housing Act of 1937 (Pub. L. 75–412) authorized the payment of rental housing assistance, often called Section 8, in the form of a voucher to private landlords to give low-income

households access to housing. Because of the limited level of housing assistance, most families and individuals seeking housing assistance are placed on long waiting lists with an average wait of 35 months (U.S. Conference of Mayors, 2007). Excessive waits for public housing mean that people must remain in shelters or inadequate housing arrangements for long periods (U.S. Conference of Mayors, 2007).

People experiencing homelessness face many challenges, including lack of safety, insufficient money for prescriptions, chronic pain, and lack of sleep (Crawley et al., 2013). For many people who are homeless, the priorities of daily survival take precedence over the development of health-promoting habit and routines. Many homeless Americans lead a nomadic life that responds to seasons, seasonal work, and access to social supports (Davis, 1996).

In a study by Crawley et al. (2013), homeless participants described the barriers they experienced to obtaining health, housing, and social services. They cited personal struggles with addiction, lack of transportation, and the perceived stigma they experienced at assistance agencies. The case example of a homeless veteran, Martin, illustrates many of these issues.

Case Example: Martin

Martin was a 26-year-old man who served in the U.S. Army in Afghanistan and was discharged with a diagnosis of posttraumatic stress syndrome. He reported that since his combat experience, he had poor attention, chronic headaches, difficulty being organized, and trouble sleeping. He had not been able to keep a job and could not afford housing, so he had been sleeping in his car in a department store parking lot. One night, Martin was very drunk and walking in the middle of the street. He was hit by an automobile and suffered a traumatic head injury and multiple fractures and contusions.

Martin was treated in the local hospital and then transferred to the rehabilitation hospital for therapy. There, the occupational therapist faced many challenges in attempting to treat Martin. He distrusted people he did not know and did not initiate even basic tasks such as dressing or bathing. He was not able to meet the schedule demands in the rehabilitation center without support, so Martin's occupational therapist set alarm clocks for him for everything he had to do, from getting out of bed and bathing to attending therapies. Although use of alarms improved his initiation of tasks from a baseline of 7% to 80%, he continued to be impulsive and had poor safety awareness in all activities. Martin refused to participate in many routine rehabilitation tasks, such as cooking and doing light housework.

The most distressing aspect of working with Martin for the occupational therapist was his lack of interest in moving into any community living arrangement on discharge. The whole rehabilitation team worked hard to convince Martin to use community resources for supported employment and group housing. Martin politely refused all of the options presented to him, stating that it was his intention to return to living in his car and "having some privacy."

Respecting his preferences, his occupational therapy goals centered on building routines such as integrating the use of medication reminders (alarms), establishing schedules for regular sponge baths using public restrooms, and increased participation in local support groups for veterans. Martin felt that his interests had been heard and respected when cooking and housework were removed from his list of goals. This affirmation of his values was reflected in greater engagement in the goals he valued more highly. Martin gained success in medication management and personal hygiene while working with the occupational therapist. Because Martin would be discharged back to homelessness, an additional focus was on assisting him in finding shelters, soup kitchens, and free or affordable dental, mental health, and medical care.

This case challenged the values typically held by occupational therapy practitioners. Martin valued his privacy and independence but expressed no interest in employment, subsidized housing, or participation in typical adult life roles. He had significant cognitive impairments and would typically have been discharged into supervised care, but he refused all efforts to build safety and social supports to accommodate his condition. The occupational therapist was able to help Martin understand his impairments and provide aids to the performance of important activities of daily living but was largely unable to support the performance of instrumental activities of daily living because of Martin's disinterest. When Martin was discharged back to living in his car, the rehabilitation team feared for his safety and called adult protective services to report his self-neglect and poor safety awareness.

We often think of culture in terms of specific ethnic or regional groups, but people experiencing homelessness come from a wide range of backgrounds. There is no coherent culture of homelessness, but it is important to recognize that each person's diverse experiences, values, and beliefs influence how he or she obtains health care and homeless services. Martin's case involves some of the alienation that was reflected in the case of Angel and her father. It also illustrates the complexities of managing a chronic health condition without the resources of a supportive home, family, and community. Sometimes occupational therapy practitioners are not able to address all of the issues that limit clients' participation in daily occupations. In cases such as that of Martin, the practitioner can only offer information and resources, including strategies to obtain supports at a later date when the client is more open to change.

Reflection 18.2. Responding to Authority

People who have had negative experiences with authority groups may feel alienated and be reluctant to trust or disclose information about their daily occupations and life choices. Consider a time when you were questioned by a person in authority (e.g., teacher, employer, parent, police officer).

- Were you more guarded or careful than usual in wording your answers?
- Did you omit some facts to protect yourself?
- Think how easily this pattern could cascade into a reluctance to disclose anything to strangers.

Poverty and Values: Discussion of the Cases

Lifestyle is understood as the way of life of an individual, group, or culture. Individual contexts, including available resources, geography, attitudes, values, and worldviews, are reflected in a person's lifestyle. Lifestyle, culture, and poverty intersect as the person builds a sense of identity based on his or her experiences. In the case of Angel, her father's traditional Appalachian values of self-sufficiency and privacy resulted in his alienation from and lack of communication with school personnel who were concerned about what he believed were his own private affairs, namely the feeding of his child. He knew himself to be a competent and compassionate parent and did not consider that outsiders might view him differently.

Ruby, in the case illustrating a low-income urban lifestyle, had a strong identity as a helper and leader in her faith community even though she was unemployed. Ruby's social and personal connections were a source of both meaning and comfort. Her commitments also included an expectation that she share meals with her colleagues. With the exacerbation of her diabetes, this sharing of meals became problematic. The challenge for her occupational therapist was to help Ruby manage her health while retaining the valued aspects of her lifestyle.

In both Angel's and Ruby's case, the client's lifestyle was influenced by limited financial resources and a strong sense of social identity with a group that may view health care providers as outsiders to be distrusted. With such clients, occupational

therapy practitioners must take the time to really explore their story and values. Using a communication style that is respectful and interested can remove the initial barriers to intervention.

In the cases of Dulakshi and Martin, the clients' values and life choices not only were different from those of the American mainstream but also reflected beliefs and social behaviors that many people do not consider acceptable. Dulakshi's family chose to follow their cultural beliefs rather than scientific or medical information in caring for their daughter. Belief in Vedic astrology remains prevalent in their country of origin, Sri Lanka, but even there, though Vedic beliefs are traditional, the mainstream viewpoint includes the application of scientific evidence and the use of Western medical resources. This family's choices could lead them into conflicts with school and medical authorities and potentially result in an allegation of child abuse.

The role of the occupational therapist was central in this case. By choosing to work around the Vedic beliefs, staying within what the family deemed acceptable without criticism, the beginning of a dialogue was established. Communication that is culturally safe and sensitive was the best support for Dulakshi and her family both to enhance Dulakshi's participation in daily occupations and to support the cohesion and comfort of the family as it adjusted to tremendous cultural and social challenges.

In the case of Martin, even more complex issues came into play. Although it is clear in all of these cases that not all aspects of a lifestyle are voluntary, Martin was actively choosing a path that was uncomfortable for his occupational therapist. Martin's homelessness may initially have been secondary to his disability and difficulty managing employment. Having resigned himself to chronic unemployment, however, Martin actively preferred living out of his car because of the privacy and freedom to maintain his own schedule and routines. Standard rehabilitation practice focuses on returning people to safe and supportive community environments. Martin's refusal to cooperate in seeking subsidized housing, to work with groups that assist people who are homeless, and to consider supported employment all created a difficult situation for his rehabilitation team.

Responding to the reality of Martin's life choices, the occupational therapist worked to help him within the scope of his chosen lifestyle. By offering support strategies to help Martin meet his basic needs, such as obtaining food, shelter, and a place to rest, the therapist was supporting his potential to look beyond the immediate to consider his health and housing situation. Nickasch and Marnocha (2009) consistently found that only after their basic needs were confidently met were people willing and able to deal with health maintenance and prevention activities.

Reflection 18.3. Lifestyle and Values

Lifestyle, particularly lifestyle limitation imposed by poverty, greatly affects people's ability to achieve a desirable balance in their patterns of occupational engagement. Consider your own lifestyle.

- What things do you do that are most important to you?
- What do you do when daily life demands make it hard to engage in your valued activities?
- Consider the social and economic resources that allow you to pursue the things that are important to you.

Implications for Occupational Therapy Practice

Improving Communication Skills

Central to all four case examples described in this chapter is communication. Building skills in culturally sensitive and nonjudgmental communication is an essential practice tool for all health care providers. *Linguistic competence* is the capacity to convey information in a manner that is easily understood by diverse audiences, including people who are not native speakers of the predominant language, who have low literacy skills, and who have cognitive or physical impairments that affect communication.

The National Center for Cultural Competence (2014) has emphasized the need for linguistic competence; the focus of this initiative is to meet the needs of the increasingly racially, ethnically, culturally, and linguistically diverse populations residing in the United States. In the cases presented in this chapter, linguistic competence does not entail a need to speak a different language but rather to use language in a way that is understandable, comfortable, and meaningful to the client.

Understanding the Aspiration Trap

Although the theory that there is a "culture" of poverty has been questioned, and arguably refuted, there is evidence indicating that people caught up in a cycle of poverty, or poverty trap, are likely to have lowered expectations for both themselves and their families. This pattern of thought has been called an *aspiration trap* (Flechtner, 2014) to denote a cycle of experiences and thoughts that lead people to become passive and accepting of unacceptable or unjust life circumstances. The aspiration trap is illustrated in Figure 18.3.

The quotation by the philosopher Khalil Gibran that introduces this chapter was included to challenge the idea that a lack of financial resources may limit life experiences and may ultimately lead people to believe that they cannot improve their situation. This cycle may result in a lack of aspiration for change or improved circumstances. Not only is this negative for the individual, it is negative for the society because people who lack aspiration do not seek to improve or change and this results in a lack of competition and resources for the larger society. Gibran's challenge for us is to look beyond the poverty to the person and to support not only skills but also the development of aspirations to improve occupational engagement and movement away from the "aspiration trap" of poverty.

Evidence supporting the existence of an aspiration trap comes from studies showing that people living in poverty are more likely to underestimate their abilities in all areas of occupation, including educational achievement and professional success, and their capacity to cause positive change in their health or their lifestyle (Flechtner, 2014). Flechtner (2014) noted that women and members of minority groups in particular may have been "brought up to believe that they cannot do certain things that other people can do. They internalize their second class status in ways that cause them to make choices that perpetuate their disempowered status" (p. 1). People in the aspiration trap may lack the confidence to challenge the status quo or to assert themselves in interpersonal interactions.

Promoting Occupational Justice

Wilcock and Townsend (2014) described *occupational justice* as that aspect of social justice that pertains to access to and participation in the full range of meaningful occupations afforded to others. Lack of

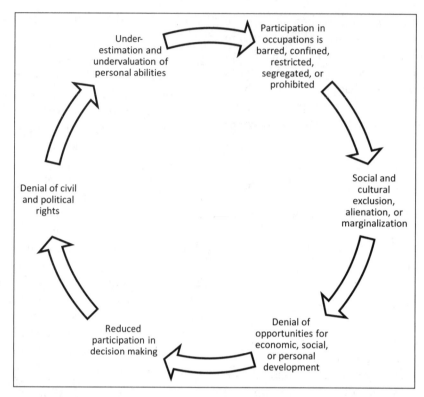

Figure 18.3. Cycle resulting in the aspiration trap.

resources, as in the case of poverty, can result in occupational injustice. Patterns of occupational injustice include alienation, deprivation, and marginalization. These patterns are evident in the cases presented in this chapter. To promote occupational justice, occupational therapy practitioners can support skills in self-advocacy and the setting of aspirational goals within the context of the therapy process.

The occupational therapy practitioner's role in supporting clients with limited financial means and significant lifestyle challenges should have an occupational justice foundation. The practitioner should consider issues that prevent the client's occupational engagement and focus on both environmental and systems barriers. Barriers commonly experienced by people living in poverty include lack of access to safe and convenient transportation, lack of access to healthy foods, easy access to unhealthy products such as tobacco and alcohol, limited availability of gratifying leisure occupations, and lack of leisure time because they must devote a greater proportion of the day to completing daily activity tasks with limited physical resources. People living in poverty may not feel comfortable or confident expressing themselves or interacting with health professionals who have no experience with the challenges of their lifestyle. The

role of the occupational therapy practitioner in these situations includes serving as an advocate in building relationships, serving as a broker between the client and social services agencies, assisting the client in finding needed supports in the community, and providing effective cultural intervention.

Reflection 18.4. Occupational Justice

- Consider this quotation offered earlier in the chapter: "You're going to lose your language and culture faster in poverty than you will in economic development" (Chief Clarence Louie, as quoted in Rose, 2013, p. 36). Explain what you think the speaker meant using the terminology of occupational justice. Read the whole article at http://bit.ly/1T7Luol and compare your interpretation with the author's.

Considering Disability With Poverty

People with disabilities are much more likely to live in poverty than their peers without disabilities. In 2012, more than 30% of adults in the United States who had a recognized work limitation had family incomes below the poverty line (Disabilitystatistics.org, 2014). Occupational therapy practitioners are likely to work with people who have disabilities and are affected by poverty and the lifestyle limitations that result from a shortage of basic resources. Understanding how poverty affects culture and lifestyle is essential to providing client-centered care to people with disabilities that is effective and supports the ideal of occupational justice.

Reflection 18.5. Considering Implications for Practice

Reflect on an experience from your own life when you experienced, or observed someone else experience, a major life change such as serious illness, divorce, or unexpected unemployment.

- How did the significant negative event affect your work, play, leisure, and self-care?

Consider how occupational therapy might offer tools that could help a client respond to the disruption of lifestyle balance caused by the event.

Summary

Poverty influences lifestyles in a way that limits people's options for participating in desired occupations in a culturally valued manner. Poverty should be given special consideration in occupational therapy evaluation and intervention because of the stigma and health disparities faced by people who are born, grow, work, live, and age in conditions of limited resources. Some of the lifestyle impacts associated with poverty are limited access to acceptable housing, limited social and geographic mobility, low motivation toward performance of behaviors (e.g., participation in education or health practices), and limited personal aspirations. Occupational therapy practitioners may encounter circumstances in which clients' observed behaviors and attitudes make them feel uncomfortable or frustrated. In these cases, it is often easy to judge the person as unmotivated or noncompliant.

People living in poverty often have behaviors and attitudes that differ from the social norm. They also tend to have significant occupational need. Occupational therapy practitioners working to support and intervene with clients experiencing poverty should develop skills such as cultural safety, linguistic competence, and motivational interviewing that help them value these individuals rather than judge them.

References

American Occupational Therapy Association. (2014). *Occupational therapy practice framework: Domain and process* (3rd ed.). *American Journal of Occupational Therapy, 68*(Suppl. 1), S1–S48. http://dx.doi.org/10.5014/ajot.2014.682006

Behringer, B., & Friedell, G. H. (2006). Appalachia: Where place matters in health. *Preventing Chronic Disease, 3*(4), A113. Retrieved from http://www.cdc.gov/pcd/issues/2006/oct/06_0067.htm

Benedek, E. (1998). *Beyond the four corners of the world.* Norman: University of Oklahoma Press.

Brobeck, E., Bergh, H., Odencrants, S., & Hildingh, C. (2011). Primary healthcare nurses' experiences with motivational interviewing in health promotion practice. *Journal of Clinical Nursing, 20,* 3322–3330. http://dx.doi.org/10.1111/j.1365-2702.2011.03874.x

Copestake, J., & Camfield, L. (2010). Measuring multidimensional aspiration gaps: A means to understanding cultural aspects of poverty. *Development Policy Review, 28,* 617–633. http://dx.doi.org/10.1111/j.1467-7679.2010.00501.x

Crawley, J., Kane, D., Atkinson-Plato, L., Hamilton, M., Dobson, K., & Watson, J. (2013). Needs of the hidden homeless—No longer hidden: A pilot study. *Public Health, 127,* 674–680. http://dx.doi.org/10.1016/j.puhe.2013.04.006

Daniels, S. (2014). Stay here anyway. *Journal of Appalachian Studies, 20,* 136–138. http://dx.doi.org/10.5406/jappastud.20.2.0136

Davis, R. (1996). Tapping into the culture of homelessness. *Journal of Professional Nursing, 12,* 176–183. http://dx.doi.org/10.1016/S8755-7223(96)80042-1

Demetry, D., Thurk, J., & Fine, G. A. (2015). Strategic poverty: How social and cultural capital shapes low-income life. *Journal of Consumer Culture, 15,* 86–109. http://dx.doi.org/10.1177/1469540513493205

Disabilitystatistics.org. (2014). *Poverty rate.* Retrieved from http://www.disabilitystatistics.org/reports/cps.cfm?statistic=poverty

Farrigan, T., & Parker, T. (2012, December). The concentration of poverty is a growing rural problem. *Amber Waves.* Washington, DC: U.S. Department of Agriculture, Economic Research Service. Retrieved from http://www.ers.usda.gov/amber-waves/2012-december/concentration-of-poverty.aspx#.UfVlMG2DLYQ

Flechtner, S. (2014). Aspiration traps: When poverty stifles hope. *Inequality in Focus, 2*(4), 1–4. Retrieved from http://www.worldbank.org/content/dam/Worldbank/document/Poverty%20documents/inequality-in-focus-january2014-final.pdf

Gibran, K. (1918). *The Madman, his parables and poems.* New York: Alfred A. Knopf.

Housing Act of 1937, Pub. L. 75–412, 42 U.S.C. §§ 1437ff.

Jull, J., & Giles, A. (2012). Health equity, Aboriginal peoples and occupational therapy. *Canadian Journal of Occupational Therapy, 79*(2), 70–76. http://dx.doi.org/10.2182/cjot.2012.79.2.2

Lewis, O. (1959). *Five families: Mexican case studies in the culture of poverty.* New York: Basic Books.

Lewis, O. (1966). The culture of poverty. *American, 215*(4), 19–25. Retrieved from http://hiebertglobalcenter.org/blog/wp-content/uploads/2013/04/Reading-8-Lewis-The-Culture-of-Poverty.pdf

Logan, J. R., & Stults, B. J. (2011). *The persistence of segregation in the metropolis: New findings from the 2010 Census.* Providence, RI: US2010 Project. Retrieved from http://www.s4.brown.edu/us2010/Data/Report/report2.pdf

Lohmann, R. (1990). Four perspectives on Appalachian culture and poverty. *Journal of the Appalachian Studies Association, 2,* 76–91. Retrieved from http://www.jstor.org/stable/41445586

Marcum, C. (2008). *Appalachian cultural awareness and community development.* West Virginia University Extension Service. Retrieved from http://fh.ext.wvu.edu/r/download/23466

Mills, C. (2015). The psychiatrization of poverty: Rethinking the mental health–poverty nexus. *Social and Personality Psychology Compass, 9,* 213–222. http://dx.doi.org/10.1111/spc3.12168

National Alliance to End Homelessness. (2012). *Snapshot of homelessness.* Retrieved from http://www.endhomelessness.org/section/about_homelessness/snapshot_of_homelessness

National Alliance to End Homelessness. (2014). *The state of homelessness in America 2013.* Retrieved from http://www.endhomelessness.org/page/-/files/SOH_2013.pdf

National Alliance to End Homelessness. (2015). *The state of homelessness in America 2014.* Retrieved from http://www.endhomelessness.org/page/-/files/State_of_Homelessness_2015_FINAL_online.pdf

National Center for Cultural Competence. (2014). *The compelling need for cultural and linguistic competence.* Retrieved from http://nccc.georgetown.edu/foundations/need.html

National Coalition for the Homeless. (2009). *Foreclosure to homelessness: The forgotten victims of the subprime crisis.* Retrieved from http://www.nationalhomeless.org/factsheets/foreclosure.html

National Low Income Housing Coalition. (2013). *Out of reach, 2013.* Washington, DC: National Low Income Housing Coalition. Retrieved from http://nlihc.org/oor/2013

Nettle, D. (2010). Why are there social gradients in preventative health behavior? A perspective from behavioral ecology. *PLOS One, 5*(10), e13371. http://dx.doi.org/10.1371/journal.pone.0013371

Nickasch, B., & Marnocha, S. K. (2009). Healthcare experiences of the homeless. *Journal of the American Academy of Nurse Practitioners, 21,* 39–46. http://dx.doi.org/10.1111/j.1745-7599.2008.00371.x

O'Connor, A. (2001). *Poverty knowledge: Social science, social policy, and the poor in twentieth-century U.S. history.* Princeton, NJ: Princeton University Press.

Patient Protection and Affordable Care Act, Pub. L. 111–148, 42 U.S.C. § 18001 (2010).

Rose, A. (2013). People can't protect their culture when they're on welfare. *Canadian Business, 86*(3), 35–38. Retrieved from http://www.canadianbusiness.com/economy/people-cant-protect-their-culture-when-theyre-on-welfare/

Rosemblatt, K. (2009). Other Americas: Transnationalism, scholarship, and the culture of poverty in Mexico and the United States. *Hispanic American Historical Review, 89,* 603–641. http://dx.doi.org/10.1215/00182168-2009-047

Sampson, R. J. (2008). Moving to inequality: Neighborhood effects and experiments meet social structure. *American Journal of Sociology, 114,* 189–231. Retrieved from http://scholar.harvard.edu/files/sampson/files/2008_ajs_moving_to_inequality.pdf

Shavitt, S., Torelli, C. J., & Riemer, H. (2011). Horizontal and vertical individualism and collectivism: Implications for understanding psychological processes. In M. J. Gelfand, C. Chiu, Y. Hong, M. J. Gelfand, C. Chiu, & Y. Hong (Eds.), *Advances in culture and psychology* (Vol. 1, pp. 309–350). New York: Oxford University Press.

Small, M., Harding, D. J., & Lamont, M. (2010). Reconsidering culture and poverty. *Annals of the American Academy of Political and Social Science, 629,* 6–27. http://dx.doi.org/10.1177/0002716210362077

Smith, S. G., Curtis, L. M., Wardle, J., von Wagner, C., & Wolf, M. S. (2013). Skill set or mind set? Associations between health literacy, patient activation and health. *PLOS One, 8*(9), e74373. http://dx.doi.org/10.1371/journal.pone.0074373

Thomas, J. E. (2011). Review of "Social sources of disparities in health and health care and linkages to policy, population concerns and providers of care." *Gender and Society, 25*(6), 789–791. http://dx.doi.org/10.1177/0891243211400599

U.S. Conference of Mayors. (2007). *A status report on hunger and homelessness in America's cities: A 23-city survey.* Retrieved from http://usmayors.org./HHSurvey2007/hhsurvey07.pdf

U.S. Conference of Mayors. (2015). *A status report on hunger and homelessness in America's cities.* Retrieved from https://www.usmayors.org/pressreleases/uploads/2015/1221-report-hhreport.pdf

U.S. Department of Housing and Urban Development. (2015). *The 2015 annual homeless assessment report (AHAR) to Congress.* Retrieved from https://www.hudexchange.info/resources/documents/2015-AHAR-Part-1.pdf

Wilcock, A. A., & Townsend, E. A. (2014). Occupational justice. In B. A. B. Schell, G. Gillen, & M. Scaffa (Eds.), *Willard and Spackman's occupational therapy* (12th ed., pp. 541–552). Philadelphia: Lippincott Williams & Wilkins.

Williams, R. (1999). Cultural safety—What does it mean for our work practice? *Australian and New Zealand Journal of Public Health, 23,* 213–214. http://dx.doi.org/10.1111/j.1467-842X.1999.tb01240.x

World Health Organization. (2015). *Social determinants of health.* Retrieved from http://www.who.int/social_determinants/en/

Chapter 19.

ADDRESSING LANGUAGE BARRIERS IN PATIENT CARE: EVIDENCE-BASED STRATEGIES

Cheryl J. Hickey, EdD, MPT, and Jacqueline Thrash, MS, OTR

Communication and language are intertwined with and are inseparable from culture. The ability to communicate effectively, therefore, is an exceptionally important variable when working cross-culturally.
Ronnie Leavitt (2010, p. 61)

Chapter Highlights

- Effects of Language Barriers
- Translator Choice and Issues of High- and Low-Context Communication
- Evidence-Based Solutions for Addressing Language Barriers in Clinical Settings

Key Terms and Concepts

✧ Anthropology
✧ Campinha-Bacote model
✧ Case-based learning
✧ Cultural anthropology
✧ Culturally and linguistically appropriate services
✧ Family dynamics
✧ High-context communication
✧ Inquiry-based learning
✧ Language barriers
✧ Linguistics

✧ Low-context communication
✧ Mind–body connection
✧ Occupation-specific language
✧ Occupational language
✧ Occupational language courses
✧ Occupational language/native language concordance
✧ Patient–therapist interaction
✧ Psychoneuroimmunology
✧ Purnell model
✧ Translator choice

Effective communication is the foundation of a therapeutic relationship and is especially important when patients and therapists come from different cultural backgrounds (Huttlinger et al., 1992). Language barriers hinder effective communication and can create difficulty in the delivery of patient care and lessen the chance of optimal outcomes (Fortier, Strobel & Aguilera, 1998; Mui, Kang, Kang, & Domanski, 2007; Ponce, Hays, & Cunningham, 2006; Timmins, 2002).

This chapter provides a brief background on the effects that language barriers can have on treatment and current strategies that address this issue, including the application of contemporary models and theories using a case-based learning approach.

Effects of Language Barriers

Language barriers occur when the patient and therapist do not share the same language and are unable to verbally communicate to establish rapport or conduct treatment. Language barriers correlate with less effective patient care. A systematic review by Timmins (2002) highlighted three areas that language barriers affect: (1) access to health care, (2) quality of health care, and (3) health status and outcomes. Almost 90% of the studies examined in this review showed significant negative outcomes associated with the presence of language barriers. Similar evidence has been found for allied health care providers (Hickey & Pinzon-Perez, 2013).

Other studies have found, in addition to the effects highlighted by Timmins, problems related to use of translators, including violation of confidentiality and lack of qualifications or training (Flores, 2005; Graham, Jacobs, & Kwan-Gett, 2008; Ponce et al., 2006). A study involving Hispanic patients with limited English proficiency found that, compared to patients without a language barrier, they had less access to care, including preventive care, longer hospitalizations, higher costs, and poorer health-related outcomes for chronic diseases (Galbraith, Semura, McAninch-Dake, Anderson, & Christakis, 2008).

Children covered by Medicaid were found to be less likely to receive timely and routine care if their parents' primary language was not English (Gresenz, Rogowski, & Escarce, 2009). English proficiency was related to poorer health in several outcomes, including quality of life, health behaviors, and access to care, for Chinese and Korean elders with low or no English language proficiency (Mui et al. 2007).

Hickey (2012) explored the patient–therapist interaction and the perception therapists have about the effects language and cultural barriers have on treatment outcomes among physical therapists. *Patient–therapist interaction* includes any interaction that occurs surrounding the patient's treatment. Results from this study indicated that physical therapists perceived that language and language-related barriers affected treatment outcomes, such as patients' understanding of what they needed to do and therapists' understanding of patients' responses, progress made during treatment, and patient compliance with treatment. The therapists surveyed also believed that absence of a translator negatively affected their ability to bond with their patients. The lower level of bonding and the language barrier increased the therapists' frustration when treating patients with a language barrier.

Hickey and Pinzon-Perez (2013) explored whether clinically measurable outcomes, particularly those used for reimbursement, could detect disparities related to language barriers. It was hypothesized that first-generation American immigrant patients who designated a language other than English as their primary language, and who spoke little or no English would be vulnerable to having lower FIM® scores compared to non-immigrant primary English-speaking patients. This study found that patients from Southeast Asia, who potentially immigrated as adults with no formal English training, showed lower FIM scores compared to non-immigrant primary English-speaking patients. It also confirmed that immigrant Spanish-speaking patients show lower FIM scores than non-immigrant primary English-speaking patients.

Hickey and Pinzon-Perez (2013), who studied speakers of English, Spanish, and Southeast Asian languages, found significant differences between the three groups in FIM scores (Uniform Data System for Medical Rehabilitation [UDS], 2015), which measure disability levels and rehabilitation outcomes. They also examined other variables, including age, comorbidities, and treatment duration. While they did not find significant differences based on language (with respect to the comorbidities and additional variables), they did find that therapists rated patients' disability level higher when a language barrier was present during the initial evaluation and the therapists set lower goals for discharge. These patients also achieved lower rehabilitation outcomes than patients who spoke fluent English.

Although the study did not offer proof of causal effect, it suggested that good communication is crucial to rehabilitation outcomes. Practitioners in allied health fields, including occupational therapy, must consider how language barriers affect patient outcomes and examine evidence-based ways to overcome these barriers.

Standards

The U.S. Office of Minority Health, prompted by evidence linking poorer patient outcomes with language barriers and the lack of guidelines to address these barriers, established 14 standards for providing *culturally and linguistically appropriate services* (CLAS; Office of Minority Health, 2013) with the aim of ensuring equitable treatment of patients. Standards 1 through 3 address culturally competent care and Standards 4 through 7 address language services. By law, these standards must be provided by all recipients of federal funding. The other standards are seen as Office of Minority Health recommendations or guidelines. These standards (8 through 14) address organizational supports for cultural competence but are not legal requirements (Leavitt, 2010).

Standard 4 requires health care providers to extend timely language services—such as interpreters (working in person or by phone) or bilingual staff—without cost to the patient. Standard 5 requires providers to inform patients, in writing and verbally, of their right to language assistance in their preferred language. Standard 6 requires providers to ensure the competency of those who provide language services and indicates that family and friends should not provide these services unless the patient so requests. Standard 7 requires providers to supply patient material and patient-related signage in languages commonly spoken by their patients (Office of Minority Health, 2013).

Policy

The CLAS standards apply to all U.S. states. They are rooted in Title VI of the 1964 Civil Rights Act. The U.S. Department of Health and Human Services (DHHS) U.S. Office of Civil Rights enforces laws relating to discrimination in the provision of medical treatment and has authority over any organization or individual receiving DHHS funding.

It is most likely that DHHS's oversight power, and ability to withhold funding, has led to the creation and proliferation of many of the top hospital-developed interpreter programs in the United States (Chen, Youdelman, & Brooks, 2007). However, the interplay between federal and state law does have some variation. As of January 2006, at least 43 states had established one or more laws addressing language access for patients (State of California Department of Developmental Services, 2016). California has more laws regarding language access than any other state, estimated to be more than 70 (Chen et al., 2007).

There has been a lag between implementation, understanding, and interpretation of some of these laws. For example, in 2003, California, one of the most ethnically and linguistically diverse states, with 42.6% non-English-speaking homes (U.S. Census Bureau, 2010), passed a law requiring health insurance plans to provide translation services (California Department of Human Resources, 2015; California Department of Managed Healthcare, 2016; U.S. Census Bureau, 2010). California law requires, at a minimum, that patients must have access to a translator by telephone or online video conferencing. This law took effect in January 2009, but its implementation was affected by unequal preparation of translator training (such as different levels of training and certification as well as lack of certification), budget-related staff layoffs at major medical facilities, the state deficit, and translator program cutbacks (Mohajer, 2009).

Translator Choice and Issues of High- and Low-Context Communication

Research shows that *translator choice* affects patient outcomes. Problems can arise during translation—especially if provided by a family member, friend, nonmedical employee, or poorly trained translator. These can include breaches of confidentiality, lack of informed consent, misinformation, and lack of acknowledgment of or respect for the patient's place in the culture (Flores, 2005;

Kaufert & Putsch, 1997; Lattanzi & Purnell, 2006; Ponce et al., 2006). Many translator issues such as misinformation and lack of acknowledging respect for the patient's place in the culture are related to the concepts of high- versus low-context communication.

High- and low-context communication relates to the idea that certain similar communication patterns are related to geographic regions. *Low-context communication* cultures include North America, Northern and Western Europe, Australia and New Zealand, and Scandinavia and focus on competition, direct communication, and emphasize content in their communication. These cultures prefer linear logic and favor flat organization structure. *High-context communication* cultures include Asia, the Middle East, Africa, the Mediterranean, and Central and South America and have a different communication emphasis. These cultures value relationships and collaboration over competition, and use indirect, circular reasoning. They also value hierarchical structures, silence, and meditation (Leavitt, 2010).

Low-context cultures align well with a Western medicine type of communication style (e.g., factually driven, bottom-line approach, explicit communication). This style may create problems when there is a mismatch between the translator or health provider and patient or family.

Practitioners must consider, for example, whether, when a family member or friend assists with translating, the patient's confidentiality is protected. Even a skilled professional translator may not be sufficiently immersed in the patient's culture to accurately convey his or her culturally influenced responses and meanings, particularly when there is a mismatch in communication contexts.

Evidence-Based Solutions for Addressing Language Barriers in Clinical Settings

Clinical case examples can illustrate how language barriers can affect practitioners' ability to understand patients' culture, values, and goals and thus contribute to poorer outcomes. Two such examples are provided in this section, followed by evidence-based strategies to address these challenges.

Reflection 19.1. Family Influence

- How did Mr. Mou's family's influence, presence, and beliefs affect communication and rapport with his therapist?

Combining Cultural Competency Models and Case-Based Learning

Therapists can apply contemporary models to their own clinical encounters, if the encounters can be viewed from the perspective of *case-based-learning*, which aims to prepare an individual for improved clinical practice through the use of real clinical cases, and it links practice with theory through inquiry type methods (Thistlethwaite et al., 2012). *Inquiry-based learning* is similar to problem-based learning in that it focuses on the student learning by proposing a problem that requires questioning, gathering information for discussion and inquiry, and reflecting for the purpose of new knowledge. However, in inquiry-based learning, as opposed to problem-based learning, the person leading is both a facilitator and provider of information in the process (Walker, Leary, Hmelo-Silver, & Ertmer, 2015).

A case-based inquiry method, paired with tested models such as those described below, facilitates discussion among colleagues, sharing of experiences, and development of more effective strategies to promote optimal outcomes of care. In this case, a culturally competent person would facilitate higher understanding based on past clinical experiences or cases with a less culturally aware clinician.

Campinha-Bacote (1999, 2002) and Purnell (2002) have proposed models of cultural competency that are widely respected in the field of nursing and have been used in other health care fields as well. The *Campinha-Bacote model* sees cultural competency as a lifelong process in which the health care provider works toward achieving different stages of cultural competency.

The *Purnell model* views cultural competency as a holistic understanding of the patient through 12 cultural domains:

1. Heritage,
2. Communication,
3. Family roles and organization,

Case Example 19.1. Mr. Mou, a Patient

An inexperienced, English-only-speaking therapist is assigned to work with Mr. Mou, who was admitted to the rehabilitation unit after a brief stay on the medical floor following a stroke that resulted in paralysis of his right side. Mr. Mou speaks only Hmong. He is always surrounded by family members, who are very attentive to his needs—but none of them speaks English, except for his adult son, who also seems to be the primary decision maker. The son works and is not present very often during treatments.

The therapist has difficulty finding a Hmong translator, and the hospital does not have remote translator services. The therapist can usually make connections with patients and their families, but Mr. Mou is different. He appears indifferent to her presence and makes little or no effort to interact with her. The therapist is unable to understand Mr. Mou's true goals because she cannot communicate effectively with him. She feels she has no connection with him because he makes no eye contact when they interact, yet she has seen him make eye contact and talk animatedly with family members in his own language.

The therapist helps to improve Mr. Mou's transfer skills, but walking remains difficult for him. As ambulation therapy continues, an ankle-foot orthosis (brace) is incorporated. At this point, Mr. Mou becomes increasingly distant. It seems odd to the therapist that he expresses very little happiness at being able to walk better following use of the brace, although it is a huge functional milestone.

Although the therapist does not realize it first, the family views her as an expert whose decisions, according to their cultural values, should not be questioned. It was not until a discussion with the son near the end of the Mr. Mou's stay that she becomes aware of this. The son also shares that Mr. Mou had been a general in the Vietnamese military, highly respected and decorated. However, in America, he was unable to find work.

A few days later, Mr. Mou's son accompanies him to therapy. The son tells the therapist that he does not want to upset her but he wishes that she would not order the brace. He means no disrespect, and he appreciates all she has done to help his father, but his father believes the brace could invite evil spirits to enter him. If lack of a brace makes it harder to walk, even if he needs another person to help him walk at home, that is fine—the family will do whatever they have to do. The son assures the therapist that the family will take care of Mr. Mou and make sure that two people are always available to help him. Everyone will learn how to help him walk, no matter how difficult it is.

The therapist realizes she has to use this information to truly prioritize Mr. Mou's treatment goals. Until now she has relied on assumptions that she was not able to confirm. Unfortunately, the goals she set were dictated by her own life experience and her limited exposure to different patient experiences and beliefs. Her experience had been that everyone wants to walk and that patients' families will always prefer care that is easier and takes less time from their busy lives. It had never occurred to her that Mr. Mou and his family would not want the brace.

4. Workforce issues,
5. Bicultural ecology,
6. High-risk behaviors,
7. Nutrition,
8. Pregnancy and childbearing,
9. Death rituals,
10. Spirituality,
11. Health care practices, and
12. Health care practitioner.

This model allows the therapist to view the interplay between these domains as they occur within the context of the patient's global, local community (area where he or she lives and interacts regularly), family, and personal levels. It also allows for assessment of the therapist's level of cultural awareness in terms of these domains (Purnell, 2002).

Applying Theory to Practice

Understanding theory does not mean practice or internalization of the proposed theoretical framework (Sumpter & Carthon, 2011). Understanding theory also does not always translate into improved patient outcomes. Students need didactic, curricular knowledge as well as experience and the ability to discuss their experiences and perceptions, such as in case-based learning (Delgado et al., 2013; Giddens, North, Carlson-Sabelli, Rogers, & Fogg, 2012; Sumpter & Carthon, 2011; Thistlethwaite et al., 2012).

Therefore, in the example of Mr. Mou, students can be taught didactically that cultural competency is important, that it carries federally mandated guidelines with respect to funding, that it is part of our professional code of ethics, and that there are models (e.g., Purnell's, Campinha-Bacote) to explain it. However, understanding the intangible effects and actually showing growth toward being more culturally competent may not be realized until applied in a more case-based inquiry approach where students are forced to reflect on a high level of real-life conflicts and resolutions (Choon-Huat Koh, Khoo, Wong, & Koh, 2008).

How Do Language Barriers Lead to Cultural Barriers?

The evolution of cultural competency in Mr. Mou's therapist illustrates the stages of the Campinha-Bacote model—from a starting point of minimal awareness and unconscious cultural bias, to cultural knowledge (having some basic understanding of the culture of her patient), to cultural skill (knowing what to do with this understanding). This case emphasizes how language barriers can intensify other types of cultural barriers with respect to cultural knowledge, cultural skills, and cultural encounters (Campinha-Bacote, 2002).

Purnell's 12 cultural domains include spirituality, health care practices, communication, family roles, and the workforce—all areas of conflict for Mr. Mou. Spirituality was critical: Mr. Mou could not articulate, in English, his beliefs about evil spirits. The therapist also did not understand various family members' roles because of the communication barrier.

In traditional Hmong culture, inanimate objects and experiences can provide an inlet for spirits; the elder members of a clan are the decision makers and hold more authority than younger members (Fadiman, 1997). Mr. Mou had been stripped of his authority during the rehabilitation process in many ways; his son had become the decision maker because he understood English. Thus, the language barrier created significant conflict.

Family Dynamics

The Purnell model's domains include *family dynamics,* which are the family roles and the organization of culturally dictated relationships among family members and outside individuals. Some examples of family dynamics would include designated head of the household, gender roles, family goals, the role of the elderly and extended family members, and the family's social status relative to the community (Lattanzi & Purnell, 2006).

Mr. Mou's case illustrates the differences between high-context and low-context cultures and between the life experiences of the therapist and Mr. Mou's family. The therapist underestimated the family's willingness to provide the level of care that Mr. Mou would need if he did not use the leg brace (at least 2 people to assist him at all times). In fact, Mr. Mou's son mentioned that his niece would stop attending college, if necessary, to help him. This is an example of the nonindividualistic, group mentality that is associated with high-context communication cultures. People in high-context cultures have elaborate networks among family and friends; are highly involved in close personal relationships (i.e., collectivist); and are not individualistically driven in nature, relative to life situations and prioritization (Leavitt, 2010).

The family also expressed a desire to honor the patient's traditional beliefs at home, because that is what is done for an elder and a member of the group, even if the care required was physically taxing and time consuming. This idea was not only foreign to the therapist but also not initially apparent to her because of the language barrier.

Reflection 19.2. Applying Models to the Case of Mr. Mou

Purnell's model includes 12 cultural domains from which one can view individuals and their life contexts.

- Which domains do you currently use to view people?
- Are there other domains that might help you understand others?
- Why would these domains be helpful, and how would a language barrier affect your understanding of each?

Case Example 19.2. Jane, an Occupational Therapist

Jane works in a skilled nursing facility in southern California. She treats non-English-speaking patients whose languages include Chinese (Cantonese and Mandarin), French, German, Japanese, Punjabi, Spanish, and Vietnamese. She does not speak more than a few words of any of these languages (for example, "hi" and "bye"). When she is unable to effectively communicate with patients due to a language barrier, she feels like she cannot develop a good rapport with them.

Jane notices that her Russian-speaking patient seems to light up when working with another therapist who speaks Russian. Jane decides to enroll in an introductory Russian language course and learn Russian phrases. As she continues to work with the patient, she feels brave enough to use some of the words that she learned in some of their treatment interactions, such as, "You have a pretty smile." She immediately notices that if she uses the few Russian words that she can work into relative conversation, such as simple greetings or a compliment, the patient shows a physical reaction, including better eye contact and more frequent smiling.

Jane begins to make an effort to learn more and more phrases in Russian. She starts with simple greetings, then starts to learn more therapy-related words such as "Please sit here," "Step to your right," and "Push with your left hand." She believes that learning the therapeutic phrases pertinent to her occupational therapy treatment created a more effective therapy relationship. Jane begins to use phrases with more of her Russian patients.

Initially, many patients seemed surprised that she would take the time to learn and use their language. Jane begins to see a difference in how the patients who have a language barrier with her react compared to how they reacted before she tried to speak a few words in their language. They seem more relaxed and open to therapy and more willing to interact; they smile and laugh during the treatments, which was behavior she had rarely seen prior to using their language. For example, she began to informally track how many times her patients with

language barriers refused therapy and compared it to an average week prior to the language course. She finds a decrease in refusals as language skills in the patients' common language improved.

Sometimes patients correct Jane's pronunciation, but even this becomes a bonding experience, as they show that they care enough to help Jane use their language correctly. By the time they are discharged, many patients express appreciation, thanking her either directly or through a family member. She is consistently thanked for her willingness to use the patients' languages and for making an effort that made the patient feel more comfortable, accepted, and included.

Jane begins to notice that whenever therapists talk to patients in their native language the patients become more animated and positive. Jane thinks back to the Russian-speaking patient who first helped her make this connection. She remembers that when the Russian-speaking therapist wasn't there, the patient appeared isolated by the language barrier and often more withdrawn and depressed. Jane starts to believe there is a connection between use of a patient's native language and the patient's physical and emotional state. Jane decides to continue to informally test her theory that using the patient's native language changes their physiological and cognitive disposition, their responses (more smiling and laughing, acting less withdrawn), and their treatment compliance (fewer treatment refusals), as well as that learning more therapy-specific phrases makes the treatment more effective.

Over the next several months, Jane continues to test her theory by applying it to Spanish-speaking patients. She at first learns simple words such as "pretty smile," "good job," and "thank you for your hard work." Patients' reactions are similar to those of her Russian-speaking patient: they are more relaxed in their positions, more animated, and listen to her more intently. They often make more eye contact and seem to have more of an emotional connection to her. They share more personal information, such as showing her family photos or telling her about their grandchildren or children. She also confirms a trend of fewer treatment refusals.

Clinical Application of Evidence-Based Strategies

By combining the case-based approach with respected cultural competency models (such as Campinha-Bacote's and Purnell's) as a frame for discussion, and applying them to the issue of language barriers, clinicians can begin to explore the impact of language barriers on treatment, and more important, propose effective ways to address them under the guidance of more culturally competent therapists who have had success.

Addressing the Mind–Body Connection

Sze-Mun Lee, Sullivan, and Lansbury (2006) discussed the psychological and physical stress experienced in the hospital environment and the increase in stress that can occur from a communication barrier. Language may be such a powerful determinant of state of mind and decisions that it has been suggested that decision making differs when bilingual individuals process decisions in two languages (Lazar, Stern, & Cohen, 2014). Additional research has examined the phenomenon of reduction in emotional reactivity with the use of different languages by bilingual individuals (Keysar, Hayakawa, & An, 2012). Reduction in emotional reactivity is the demonstration of greater cognitive and emotional distance in a situation when a person is forced to communicate in a foreign language because of the cognitive load created by using a non-native language. In the case of the patient, this cognitive and emotional distance may be increased in treatment situations when the patient cannot communicate in his or her native language.

Given language's importance in the context of care, language has a place in influencing the *mind–body connection.* A patient's inability to use his or her native language to communicate and inability to understand communication with the therapist because the therapist uses a foreign language can create negative emotional reactions in the patient's cognitive state. This may translate into physiological responses and behaviors (e.g., feelings of depression [serotonin levels], isolation, withdrawal and frustration [changes in heart rate, blood pressure, and respiration]).

It has already been demonstrated that physiological stressors can create emotional barriers. For example, Spiegel (2012) found that the stress of managing cancer contributed to endocrine, immune, and autonomic dysfunction in cancer patients. Nelson et al. (2013) additionally demonstrated that mind–body therapies (e.g., hypnosis, guided imagery, relaxation techniques) may contribute to more positive postsurgical outcomes.

Thrash (2010) argued that it is critical to bridge language barriers between therapists and patients, not only to improve rapport and communication but also to decrease stress, which can interfere with healing. Key theoretical frameworks for doing this include increasing understanding of the use of *cultural anthropology, psychoneuroimmunology,* and occupation-specific language. *Psychoneuroimmunology* refers to the mind–body connection and the effect that one's state of mind can have on neurological and immune responses. *Cultural anthropology* involves comparative study of how language shapes life in society and how practices of language use create patterns of communication. These patterns influence the formation of social identity, group membership, and, subsequently, broad cultural beliefs and ideologies. Language practices equip people with common cultural practices (Nelson et al., 2013; Society for Linguistic Anthropology, 2016), coupled with influences of *occupational language* (i.e., the therapist speaking the patient's native language that is context-specific to therapy situations).

Psychoneuroimmunology concerns the mind–body connection, such as the fight-or-flight response, while the anthropological–linguistic relationship involves personal experiences, emotional connections, and the impact that native language communication can have on an individual's processing and state of mind (Keysar et al., 2012; Lazar et al., 2014). The occupational language suggests that learning just any words of a patient's language may not be as effective as learning words that are critical to the shared social context, which in this case is the therapy treatment. For example, an occupational therapist learning how to say "Lift your right arm" would be better than learning "Thank you for the cup of coffee." Learning random words in another language is not as helpful as taking into consideration the context in which the learned language is used. For example, a language barrier between a store clerk and a customer is not comparable to a language barrier between a therapist and a patient, because the environmental context and the gravity of what is being communicated are different.

Consideration must be given to the environment of the occupational therapy practice. Therapists, for example, who enroll in a basic Spanish class may not be as successful countering a language barrier with Spanish-speaking patients as they would if they enrolled in a course that taught occupational therapy–specific Spanish terms and phrases—which, previously, was not necessarily available.

A patient's psychological state can have an immediate effect on the nervous system and subsequently on the immune system, so that feelings such as fear and isolation can actually impede the healing process (Freeman, 2009). A language barrier, which aggravates such feelings, can thus greatly interfere with therapeutic outcomes. Fight-or-flight mode is not conducive to healing (Thrash, 2010). In contrast, when patients feel relaxed, valued, and included in treatment, they are better able to heal.

Interaction Among Occupational Therapy, Anthropology, and Occupational Language

Figure 19.1 illustrates how occupational therapy (both the therapist and the clinical setting) overlaps with the anthropology, linguistics, and occupational language circle and the psychoneuroimmunology circle. *Anthropology* includes the study of people and the way they classify and express their experiences; *linguistics* includes the study of language, both its semantics and its pragmatic use; and *occupational language* emphasizes the use of occupation specific phrases pertinent to that field instead of academic or daily life, situational language. Psychoneuroimmunology emphasizes the mind–body

connection and how the psyche affects the body's physiological functions.

As demonstrated in Jane's case, using simple greetings positively affected patients' psychoneurological responses. By improving her ability to speak Russian, Jane could prolong this positive response. She became more effective at giving directions in the patient's native language, in asking simple "yes" and "no" questions, and in providing positive feedback and encouragement in the patient's native language.

Occupational language courses, like Thrash's (2010), provide one way to address language barriers. This course differed from other courses in that the phrases were specific to occupational therapy. Traditional language courses focus more on everyday language such as naming common objects and asking where a particular place is. Lack of phrases pertinent to the therapeutic situation can be a major drawback in improving communication.

Reflection 19.3. Personal Experiences of the Mind–Body Connection

Emotions can have a powerful effect on physiological functions.

• Name 3 times in your life when you have experienced this effect (such as nervousness about public speaking giving you an upset stomach).
• If your patient experienced physical problems due to psychological stress, what could you do to help?

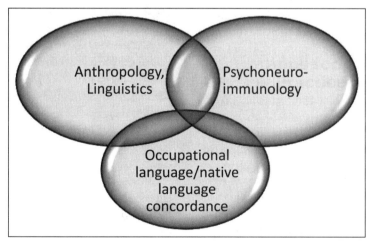

Figure 19.1.   Interaction among language-related issues affecting therapy.
Source. Adapted from Thrash, J. (2010). *Functional communication: Spanish for occupational therapy: A weekend course.* Unpublished course data, San Jose State University.

Clinical Application of Evidence-Based Strategies

The absence of *occupational language/native language concordance*, and the resulting inability to communicate, can exacerbate the distress patients feel when they experience frightening or painful circumstances. This distress can produce a physiological reaction, for example, suppressing a patient's immunological response or diminishing the patient's self-efficacy and therapeutic outcome.

Summary

The growing diversity of patient populations makes language barriers a prominent contemporary issue that therapists must confront. A large body of research on the impact of language barriers and strategies to address them exists in nursing and medicine. Allied health professionals, such as occupational therapists, also carry out discipline-specific research, and more is needed. Simply providing a translator does not resolve all obstacles a language barrier creates or facilitate building rapport and subsequently achieving good patient outcomes.

This chapter presented two strategies to address language barriers. The first strategy uses cultural competency models coupled with a case-based learning approach that can be carried out by novice and experienced clinicians working together. The second strategy uses the psychoneuroimmunology approach, coupled with an occupational-language strategy that could also be presented in a case-based learning approach, to heighten therapists' awareness of the effects of a language barrier. Because language barriers affect every aspect of care and go to the heart of how therapists establish rapport, strategies that incorporate shared clinical experiences, framed by case-based learning and cultural competency models, can be very effective (Thistlethwaite et al., 2012).

References

California Department of Human Resources. (2015). *Bilingual services program.* Retrieved from https://www.calhr.ca.gov/state-hr-professionals/Pages/Bilingual-Services.aspx

California Department of Managed Healthcare. 2016. *Language assistance.* Retrieved from https://www.dmhc.ca.gov/HealthCareinCalifornia/YourHealthCareRights/LanguageAssistance.aspx#.V7t711srKxg

Campinha-Bacote, J. (1999). A model and instrument for addressing cultural competence in health care. *Journal of Nursing Education, 38,* 203–207. http://dx.doi.org/10.3928/0148-4834-19990501-06

Campinha-Bacote, J. (2002). The process of cultural competence in the delivery of healthcare services: A model of care. *Journal of Transcultural Nursing, 13,* 181–184. http://dx.doi.org/10.1177/10459602013003003

Chen, A., Youdelman, M. K., & Brooks, J. (2007). The legal framework for language access in healthcare settings: Title VI and beyond. *Journal of General Internal Medicine, 22*(2), 362–367. http://dx.doi.org/10.1007/s11606-007-0366-2

Choon-Huat Koh, G., Khoo, H., Wong, M. L., & Koh, D. (2008). The effects of problem-based learning during medical school on physician competency: A systematic review. *Canadian Medical Association Journal, 178*(1), 34–41.

Delgado, D., Ness, S., Ferguson, K., Engstrom, P. L., Gannon, T. M., & Gillett, C. (2013). Cultural competence training for clinical staff: Measuring the effect of a one-hour class on cultural competence. *Journal of Transcultural Nursing, 24*(2), 203–213. http://dx.doi.org/10.1177/1043659612472059

Fadiman, A. (1997). *The spirit catches you and you fall down: A Hmong child, her American doctors, and the collision of two cultures.* New York: Farrar, Straus, & Giroux.

Flores, G. (2005). The impact of medical interpreter services on the quality of health care: A systematic review. *Medicinal Research Reviews, 62*(3), 255–299. http://dx.doi.org/10.1177/1077558705275416

Fortier, J., Strobel, C., & Aguilera, E. (1998). Language barriers to health care: Federal and state initiative, 1990–1995. *Journal of Health Care for the Poor and Underserved, 9,* 81–101. http://dx.doi.org/10.1353/hpu.2010.0692

Freeman, L. (2009). *Mosby's complementary and alternative medicine: A research-based approach.* Atlanta: Elsevier.

Galbraith, A., Semura, J., McAninch-Dake, R., Anderson, N., & Christakis, D. (2008). Language disparities and timely care for children in managed care Medicaid. *American Journal of Managed Care, 14*(7), 417–426.

Giddens, J., North, S., Carlson-Sabelli, L., Rogers, E., & Fogg, L. (2012). Using a virtual community to enhance cultural awareness. *Journal of Transcultural Nursing, 23*(2), 198–204. http://dx.doi.org/10.1177/1043659611434061

Graham, E., Jacobs, T., Kwan-Gett, T., & Cover, J. (2008). Health services utilization by low-income limited English proficient adults. *Journal of Immigration and Minority Health, 10,* 207–217. http://dx.doi.org/10.1007/s10903-007-9069-3

Gresenz, C., Rogowski, J., & Escarce, J. (2009). Community demographics and access to health care among U.S. Hispanics. *Health Services Research, 44*(5), 1542–1562. http://dx.doi.org/10.1111/j.1475-6773.2009.00997.x

Hickey, C. (2012). Physical therapists' perceptions regarding language and language-related barriers in clinical settings. *Physical Therapy Journal of Policy, Administration and Leadership, 12*(3), 1–12.

Hickey, C., & Pinzon-Perez, H. (2013). Retrospective analysis of language-related cultural disparity trends in acute rehabilitation: Implications for health communication. *Salud Uninorte, 29*(2), 201–213. Retrieved from http://www.redalyc.org/html/817/81730430006/

Huttlinger, K., Krefting, L., Drevdahl, D., Tree, P., Baca E., & Benally, A. (1992). "Doing battle": A metaphorical analysis of diabetes mellitis among Navajo people. *American Journal of Occupational Therapy, 46*(8), 706–712. http://dx.doi.org/10.5014/ajot.46.8.706

Kaufert, J., & Putsch, R. (1997). Communication through interpreters in healthcare: Ethical dilemmas arising from differences in class, culture, language, and power. *Journal of Clinical Ethics, 8,* 71–87.

Keysar, B., Hayakawa, S. L., & An, S. G. (2012). The foreign-language effect: Thinking in a foreign tongue reduces decision biases. *Psychological Science, 23,* 661–668. http://dx.doi.org/10.1177/0956797611432178

Lattanzi, J., & Purnell, L. (2006). *Developing cultural competence in physical therapy practice.* Philadelphia: F. A. Davis.

Lazar, J., Stern, A., & Cohen, R. (2014). Decision making in foreign language reduces emotional arousal. *Psychology, 5,* 2180–2188. http://dx.doi.org/10.4236/psych.2014.519220

Leavitt, R. (2010). *Cultural competence: A lifelong journey to cultural proficiency.* Thorofare, NJ: Slack.

Mohajer, S. (2009, January 14). Translator law helps patients avoid medical confusion. *Santa Rosa Press Democrat,* p. B7.

Mui, A., Kang, S., Kang, D., & Domanski, M. (2007). English language proficiency and health-related quality of life among Chinese and Korean immigrant elders. *Health and Social Work, 32*(2), 119–127. http://dx.doi.org/10.1093/hsw/32.2.119

Nelson, E., Dowsey, M. M., Knowles, S. R., Castle, D. J., Salzberg, M. R., Monshat, K., Dunin, A. J., & Choong, P. F. M. (2013). Systematic review of the efficacy of pre-surgical mind-body based therapies on post-operative outcome measures. *Complementary Therapies in Medicine, 21*(6), 697–711. http://dx.doi.org/10.1016/j.ctim.2013.08.020

Office of Minority Health, U.S. Department of Health and Human Services. (2013). *National standards for culturally and linguistically appropriate services in health care.* Retrieved from http://minorityhealth.hhs.gov/assets/pdf/checked/finalreport.pdf

Ponce, N., Hays, R., & Cunningham, W. (2006). Linguistic disparities in health care access and health status among older adults. *Journal of Internal Medicine, 21,* 786–791. http://dx.doi.org/10.1111/j.1525-1497.2006.00491.x

Purnell, L. (2002). The Purnell model for cultural competence. *Journal of Transcultural Nursing, 13*(3), 193–196. http://dx.doi.org/10.1177/10459602013003006

Society for Linguistic Anthropology. (2016). *About the Society for Linguistic Anthropology.* Retrieved from http://linguisticanthropology.org/about/

Spiegel, D. (2012). Mind matters in cancer survival. *Psycho-Oncology, 21,* 588–593. http://dx.doi.org/10.1002/pon.3067

State of California Department of Developmental Services. (2016). *Dymally-Alatorre Bilingual Services Act.* Retrieved from http://www.leginfo.ca.gov/cgi-bin/displaycode?section=gov&group=07001-08000&file=7290-7299.8

Sumpter, D., & Carthon, J. (2011). Lost in translation: Students perceptions of cultural competence in undergraduate and graduate nursing curriculum. *Journal of Professional Nursing, 27,* 43–49. http://dx.doi.org/10.1016/j.profnurs.2010.09.005

Sze-Mun Lee, T., Sullivan, G., & Lansbury, G. (2006). Physiotherapists' communication strategies with patients from culturally diverse backgrounds. *Advances in Physiotherapy, 8,* 168–174. http://dx.doi.org/10.1080/14038190600845602

Thistlethwaite, J. E., Davies, D., Ekeocha, S., Kidd, J. M., MacDougall. C., Matthews, P., Purkis, J., & Clay, D. (2012). The effectiveness of case-based learning in health professional education: A BEME systematic review. BEME Guide no. 23. *Medical Technology, 34*(6), 421–444. http://dx.doi.org/10.3109/0142159X.2012.680939

Thrash, J. (2010). *Functional communication: Spanish for occupational therapy: A weekend course.* Unpublished course data, San Jose State University.

Timmins, C. (2002). The impact of language barriers on the health care of Latinos in the United States: A review of the literature and guidelines for practice. *Journal of Midwifery and Womens' Health, 47*(2), 80–96. http://dx.doi.org/10.1016/S1526-9523(02)00218-0

Uniform Data System for Medical Rehabilitation. (2015). *About the FIM System.* Retrieved from http://www.udsmr.org/WebModules/FIM/Fim_About.aspx

U.S. Census Bureau, United States Department of Commerce. (2010). *Quickfacts.* Retrieved from http://www.census.gov/quickfacts/table/PST045215/06

Walker, A., Leary, H., Hmelo-Silver, C., & Ertmer, P. (2015). *Essential readings in problem based learning.* West Lafayette, IN: Purdue University Press.

Chapter 20.

INTEGRATING HEALTH PROMOTION, CULTURE, AND OCCUPATIONAL THERAPY

Jami E. Flick, MS, OTR/L

> *The only way to keep your health is to eat what you don't want,*
> *drink what you don't like, and do what you'd druther not.*
> **Mark Twain (1897, p. 151)**

Chapter Highlights

- Health Promotion Models
- Integrating Practice, Theory, and Health Promotion

Key Terms and Concepts

✧ Change theory
✧ Explanatory theory
✧ Health Belief Model
✧ Health disparity
✧ Health promotion
✧ Health promotion model
✧ Health promotion theory

✧ Perceived barriers
✧ Perceived benefits
✧ Perceived severity
✧ Perceived susceptibility
✧ Person–Environment–Occupation (PEO) model
✧ Self-efficacy

Whether a community is urban or rural, occupational therapy practitioners must appreciate its diversity and uniqueness. To deliver culturally effective care, a practitioner should provide occupation-based services that will influence healthy behavior changes and also promote the client's well-being. Blending health promotion concepts with occupational therapy practice provides a more holistic approach to care and promotes potential long-term improvements to clients' health and well-being.

To deliver optimal occupational therapy services, practitioners should consider integrating occupational therapy theory with health promotion models. This chapter explores how to infuse health promotion and prevention into traditional occupational therapy service delivery using the Health Belief Model and occupation-centered theory. Strategies for incorporating health and wellness into daily practice are highlighted in case examples.

Health Promotion Models

Health promotion is defined by the World Health Organization (WHO, 1986) as a "process of enabling people to increase control over, and to improve their health" (para. 4). According to the *Occupational Therapy Practice Framework: Domain and Process,* health promotion is an approach "that does not assume a disability is present or that any aspect would interfere with performance" (American Occupational Therapy Association, 2014, p. S48). Therefore, occupational therapy practitioners can provide holistic and contextually relevant experiences that will engage people in occupation and empower them to control and improve their health and well-being.

Reitz (2014) defines occupational therapy–directed health promotion as "the client-centered use of occupations, adaptations to context, or alteration of context to maximize individuals,' families,' communities,' or groups' pursuit of health and quality of life" (p. 575). For example, teaching a stretching program and ergonomic principles to office workers who sit for prolonged periods during the workday can promote positive health behaviors and may prevent health issues associated with sedentary positions.

To carry out health promotion in daily practice, an occupational therapist needs to understand the theory behind health behavior choices and strategies for intervention. A **health promotion model,** or theory, can be broadly understood as a "systematic way to think about" addressing health needs of individuals, groups, or communities (National Cancer Institute [NCI], 2005). **Health promotion theory** attempts to address the behavioral changes people must make to follow through with healthy lifestyle modifications (NCI, 2005; Scaffa, Reitz, & Pizzi, 2010).

Health promotion theory is divided into two major theory types: (1) explanatory and (2) change. **Explanatory theory** provides the occupational therapist with the means to define and describe why health problems are occurring within an individual, group, or community (NCI, 2005). **Change theory** provides a guide to health intervention planning and development to address health concerns of a person, group, or community (NCI, 2005). Traditional occupational therapy theory can be used for health promotion, especially when combined with explanatory or change theory.

Person–Environment–Occupation Model

Occupational therapists understand that if consumers are to achieve health and well-being, they need to balance their personal needs and occupations with the context and environment. For example, the **Person–Environment–Occupation (PEO) model** (Law et al., 1996) stresses the importance of a balanced fit among a person, environment, and occupation for health and participation. Matching the occupation and environment to the person's ability and capacity as well as adjusting the demands of the environment and occupation create an optimal fit that enhances a person's occupational performance and well-being (Law et al., 1996; Scaffa & Reitz, 2014; Stewart et al., 2003).

Incorporating the traditional PEO model with a health promotion model has the potential to increase the client's knowledge and understanding of the importance of health and prevent disability (Scaffa & Reitz, 2014; Scaffa, Reitz, & Pizzi, 2010).

Health Belief Model

When working with diverse populations, practitioners must be aware that society members may experience declining health because of social determinants of health and health disparities. A **health disparity** is

A particular type of health difference that is closely linked with social, economic, and/or environmental disadvantage. Health disparities adversely affect groups of people who have systematically experienced greater obstacles to health based on their racial or ethnic group; religion; socioeconomic status; gender; age; mental health; cognitive, sensory, or physical disability; sexual orientation or gender identity; geographic location; or other characteristics historically linked to discrimination or exclusion. (U.S. Department of Health and Human Services [DHHS], 2008, p. 28)

Global citizens are affected by social determinants of health, which are all of the external factors that can influence health, such as income, access to resources and health care, and education (Tarlov, 1996). As society's health needs become increasingly multifaceted and dependent on the external environment, the delivery of occupational therapy services becomes more complex.

To address this complexity, an occupational therapist could integrate the health belief model, an explanatory theory, with the PEO model. The *Health Belief Model* consists of multiple concepts that address consumers' beliefs about health and how current behaviors can influence health (Janz, Champion, & Strecher, 2002). The Health Belief Model was originally created by social psychologists in the public health discipline during the 1950s (NCI, 2005). The first concept, *perceived susceptibility,* occurs when the client has a belief or subjective impression of the risk for disease, illness, or trauma (Rosenstock, 1966; NCI, 2005). The client's perceived susceptibility can be skewed by lack of or erroneous information about health conditions and consequences.

Next, the health belief model addresses *perceived severity,* or a client's perception of how severe the consequences will be for disability, injury, or trauma (NCI, 2005; Rosenstock, 1966). The Health Belief Model also examines how the consumer weighs perceived benefits versus perceived barriers. *Perceived benefits* are the client's belief that possible actions are available, effective, or available and effective to address a health need (NCI, 2005; Rosenstock, 1966). *Perceived barriers* are the costs or negative repercussions that may result from engaging in specific or preventive behaviors (NCI, 2005; Rosenstock, 1966). If clients perceive or expect barriers, then they may need a "cue to action" or the "just-right" circumstance to support behavior changes (NCI, 2005; Rosenstock, 1966). Occupational therapy practitioners could provide the cue to action based on an understanding of the client's health perceptions, health needs, and occupational performance.

The Health Belief Model supports *self-efficacy,* or building confidence to make the best decisions for health and well-being (NCI, 2005; Rosenstock, 1966). Practitioners can apply the Health Belief Model to help clients remove barriers and identify benefits to health. The Health Belief Model is only one example of the many types of health promotion theory available to occupational therapists; therefore, further education in this area is highly encouraged.

Integrating Practice, Theory, and Health Promotion

To illustrate the integration of holistic occupational therapy practice, theory, and health promotion, consider the process of occupational therapy for a premature infant discharged from a neonatal intensive care unit (NICU) in Memphis, Tennessee. Whether the infant and family are followed in the home or on an outpatient basis, the occupational therapy practitioner should go beyond motor acquisition skills and focus on caregiver participation and support to reduce the child's risk for disability and increase the overall health of the child and family.

Raising a child is a culturally driven and unique life role. In certain geographical areas, poverty, limited education, and external stressors, such as neighborhood crime and violence, can hinder roles and occupations. Imagine the difficulty of absorbing recommendations from physicians and allied health providers when trying to balance safety and survival within a particular environment and context.

In this scenario, we will explore opportunities for providing culturally effective care to an infant and her family by balancing the cultural needs of the consumers, their occupations, and their environmental limitations with the PEO model. In addition, we will use the Health Belief Model to address parenting skills, breastfeeding, and demystifying the cause, susceptibility, and complications of prematurity.

Reflection 20.1. What Are Your Health Beliefs?

Think about a time in your life or a loved one's life where you or your loved one had to make a critical decision about health and wellness, for example, deciding whether to remove fast food from your diet or whether to have an elective surgery. Envision yourself in that moment and apply the Health Belief Model.

- How susceptible or vulnerable to the health issue or risks did you feel in that moment?
- Did the potential outcome of the decision seem too severe, or did it seem like a suitable risk to take to improve your health?
- Did the benefits of your health decision outweigh the risks? Why or why not?
- What barriers did you face? Were you able to overcome them by yourself, or did you need help?
- How empowered did you feel to make the decision and follow through with it?

Phase 1: Problem Setting (Occupational Profile)

Client's Referral Information

- The client is a 3-month-old (chronological age) African American female.
- The child's medical history: born at 30 weeks' gestational age with respiratory distress syndrome, poor feeding status, Grade I intraventricular hemorrhage, and increased risk for developmental delay.
- Maternal history consists of no prenatal care, marijuana use, and premature labor.

General Cultural Knowledge: African American Culture

- Extended and multigenerational family structures are important to the daily routine and family dynamics (Bigby & American College of Physicians [ACP], 2003; Black & Wells, 2007).
- Elders should be addressed by title and last name (e.g., Mrs. Jones) unless otherwise stated by the family member, or ask permission before using an informal first name (Bigby & ACP, 2003; Black & Wells, 2007).
- Eye contact during dialogue is important for building rapport; however, the caregiver's level of eye contact can vary. A family member may limit eye contact when information is being received or processed (Bigby & ACP, 2003).
- The family should be allowed to guide the formality and focus of conversations, especially if personal issues or family dynamics are too sensitive to discuss with outsiders (Bigby & ACP, 2003; Black & Wells, 2007).
- Family members may have different perceptions of disability that may be culturally, socially, or spiritually influenced; these perceptions may support or hinder participation in continued therapy services (Black & Wells, 2007; Terhune, 2005).

General Cultural Knowledge: Poverty

- Emphasis may be on immediate needs rather than long-term goals (Black & Wells, 2007).
- Physical context may be influenced by poverty and could include unsafe neighborhoods, low-income housing, or lack of access to transportation.
- Community resources and access to resources may be limited.

Initial Response

- Try to use a casual, nonthreatening, and informal therapeutic manner or style.
- Involve extended family in the appointment, especially the family member believed to be or identified as the decision maker or the mother's primary mentor (Black & Wells, 2007).
- Be specific and transparent about what services are being offered and their purpose.
- Encourage caregivers to identify the problems or areas of concern from their perspective through a narrative expression of thoughts and ideas.
- Concentrate on the present condition and situation until the family indicates readiness for long-term planning. For example, focus on addressing safety, such as encouraging the parent to use a crib rather than share a bed and having the infant sleep on her back to prevent potentially fatal respiratory conditions. Infant mortality is a public health concern, and statistics show that non-Hispanic Black infants have a high risk of death due to sudden infant death syndrome (SIDS), with the syndrome affecting 99 of every 100,000 live births (American Academy of Pediatrics [AAP], 2011). SIDS has been attributed to the lack of adherence to AAP recommendations regarding infants sleeping on their backs during the first year of life, bed sharing, and the proper use of bedding materials (AAP, 2011).
- Encourage family members to choose their location or position in the room. For example, allow the caregivers to choose to sit in chairs versus on the floor or a mat, even though the treatment session may take place on the floor. The AAP (2008)

Reflection 20.2. Be a Scholar of Culture

- How do you learn about a client's culture?
- Are you interpreting cultures through your personal lens, or are you objectively interpreting cultures as an outsider looking in?

Sit on a park bench and become a humble observer of your peers. Take note of what you see, but also write your initial responses to your observations. This practice may help improve self-awareness of personal biases and will help you practice objectively learning about other cultures.

suggests that practitioners should respect a family that may live in a low-income area and may not have suitable space for a child to play while still encouraging supervised tummy time to decrease the risk of positional plagiocephaly and promote normal motor development (AAP, 2011).

Phase 2: Framing and Delineating the Problem (Analysis of Occupational Performance)

Client's Presenting Information

- The child lives with her 15-year-old biological mother, maternal grandmother, and 2 cousins on the first floor of a low-income-housing apartment complex.
- The mother is a sophomore in high school. She expresses the desire to finish high school and pursue a career as a hair stylist.
- The father is involved 1–2 times a week, depending on his school and work schedule. The father is a 17-year-old African American and senior in high school.
- The child's maternal grandmother performs most of the caregiver responsibilities and determines the extent to which the child's mother can be involved in daily care.

Specific Cultural Knowledge

- Family members live in urban Memphis, Tennessee.
- Community is predominantly African American with a low socioeconomic status but is very community-, neighborhood-, and spiritually oriented.
- Caregivers and family members present in the home will attend appointments when they are available. Caregivers, family members, or both are frequently contacted by phone during the appointment, especially if the mother does not feel confident in reporting new information about the child's medical status.
- Family members are Southern Baptist and attend church every Sunday.
- Multigenerational care of the child is used to distribute family responsibilities and to mentor the young mother. The elder family member, the maternal grandmother, ultimately decides parenting roles and methods. Cultural strengths are the intergenerational support from extended family members (e.g., grandmothers, aunts, cousins) and

their motivation to integrate the child's health and routine into their daily life patterns and routines (Flaherty & Sadler, 2010).
- The dual role of being a teenager and a new parent can be a potential barrier. Healthy attachment and bonding with the infant may be affected by the parents' own adolescent developmental needs (Flaherty & Sadler, 2010).
- The infant mortality rate for Shelby County and Memphis, Tennessee, is 10.3 infant deaths per 1,000 births (Urban Child Institute, 2012). The rate is 50% more than the national average; promoting the child's health and safety is key for the child's survival (Lewallen & Street, 2010).
- Feeding can be a particularly sensitive subject matter, especially breastfeeding. Feeding practices are typically guided by the family's beliefs on breastfeeding, the introduction of solids, and the use of bottles and cups. Family reasoning can range from a desire to allow the young mother to return to school, past family experiences with breastfeeding, breastfeeding pain, and the young woman's self-image.

  African American women are less likely to initiate and sustain breastfeeding compared with Hispanic and Caucasian women (Hall Smith, Coley, Labbock, Cupito, & Nwokah, 2012; Hurley, Black, Papas, & Quigg, 2008; Lewallen & Street, 2010). In addition, African American young girls and women reportedly demonstrate decreased compliance with the AAP's recommendation to exclusively breastfeed until 4 months and then initiate additional nutritional supports (DHHS, 2011). However, recent clinical guidelines from the American College of Obstetricians and Gynecologists (ACOG, 2013) recognize the barriers women experience with breastfeeding and recommend that health care providers should be sensitive to the needs of women, regardless of whether or not they choose to breastfeed. Health care providers should aim to support women in the vulnerable postpartum period and encourage and assist women who choose to breastfeed and accept the decision of women who choose not to breastfeed (p. 1).

  Barriers to breastfeeding include the stigma associated with being a teen mother, the teen's lack of parenting readiness, a lack of support from family members, the effect of peer pressure on self-image, and dependence on social supports, such as friends and peers (Hall Smith et al., 2012).
- Multiple outside stressors affect family participation and acceptance of interventions. Stressors can be

external and environmental secondary to neighborhood safety and crime, poverty, limited education, and inadequate transportation. Internal stressors can be related to the demands of parenting, the individual's ability to cope with stress, interfamily dynamics, peer relations, and adolescent self-image.

Professional Knowledge

- The child was discharged from the NICU 2 months ago.
- The child presents with difficulties regulating responses to sensory environment, difficulties regulating emotional responses when stressed, decreased eye contact and visual fixation, fair oral–motor control when feeding on bottle, and decreased cervical strength for head and neck extension in prone.
- The standard treatment approach is to provide external supports through environmental modifications, appropriate stimulation for sensory and motor development, and interventions to improve feeding abilities and patterns.

Preliminary Delineation of Problems

- Gross and fine motor delay
- Impaired emotional and sensory regulation
- Delayed feeding skills and nutritional insufficiency
- Impaired visual–motor integration skills
- At risk for developmental delay—physical, cognitive, emotional, and sensory
- Cultural conflicts

Phase 3: Forming Hypotheses and Developing Intervention Plans (Intervention Process)

Forming Hypotheses

- The client will demonstrate increased cervical strength to perform lateral rotation to clear airways in prone position, to hold head in midline with chin tucked in supine, and to sustain extension in prone for 3–5 seconds.
- The client will demonstrate increased self-regulation behaviors for self-soothing with environmental supports.
- The client will visually fixate and track into vertical and horizontal planes.
- The client will demonstrate improved oral–motor control for suck/swallow/breath pattern on bottle or nipple.

- The client will demonstrate increased tolerance of supervised prone positions (i.e., tummy time) on caregiver's chest, floor, or appropriate equipment/furniture.

Developing Cultural Intervention Strategies

- Involve the family in the treatment process. Use the Health Belief Model to understand the clients' perceptions regarding susceptibility and severity of developmental delays. Encourage the family to identify their perceptions regarding benefits and barriers to healthy behavior changes. Provide opportunities for family members to prioritize goals and interventions, which will ensure that goals are client-centered but will also help promote self-efficacy.
- Use task-specific or activity-guided interventions during the session to provide concrete examples and feedback for the family. Incorporating health education interventions will encourage self-efficacy and ensure a balanced fit of person, occupation, and environment when the family implements these strategies at home.
- Provide appropriate resources that appeal to each generation's needs as well as respect each member's literacy level. Examples include websites, videos, or visual handouts for the young mother. Nelson (2009) recommends engaging teen mothers in active learning opportunities, such as facilitating Internet searches on breastfeeding to empower the mother to explore and discover the information and make informed decisions. Elder members may prefer resources in text or written formats. Present options to family members, and let them choose their preferred resource.
- Build rapport before discussing long-term implications of prematurity.
- Promote the importance of safe, supervised prone play and exposure to a variety of experiences for brain development. Address any concerns about protecting the infant from injury, illness, or germs. Explore alternatives for floor play if the floor is not acceptable or safe for the child (e.g., prone play on the caregiver's chest).
- Refer the family to community or faith-based services or both for additional resources. Even if occupational therapy is home based, the mother must have peer models and support in comfortable and familiar settings (Black & Wells, 2007).

Phase 4: Implementing the Intervention Plan (Targeting Outcomes)

Reevaluate and modify the treatment as needed to reflect the client and caregiver's performance, lifestyle, and culture.

Reflection 20.3. Apply Cultural Context

Reflect on a past client or create a case study. How would you apply your cultural knowledge during the occupational therapy process? How could you improve your therapeutic use of self to provide culturally competent services? Think of ways to use the Health Belief Model in addition to your preferred occupational therapy theory and approach.

Case Summary

In this case example, the family's health risks were identified and addressed. The increased risk for infant mortality in the Memphis area was acknowledged by the occupational therapy practitioner and incorporated into the family's education on co-occupations. Providing comprehensive knowledge to the family in a culturally effective way may have saved the infant's life and decreased the child's risk for disability. The family was empowered by health promotion knowledge and educated by the occupational therapist on how to incorporate these strategies into their daily routines. For example, the entire family implemented "tummy time" and prone positions on the mother's chest before and after school for 10–15 minutes 2–3 times a day. This increase in prone play improved the parents' and grandparents' ability to bond with the infant while supporting her developmental needs.

Another example of incorporating a public health initiative with engagement in occupation comes from the promotion of the Urban Child Institute's Touch, Talk, Read, and Play campaign. This public health initiative promotes critical brain development for the infant (Urban Child Institute, 2013). With mutual exploration of potential opportunities for touching, talking, reading, and playing, the family was able to discover the best times for implementing each of these occupations during their daily routines. This family found their caregiving rhythm with gentle guidance, or cues to action, from the occupational therapist, which supported their infant's developmental needs.

The child's developmental outcomes improved significantly with the achievement of all therapeutic goals that were set through family and occupational therapist collaboration. In pediatrics, the child's outcomes are dependent on their caregivers and the environmental supports. Occupational therapy practitioners must meet the clients where they are and be mindful of their culture and unique life experiences. In places such as Memphis, Tennessee, promoting comprehensive health and development may save a child's life.

Summary

The Health Belief Model is just one theory to use to help clients improve their health. A variety of health promotion theories can be incorporated, but focusing on the big picture of health and well-being when delivering occupational therapy services can improve a client's quality of life. Health behaviors are closely correlated to culture, lifestyle, and context; thus, an occupational therapist's impact can manifest beyond any setting.

Occupational therapy practitioners can use theoretical and practice frameworks from health promotion and occupational therapy to strengthen their cultural knowledge, to enhance their ability to evaluate and produce successful interventions, and to educate consumers. Using health promotion theory, occupational therapy practice, and cultural knowledge can help clients achieve the definition of *health*, which is "a complete state of physical, mental, and social well-being, and not merely the absence of disease or infirmity" (WHO, 1947, p. 29).

Acknowledgments

Special thanks to Dr. Anne Zachry of the University of Tennessee Health Science Center for providing guidance and feedback, and sincere thanks to Joshua Thomas of the Memphis Public Library for tracking down the Mark Twain reference for this chapter.

References

American Academy of Pediatrics. (2011, November). SIDS and other sleep-related infant deaths: Expansion of recommendations for a safe infant sleeping environment. *Pediatrics, 128*(5), 1341–1367. http://dx.doi.org/10.1542/peds.2011-2285

American Academy of Pediatrics. (2008). Theme six: Promoting physical activity. In J. F. Hagan Jr., J. S. Shaw, & P. Duncan (Eds.), *Bright futures: Guidelines for health supervision of infants, children, and adolescents* (3rd ed., pp. 147–154). Elk Grove Village, IL: American Academy of Pediatrics.

American College of Obstetricians and Gynecologists. (2013). Committee opinion No. 570: Breastfeeding in underserved women: Increasing initiation and continuation of breastfeeding. *American Journal of Obstetrics and Gynecology, 122*(2), 423–427. http://dx.doi.org/10.1097/01.AOG.0000433008.93971.6a

American Occupational Therapy Association. (2014). Occupational therapy practice framework: Domain & process (3rd ed.). *American Journal of Occupational Therapy, 68*(Suppl. 1), S1–S48. http://dx.doi.org/10.5014/ajot.2014.682006

Bigby, J. A., & American College of Physicians–American Society of Internal Medicine. (2003). *Cross-cultural medicine.* Philadelphia: American College of Physicians.

Black, R. M., & Wells, S. A. (2007). *Culture and occupation: A model of empowerment in occupational therapy.* Bethesda, MD: AOTA Press.

Flaherty, S. C., & Sadler, L. S. (2010). A review of attachment theory in the context of adolescent parenting. *Journal of Pediatric Health Care, 25*(2), 114–121. http://dx.doi.org/10.1016/j.pedhc.2010.02.005

Hall Smith, P., Coley, S. L., Labbock, M. H., Cupito, S., & Nwokah, E. (2012). Early breastfeeding experiences of adolescent mothers: A qualitative prospective study. *International Breastfeeding Journal, 7*(13), 1–14. http://dx.doi.org/10.1186/1746-4358-7-13

Hurley, K. M., Black, M. M., Papas, M. A., & Quigg, A. M. (2008, April). Variation in breastfeeding behaviours, perceptions, and experiences by race/ethnicity among a low-income statewide sample of Special Supplemental Nutrition Program for Women, Infants, and Children (WIC) participants in the United States. *Maternal and Child Nutrition, 4*(2), 95–105. http://dx.doi.org/10.1111/j.1740-8709.2007.00105.x

Janz, N. K., Champion, V. L., & Strecher, V. J. (2002). The health belief model. In K. Glanz, B. K. Rimer, & F. M. Lewis (Eds.). *Health behavior and health education: Theory, research, and practice* (3rd ed., pp. 45–66). San Francisco: Jossey-Bass.

Law, M., Cooper, B., Strong, S., Stewart, D., Rigby, P., & Letts, L. (1996). The Person–Environment–Occupation Model: A transactive approach to occupational performance. *Canadian Journal of Occupational Therapy, 63*(1), 9–23. http://dx.doi.org/10.1177/000841749606300103

Lewallen, L. P., & Street, D. J. (2010, November/December). Initiating and sustaining breastfeeding in African American women. *Journal of Obstetrical Gynecology Neonatal Nursing, 39*(6), 667–674. http://dx.doi.org/10.1111/j.1552-6909.2010.01196.x

National Cancer Institute, U.S. Department of Health and Human Services, & National Institute of Health. (2005). *Theory at a glance* (2nd ed.). Bethesda, MD: National Institutes of Health.

Nelson, A. M. (2009). Adolescent attitudes, beliefs, and concerns regarding breastfeeding. *American Journal of Maternal Child Nursing, 34*(4), 249–255. http://dx.doi.org/10.1097/01.NMC.0000357918.18229.25

Reitz, S. M. (2014). Health promotion theories. In B. A. Boyt Schell, G. Gillen, M. E. Scaffa, & E. S. Cohn (Eds.). *Willard and Spackman's occupational therapy* (12th ed., pp. 574–587). Philadelphia: Lippincott Williams & Wilkins.

Rosenstock, I. (1966). Why people use health services. *Milbank Memorial Fund Quarterly, 44*(3), 94–124. http://dx.doi.org/10.1111/j.1468-0009.2005.00425.x

Scaffa, M. E., & Reitz, S. M. (2014). *Occupational therapy in community-based practice settings* (2nd ed.). Philadelphia: F. A. Davis.

Scaffa, M. E., Reitz, S. M., & Pizzi, M. A. (2010). *Occupational therapy in the promotion of health and wellness.* Philadelphia: F. A. Davis.

Stewart, D., Letts, L., Law, M., Cooper, B., Strong, S., & Rigby, P. J. (2003). The Person–Environment–Occupation model. In E. B. Crepeau, E. S. Cohn, & B. A. Boyt Schell (Eds.). *Willard and Spackman's occupational therapy* (10th ed., pp. 227–233). Philadelphia: Lippincott Williams & Wilkins.

Tarlov, A. R. (1996). Social determinants of health: The sociobiological transition. In D. Blane, E. Brunner, & R. Wilkinson (Eds.). *Health and social organization: Towards a health policy for the twenty-first century* (pp. 71–93). London: Routledge.

Terhune, P. S. (2005). African-American developmental disability discourses: Implications for policy development. *Journal of Policy and Practice in Intellectual Disabilities, 2*(1), 18–28. http://dx.doi.org/10.1111/j.1741-1130.2005.00004.x

Twain, M. (1897). *Following the equator: A journey around the world* (Ch. 13, Vol. 2). Hartford, CT: American Publishing Co.

Urban Child Institute. (2012). Chapter four: Health. In J. Kmet, & K. Morrell (Eds.). *The state of children in Memphis and Shelby County: Data book* (7th ed., pp. 30–43). Memphis, TN: Urban Child Institute.

Urban Child Institute. (2013). *Touch, talk, read, and play.* Retrieved from http://www.urbanchildinstitute.org/key-initiatives/touch-talk-read-play

U.S. Department of Health and Human Services. (2008). *The secretary's advisory committee on national health promotion and disease prevention objectives for 2020. Phase I report: Recommendations for the framework and format of Healthy People 2020.*

Retrieved from http://www.healthypeople.gov/sites/default/files/PhaseI_0.pdf

U.S. Department of Health and Human Services. (2011). *The surgeon's general call to action to support breastfeeding*. Washington, DC: U.S. Department of Health and Human Services, Office of the Surgeon General.

World Health Organization. (1947). Preamble to the Constitution of the World Health Organization. *Chronicle of the World Health Organization, 1*(1), 29–40.

World Health Organization. (1986). *The Ottawa charter for health promotion*. Retrieved from http://www.who.int/healthpromotion/conferences/previous/ottawa/en/

Chapter 21.

INFLUENCE OF CULTURE ON FOOD IN OCCUPATIONAL THERAPY INTERVENTION

Toni Thompson, OTR/L

Food is a central activity of mankind and one of the single most significant trademarks of a culture.
Mark Kurlansky (Allhoff & Monroe, 2007, p. 11)

Chapter Highlights

- Understanding Clients' Cultures Related to Food
- Evaluations Incorporating Food
- Feeding Choice Influences
- Universal and Unique Foods
- Food as Prevention and Remedy
- Mechanical Components of Eating Addressed in Evaluation and Intervention
- Need for Evidence-Based Interventions With Food

Key Terms and Concepts

- ✧ Comfort foods
- ✧ Curanderos
- ✧ Finger foods
- ✧ Folk medicine
- ✧ Hakim system
- ✧ Halal preparation
- ✧ Herbal medicine

- ✧ Hot and cold illnesses and conditions
- ✧ Jain religion
- ✧ Jhatka process
- ✧ Kashrut
- ✧ Lent
- ✧ Sawm
- ✧ Yin–yang system

Food plays a central role in the daily occupation of every person in every culture. As a nutrient source, medicine, social bond, socioeconomic divider, mood moderator, and psychological stressor, food encompasses an integral component in intervention and falls under the scope of occupational therapy (American Occupational Therapy Association, 2007). Occupations of food acquisition, selection, preparation, presentation, self-feeding, and rituals form part of individual and group activities for clients in all practice areas across the continuum of care, but evidence-based research focuses on evaluation and implementation of feeding practices using Western-style utensils and seating positions. Current practice tools reflect a lack of evidence-based research into diversity of utensils, postures, and foods. By incorporating awareness of diversities and knowledge of the cultural aspects of food, occupational therapy practitioners can develop the cultural skills to affect meaningful, individualized interventions.

This chapter discusses the variety of cultural and personal components inherent in the daily occupation of food and the breadth of food in daily living skills. Exploring some of the many subtle cultural differences encompassed by food can offer better ways to address a client's success in occupations involving food.

Understanding Clients' Cultures Related to Food

Consider the case of a 10-year-old girl with cerebral palsy and right-side hemiplegia who showed progress in cutting meat and using utensils with her left hand. Instead of showing pleasure at their child's progress, the parents gave nonverbal signs of distress. What was going on?

The father confided that they used the right hand for eating and the left hand for toileting. Moreover, they did not use utensils in their home. They ate semisolid food with their fingers and soft breads, and they used spoons, forks, and knives in public. The treatment plan was modified to focus on the use of adaptive equipment and techniques so the girl could feed herself with her right hand using her fingers, soft breads, and Western utensils.

Cultural and individualized aspects of feeding skills are often not addressed in standard evaluations. To address the cultural element of foods,

occupational therapists must strive to understand the food selection, preparation, presentation, serving styles, rituals, and utensil use in each client's culture. Literature reviews reveal extensive information about cultural aspects of food in popular culture, including recipes, exploration of travel destinations, and culinary adventures.

Spector (2012) catalogued extensive information on foods, herbs, nutritional regimens, and customs in various cultures and religions, focusing on their impact in health care practices. However, the field of occupational therapy has a void in evidence-based research and its practice of incorporating cultural aspects into the use of food as a treatment intervention modality.

Evaluations Incorporating Food

Occupational therapy practitioners use standardized assessment tools, nonstandardized measures, and observations when evaluating feeding skills. Standardized assessments tend to use specific foods, techniques, utensils, and methods to maintain reliability and validity. Most standardized assessments require specific foods, procedures, and techniques.

For example, the Kitchen Task Assessment (KTA; Baum & Edwards, 1993), using boxed chocolate pudding, formed the basis for the Executive Function Performance Test (EFPT; Baum, Morrison, Hahn, & Edwards, 2007), which involves the preparation of oatmeal. The KTA and the EFPT have been proven reliable and valid for their diagnostic conditions but lack flexibility for cultural diversity (Baum, 1993, 2007a, 2007b). Subjective eating assessment tools allow for more flexibility at the risk of objective measurement.

The Children's Eating Behavior Inventory (CEBI; Archer, Rosenbaum, & Streiner, 1991) addresses 40 items and the Behavioral Pediatrics Feeding Assessment (BPFA; Crist & Napier-Phillips, 2001) addresses 35 items related to parental reports of behavioral feeding aspects. These allow for consideration of individualized feeding elements but lack the reliability and validity of structured objective tools (Archer et al., 1991; Crist & Napier-Phillips, 2001). The Activity Configuration Log provides a pen-and-paper or computer-based method to track and rate daily activities for assessment and intervention purposes. This subjective tool, not yet standardized, offers opportunity for the client to include individualized aspects of feeding (Söderback, 2009).

For outcomes and reimbursement, most intervention settings require the use of evidence-based assessment tools and interventions. The lack of culturally sensitive assessments leaves a void—even a conflict—in carrying out effective client-centered therapy. The challenge of intervention using food lies in incorporating the client's personal choices amid medical conditions, medications, and availability options—in other words, accounting for the client's unique culture (see Case Example 21.1).

Case Example 21.1. Making Meals

A retired elderly gentleman with a diagnosis of mild cerebral vascular accident in a rehabilitation center received occupational therapy with the goal of returning to his home, where he had lived independently. He consistently refused to perform the kitchen skills activities for evaluation or treatment purposes. He also stated he would not allow outsiders to provide household help. An occupational therapy intern was asked to work with the client. The intern asked, "What do you want to do in the kitchen?" This simple question evolved into a long dialogue about his dislike for the packaged and processed foods in the rehabilitation center and his desire to make meals from "real food." In response to their conversation, the intern had the gentleman prepare tomato sauce from fresh tomatoes and herbs as well as make several creative meals. A simple dialogue formed the basis for this intervention that increased the client's level of independence in his post-discharge living situation.

Reflection 21.1. Evaluation and Food

- Review the case of a previous client whom you treated for an intervention involving food, or imagine that you have received a referral for a feeding evaluation typical to your setting. Visualize how you typically set up for the evaluation. Identify 3 components that reflect assumptions about the client's culture: food choices, religious beliefs, posture, utensils, personal choices, and medical concerns.

Feeding Choice Influences

Feeding choices are influenced by many factors, including the client's medical considerations; culture-related interpretations of health; religion, spirituality, and ethics; awareness of weight and fitness; and rituals, holidays, and comfort foods. Considering these cultural influences on clients' food selection can lead to more effective assessment and intervention.

Medical Considerations

Successful intervention relies on the practitioner's ability to observe and verbally ascertain individual medications, conditions, allergies, sensitivities, and beliefs surrounding health and incorporate these into the intervention. Many people with autism spectrum disorder report achieving symptom reduction by eliminating specific foods, such as sugar, artificial colors, food dyes, preservatives, and other foodstuffs (Food for the Brain, 2012).

Some individuals encounter difficulty managing specific food textures and consistencies. Clients of all ages may require pureed diets or G-tube feedings. The intervention areas of eating disorders and other mental health conditions such as obsessive–compulsive disorders present additional unique challenges to the medical team to ensure adequate nutrition with healthy attitudes toward food (Martin, 2000; Anderson, 2005).

Interpretations of Health

Some cultures that incorporate health beliefs combine foods, herbs, and beverages such as the Asian *yin–yang system.* Some follow these guidelines on a daily basis with increased adherence to the system during health challenges, illnesses, and emotional difficulties. More than 4,500 years ago, Huang-ti Nei Ching wrote *The Yellow Emperor's Classic of Internal Medicine* to describe the yin–yang system. *Yang* tends to be dominant and masculine, and *yin* tends to be passive and feminine. Yang foods are hot, spicy, well cooked, and orange, red, and yellow in color, while yin foods are raw or cooked at a low temperature, bland, and white or light green in color. Based on yin and yang characteristics, foods, beverages, and herbs like ginseng coordinate with various medical conditions and daily occupations to achieve emotional and physical homeostasis (Civitello, 2008; Spector, 2009).

Many Hispanic cultures in Latin America adhere to interpretations of *hot and cold illnesses and conditions.* Specific conditions and illnesses are traditionally defined as "hot" or "cold," and foods, herbs, and treatments are given to balance the temperature. Cold conditions and illnesses require hot beverages and foods, and vice versa. For example, pregnancy is a cold condition, while the postpartum period is a hot condition. The hot–cold system evolved from the four elements or humors of hot, cold, wet, and dry. Blood represented hot and wet elements; yellow bile constituted hot and dry elements; phlegm represented cold and wet elements; and black bile constituted cold and dry elements (Foster, 1994; Spector 2009).

Many people in Northern India and educated residents of Karachi, Pakistan, subscribe to treatment in the *hakim system,* an Arabic system of health modified by Indian practitioners, based on the four elements or humors and four qualities (Kittler & Sucher, 2008). Similar attention to hot–cold and humors exists among people from Cambodia, Laos, the Philippines, and the Middle East as well as the Hmong population (Kittler & Sucher, 2008).

Curanderos, or healers, offer herbal treatments for medical conditions to believers in Mexico, Central America, and northern South America (Spector, 2009). Some believe that if a pregnant woman does not eat every food she craves, the pregnancy could result in a miscarriage or congenital anomalies. Some Mexican women believe that the child may be born with a strawberry-like birthmark if the woman does not eat strawberries when she craves them (Dinsmore, 2000; Spector, 2009).

Religion, Spirituality, and Ethics

Effective intervention may incorporate spiritual use of food that is not addressed in evidence-based research. Many people subscribe to religious standards that exclude certain foods and include specific ritual foods. Ethical considerations for animal welfare lead some people to adopt vegan, vegetarian, or Jainism regimes. Followers of the *Jain religion* do not eat foods that are pulled out of the ground to prevent killing the plant and surrounding microorganisms (Jain, 2000). Followers of Sikhism, a religion founded in India, eat meat prepared by the *Jhatka process* with a quick blow to the animal's head to avoid

Reflection 21.2. Practitioner Reflection: Avoiding Cultural Food Stereotypes

My husband and I traveled to Kerala in South India for the All India Occupational Therapists' Association Conference. We enjoyed the opportunity to share daily meals and tea in a communal setting with participants and family members. At our first meal, we observed many people eating with their fingers. They used soft flat breads, like *naan* and *paratha,* to collect food the consistency of a stew; they used their fingers to manage *avial,* a vegetable dish spiced with curry and coconut. By the second day, we embraced the local custom and ate with our fingers, using the breads to manage the food. A few people used silverware. We observed that the use of fingers in lieu of silverware was prevalent in the southern part of India. Then we dined at a very exclusive Indian restaurant. The waiters served us with impeccable attention. They informed us that there was no silverware and the food was to be eaten in the real Indian style with the fingers. Had we only ventured to the conference, we would have assumed that most people in India eat all foods with their fingers. Had we dined only in major cities, we would have concluded that everyone in India uses silverware. Had we dined in only the exclusive restaurant, we would have concluded that everyone in India eats all their food with their fingers.

—*Toni Thompson, OTR/L (used with permission)*

suffering, and they do not eat meat that has been prepared for sacrifice (Brar, 2011).

Roman Catholics adhere to the practice of no meat on Fridays during *Lent,* a season of 40 days before Easter. Colored hard-boiled eggs are used in the Christian celebration of Easter. Many Christian denominations offer flat wheat wafers and red wine for Communion services.

Muslims refrain from consuming pork products, and all other meats must undergo a *halal preparation* process. In the halal process, "meat of an animal that was slaughtered when any name besides God's was mentioned is prohibited" (Kittler & Sucher, 2008, p. 98). During Ramadan, Muslims observe a month of *sawm* and refrain from food, beverage, and physical activity from sunrise to sunset (Civitello, 2008; Harris, Lyon, & McLaughlin, 2005).

Followers of the Jewish faith refrain from eating pork and shellfish. They observe **kashrut,** or "keeping kosher," with specific preparation of foods, including the separation of milk products from meat products in storage, preparation, and serving (Buller, 2005; E. Goldin, personal communication, November 25, 2012). Jews typically observe Passover by sharing unleavened bread and bitter herbs.

Hindus traditionally observe a vegetarian diet, although some younger Hindus eat meat, except meat from cows, the sacred animal. Christian Scientists and Seventh-day Adventists often follow a vegetarian diet. Navajo American Indians refrain from fish consumption (Ferris, 2013).

Followers of the Church of Jesus Christ of Latter-Day Saints refrain from "strong liquids," meaning alcohol, and "hot liquids," often interpreted as coffee and tea (Church of Jesus Christ of Latter-Day Saints, 2012).

Many religions observe commemorative events and celebrations with specific foods. Indian women in Trivandrum celebrate the festival of Pongala with 20 hours of chanting and ritual offerings of rice balls prepared with coconut and molasses ("Hearths ready," 2013).

Awareness of Weight and Fitness

Awareness of weight and fitness affects voluntary adherence to food regimens that can present challenges in food-based therapeutic activities. Clients may adopt mainstream or unique regimens for weight loss, weight gain, bodybuilding, high-level athletic training, preventive health reasons, or medical healing. Some specific regimens focus on high-protein, macrobiotic, or raw foods, while other options are plan based, such as the Atkins Diet, South Beach, Diet, 4-Hour Body, and WeightWatchers (Atkins Diet, n.d.; South Beach Diet, 2016).

Many people use food pyramids to guide food selection; the pyramid's large base is composed of essential food groups with smaller levels ascending to less important food groups. Some food group pyramids include the Asian Diet Pyramid, Vegetarian Diet Pyramid, Mediterranean Diet Pyramid, and the Latin America Diet Pyramid (Civitello, 2008). To augment or replace regular meals, many people consume nutritional supplements, including vitamins, minerals, protein powders, herbs, and energy or sports drinks, all of which bear varying levels of approval by the U.S. Food and Drug Administration.

Rituals, Holidays, and Comfort Foods

Food choices are also influenced by culture-related rituals, holidays, and comfort foods. Most cultures mark specific holidays and events with rituals and specific foods. Christian Scientists and some other religions do not call attention to individual birthdays, but many cultures celebrate birthdays, religious events, secular holidays, and weddings with special dishes and sweets in the form of puddings, cakes, or other favorites.

Religious and cultural holidays abound with specific foods, such as *latkes* (potato pancakes) for the Jewish celebration of Hanukah, and turkey and pumpkin pie for the North American Thanksgiving. Muslims celebrate the end of their month-long fast with Eid al-Fitr and a variety of sweet and savory preparations based on regional and family preferences, such as Pakistani *zarda* (a sweet rice dish), Middle Eastern *roz bil halib* (rice pudding), or Somali *cambaabur* (crepes; Collins, 2010).

Foods associated with sentimental experiences become one's personal ***comfort foods*** that provide physical and psychological relief. Comfort foods, unique to each person, often relate to specific loved family members or childhood rituals. In times of illness or sadness, one may find comfort in grandma's chicken soup or *biriyani* (spicy rice) or tortillas, meatloaf, egg salad, or pasta. During celebrations, one may expect foods such as birthday cake, ice cream, or chocolate.

Another form of comfort food, sweets can be made of sugar and flour with fruit, as in apple pie, or with walnuts and cream, as in the Slovenian specialty *prekmurska gibanica*. Most cultures enjoy a form of frozen dessert from milk-based ice cream, gelato, dairy-free *granita*, Indian *kulfi*, or *cassata gelata* of Middle Eastern origin. While children in the United States might eat raw chocolate chip cookie dough, youngsters in Venezuela might eat handfuls of powdered milk or single-serving size containers of condensed milk.

Action 21.1. Religion and Food Customs

- Talk to someone of a different religion about food customs for every day, holidays, and special occasions. Ask an individual with whom you feel comfortable or a religious authority at a place of worship.

Universal and Unique Foods

Some foodstuffs are universal to many cultures, and other foods are found only in specific cultures. This section explores unique preparations, uses, and evolutions of the world's basic foods across different cultures, countries, regions, provinces, states, and homes as elements to explore in food intervention. For example, staple tea and coffee beverages vary according to culture and individual choice.

Rice, Corn, and Wheat

Rice, corn, and wheat comprise up to 60% of the world's food energy (Buller, 2005). The array of food created from these basic grains varies immensely with unique regional preparations. Many people use various breads to mobilize the food to the mouth; examples include African wheat *chapattis*, Indian lentil *dosa* or wheat *naan*, African millet *ngome*, Mid-Eastern pita, and Brazilian *cassava*. Corn is served as grits in the Southern United States, polenta in Italy, soup in Asia, and *ugali* in Africa. Many cultures enjoy food "pockets" filled with prepared vegetables, meats, cheeses, almonds, or fruits. These pockets include *empanadas* of corn or wheat from Latin America, *manti yougurt pastry* from Iran and Uzbekistan, *b'stilla* from Morocco, *momo noodles* from Tibet, *kolodny* from Poland, *wonton* and *bao* from China, *samosas* from Asia, pastries from England, *pel'meni* from Russia, and dumplings from the United States (Civitello, 2008).

Animals

People in some areas dine on delicacies of grasshoppers and other insects, while other people find such consumption unsettling, even repulsive. People in Cambodia may enjoy deep-fried tarantulas. Chinese food markets offer a variety of scorpions (Anderson, 2005).

Although people across the globe dine on the same animals, they savor different parts. In China, many people eat all parts of the animal, including deer penis, while Uruguayans feast on sweetbreads made from the thymus and pancreas glands of beef cattle. Guinea pig, called *cuy*, holds a long history in the Andean countries of Peru and Ecuador, and connoisseurs enjoy eating every part, including ears and tongue. More than 50 years ago, sweetbreads, brains, and organ meats formed part of the U.S. diet but have now become less popular, although some enjoy chitlins (intestines), and others add chicken necks or fish eyeballs into soups and stews.

Evolution of Food

Foods evolve and show a long migratory history alongside immigrants and through traders and travelers. Chocolate was originally cultivated by the Mayans about 2,000 years ago and was reserved for royalty; it was gradually integrated into most cultures, shifting to medicinal use, and eventually developed by Europeans into a variety of sweets (Civitello, 2008, p. 106). Currently, nutritionists stress the antioxidant powers of chocolate, especially dark chocolate (Maskarinec, 2009). In Mexico and Central America, chocolate combined with chili powder remains a main ingredient in savory dishes such as *molé* (Field Museum, n.d.; Tannahill, 1988).

Tapioca has been used in various forms in various cultures for centuries. It is used as flour for breads in Latin America, Africa, and Asia and in the gelatinous parts of many sweets and puddings. In the past decade, Asian tapioca drinks, such as *boba* and bubble tea, have invaded international markets.

Many people may not understand or may disagree on the historical development of the foods typical of their culture. Peruvians and Ecuadorians argue over who invented *ceviche,* a specialty made of various varieties of raw fish marinated in lemon juice and local spices, including cilantro. Some historians believe the origin lies with the Japanese immigrants who used their customs for fish preparation in areas where cooking was not always available, adapting to the spices of Peru (N. LaPuente, personal communication, 2013; "Peruano," 2013; Rodriguez, Zimmerman, Hirsheimer, & McAndrews, 2010).

U.S. Regional Differences

The diverse cultures of, established ethnic groups in, and recent immigrants to the United States offer a multitude of regional differences in food preparations, selections, and names (Kurlansky, 2009; Smith, 2007; Stern & Stern, 2011).

Some foods are universal with a few ingredient changes and diverse names. Eames and Robboy (1967) defined more than 13 names for the sandwich popularized by the Subway and Blimpie food chains. The sandwich goes by *sub, subway,* and *blimpie* in New Jersey; *hero* in New York; *hoagie* and *grinder* in New England; *Jackson's gambit* and *poor boy* in St. Louis, *po'-boy* in Louisiana; and *Cuban* in Florida (Stern & Stern, 2011).

Stern and Stern (2011) note that in the United States, "devoted aficionados say that barbecue is like DNA: No two examples are precisely alike" (p. 7). Major differences include regional and personal preferences in meats, cuts, preparation, and an array of sauce mixtures.

With the advent of technology and the immigration of new ethnic groups into all regions of the United States, diverse foods are becoming more common on restaurant menus, as food truck offerings, and as home-cooked options.

Texans along the Mexican border distinguish their Mexican cuisine of tamales, beans, and meat preparations from central Texas's Tex-Mex. Often, Southern cuisine conjures up visions and smells of cornbread, collard greens, shrimp and grits, fried chicken, and hot sauces. The mint julep calls Kentucky home. Florida is home to key lime pie, Georgia boasts peaches, and pecans are present in various creations throughout the Southeast (Kurlansky, 2009; Smith, 2007).

Midwestern foods reflect the influence of Native Americans and diverse immigrant groups from Italy, Poland, Greece, Germany, and the United Kingdom. Kurlansky (2009) defined the influence on meals from the Norwegian and Swedish settlers. Cold-climate fruits of apples and berries find their way into pies and tarts. Although the U.S. dairy industry originated in the Northeast, Wisconsin holds the title of America's Dairyland for developing cheese standards, the first American cheeses, gourmet cheeses, and processed cheeses (Smith, 2007).

Originating in the area of the Hudson and Ohio rivers, the fish fry has filtered out to many Catholic communities, but the fish boil remains characteristic of Door County, Wisconsin. St. Louis hosts the gooey butter cake, the result of a baker's mistake during the Depression (Stern & Stern, 2011). Nebraska boasts the record for popcorn production (Kurlansky, 2009), just one of the many uses for corn in the Midwest.

The cuisine of the Northeast uses seafood from the coast with Boston and Maine lobsters. Kurlansky (2009) details diverse preparations of clams and oysters in this region.

Southwestern cuisine combines the influence of Native Americans, cowboys, and Mexican immigrants. Beans provided the original dietary staple. "New Mexicans honor chili and pinto beans as

their state vegetables" (Smith, 2007, p. 557). The emergence of Texas barbecue married with the New Mexican foods emerged into Tex-Mex cuisine.

Mormons from Utah retain several years of canned foods in food cellars and have traditionally been known for funeral potatoes, a casserole of cream soup, cheese, and sliced potatoes (Hill & Popp, 1988). Rocky Mountain fare includes bison, smoked meats, and fish. Tlingit cuisine in the Pacific Northwest uses kale, fresh and preserved herring, hooligan, salmon, and beach seafood topped with Nanaimo custard for dessert. Hawaiian cuisine features various fish and tropical fruits with influences from Asia and other islands, the Pennsylvania Dutch, and dynamic cuisines of major cities.

Reflection 21.3. Hands-On Ways to Learn About Cultural Components

Visit a store or shop that sells unfamiliar food or herbal products. Ask the staff to explain the items and guide you through the store.

- What questions can you ask about the sources of and uses for the foods and products?

Food as Prevention and Remedy

Using foods, beverages, spices, and herbs to prevent illness and to remedy a variety of health conditions has been done for centuries. As in food preparations for meals and snacks, various cultures define these preparations in unique ways. Often individuals cannot define the etiology of the methods, despite adhering to the techniques. Awareness of the role of food in health and illness can enhance food interventions.

Spices

International spice trade forms one of the largest international commerce bases (Natural Products Insider, 2014). Besides enhancing a food's flavor and aroma, some spices provide health properties, including fighting off infections, parasites, and fungi. Numerous spices, like cinnamon, cardamom, fennel seeds, ginger, allspice, mace, licorice, basil, oregano, vanilla, cloves, dill, coriander, caraway, and many more offer unique flavors; many offer health properties. Turmeric, though offering minimal flavor, provides a rich yellow color to dishes and offers high levels of antioxidants.

Many cultures incorporate hot sauces from various chili peppers cooked or marinated in sugar, vinegar, or fruit or a combination of those. The tropical islands of Oceania offer the Portuguese *piri piri* sauce, the West Indies use the scotch bonnet pepper blended with tropical fruits, and *sos cili* sauce is popular in Brunei and Malaysia (Oceania Cuisine, 2011). Chili peppers contain capsicum, and its derivative capsaicin, which is used topically as an analgesic and taken orally to clear the sinuses. Spices, like basic foods of corn and wheat, are used to make unique tastes in each culture and each kitchen. Although Indian food and Caribbean dishes incorporate turmeric, cilantro, and cumin, they result in unique dishes, tastes, and presentations.

Folk Medicine

Some foods may have specific meanings and uses for members of certain groups. *Folk medicine,* often called natural folk medicine, "utilizes herbs, plants, minerals, and animal substances to prevent and treat illnesses" (Spector, 2012, p. 104). Spector (2012) also describes occult or "magico-religious folk medicine . . . the use of charms, holy words, and holy actions" (p. 104). Almost all cultures have developed folk medicine uses of foods for remedies and health maintenance, with members subscribing at different levels of incorporation.

Spector (2009, 2012) describes foods that may have special meaning for remedies within certain cultural groups. Black Baptists, Native American tribes, Swedish Protestants, and Nova Scotian Catholics often use molasses for health purposes, especially a sore throat. Iranians, German Catholics, Irish Catholics, Eastern European Jews, and French Canadian Catholics employ honey and lemon alone or in various tea preparations to ease the symptoms of colds and sore throats and to enhance immunity. Norwegians often draw on hot peppermint tea for sore throat relief. German Catholics might also use salt water. Irish Catholics tend to add some whiskey to that concoction for health, while other cultures rub whiskey or other alcohol on the gums of teething babies.

Many groups use baking soda for indigestion relief, fueled by industry advertising. English Catholics might use onions boiled with sugar for health. Many groups use garlic for a variety of health conditions, especially heart health. Ginger ale often serves as a source of electrolytes and fluid when one is suffering from a stomachache, cold, or the flu. Eastern European Jews and Polish Catholics eat chicken soup for colds. Some factions may wear food items, as garlic, on a string around their neck. Black Baptists may don an onion around their neck, while Swedish Protestants might chose a herringbone wrapped in flannel.

Some food items may be used topically. Italians and English Catholics may heat cod liver oil or olive oil and allow it to set in the ears of someone with an earache. Many Asians use coconut oil for a variety of skin conditions and other disorders. Some people try potato slices or onion slices to heal wounds or treat warts. German Catholics often use hot mustard plasters for backache, while occupational and physical therapists recommend bags of frozen peas for use as a cold pack for various body injuries.

Herbal medicine, the use of a plant's seeds, berries, roots, leaves, bark, or flowers for prevention and medical treatment, is increasing in all parts of the world. Native Americans and Asian cultures have maintained a long tradition of extensive herb use for medicine and cultural rituals. Many herbs, including the use of ginseng as a digestive, restorative, and sedative, migrated from China to the Western world many years ago (Spector, 2009).

Mechanical Components of Eating Addressed in Evaluation and Intervention

In addition to unique food and beverage preparations and uses, people throughout the world prepare and eat food in many styles. Before food intervention, practitioners should consider unique cultural and personal use of tools, utensils, and fingers as well as postures and positions for success.

Food Preparation

Occupational therapy research offers no evidence-based study of food acquisition or preparation. Foods may be fresh, canned, packaged, or frozen and consist of vegetables, fruits, meats, seafood, and prepared options. Preparation considerations include the use of cooked and uncooked foods. Traditionally no-cook meal prep activities are the first step in progressively graded meal preparation intervention. For the individual who maintains a raw foods regimen, this step may be considered the final goal rather than a short-term goal.

Meal preparation tools can be electrical appliances including mixers, food processors, or manually operated wood, metal, or plastic implements with a variety of stirrers, spoons, whisks, and spatulas. Preparation tools vary from basic wooden stirring devices formed from sticks to an array of gadgets designed to perform every conceivable kitchen task.

Serving styles include finger foods, servings on one's individual plate, buffet serving, servings taken from communal dishes to an individual plate, or fingers continuously dipped into one communal serving bowl.

Posture and Positioning

Occupational therapy feeding evaluations address positioning in a chair seated at a table or in a high chair or booster seat for children. Adapted seating may be included for those with postural deficits. Literature reviews show no evidence of interventions in alternative postures, which is especially important in community-based rehabilitation.

Feeding during meals, snacks, informal settings, and formal events includes the positions of sitting at a table, sitting on one's haunches, sitting cross-legged on the floor, sitting on a bed, or standing. Some people eat in a rushed manner while driving a car or animal-powered cart or on public transport of train, subway, bus, motorcycle, or even horseback. Occupational therapy practitioners often address positioning for feeding with a variety of adaptations, such as sitting in a wheelchair or other device to provide support. Babies often eat while held in arms or sitting in a feeder seat. Alternative postures in feeding offer an array of opportunities for further study.

Utensils

Practitioners often employ a variety of adapted utensils and handles on silverware, such as built-up handles, curved handles, weighted handles, and long-handled devices. Hands-free feeders, from low-tech self-powered to high-tech electronic, offer options for those who cannot use their hands for self-feeding. These options often exclude the variety of or lack of utensil options that people use throughout the world.

Many people eat all forms and consistencies of foods with their fingers and sometimes incorporate various breads to facilitate feeding. People in India use *naan,* a wheat bread, and *dosa,* a lentil bread, while people in Africa use wheat *chapattis.* Knives, forks, and spoons are the preferred utensils in most modern settings. People of all social strata in Vietnam, Cambodia, Laos, Thailand, Korea, China, Japan, and Southeast Asia use chopsticks (Luitel, 2006). Chopsticks adapted with rubber bands on the proximal end provide a learning tool for children to master this skill. Most cultures use a type of stick or skewer for cooking meat or vegetable pieces or for serving pieces of raw foods. Some cultures adhere to the principle of eating with the right hand and using the left hand for personal self-care and toileting, which may present difficulties for clients with right hemiplegia and other unilateral upper-extremity difficulties.

Most cultures have some foods savored with fingers, often called *finger foods.* Some foods are retrieved from a serving piece with fingers, toothpicks, or tongs. Feeding options vary by setting formality. For example, cooked chicken on the bone is often eaten with fingers in an informal picnic setting, eaten with a fork and knife in a formal dining setting, and can be eaten in either style during informal dining at home or in a casual restaurant.

Europeans tend to use the left hand to hold the fork and the right hand to manage the knife, and people in the United States and many Latin American countries tend to cut with a knife in the right hand and then switch the fork to the right hand for mobilizing the food from the plate to the mouth. Left-handers reverse the use of hands for fork and knife management in the latter setting.

Action 21.2. Dining Out

- Dine at a restaurant of an ethnicity different than your own. Observe the other diners and their approach to the food. Participate in the postures, utensil use, and other elements that are unique to that culture.

Need for Evidence-Based Interventions With Food

Areas that merit further discussion and research are the use of client-centered and culturally relevant foods, utensils, positioning, and meaningfulness in food-related evaluation and treatments. Research may cover the effectiveness of basic additions for information to initial forms and interview tools, including favorite foods, least-liked foods, utensil use, and positioning during meals and snacks. Other research may consider specific questions on satisfaction surveys to address the accuracy and effectiveness of foods and food components during treatments.

More extensive research can focus on adaptions of specific standardized assessment tools, individual interventions, and group treatments to accommodate medical, cultural, and individual food concerns.

Action 21.3. Cooking Class

Take a cooking class in a food that is unique to you. Research the food and region of the food before the class. Pay attention to the food preparation process. Engage the presenter(s) in conversation about the history, meaning, and uses of the foods.

- How do these conversations challenge the way you select, prepare, serve, and eat foods?

Summary

Occupational therapy practitioners must consider a wide variety of cultural and, more important, individual variables in selecting foods to affect successful intervention. After a review of each client's medical conditions, medications, allergies, and food preferences, practitioners should be aware of the meanings of and uses of foods. They can develop awareness of foods in cultural contexts.

The best practice of occupational therapy focuses on the individual's specific culture to develop unique goals and an individualized approach for each client to meet functional goals. One can begin with a simple dialogue about what and how the client likes to eat. This information forms the basis of new evidence for research to expand more effective use of food in occupational therapy interventions.

References

Allhoff, F., & Monroe, D. (Eds.). (2007). *Food and philosophy: Eat, drink, and be merry.* Hoboken, NJ: Wiley-Blackwell.

American Occupational Therapy Association. (2007). Specialized knowledge and skills in feeding, eating, and swallowing for occupational therapy practice. *American Journal of Occupational Therapy, 61*(6), 686–700. http://dx.doi.org/10.5014/ajot.61.6.686

Anderson, E. N. (2005). *Everyone eats.* New York: New York University Press.

Archer, L., Rosenbaum, P., & Streiner, D. (1991). The Child Eating Behavior Inventory (CEBI). *Journal of Pediatric Psychology.* http://dx.doi.org/10.1093/jpepsy/16.5.629

Atkins Diet. (n.d.). Retrieved from http://www.atkins.com/

Baum, C., & Edwards, D. F. (1993, May). Cognitive performance in senile dementia of the Alzheimer's type: The Kitchen Task Assessment. *American Journal of Occupational Therapy, 47*(5), 431–436. Retrieved from http://ajot.aotapress.net/content/47/5/431.full.pdf

Baum, C., Morrison, T., Hahn, M., & Edwards, D. (2007a). *Executive Function Performance Test: Test protocol booklet.* Unpublished program in Occupational Therapy, Washington University School of Medicine, St. Louis.

Baum, C., Morrison, T., Hahn, M., & Edwards, D. (2007b). *Executive Function Performance Test.* Retrieved from http://www.rehabmeasures.org/Lists/RehabMeasures/DispForm.aspx?ID=944

Brar, S. S. (2011). *Misconceptions about eating meat.* Retrieved from http://www.sikhs.org/meat.htm

Buller, L. (2005). *Food.* New York: DK Publishing.

Church of Jesus Christ of Latter-Day Saints. (2012). Retrieved from http://www.lds.org/

Civitello, L. (2008). *Cuisine and culture.* Hoboken, NJ: John Wiley & Sons.

Collins, A. (2010, September 9). *Celebrate Eid ul-Fitr with food from around the Muslim world.* WNYC. Retrieved from http://www.wnyc.org/story/93908-food-traditions-eid-ul-fitr/

Crist, W., & Napier-Phillips, A. (2001). Mealtime behaviors of young children: A comparison of normative and clinical data. *Journal of developmental and behavioral pediatrics, 22*(5), 279–286. http://dx.doi.org/10.1097/00004703-200110000-00001

Dinsmore, C. (2000). *Traditional beliefs of Mexican-American women: Implications for health care.* Retrieved from http://www.instituteofmidwifery.org/MSFinalProj.nsf/a9ee58d7a82396768525684f0056be8d/a66f5bafd9f749918525699d007bdc6d?OpenDocument

Eames, E., & Robboy, H. (1967, December). The submarine sandwich, lexical variations in a cultural context. *American Speech, 42*(4), 279–288. http://dx.doi.org/10.2307/452990

Field Museum. (n.d.). *Chocolate history at a glance.* Retrieved from http://archive.fieldmuseum.org/Chocolate/history_intro2.html

Food for the Brain. (2012). *About autism.* Retrieved from http://www.foodforthebrain.org/nutrition-solutions/autism/about-autism.aspx

Foster, G. M. (1994). *Hippocrates' Latin American legacy: Humoral medicine in the New World.* Langhorne, PA: Gordon & Breach.

Harris, P., Lyon, D., & McLaughlin, S. (2005). *The meaning of food*. Guilford, CT: Pie in the Sky Productions.

Hearths ready, city on a Pongala high. (2013, February 26). *The Hindu*. Retrieved from http://www.thehindu.com /todays-paper/hearths-ready-city-on-a-pongala-high/article 4454157.ece

Hill, J. M., & Popp, R. L. (May 1988). Toward a Mormon cuisine: A light-hearted enquiry into the cultural significance of food. *Sunstone Magazine, 33–35*. Retrieved from https:// www.sunstonemagazine.com/pdf/065-33-35.pdf

Jain, P. K. (2000). *Dietary code of practice amongst Jains*. International Vegetarian Union. Retrieved from http://www.ivu .org/congress/2000/jainism.html

Kittler, P. G., & Sucher, K. (2008). *Food and culture* (5th ed.). Belmot, CA: Thomson Higher Education.

Kurlansky, M. (2009). *The food of a younger land*. New York: Riverhead Books.

Luitel, A. (2006). *Food and eating customs differ around the world*. Retrieved from http://silverinternational.mbhs.edu /v202/V20.2.05a.eatingcustoms.html

Martin, J. (2000). *Eating disorders, food and occupational therapy*. London: Whurr Publishers.

Maskarinec, G. (2009). Cancer protective properties of cocoa: A review of the epidemiologic evidence. *Nutrition and Cancer, 61*(5), 573–579. http://dx.doi.org/10.1080/01635580902825662

Natural Products Insider. (2014, March 24). *Seasonings, spice market to reach $16 billion by 2019*. Retrieved from http:// www.foodproductdesign.com/news/2014/03/seasonings-spices -market-to-reach-16-billion-by-2.aspx

Oceania Cuisine. (2011). Retrieved from http://www.world widewebawards.net/Food/Oceania.html

Peruano. (2013, March 25). CNN En Español.

Rodriguez, D., Zimmerman, L., Hirsheimer, C., & McAndrews, C. (2010). *The great ceviche book*. Berkeley, CA: Ten Speed Press.

Smith, A. (2007). *American food and drink*. New York: Oxford University Press.

Söderback, I. (2009). *International handbook of occupational therapy interventions*. New York: Springer Science+Business Media.

South Beach Diet. (2016). Retrieved from http://www.south beachdiet.com

Spector, R. (2009). *Cultural diversity in health and illness* (7th ed.). Upper Saddle River, NJ: Pearson/Prentice Hall.

Spector, R. (2012). *Cultural diversity in health and illness,* (8th ed.). Upper Saddle River, NJ: Pearson/Prentice Hall.

Stern, J., & Stern, M. (2011). *The lexicon of real American food*. Guilford, CT: Lyons Press.

Tannahill, R. (1988). *Food in history*. New York: Three Rivers Press.

Section IV.

CULTURE AND EDUCATION

Chapter 22.

EDUCATING FOR CULTURAL EFFECTIVENESS

Roxie M. Black, PhD, OTR/L, FAOTA

> *Hope is something shared between teachers and students. The hope that we can learn together, teach together, be curiously impatient together, produce something together, and resist together the obstacles that prevent the flowering of our joy.*
> **Paulo Freire (1998, p. 69)**

Chapter Highlights

- Pedagogy Considered
- Teaching Philosophy and Strategies

Key Terms and Concepts

- ✧ Active learning
- ✧ Affective learning
- ✧ Banking method
- ✧ Classroom climate
- ✧ Curricular fit
- ✧ Dialogic classroom
- ✧ Dialogue
- ✧ Endullment
- ✧ Engaged learning

- ✧ Internalized oppression
- ✧ Openness
- ✧ Pedagogy
- ✧ Safe classroom
- ✧ Self-fulfilling prophecy
- ✧ Service learning
- ✧ Transformative curriculum
- ✧ Transformative education
- ✧ Transformative learning

Recognition of the importance of cultural effectiveness when providing therapy services has developed significantly over the past two decades, and aspects of culture are now addressed in many occupational therapy documents, including the

Occupational Therapy Practice Framework: Domain and Process (American Occupational Therapy Association [AOTA], 2014), the accreditation standards (Accreditation Council for Occupational Therapy Education, 2012), and the *Occupational Therapy*

Code of Ethics (AOTA, 2015). The implication, of course, is that occupational therapy educational program curricula must incorporate content about culture and diversity. However, the documents previously listed do not guide how to teach this content. Pedagogical approaches used to teach culture effectiveness throughout the United States are wide and varied; many are quite exciting and very effective. Several such programs are described in the subsequent chapters of this section.

Health care literature includes compelling evidence that teaching about diversity enhances student learning and critical thinking (Edmonds, 2010; Long, 2012; Merryfield, 2003). Occupational therapy literature supports this premise and offers numerous suggestions for conceptualization of content and effective teaching and learning strategies (Mu, Coppard, Bracciano, Doll, & Matthews, 2010). Yet, questions remain: How do I educate my students for cultural effectiveness? Are there models I can apply? What kinds of teaching strategies would be best for my students? Do I know enough to be able to appropriately present this content, and what are my goals in doing so? What kind of electronic support is out there?

Answers to these questions depend on the context of the curricular fit of the diversity content; the interests, skills, and knowledge of the faculty; and the demographics of the student population. This chapter begins to address these questions by identifying which of the many pedagogical approaches might be right for you and your program.

Pedagogy Considered

Pedagogy is commonly understood as the teaching methods a teacher selects, but it also includes one's educational philosophy; specific curriculum content and design, including face-to-face, blended, or electronic delivery; classroom strategies; techniques and methods; and evaluation. These aspects of educational practice influence what happens in classrooms or online.

> Together, they organize a view of how teachers work within an institutional context which specifies a particular version of what knowledge is of most worth, what it means to know something, and how we might construct representations of ourselves, others, and our physical and social environment. (Simon, 1987, p. 370)

Reflection 22.1. Faculty Reflection: Pedagogy

Faculty: Consider the various aspects of pedagogy listed above.

- Are there areas that you need to explore further or learn more about?
- To whom can you go to find answers?
- Might you develop a small study group with which to collaborate on approaches to your teaching?

The editors of this text support a model of intercultural education that promotes empowerment and transformation. According to Mezirow (2000), ***transformative learning*** is the "process by which we transform our taken-for-granted frames of reference (meaning perspectives, habits of mind, mind-sets) to make them more inclusive, discriminating, open, emotionally capable of change, and reflective so that they may generate beliefs and opinions that will prove more true or justified to guide action" (pp. 7–8). Lee and Greene (2004) suggest that transformative learning "emphasizes the creation of a learning context that facilitates students revisiting, examining, questioning, expanding, and transforming their taken-for-granted frames of reference and assumptions" (p. 3).

Transformative curriculum is defined by Vera (n.d.) as a curriculum that is "organized around significant problems and issues" (slide 3) and where learning is "diversified, lifelong and inquiry based" (slide 2). When focused on culturally effective practice, transformative curricula cannot be constructed by merely adding content about ethnic and other diverse groups to an existing Eurocentric curriculum or by integrating or infusing diverse content into a mainstream curriculum (Banks, 1994). Such an additive approach does not challenge or substantively change the basic assumptions, perspectives, and values of the dominant culture or curriculum. Rather, ***transformative education*** is thoughtfully constructed and intentionally delivered and is comprehensive in scope, addressing all aspects of the thinking–teaching–learning process.

Classroom Climate

Classroom climate is

> the intellectual, social, emotional, and physical environments in which students learn. Climate is determined by a constellation

of interacting factors that include faculty–student interaction, the tone instructors set, instances of stereotyping or tokenism, the course demographics (for example, relative size of racial and other social groups enrolled in the course), student–student interaction, and the range of perspectives represented in the course content and materials. (Ambrose, Bridges, DiPietro, & Lovett, 2010, p. 170)

Teaching about beliefs related to culture and diversity may become personal and is often quite emotional for students. Because a climate of emotional safety is vital, the tone or climate of the classroom must be a first consideration when teaching about these issues. Foss (1991) defines a **safe classroom** as a place where everyone experiences equality in terms of personal value, where students and the professor have equal respect for each other as people, and where this respect affects all aspects of the interaction and learning in the class.

Evans, Harvey, Buckley, and Yan (2010) indicate that a classroom's emotional climate is extremely important in the overall classroom environment. Educators establish this open and accepting climate by treating each student and his or her ideas and beliefs with respect. Students must be told, and believe, that their ideas, beliefs, and comments will be heard and respected, even if they do not align with the prevailing attitudes of the majority of the class. Instructors should encourage students to challenge and discuss ideas but also make clear that personal attacks, humiliating remarks, name calling, accusations, and ridicule are never appropriate and are not acceptable in the classroom.

Reflection 22.2. Classroom Climate

Students:

- What do you need in a classroom setting to make you feel safe when talking about personal issues such as values and biases?
- If you don't feel safe to express your viewpoints, are you able to discuss this with the instructor?

Faculty:

- If students approach you to say they don't feel comfortable expressing themselves during classroom discussions, what steps can you take to improve the safety in the classroom?

Confidentiality

One important aspect of classroom safety is confidentiality. Students must believe that whatever is discussed or disclosed will not be revealed outside of the classroom. If instructors assign reaction papers in response to classroom discussions that elicit personal feelings or reactions, they must remind students not to share the contents of their papers with friends or leave them lying around where others may read them. To further ensure confidentiality in written work, classmates' full names should never be used. Instructors should discuss climate and confidentiality issues at the beginning of the course and elicit consensual agreement about classroom safety from each class member.

Instructor Attitude

Classroom climate is strongly influenced by instructors' attitudes. They must model and create an open and accepting atmosphere that encourages a willingness to share ideas and beliefs, to explore values, and to confront and grapple with concepts that may be new, uncomfortable, and possibly frightening. When students are compelled to examine ideas that conflict with lifelong family and personal values, they may experience anxiety and discomfort. Instructors must present information and respond to each student in a way that provides a model of behavior for all students to emulate.

Pedagogical Assumptions

Educators' assumptions about diversity play an important role in intercultural education. For the educational process to be empowering or transformative, consider adopting these pedagogical assumptions:

- Each student has a unique and equal capacity to learn.
- Students must be actively engaged participants in the learning process.
- Effective teaching and learning is dialogic.
- Learning is facilitated in an affective classroom.

Fostering Students' Unique and Equal Capacity to Learn

Faculty expectations influence a student's academic performance. Two decades ago, Nieto (1996) summarized numerous research studies illustrating that teachers' low expectations of students on the basis of gender, race, or class results in lower academic performance. Still present today, this phenomenon exemplifies the **self-fulfilling prophecy** concept Merton identified in 1948. If an educator believes a student does not have the capacity to learn because of some inherent quality, the educator will not expect that student to perform at the same level as other students.

Educators then (often unconsciously) treat the student differently than other students, causing the student to believe that he or she cannot learn as well as others, a reaction known as **internalized oppression,** resulting in a loss of self-esteem and diminished academic performance. The student's subsequent less-than-stellar performance affirms to the teacher that the initial assumption of the student's abilities was correct and justifies the lowered expectations. And the cycle continues.

Having high expectations for all students supports their potential, resulting in improved academic performance, increased success, and a sense of empowerment. According to LaBelle and Ward (1994), "Attention to increasing student achievement, including enhancement of basic skills, is a vital component of an empowerment curriculum model" (p. 170).

Encouraging Active and Engaged Student Participation

The traditional approach to college teaching emphasizes the lecture method, where the all-knowing professor fills students' minds with knowledge as if they were empty vessels. In this model, students are passive recipients of this wisdom, taking in information and regurgitating it on an exam in a process that Shor (1992, p. 20) labels **endullment**—the dulling of students' minds as a result of nonparticipation.

Paulo Freire (1968/1986), a Brazilian educator and philosopher who was a leading advocate for critical pedagogy, called this process the **banking method** of education, where instead of "communicating the teacher issues communiques and makes deposits that the students patiently receive, memorize and repeat. . . . The scope of action allowed to the students extends only as far as receiving, filing, and storing the deposits" (p. 58). Freire sees the banking method as oppressive to students, establishing teachers as the knowledgeable authorities and keepers of wisdom and the students as knowing nothing except what teachers choose to impart to them.

Engaged Learning. **Engaged learning** was identified as an effective approach to higher education more than a decade ago (Krause, 2005). Although Krause (2005) believed that it "has become a catch-all term most commonly used to describe a compendium of behaviours characterizing students who are said to be more involved with their university community than their less engaged peers." (p. 3), others have defined *engaged learning* as "the things students do on their own initiative that will make their college experience most valuable" (Pace, 1984, as cited in Garrett, 2011, p. 4; see Figure 22.1).

Engaged learning is an important aspect of an occupational therapy educational curriculum. Learning labs where specific skills are taught and practiced are a standard and expected part of the chosen pedagogy. In addition to participating in lab situations, students engage in discussion groups, case studies, problem-based learning, role-play experiences, research and presentations, and simulated and real client–practitioner interactions in the classroom and as fieldwork (Hooper, 2006). An occupational therapy education is definitely not passive!

Active Learning. Some authors have equated engaged learning with student involvement (Astin, 1985) or have called it **active learning** (Warren, 1997). Barkley (2010) proposes, "Student engagement is a process and a product that is experienced on a continuum and results from the synergistic interaction between motivation and active learning" (as cited in Garrett, 2011, p. 5).

Active (or engaged) learning is not a new concept and is recognized as a more empowering approach to education. Actively engaging students in the learning process is crucial because action is essential in gaining knowledge and developing intelligence (Shor, 1992). Decades ago, educational theorists Jean Piaget and John Dewey wrote about the importance of action for learning. According to Piaget (1969/1979), "Knowledge is derived from action . . . To know an object is to act upon it and to transform it" (p. 28). Dewey (1938/1963) argued that participation in school is crucial to learning; he is often credited with the notion that "learning is doing."

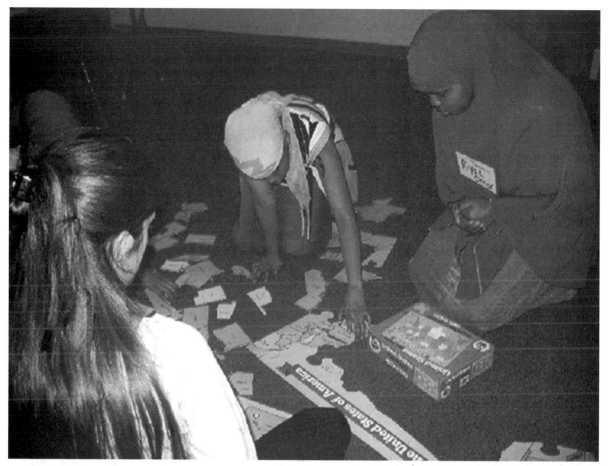

Figure 22.1. Occupational therapy student engaging with Somali girls as part of a service learning project.
Source. Photo by author with permission.

Fortunately, most occupational therapy educational programs now embrace a curriculum that enhances learning through active engagement of the students.

Service Learning. **Service learning** is a pedagogical approach that engages students with the community outside of the classroom for the purpose of "the accomplishment of tasks that meet genuine human needs in combination with conscious educational growth" (Stanton, Giles, & Cruz, 1999, as cited in O'Grady, 2000, p. 6). O'Grady (2000) states that integrating service learning with intercultural education is a natural and effective teaching–learning

---

Reflection 22.3. Engaged Learning

Faculty:

- Do you develop learning strategies that give students the opportunity to be actively engaged in their learning?
- If not, what are the reasons for not doing so? If you want to increase the level of engagement in your classes, do you know where and to whom you can go to discuss this or get ideas?

Are you comfortable seeking out a peer who might brainstorm ideas with you?

Students:

- Do you learn better from lectures or from class activities?
- What are your favorite kinds of class activities?
- Does the faculty give you enough opportunities to actively engage in your learning? If not, do you feel you can express this?

Exhibit 22.1. Definition of *Service Learning* as a Method

Service learning is a method of learning with the following characteristics:
- It allows students to learn and develop through active participation in thoughtfully organized service experiences that meet community needs and are coordinated in collaboration with the school and the community.
- It is integrated into the students' academic curriculum or provides structured time for a student to think, talk, or write about what the student did and saw during the service activity.
- It provides students with opportunities to use newly acquired skills and knowledge in real-life situations in their own communities.
- It enhances what is taught in the classroom by extending students' learning beyond the curriculum and into the community and helps to foster the development of a sense of caring for others.

Sources. National Service Act of 1993; O'Grady (2000).

strategy. Flecky and Gitlow (2009) have also written of its effectiveness in occupational therapy education.

The federal definition of service learning, as outlined in Exhibit 22.1, includes the four main themes of (1) community collaboration, (2) importance of reflection, (3) active or engaged learning, and (4) caring. This approach meets several of the requirements for intercultural education.

Encouraging Dialogue

The next pedagogical assumption is to establish a practice of dialogue in the classroom. Students learn best when teachers talk *with* them rather than *at* them. Mutual discussion is the heart of the dialogic classroom (Bowers, 2005; Warwick, Hennessy, & Mercer, 2011). *Dialogue* is a conversation between two or more people and implies that at least two voices will be heard. A *dialogic classroom,* therefore, is one that is "collective, supportive and genuinely reciprocal; it uses carefully structured extended exchanges to build understanding through culmination; and throughout, [students'] own words, ideas, speculations and arguments feature much more prominently" (Alexander, 2005). A dialogic classroom encourages students to have a voice, share ideas and opinions, and generally have a say.

Within the context of a climate of safety, students who often are silent and silenced in traditional classrooms gain the courage and feel empowered to present their ideas and questions, and actively enter the conversation in a dialogic classroom. For shy or introverted students, small-group discussions, as shown in Figure 22.2, or conversations in dyads provide forums for their voices to be heard and included. A dialogic classroom, therefore, results in an increased sharing of diverse ideas and facilitates learning.

Shared interaction among students and teachers results in mutual learning, in which all reflect together on the meaning of their experience and knowledge (Shor, 1992), an important aspect of cultural effectiveness.

For dialogue to be effective, each person must enter the conversation with an attitude of openness and willingness to learn. Freire (1998) discussed the condition of *openness* in this way:

> To live in openness toward others and to have an open-ended curiosity toward life and its challenges is essential to educational practice. To live this openness toward others respectfully and, from time to time, when opportune, critically reflect on this openness, ought to be an essential part of the adventure of teaching. (p. 121)

Although some may see such openness and willingness to learn from students as diminishing the authority of educators, placing them in a more horizontal rather than hierarchical position *vis-à-vis* the student (Freire, 1970/1986), true dialogue transforms teachers' unilateral authority to a shared authority. It calls on them to relinquish some authority to become co-learners in the classroom and empowers students to co-develop a joint learning process.

Developing an Affective Classroom

Although many occupational therapy practitioners have addressed curricular issues related to educating about culture and diversity, few have written about awareness of *affective learning,* or using emotions in the process of constructing knowledge. However, many authors believe that cognitive learning is linked with affective learning and

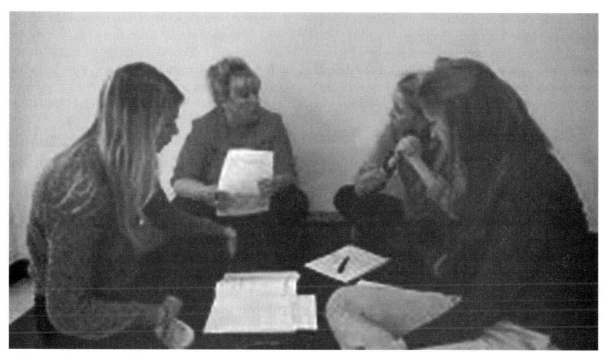

Figure 22.2. Students working together on a project.
Source. Photo by author with permission.

supports students' engagement in the learning process (Felten, Gilchrist, & Darby, 2006; Hooks, 1994; Shor, 1992).

Research suggests that emotion is not a separate process from cognition (Felten et al., 2006). Shor (1992) does not discriminate between empowering and traditional pedagogies by the emotions they elicit:

> In traditional classrooms, negative emotions are provoked in students by teacher-centered politics. Unilateral teacher authority in a passive curriculum arouses in many students a variety of negative emotions: self-doubt, hostility, resentment, boredom, indignation, cynicism, disrespect, frustration, [and] the desire to escape. (p. 23)

Shor believes that negative emotions interfere with learning. In contrast, he believes that in a participatory class, "some of the positive effects which support student learning include cooperativeness, curiosity, humor, hope, responsibility, respect, attentiveness, openness, and concern about society" (p. 24).

A sense of joy is another emotion that can be found in some classrooms. There can be joy in the discovery and mutual construction of knowledge. Freire (1998) discusses the importance of joy in the classroom and its relationship with hope: "Hope is something shared between teachers and students. The hope that we can learn together, teach together, be curiously impatient together, produce something together, and resist together the obstacles that prevent the flowering of our joy" (p. 69).

Reflection 22.4. Affective Classrooms

Faculty:

- Are you comfortable with students expressing strong emotions in the classroom?
- How do you feel when a student gets loud or begins to cry?
- Do you know how to effectively interact in this situation?
- What resources are on your campus that will help you respond in these situations?

Students:

- Have you been in classrooms where a variety of emotions is allowed or encouraged? If so, were you comfortable?
- How might you feel in a practice situation where your client expresses strong emotions?

Teaching for cultural effectiveness may evoke strong emotions because it often challenges students' (and faculty members') personal values and beliefs. Faculty should allow the expression of feelings, even though passionately debating issues of oppression, bias, and discrimination may be uncomfortable for students and teachers alike. Many educators have been taught that a dispassionate, objective stance is the appropriate and rational way to examine ideas. Intercultural education strongly refutes that philosophy. Transformative intercultural content is inherently emotive, personal, conflictual, and engaging. Consequently, students must be given ample opportunities to express their beliefs and emotions, to interact with their classmates, and "to express rage or pride when multicultural issues are discussed" (Banks, 1994, p. 96).

Teaching Philosophy and Strategies

After the classroom climate has been established and the pedagogical assumptions identified, faculty must determine which philosophical or theoretical model they will use. Some teachers may base their teaching on a foundation of occupational and social justice, "getting students to understand notions of power, privilege, prejudice, and whiteness" (Gupta, 2008, p. 3). Others may focus on the development of cultural competence, following published guidelines (Nochajski & Matteliano, 2008) and aiming to develop cultural awareness and attitudes, cultural knowledge, and cultural skills (Black & Wells, 2007) in their students. Some may focus on a curriculum of inclusion (Trentham, Cockburn, Cameron, & Iwama, 2007).

Curricular fit and integration of intercultural content are determined by the

- Philosophy of the institution in which the occupational therapy program is located,
- Model and structure of the program's curriculum,
- The interests and desires of the program director and faculty, and
- Demographics of the student body.

Curricular fit (i.e., developing teaching strategies that support the curricular goals and student outcomes) determines whether one chooses to teach a separate course focusing on diversity or cultural content; to include an intercultural module within a course; to provide an individual class, lecture, or short workshop devoted to diversity issues; to include a service learning experience with a diverse population; to integrate or infuse multicultural content throughout the curriculum; or to provide a combination of approaches (see Black & Wells, 2007, for a more thorough discussion of these strategies).

Summary

Occupational therapy is trending as one of the fastest growing fields in health care (Career Cast, 2016), and most educational programs are seeing an increase in the number of applicants. At the same time, however, many institutions of higher learning, particularly public facilities, are struggling with limited resources, including diminishing budgets, insufficient faculty, and fewer fieldwork settings. This conundrum, coupled with increasing pluralism in the United States and beyond, challenges occupational therapy educators to develop and teach cultural content in the most efficient and effective way possible to meet the needs of the students, the programs, and the centennial goals of the profession.

This chapter suggested multiple ways to incorporate learning strategies and practices that support the development of cultural self-awareness, cultural knowledge, cultural skills, and critical reflection within the classroom setting, all components necessary for culturally effective practice.

References

Accreditation Council for Occupational Therapy Education. (2012). 2011 Accreditation Council for Occupational Therapy Education (ACOTE®) standards. *American Journal of Occupational Therapy, 66*(6, Suppl.), S6–S74. http://dx.doi.org /10.5014/ajot.2012.66S6

Alexander, R. (2005). *Teaching through dialogue: The first year.* London: London Borough of Barking and Dagenham.

Ambrose, S. A., Bridges, M. W., DiPietro, M., & Lovett, M. C. (2010). *How learning works: Seven research-based principles for smart teaching.* San Francisco: Jossey-Bass.

American Occupational Therapy Association. (2014). Occupational therapy practice framework: Domain and process (3rd ed.). *American Journal of Occupational Therapy, 68,* S1– S48. http://dx.doi.org/10.5014/ajot.2014.682006

American Occupational Therapy Association. (2015). Occupational Therapy Code of Ethics. *American Journal of Occupational Therapy, 69*, 6913410030p1–6913410030p8. http://dx.doi.org/10.5014/ajot.2015.696S03

Astin, A. W. (1985). *Achieving educational excellence: A critical assessment of priorities and practices in higher education.* San Francisco: Jossey-Bass.

Banks, J. A. (1994). *An introduction to multicultural education.* Newton, MA: Allyn & Bacon.

Barkley, S. G. (2010). *Quality teaching in a culture of coaching.* Lanham, MD: Rowman & Littlefield Education.

Black, R. M., & Wells, S. A. (2007). *Culture and occupation: A model of empowerment in occupational therapy.* Bethesda, MD: AOTA Press.

Bowers, R. (2005). Freire (with Bakhtin) and the dialogic classroom seminar. *Alberta Journal of Educational Research, 51*(4), 368–378. Retrieved from http://ajer.synergiesprairies.ca/ajer/index.php/ajer/article/view/592/577

Career Cast (2016). *Jobs rated report 2015: Ranking the top 200 jobs.* Retrieved from http://www.careercast.com/jobs-rated/jobs-rated-report-2015-ranking-top-200-jobs

Dewey, J. (1963). *Experience and education.* New York: Collier. (Original work published 1938.)

Edmonds, M. L. (2010). The lived experience of nursing students who studied abroad: A qualitative inquiry. *Journal of Studies in International Education, 14*(5), 545–568. http://dx.doi.org/10.1177/1028315310375306

Evans, I. M., Harvey, S. T., Buckley, L., & Yan, E. (2010). Differentiating classroom climate concepts: Academic, management, and emotional environments. *Kōtuitui: New Zealand Journal of Social Sciences Online, 4*(2). http://dx.doi.org/10.1080/117708 3X.2009.9522449

Felten, P., Gilchrist, L. Z., & Darby, A. (2006, Spring). Emotion and learning: Feeling our way toward a new theory of reflection in service-learning. *Michigan Journal of Community Service Learning, 12*(2). Retrieved from http://quod.lib.umich.edu/m/mjcsl/3239521.0012.204/1

Flecky, K., & Gitlow, L. (2009). *Service-learning in occupational therapy education: Philosophy and practice.* Sudbury, MA: Jones & Bartlett.

Foss, S. K. (1991). *What is feminist pedagogy?* Paper presented at the annual meeting of the Organization for Research in Gender and Communication, San Antonio, TX.

Freire, P. (1968/1986). *Pedagogy of the oppressed.* New York: Continuum.

Freire, P. (1998). *Pedagogy of freedom: Ethics, democracy, and civic courage.* New York: Rowman & Littlefield.

Garrett, C. (2011). Defining, detecting, and promoting student engagement in college learning environments. Transformative Dialogues. *Teaching & Learning Journal, 5*(2), 1–12. Retrieved from http://www.kpu.ca/sites/default/files/Teaching%20and%20Learning/TD.5.2.5.Garrett_Student_Engagement.pdf

Gupta, J. (2008). Reflections of one educator on teaching cultural competence. *Education Special Interest Section Quarterly, 18*(3), 3.

Hooks, B. (1994). *Teaching to transgress.* New York: Routledge & Kegan Paul.

Hooper, B. (2006). Beyond active learning: A case study of teaching practices in an occupation-centered curriculum. *American Journal of Occupational Therapy, 60*, 551–562. http://dx.doi.org/10.5014/ajot.60.5.551

Krause, K.-L. (2005). *Understanding and promoting student engagement in university learning communities.* Melbourne, Australia: University of Australia. Retrieved from http://www.liberty.edu/media/3425/teaching_resources/Stud_eng.pdf

LaBelle, T. J., & Ward, C. R. (1994). *Multiculturalism and education: Diversity and its impact on schools and society.* Albany: State University of New York.

Lee, M. Y., & Greene, G. J. (2004). A teaching framework for transformative multicultural social work education. *Journal of Ethnic and Cultural Diversity in Social Work, 12*(3), 1–28. http://dx.doi.org/10.1300/J051v12n03_01

Long, T. B. (2012). Overview of teaching strategies for cultural competence in nursing students. *Journal of Cultural Diversity, 19*(3), 102–108.

Merryfield, M. (2003). Like a veil: Cross-cultural experiential learning online. *Contemporary Issues in Technology and Teacher Education, 3*, 146–171. Retrieved from http://www.citejournal.org/volume-3/issue-2-03/social-studies/like-a-veil-cross-cultural-experiential-learning-online/

Merton, R. (1948). The self-fulfilling prophecy. *Antioch Review, 8.* Retrieved from http://www.jstor.org/stable/4609267

Mezirow, J. (2000). Learning to think like an adult: Core concepts of transformation theory. In J. Mezirow and Associates (Eds.), *Learning as transformation: Critical perspectives on a theory in progress* (pp. 3–33). San Francisco: Jossey-Bass.

Mu, K., Coppard, B. M., Bracciano, A., Doll, J., & Matthews, A. (2010). Fostering cultural competency, clinical reasoning, and leadership through international outreach. *Occupational Therapy in Health Care, 24*(1), 74–85. http://dx.doi.org/10.3109/07380570903329628

Nieto, S. (1996). *Affirming diversity: The sociopolitical context of multicultural education* (2nd ed.). White Plains, NY: Longman.

Nochajski, S. M., & Matteliano, M. A. (2008). *A guide to cultural competence in the curriculum: Occupational therapy.* Buffalo, NY: Center for International Rehabilitation Research.

O'Grady, C. R. (Ed.). (2000). *Integrating service learning and multicultural education in colleges and universities.* Mahwah, NJ: Lawrence Erlbaum.

Pace, C. R. (1984). *Measuring the quality of college student experiences. An account of the development and use of college student experience questionnaire.* Los Angeles: University of California, Higher Education Research Institute.

Piaget, J. (1979). *Science of education and the psychology of the child.* New York: Penguin. (Original work published 1969.)

Shor, I. (1992). *Empowering education: Critical teaching for social change.* Chicago: University of Chicago Press.

Simon, R. (1987). Empowerment as a pedagogy of possibility. *Language Arts, 64,* 370. Retrieved from http://www.jstor.org/stable/41961618

Stanton, T. K., Giles, D. E. Jr., & Cruz, N. I. (1999). *Service-learning: A movement's pioneers reflect on its origins, practice and future.* San Francisco: Jossey-Bass.

Trentham, B., Cockburn, L., Cameron, D., & Iwama, M. (2007). Diversity and inclusion within an occupational therapy curriculum. *Australian Occupational Therapy Journal, 54*(1), 549–557. http://dx.doi.org/10.1111/j.1440-1630.2006.00605.x

Vera, E. (n.d.). *Transformative curriculum: Based on Henderson and Hathorne, 2001.* [PowerPoint presentation.] Retrieved from www.slideshare.net/evera/transformative-curriculum

Warren, R. G. (1997). Engaging students in active learning. *About Campus, 2*(1), 16–20 ERIC # EJ550318.

Warwick, P., Hennessy, S., & Mercer, N. (2011). Promoting teacher and school development through co-enquiry: Developing interactive whiteboard use in a 'dialogic classroom.' *Teachers and Teaching: Theory and Practice, 17*(3), 303–324. http://dx.doi.org/10.1080/13540602.2011.554704

Chapter 23.

LESSONS LEARNED EDUCATING FOR CULTURAL COMPETENCE: EXPERIENTIAL AND REFLECTIVE STRATEGIES

Theresa Leto, DHS, OTR/L, and Rosalie King, DHS, OTR/L

Culture makes people understand each other better. And if they understand each other better in their soul, it is easier to overcome the economic and political barriers. But first they have to understand that their neighbor is, in the end, just like them, with the same problems, the same questions.
Paulo Coelho (n.d., para. 1)

Chapter Highlights

- Preparing Culturally Competent Occupational Therapy Practitioners
- Challenges in Educating for Cultural Competence
- Example of a University's Effort to Improve Cultural Competence
- Considerations for Implementing Academic Service Learning
- Developing Reflective Practitioners
- Cultural Desire

Key Terms and Concepts

- ✧ Academic service learning
- ✧ Content-centered learning
- ✧ Constructivist learning
- ✧ Cultural desire
- ✧ Preparatory reflection
- ✧ Reflection

- ✧ Reflection in action
- ✧ Reflection on action
- ✧ Reflective practice
- ✧ Scaffolding
- ✧ Strategic questioning
- ✧ Subject-centered learning

This chapter explores one component of client-centered care—cultural competence—and considers the challenges of educating for cultural competence. We present a rationale and description of one university's strategies in educating for cultural competence in an occupational therapy program. We also share outcomes and reflections on the process.

Preparing Culturally Competent Occupational Therapy Practitioners

The American Occupational Therapy Association's (AOTA) *Vision 2025* states, "Occupational therapy maximizes health, well-being, and quality of life for all people, populations, and communities through effective solutions that facilitate participation in everyday life" (AOTA, 2016, para. 6). *Vision 2025* builds on the profession's previous vision statements in that it continues to embody the ideals of quality services for all people. "Services for all people, populations, and communities" implies provision of services for all societal needs, including culture and diversity. The educational preparation of future occupational therapy practitioners can ensure that the profession continues to move toward the realization of this vision.

Baum (2006) recognized that educational programs for occupational therapy practitioners, while meeting the minimum standards, use "vastly different approaches" (p. 612) and questioned whether these approaches to education are based on evidence. Effective educational approaches must be identified because occupational therapy practice will continue to evolve as health care evolves. A strong educational foundation will provide occupational therapy practitioners with the skills and leadership to be client centered and culturally competent practitioners.

Hooper (2010) examined the path to the AOTA's *Centennial Vision* (AOTA, 2007) through the lens of an educator and cautioned against merely adding new or advanced content to occupational therapy curricula. Additional content is associated with less learning and less transfer of learning (p. 98), so merely adding topics related to cultural competency does not ensure that students will achieve progress toward cultural competence. Hooper (2010) proposed that a curricular shift from content-centered learning to subject-centered learning may be a more effective vehicle to achieving the goals of the profession.

Content-centered learning focuses on specific topics or content that is identified as important for students to learn (Hooper, 2010). For example, the Accreditation Council for Occupational Therapy Education® (ACOTE®) identifies specific, required subject matter, such as cultural competence, for an accredited occupational therapy or occupational therapy assistant program. Another example of content in occupational therapy education may be specific topics recommended for inclusion in an occupational therapy or occupational therapy assistant program by the program's advisory board. This focus on content may create tension between meeting the mandated content standards and educating for lasting change.

In ***subject-centered learning,*** students are actively engaged with the underlying concepts of the subject versus just receiving information about the subject. Students can make a strong connection between the course topic and the curriculum's core subject (Hooper, 2010). Thus, depth of understanding and the link between content and the core subject may be sacrificed for breadth of content.

Challenges in Educating for Cultural Competence

Regardless of the educational paradigm, there are challenges in educating for cultural competence (Brown, Muñoz, & Powell, 2011). Consistent with other studies (Echeverri, Brookover, & Kennedy, 2010), occupational therapy students often cite education in cultural competence as inadequate (Murden et al., 2008).

Murden et al. (2008) examined student perceptions of cultural competence at four developmental stages: (1) entry into an occupational therapy program, (2) completion of the academic phase of education, (3) after fieldwork, and (4) following one year of professional practice. The results of this study indicated that although all respondents graduated with an understanding of the essence and components of culturally competent practice, students reported limited exposure to issues surrounding culture in both the academic and fieldwork phases of their education.

Reflection 23.1. Cultural Competence Perceptions

Students:

• How has your understanding of what constitutes culturally competent practice changed as you have gone through the phases of your professional education?

Faculty:

• How has your understanding evolved over time?

Brown et al. (2011) gathered data from 78 established occupational therapy programs throughout the United States. The study investigated the frequency of cultural content in occupational therapy programs, including knowledge, practice skills, and teaching methods.

The knowledge areas most frequently addressed, and also rated as the most important, included

• Interpersonal communication patterns,
• Culture specific information, and
• Sociopolitical influences on health and health disparities.

The practice skills most frequently identified, and also reported as the most important, were

• Interviewing strategies,
• Culturally relevant care planning,
• Interpreting verbal and nonverbal behaviors, and
• Selecting occupations with cultural meaning.

Finally, this study explored the methods used to teach cultural competency. The teaching strategies identified as the most frequently used, however, were inconsistent with those strategies identified as being the most effective. The most frequently used teaching methods were

• Case studies,
• Lectures,
• Readings, and
• Self-assessment tools.

Teaching methods identified as the most effective were

• Case studies,
• Activities that emphasize exposure to diverse populations,
• Reflective journals, and

• Interviewing someone of a different culture.

Respondents also wrote in additional teaching methods they viewed as effective. These were identified as fieldwork, activities that increase self-awareness, experiential learning, and exploration of other cultures. Less than half of the respondents indicated that an assessment method was available to evaluate the effectiveness of the curriculum's approach to teaching cultural competency (Brown et al., 2011).

The teaching methods identified as the most effective were experiential in nature. However, Brown et al. (2011) reported several obstacles to educating for cultural competence. The most frequently identified challenges included lack of diversity both in the faculty and in the student body, and lack of time. Either of these challenges would limit an educator's ability to develop and implement experiential learning opportunities.

Reflection 23.2. Teaching Methods

Students:

• Which teaching strategies were most effective in facilitating your progress toward cultural competence?

Faculty:

• How have you incorporated experiential learning to facilitate movement toward cultural competence in your students?
• How have you been a role model in this regard?

Example of a University's Effort to Improve Cultural Competence

In 2006, the occupational therapy faculty at a private Midwestern university began a coordinated effort to emphasize the importance of client-centered care, including incorporation of specific elements of culture into the curriculum. This initiative began initially based on informal observation of student outcomes. Next, a targeted needs assessment was developed and implemented. The needs assessment validated the initial observations and also identified a need to include topics addressing health care quality and health care disparities in the occupational therapy curriculum. The results of the needs assessment prompted the development of an academic curricular thread focused on client-centered care and, in particular, cultural competency as a strategy to prepare occupational therapy students to practice in an increasingly diverse society.

Defining *Culture* and *Cultural Competence*

To focus on client-centered care with attention to culture, clear learning outcomes for the proposed curriculum were established. Essentially, the overall curricular objective was to promote the development of occupational therapy practitioners who are client centered, culturally competent, and holistic. Importantly, the students needed to understand a definition of *culture* reaching beyond race and ethnicity. The following definitions were used as a foundation for the curricular thread.

Black and Wells (2007) crafted a definition of *culture* as being "the sum total of a way of living, including values, beliefs, standards, linguistic expression, patterns of thinking, behavioral norms, and style of communication that influence behavior(s) of a group of people that is transmitted from generation to generation" (p. 5). Black and Wells (2007) then define *cultural competence* as

> The process of actively developing and practicing appropriate, relevant, and sensitive strategies and skills in interacting with culturally different people. The capacity to respond to the needs of populations whose cultures are different from what might be called dominant or mainstream. (p. 278)

Wells and Black (2000) developed the Cultural Competency Education Model as a framework for students to develop the skills needed in a society that is increasingly diverse and to assess their progress toward becoming culturally competent health care providers. Self-exploration and awareness, knowledge, and skills were identified as the primary areas of focus to foster student development of cultural competence. The university's occupational therapy program built educational strategies addressing cultural competence on this model.

Threading Curricular Content and Instructional Methods

Constructivist learning argues that individuals learn best through making sense of learning experiences (Joyce, Weil, & Calhoun, 2004). Knowledge is created as new information by means of these learning experiences and is absorbed and integrated into the existing base of knowledge (p. 13), implying that knowledge is constructed over time.

Content and learning experiences specific to cultural competence were developed and threaded throughout the curriculum; the thread was strategically placed and woven intentionally. However, two core courses, "Professional Relationships in Context" and "Contextual Issues in Practice: Supporting Client-Centered Care," were designed to focus on these concepts more specifically. The initial course was offered in the first semester of the professional program (junior year), and the second course was offered the following year (senior year).

Concepts integral to cultural competence are visited and revisited at these two stages to help the student connect cultural competence to the core subject of occupation and occupational therapy practice (Hooper, 2010). The primary assignments in these two courses are described in Exhibit 23.1 to illustrate instructional methods used in the core courses. These educational strategies emphasize experiential learning and reflection. Additionally, the faculty facilitates a great deal of reflective discussions to link concepts, which is not readily apparent in the brief assignment descriptions.

Reflection 23.3. Constructivist Learning

Students:

- How might some of the experiences or assignments in Exhibit 23.1 assist you in furthering your progress as a future practitioner toward being more culturally competent?

Faculty:

- How might some of the experiences in Exhibit 23.1 better assist your students toward this end?

Curricular Effectiveness

Students' responses to the content delivered in both courses have been positive, based on formal and informal feedback and observation. An objective evaluation was conducted through student end-of-term course surveys from the 114 students (5 cohorts) who completed both courses.

Exhibit 23.1. Primary Assignments for Core Courses

Professional Relationships in Context, First Semester (Junior Year)

Academic service learning (ASL)	20 hours of service required. Service opportunities contracted with agencies serving culturally diverse populations frequently seen in occupational therapy practice. The companion assignment is an ongoing reflective journal.
ASL presentation	Students present on their ASL agency and experiences throughout the semester with specific reflection points, including preconceived ideas about the population, new understanding and awareness of the population, and how this experience can inform future occupational therapy practice.
Interpersonal role play focused on connecting with the "client"	Based on a randomly chosen brief case scenario, students role play specific components of the therapeutic relationship, that is, establishing rapport, building trust, and dealing with the difficult client. Students submit a brief reflection on their experiences.
Occupational profile	Students are randomly assigned a client at a local nursing home. Students complete an occupational profile in preparation for developing client-centered intervention. Students submit a reflection on the experience.
Poverty simulation	Students are randomly assigned roles as family members living in poverty. "Family" members are assigned specific challenges and tasks, requiring them to complete daily occupations in poverty and seek services from community agencies. This experience is facilitated by the coordinator of the local Bridges Out of Poverty program.
Interpersonal style paper	Students write a paper focusing on self-examination of style of communicating and interacting.
Personal growth activities	Students participate in numerous in-class experiences to enhance self-awareness and understand cultural identity.

Contextual Issues in Practice: Supporting Client-Centered Care, Fourth Semester (Senior Year)

Cultural object (Black & Wells, 2007, p. 13)	Students share an object reflecting their own culture to increase understanding of a broad definition of *culture*.
Cultural questionnaire	Students begin to increase awareness of their own culture through a written response to a series of questions exploring family structure, roles, values, community, and faith traditions.
Student-led discussions	Students formulate questions and lead an in-class discussion from content in the Black and Wells (2007) text.
Photo-narrative project and presentation	Students identify a community participant with a chronic health condition or challenging life situation; conduct interviews; and present a primarily visual representation of the participant's story following validation from the participant regarding the accuracy of the story.
Interaction with international students	Students join with international students to exchange information about their respective heritage and learn about each another.
Out-of-comfort-zone experience and reflection	Students immerse themselves in a totally foreign environment and provide an associated written reflection about the experience.
Reflection on own social location	Students research demographics of the community in which they were raised and become aware of their own social location.
Current events discussion board	Students post and respond to culturally related issues from the media with the expectation of increasing awareness and expressing opinions.
Films or film clips	Students view films as a basis for increased understanding and discussion regarding different populations and issues.
Poverty simulation	Students assume roles in community agencies from which the junior cohort must access services (facilitated by the coordinator of the Bridges Out of Poverty program).

Professional Relationships in Context (Junior Year)

A formal program evaluation was conducted in 2007–2008 to examine the extent to which the initial course focused on client-centered care and culture, and facilitated student movement toward cultural competence (King, 2010). The results from this first cohort revealed students perceived an increase in awareness of self and others, personal growth, communication skills, and confidence.

Of all the course components, **academic service learning (ASL)** was the most valued and viewed as the primary mechanism through which these gains were made. ASL is an experiential teaching and learning strategy that incorporates meaningful service to the community with academic instruction aimed at enhanced understanding of key course objectives (Bringle, Phillips, & Hudson, 2004). As a component of this teaching and learning method, opportunities for critical reflection in relation to the service experience contribute to skill and knowledge acquisition (see Exhibit 23.1).

Following approval from the university's Institutional Review Board, a qualitative pilot study was initiated to examine students' perceptions of developing cultural competence through the course's ASL component. ASL journals from the 2008 student cohort were de-identified and coded to identify themes in an effort to capture the student experience and personal significance of the ASL assignments (Leto, 2011). The themes that emerged indicated students increased in

- Self-awareness and recognition of stereotyping or biases,
- Awareness of others,
- Understanding of the importance of communication and the therapeutic relationship, and
- The development of self-concept and a professional identity.

A quantitative survey using a Likert scale as a measure was then developed to quantify the outcomes of the ASL experience producing the aggregated results from 2009 through 2011, as indicated in Exhibit 23.2.

Contextual Issues in Practice: Supporting Client-Centered Care (Senior Year)

The senior-level course builds on the knowledge and experiences gained in the previous year, in addition to content delivered in other courses. A qualitative survey completed by students at the semester's end gathers feedback to include

- What was meaningful,
- What was most challenging,
- Skills developed,
- Important things learned,

Exhibit 23.2. Effectiveness of Academic Service Learning*

Academic Service Learning (Likert scale: 5 = *strongly agree*; 4 = *agree*)

Survey Questions 1–6	5	4	Survey Questions 7–11	5	4
Because of service learning:					
I interact effectively with people of different cultures.	16%	72.73%	I have a better understanding of myself in relation to others.	35.24%	60.67%
I am more knowledgeable about aspects of diversity.	31.94%	58.45%	I am beginning to change the way that I do things.	26.53%	64.22%
I reflect on my experiences so I can learn from them.	31.94%	58.45%	I am beginning to understand the concepts of therapeutic use of self.	39.69%	57%
I am more aware of how I interact with others that are different from me.	59.18%	36.1%	I am aware of the connection between values and behavior.	47.36%	50.14%
I am changing the way I look at myself.	32.12%	57.36%	I am more aware of my own cultural identity.	31.68%	57.81%
I have begun to examine my personal beliefs.	17.71%	68.75%	*Full-scale results not provided given the predominance of responses in the above categories.		

- Concepts that would be used in clinical practice, and
- Areas for growth in becoming more culturally competent.

Results indicated some overlap and duplication in responses among categories, which would be expected given the nature of the survey questions. Communication, self-awareness, acceptance or tolerance of others, and the importance of attending to culture in intervention dominated the aggregated feedback (see Exhibit 23.3).

In teaching this senior course, ***strategic questioning*** is used to provoke thoughtful reflection. Strategic questioning uses open-ended questions to help the student synthesize new information with what is already known about a specific concept. In effect, the student creates new knowledge about the concept from reflecting on the question. This teaching method is an effective means to facilitate self-discovery and deeper reflection related to the course's core concepts. This is particularly true when difficult subject matter is the focus of classroom discussions. Strategic questioning prompts deeper thinking, refocuses observations, and requires active engagement with the difficult subject being discussed.

Reflection 23.4. Strategic Questioning

Students:

- If you have had a similar course, how has strategic questioning helped you to be more reflective, assertive, and confident in expressing your views?
- How has input from your instructor assisted or hindered you in this process?
- Was a safe atmosphere created in which to express your views?

Faculty:

- How have you created a climate of safety and allowed yourself to be vulnerable to facilitate growth in yourself and your students?

Exhibit 23.3. Contextual Issues in Practice: Course Evaluation Data*

Survey Questions				
Most meaningful experiences	**Biggest challenges**	**Skills developed, learned**	**Use in future practice**	**Areas for growth**
Cultural object 6.5%	Sharing or talking in class; discussing difficult subjects 54.6%	Communication 78%	Communication or interviewing and therapeutic use of self 43%	Improving communication and interview skills 26%
International students 15.4%	Reflecting, increasing self-awareness 14%	Greater self-awareness 44%	Ongoing reflection and self-awareness 24%	Ongoing reflection and self-awareness 18%
Poverty simulation 0.38%	Tolerance, acceptance of others 12.5%	Tolerance and openness 72%	Acknowledging whole person 44%	Tolerance, acceptance of others 17%
Out of comfort zone 0.59%	Acknowledging biases 17%	Importance of client-centered care or culture 41%		Willingness to learn about other cultures 61%
Photo-narrative 24.5%				
Student-led discussions 23.2%				
Current events 0.07%	* Results provided only for categories with highest percentage of responses.			

Analysis of the Effectiveness

Implementation of a curricular thread focusing on cultural competence has affected the occupational therapy students and the program. Students noted growth in developing a professional identity, improved self-confidence, and increased tolerance of others. The broad definition of the term *culture* has allowed the program to be inventive in providing learning experiences despite the homogenous nature of the community.

Results at the Student Level

In examining survey results from both courses, continuous themes emerge from Year 1 to Year 2. The emerging themes indicate progression toward cultural competence.

In the first year, students gain awareness of themselves and their developing identity as occupational therapists. They begin to attend to how they interact with the world around them and establish personal goals. Through multiple levels of experiential learning, students are exposed to novel populations and environments. Through these experiences, students have demonstrated progress toward developing skills in cultural competency consistent with the Wells and Black (2000) Cultural Competence Education Model, in that the first steps toward cultural competence are self-exploration and self-awareness (see skills developed, Exhibit 23.3). Students also identified progress toward cultural competence through tolerance of others and confidence in themselves. In the senior year, there is a developmental surge toward cultural competence as seen in greater acceptance and tolerance of differences as well as increased understanding of the importance of culture and willingness to learn more to be truly client centered.

The issue of lack of diversity in the community and the occupational therapy faculty has proved to be a double-edged sword. The university is located in a Midwest county that is 93% White (U.S. Census Bureau, 2010). A large percentage of the occupational therapy students come from small communities within a 90-mile radius of the university. At the outset, this would appear to be a disadvantage. The students may have a limited ability to imagine how people in the larger community live based on their own backgrounds. Thus, small exposures can bring large insights. One junior-level student who was confident about her abilities and skeptical of gaining new knowledge or awareness from her ASL experiences stated in her journal, "I learned that I may not have been as ready as I thought to deal with this population of people. I am middle class and white. I thought I could somewhat relate to what they are going through. The truth is I can't at all" (Leto, 2012, p. 16). Another junior-level student stated in her journal, "I realized how much I had stereotyped this population before I had given them a chance. I went into this with the thought that they were going to be so different from me and I was never going to have anything in common with them" (Leto, 2012, p. 16).

Reflection 23.5. Increasing Diversity Awareness

- How can an educator situated in a fairly homogenous community better expose his or her students to diversity and a broader understanding or experience of culture?

Results at the Program Level

Program assessment revealed several strengths and challenges. Although the occupational therapy faculty and students themselves are a uniform group, the view of cultural competence articulated by Wells and Black (2000) used as a basis for the two courses is broad and inclusive, enabling the occupational therapy program to maximize the opportunities available in the community while still offering the students learning challenges. The faculty welcomed open dialogue and discussion related to student experiences. Additionally, the faculty has interest and expertise in client-centered care and cultural competence that assist in creating learning opportunities.

Considerations for Implementing Academic Service Learning

Based on student feedback, the ASL experience facilitated the greatest growth toward cultural competence in first-year students. At the university level, the occupational therapy program has the support of the Campus Compact coordinator. This support relieves some of the time-constraint challenges in educating for cultural competence identified by Brown et al. (2011).

The Campus Compact Center maintains relationships with local nonprofit agencies throughout the university's county of residence. A faculty relationship with someone on campus who serves as a coordinator for ASL is invaluable when designing these learning experiences. The coordinator identifies service opportunities within the community and presents this information to occupational therapy faculty and students.

Direct communication between faculty and the community agencies occurs on an as-needed basis. This level of communication is preferable and strengthens the relationship between the agencies and the occupational therapy department. However, ongoing communication throughout the academic term is impractical. Despite the time limitations, the benefits of ASL far outweigh the challenges in designing and implementing a program.

The coordinator develops the service agreement that outlines the responsibilities of both the student and the hosting agency, including a waiver of liability. Students meet with the identified supervisor at the agency and negotiate mutually agreed-upon responsibilities based on the course objectives and needs of the agency. This ensures that both parties commit to the identified community need and the student learning objectives for the course.

Developing Reflective Practitioners

The skill of *reflection,* or thinking with intentional, critical consideration and applying it to occupational therapy practice, is recommended in occupational therapy and the health professions (Dunn & Musolino, 2011). Schön (1992) links intentional reflection with action and describes three specific constructs: (1) reflective practice, (2) reflection in action, and (3) reflection on action.

Reflective practice is an overarching term and is described by Schön (1992) as critical self-appraisal as a means of developing the practitioner's own abilities in the practice setting.

Reflection in action describes the competent response to unexpected and ambiguous events that occur in practice (Kinsella, 2009; Roberts, 2009). This is the fluid reflection and reasoning that occurs in the midst of practice. Schön (1992) views reflection and action as intricately linked and likens this process to artistry. This artistry allows the

practitioner to effectively address the complexities and uncertainties in everyday practice. Without this reflection, professional practice is simply "technique" (Kinsella, 2009).

Reflection in action is an unrealistic expectation of most students at this level of the professional program. However, some of the junior-level students demonstrated reflection in action during communication with clients of their respective ASL agencies. Most students demonstrated *reflection on action* throughout the experiential learning assignments. This type of reflection is retrospective in nature whereby thinking is in relation to the action that has already occurred (Kinsella, 2009). Students reflected on the actions they had taken during assignment completion, the effectiveness of the actions, and potential action in the future. Ong (2011) refers to reflection on action as "pre-action or anticipatory" reflection or, more simply stated, reflection for action. He argued that this *preparatory reflection* is a strategy for an optimal outcome in health care.

Learner Characteristics

The core courses are graded and sequenced to meet the students at the appropriate educational and developmental level. Developmentally, students at this age and stage in the professional program may be less inclined to reflect on their experiences in a way that will inform future behavior (Cole, 2012).

Prompts in the first course bring the students' attention to relevant events and interactions that they may or may not have attended to previously. In the second course, students are, in essence, required to skillfully observe and analyze relevant events with fewer cues and at more complex and personal levels. Introduction to the concepts of cultural competence combined with experiential learning allow students to discover personal meaning from their experiences. Additionally, because students are placed in the community through ASL in the junior year, the community is more accessible for the assignments required in the senior year (i.e., the photo-narrative and the out-of-comfort-zone experience).

Facilitating Reflection

Roberts (2009) stated that the extent to which an individual has a tendency to reflect is unclear. In the first semester of a professional program, students may be focusing their academic energies on courses that are acutely more challenging—anatomy or kinesiology, for example. By providing appropriate scaffolding, those who may be less inclined to reflect can progress toward the outcome of reflective practitioner (Roberts, 2009). *Scaffolding* is a framework of supports that is tailored to the student's needs and designed to move the student in small steps toward a stronger understanding of a topic.

For example, a course instructor may link a new topic to a topic previously mastered. The instructor may also link the new topic to the student's personal experiences. Thus, the prompts in the ASL journal, the strategic questioning, and the class exercises with discussion provided a structure to assist with reflection and supported the students' deeper thinking about their experiences. If we agree with the stated assumption that self-awareness is the first step toward cultural competence, then reflection is critical to the development of cultural competency. Self-awareness is a result of reflection and learning about self.

Fostering Student Reflection

Students' assignments and the course-related experiences described previously were focused on thinking about experiences and developing personal meaning from them. The assignments were carefully chosen and designed to encourage reflection. The knowledge and insights students gleaned from lectures and guided discussions based on the adopted textbooks have been instrumental in fostering growth.

An additional benefit derived from the process-focused structure of these courses has been that students report becoming closer as a cohort and more confident in publicly expressing their opinions. The course instructor facilitates the students' ability to assert a personal opinion and actively engage in discussion by creating a safe climate through encouragement, support, and sharing of personal opinions and feelings. Course instructors also model tolerance for opposing views, acknowledge personal limitations, and prompt further reflection. Students have recognized their instructors as knowledgeable but also as colleagues on a shared journey toward becoming more culturally competent, as validated

by responses to an additional survey question posed to the seniors.

The community experiences exposed the junior-level students to novel situations that illuminated concepts of cultural competency, thereby helping them understand the knowledge and skills needed for this competency. Examination of the students' reflective writing assignments, including the ASL journals, clearly demonstrates increased self-awareness and knowledge, the first two phases of the Cultural Competence Education Model (Wells & Black, 2000).

Survey results indicated that, as an assignment, the senior student-led discussions were highly valued and served to broaden perspectives on the various topics while fostering confidence in expressing opinions openly. Experiential learning and related written reflections were effective in facilitating growth for these students, as they proved to be for the juniors. Exposure to a setting and population that was foreign and uncomfortable (i.e., out of comfort zone) challenged students' stereotypes and biases as well as fostered understanding and acceptance of differences. Interaction with international students had this result as well. The photo-narrative assignment, also highly valued, allowed students to test their interviewing skills, use therapeutic use of self, establish rapport with a stranger, and communicate effectively to capture an individual's story.

Cultural Desire

Cultural desire is defined as "the motivation to 'want to' engage in the process of becoming culturally competent; not 'have to'" (Campinha-Bacote, 2008, p. 142). Campinha-Bacote (2002) designed a model for developing cultural competence that assumes "cultural competence is a process, not an event" (p. 142). This assumption reiterates concepts in the Purnell model of cultural competence (2002) in that it accounts for the needs of a constantly changing society. Unique to the Campinha-Bacote model is the concept of cultural desire, which "includes a genuine passion to be open and flexible with others, to accept differences and build on similarities and to be willing to learn from others as cultural informants" (Campinha-Bacote, 2002, p. 183).

In response to a survey question asking senior-level students to identify areas for growth, 61% of the 114 students expressed a desire and willingness to continue to learn more about other cultures. This is consistent with findings from a study completed by Hunter and Krantz (2010) measuring a specific approach to teaching cultural competence. The authors indicate that although cultural desire was not specifically taught in the course assessed, cultural desire was measured as the area showing the most significant change following the course. Cultural desire can be a product of instructing in any one of the constructs of cultural competence. Hunter and Krantz suggest that growth in any of the constructs of cultural competence will drive improvement in the other constructs, specifically cultural desire. Cultural desire would seem crucial to continued development toward cultural competence.

Summary

Our experiences with educating for cultural competence have been consistent with other research and educational literature. The example described in this chapter provided evidence that experiential learning is an effective method for progressing students toward cultural competence regardless of their developmental level. It is unrealistic to think full cultural competence can be achieved in the allotted time of an accredited program. However, beginning the process in the first semester allows students the most time to develop self-awareness and knowledge, the first phases of the Cultural Competency Education Model. Some students did progress to the skill level through exposure to cultural diversity in the community.

The development of cultural competence is an ongoing process, and skills are attained through exposure, reflection, and practice. Client-centered and culturally competent occupational therapy practice is imperative for best outcomes. We have been dedicated to facilitating the process with our students, hoping to engender in them a spirit of willingness, as described by Black and Wells (2007), to continue on the journey.

This accredited occupational therapy program's experience contributes to the investigation of effective teaching methods for cultural competency.

Research should continue to investigate and assess which teaching strategies are the most effective in training students for culturally competent practice.

Reflection 23.6. Advancing Cultural Competency

Students:

- During the evaluation phase of the occupational therapy process, the occupational therapist gathers pertinent information regarding the client's occupational history, lifestyle, goals, and priorities (AOTA, 2014). During the occupational profile, how might you structure strategic questions to gather information about the client's cultural background and perception of the hospitalization or intervention and recovery process?
- Provide specific examples of how you will consider culture during occupational therapy practice.

Faculty:

- Provide specific examples of how you can create a safe learning environment that supports student discussion of sensitive topics.
- Consider one assignment about cultural competence that would require students' active engagement with the concepts of cultural competence.
- Consider how you might developmentally progress your students in cultural competence from self-awareness to knowledge to skill acquisition.
- How might you measure the effectiveness of teaching strategies in the area of cultural competence?

References

American Occupational Therapy Association. (2007). AOTA's *Centennial Vision* and executive summary. *American Journal of Occupational Therapy, 61,* 613–14. http://dx.doi.org/10.5014/ajot.61.6.613

American Occupational Therapy Association. (2014). Occupational therapy practice framework: Domain and process (3rd ed.). *American Journal of Occupational Therapy, 68*(Suppl. 1). http://dx.doi.org/10.5014/ajot.2014.682006

American Occupational Therapy Association. (2016). *AOTA unveils vision 2025.* Retrieved from http://www.aota.org/About AOTA/vision-2025.aspx

Baum, M. C. (2006). Centennial challenges, millennium opportunities. *The American Journal of Occupational Therapy, 60*(6), 609–616. http://dx.doi.org/10.5014/ajot.60.6.609

Black, R., & Wells, S. (2007). *Culture and occupation: A model of empowerment in occupational therapy.* Bethesda, MD: AOTA Press.

Bringle, R. G., Phillips, M. A., & Hudson, M. (2004). *The measure of service learning: Research scales to assess student experiences.* Washington, DC: American Psychological Association.

Brown, E., Muñoz, J., & Powell, J. M. (2011). Multicultural training in the United States: A survey of occupational therapy programs. *Occupational Therapy in Health Care, 2–3,* 178–193. http://dx.doi.org/10.3109/07380577.2011.560240

Campinha-Bacote, J. (2002). The process of cultural competence in the delivery of healthcare services: A model of care. *Journal of Transcultural Nursing, 13,* 181–184. http://dx.doi.org/10.1177/10459602013003003

Campinha-Bacote, J. (2008). Cultural desire: 'Caught' or 'taught'? *Contemporary Nurse: A Journal of the Australian Nursing Profession, 28,* 141–148. http://dx.doi.org/10.5172/conu.673.28.1-2.141

Coelho, P. (n.d.). *Paul Coelho quotes.* Retrieved from http://www.brainyquote.com/quotes/quotes/p/paulocoelh620592.html

Cole, M. (2012). The developmental approach. In *Group dynamics in occupational therapy: The theoretical basis and practice application of group intervention* (4th ed.). Thorofare, NJ: Slack.

Dunn, L., & Musolino, G. M. (2011). Assessing reflective thinking and approaches to learning. *Journal of Allied Health, 40,* 128–136.

Echeverri, M., Brookover, C., & Kennedy, K. (2010). Nine constructs of cultural competence for curriculum development. *American Journal of Pharmaceutical Education, 74,* Article 181. http://dx.doi.org/10.5688/aj7410181

Hooper, B. (2010). On arriving at the destination of the centennial vision: Navigational landmarks to guide occupational therapy education. *Occupational Therapy in Healthcare, 24*(1), 97–106. http://dx.doi.org/10.3109/07380570903329636

Hunter, J. L., & Krantz, S. (2010). Constructivism in cultural competence education. *Journal of Nursing Education, 49,* 201–214. http://dx.doi.org/10.3928/01484834-20100115-06

King, R. (2010, May). *Efficacy of course content in facilitating cultural competence: A program evaluation.* Poster session presented at the AOTA Annual Conference, Orlando, FL.

Kinsella, E. A. (2009). Professional knowledge and the epistemology of reflective practice. *Nursing Philosophy, 11,* 3–14. http://dx.doi.org/10.1111/j.1466-769X.2009.00428.x

Joyce, B., Weil, M., & Calhoun, E. (2004). *Models of teaching* (7th ed.). Boston: Pearson.

Leto, T. (2011). *Transitioning from practitioner to researcher.* (Unpublished manuscript). University of Indianapolis, Indianapolis.

Leto, T. (2012). *Educating for cultural competence: The impact of academic service learning.* (Unpublished manuscript). University of Indianapolis, Indianapolis.

Murden, R., Norman, A., Ross, J., Sturdivant, E., Kedia, M., & Shah, S. (2008). Occupational therapy students' perceptions of their cultural awareness and competency. *Occupational Therapy International, 15,* 191–203. http://dx.doi.org/10.1002/oti.253

Ong, K. (2011). Reflection for action in the medical field. *Reflective Practice, 12,* 145–149. http://dx.doi.org/10.1080/14623943.2011.541102

Purnell, L. (2002). The Purnell model for cultural competence. *Journal of Transcultural Nursing, 13*(3), 193–196. http://dx.doi.org/10.1177/10459602013003006

Roberts, A. (2009). Encouraging reflective practice in periods of professional workplace experience: The development of a conceptual model. *Reflective Practice, 10,* 633–644. http://dx.doi.org/10.1080/14623940903290703

Schön, D. A. (1992). The theory of inquiry: Dewey's legacy to education. *Curriculum Inquiry, 22,* 119–139. http://dx.doi.org/10.2307/1180029

U.S. Census Bureau. (2010). *Profile of general population and housing characteristics: 2010.* Retrieved from http://factfinder2.census.gov/faces/tableservices/jsf/pages/productview.xhtml?pid=DEC_10_DP_DPDP1

Wells, S., & Black, R. (2000). *Cultural competency for health professionals.* Bethesda, MD: American Occupational Therapy Association.

Chapter 24.

BRIDGING CLASSROOM AND COMMUNITY: DESIGNING A CULTURALLY RESPONSIVE CURRICULUM

Nina Robins, PhD, OTR/L

> *Culture is always evolving and never stays the same. Likewise, the amount of knowledge necessary to understand different cultures is vast, and our very being in the contemporary, interconnected world requires cultural understanding as never before.*
> **Fabricio E. Balcazar, Yolanda Suarez-Balcazar, Tina Taylor-Ritzler, & Christopher B. Keys (2010, p. 301)**

Chapter Highlights

- Cultural Competence Training
- Designing a Culturally Responsive Curriculum
- Assessing Cultural Competence
- Determining Course Phases
- Classroom Learning
- Cultural Competence Models
- Service Learning and Community Collaboration
- Classroom-to-Community Learning Framework
- Outcomes Derived From the Course
- Future Steps: Recommendations

Key Terms and Concepts

- ✧ CCBMDR Cultural competence model
- ✧ Community partnerships
- ✧ Cultural brokering model
- ✧ Cultural competence training
- ✧ Culturally sensitive care
- ✧ Cultural responsiveness
- ✧ Service learning framework

This chapter discusses the design and implementation of a cultural competency course for an occupational therapy curriculum. Practical application of two cultural competency models for the purpose of increasing understanding of ethnically and culturally diverse populations is emphasized. Service learning and community collaboration with organizations traditionally not served by occupational therapy serve as the framework for this course and are described.

Cultural Competence Training

Cultural competence training has been highly associated with reduction in health disparities (American Occupational Therapy Association [AOTA], 2014; Bass-Haugen, 2009; Purnell & Paulanka, 2003). Increased awareness of multicultural issues is cited as directly affecting public policies to improve access to health care as well as facilitating effective communication between clinicians, clients, and their families (Balcazar, Suarez-Balcazar, Willis, & Alvarado, 2010; Hammell, 2013; Matteliano & Stone, 2010). In addition, training to become more culturally responsive is considered critical to identifying and reducing assumptions and prejudice and in enabling social participation and inclusion (Black & Wells, 2007; Chiang & Carlson, 2003; Hammel et al., 2008; Suarez-Balcazar et al., 2009).

Reflection 24.1. Stereotypes

The single story creates stereotypes, and the problem with stereotypes is not that they are untrue, but that they are incomplete. They make one story become the only story. (Adichie, 2009, 13.24)

- What is the significance of this statement in relation to working with people from different cultures and backgrounds?
- What potential problems emerge when health care providers have stereotypes of people from different cultures?

Tervalon and Murray-García (1998) suggest that culturally sensitive or competent care training should strive to achieve a commitment to appropriate practice and policies for diverse groups of people. To that end, numerous methods for teaching cultural competence have been implemented in an effort to increase health care professionals' confidence and competence when

working with multicultural populations (Gupta, 2012; Muñoz, 2007; Murden et al., 2008; Stepnick & Silow-Carroll, 2006; Suarez-Balcazar et al., 2009). However, the effectiveness of existing programs in achieving these objectives is inconclusive (Muñoz, 2007; Suarez-Balcazar et al., 2009).

Cultural competence training paradigms are generally theorized as incorporating the following concepts: responding with respect to people of all cultures in ways that affirm and value cultural differences; protecting and preserving the dignity of individuals; and understanding that culture influences people's beliefs, behaviors, occupational performance, and intervention outcomes (Balcazar, Suarez-Balcazar, Taylor-Ritzler, & Keys, 2010; Muñoz, 2007). These tenets served as the foundation for a course I called "OT Perspectives in Cultural Responsiveness." The class was composed of 36 master's-level occupational therapy students.

Designing a Culturally Responsive Curriculum

My challenge as a new professor was to teach cultural responsiveness in a way that allowed the students to apply the knowledge that they learned in the class, through discussion and readings, in active learning situations. I drew upon my personal experiences from graduate training, as a clinician who has been practicing for more than 20 years, and as a disability studies scholar to structure the curriculum and create the overarching framework. This involved clearly defining **culturally sensitive care.**

On the basis of my own clinical and research experiences, I envisioned cultural competency or sensitivity as providing care to people who may look, think, and behave in vastly different ways from the majority of occupational therapists who are, typically, well-educated White women with little or no personal experience with the challenges experienced by many of their clients (Kirsh, Trentham, & Cole, 2006; Stepnick & Silow-Carroll, 2006). The critical questions guiding me were

- As health care professionals, how do we form a therapeutic relationship and foster trust with people who may seem unfamiliar and foreign in multiple ways?
- In what ways can we avoid imposing our "professionalism" without causing intimidation or distrust?

• How can cultural sensitivity training incorporate sociocultural perspectives of illness or injury most effectively so occupational therapy interventions are most relevant to diverse populations?

I also believed it was important to make explicit that cultural competency training is an ongoing and lifelong learning process.

Reflection 24.2. Personal Biases

Becoming culturally competent or responsive is a process that evolves throughout one's lifetime. Being a culturally responsive health care professional requires honest self-reflection and acknowledgment of one's own biases and assumptions.

• What are your deeply held and long-standing beliefs about people different from yourself?
• Where do you think these beliefs came from?
• How does acknowledging that we all have biases contribute to being a more responsive caregiver?

Developing Clinical Reasoning Skills

Developing clinical reasoning skills informed every phase of this course by exposing students to real-life scenarios of people from different cultural backgrounds and creating opportunities for interaction and collaboration with various community organizations serving people of different cultural, ethnic, and social affiliations (Neistadt, 1987; Robertson, 2012). I adapted a model of clinical reasoning described as "classroom as clinic" (Neistadt, 1987) into a version that I conceptualized as "bridging classroom to community." The original model involved providing students with opportunities to practice evaluation skills learned in the classroom with real people with disabilities from the community. My adapted version encompassed hierarchical but interrelated steps of classroom teaching leading to community practice.

Service Learning

Community participation phases of the course were accomplished through a service learning approach that encompassed providing services and learning about community agencies serving people of multicultural backgrounds (Bazyk, Glorioso, Gordon, Haines, & Percaciante, 2010; Gitlow & Flecky, 2005; Jenkins & Sheehey, 2012). According

to Bazyk and colleagues (2010), *service learning* comprises developing empathic interpersonal skills with clients and other health care professionals and finding solutions to assist in ameliorating social injustice to marginalized populations.

Incorporating Interdisciplinary Learners

A consistent thread of interdisciplinary learning was woven throughout this course, involving faculty–researchers and two students from Disability Studies and Occupational Therapy programs from the University of Illinois at Chicago (UIC) who participated in classes. During the first class in which they participated, they introduced two cultural competency models; in the second session, during the last 2 weeks of the class, they provided feedback to the students as they created their final cultural competency project. In addition, the director and the provost for the Multicultural Affairs and Community Health and Nursing programs at Rush University enhanced the theme of interdisciplinary partnership, as did ongoing collaboration with various professionals in the community.

Facilitating consistent interdisciplinary collaborative experiences from the initial phase of the course was a deliberate effort so students would develop professional relationships and communication skills with providers from various disciplines and backgrounds. Interdisciplinary collaborative experiences are believed to provide the preparation necessary for working as part of a treatment team to provide comprehensive care (Gitlow & Flecky, 2005). From the first day of class, each course phase represented a segment of bridging the classroom to the community using a service learning model (Bazyk et al., 2010; Gitlow & Flecky, 2005).

Assessing Cultural Competence

Providing culturally competent care demands that health care providers possess an understanding of the concept cultural competence. It is critical to have validated instruments to measure this. The Cultural Competence Assessment Instrument (CCAI) was chosen as the assessment for the students to learn because it has been found to be valid and have sound psychometric properties, which is limited in the rehabilitation literature (Suarez-Balcazar et al., 2011).

Cultural Competence Assessment Instrument

To evaluate how this community collaborative service learning course affected students' perception of their cultural knowledge and skills, I administered the CCAI on the first day and the last days of class (Balcazar et al., 2008; Suarez-Balcazar et al., 2011; see Exhibit 24.1). The CCAI is an instrument designed by researchers from the UIC to measure cultural competency from rehabilitation providers' perspectives (Balcazar et al., 2008).

Exhibit 24.1. Cultural Competence Assessment Instrument

Rate your level of success in outreaching the following ethnic populations:

Ethnicity	Very Successful	Successful	Unsuccessful	Very Unsuccessful	N/A
African American/Black	4	3	2	1	0
Asian	4	3	2	1	0
Hawaiian/Pacific Islander	4	3	2	1	0
Native American/Alaskan Native	4	3	2	1	0
Hispanic/Latino	4	3	2	1	0
White	4	3	2	1	0
Other *(Please specify)*	4	3	2	1	0

Cultural Competence Assessment Instrument (CCAI)

CONSIDERING YOUR WORK OVER THE PAST YEAR	Strongly Agree	Agree	Disagree	Strongly Disagree
1. I feel that I can learn from my ethnic minority clients.	4	3	2	1
2. I am effective in my verbal communication with clients whose culture is different from mine.	4	3	2	1
3. My organization does not provide ongoing training on cultural competence.	4	3	2	1
4. I feel confident that I can learn about my clients' cultural background.	4	3	2	1
5. I am effective in my nonverbal communication with clients whose culture is different from mine.	4	3	2	1
6. I feel that I have limited experience working with ethnic minority clients.	4	3	2	1
7. It is difficult to practice skills related to cultural competence.	4	3	2	1
8. I am sensitive to valuing and respecting differences between my cultural background and my clients' cultural heritage.	4	3	2	1
9. I have opportunities to learn culturally responsive behaviors from peers.	4	3	2	1
10. I do not feel that I have the skills to provide services to ethnic minority clients.	4	3	2	1
11. I examine my own biases related to race and culture that may influence my behavior as a service provider.	4	3	2	1
12. I actively strive for an atmosphere that promotes risk-taking and self-exploration.	4	3	2	1
13. I would find it easy to work competently with ethnic minority clients.	4	3	2	1
14. I learn about different ethnic cultures through educational methods and/or life experiences.	4	3	2	1

Note. Sample content.
Source. From *Cultural Competence Assessment Instrument (CCAI)*, by F. Balcazar et al., 2008, Chicago: Center for Capacity Building on Minorities with Disabilities Research. Copyright © 2008 by University of Illinois at Chicago. Adapted with permission.

The self-report format of the CCAI was developed within the context of occupational therapy and encompasses a cognitive component (awareness or knowledge), a behavioral component (i.e., skills), and a contextual component (organizational support) that the authors found to be critical to cultural competency training (Balcazar, Suarez-Balcazar, & Taylor-Ritzler, 2009; Suarez-Balcazar et al., 2011). Moreover, the CCAI has been found to have strong psychometric properties and is one of only a few instruments that have been validated in the rehabilitation research for cultural competence (Suarez-Balcazar et al., 2011).

Personal communication with one of the researchers who developed this assessment confirmed the feasibility of using it with students who have not yet been practicing as therapists (F. Balcazar, personal communication, November 9, 2012). Administering the CCAI enabled me to obtain preliminary information about how this course affected students' perceptions of how culturally competent they felt as a result of their experiences in this course (Balcazar et al., 2008; Suarez-Balcazar et al., 2011).

For example, in response to whether one feels their nonverbal communication is effective when working with clients from cultures different from their own (see Exhibit 24.1), 34 of 36 students disagreed initially. At the end of the course, 32 students strongly agreed with this statement, and 4 students agreed.

Similarly, in response to whether one believes they do not have the skills to provide services to ethnic minority clients (see "Phase One" description in Appendix 24.A), 35 students indicated that they strongly agreed initially, but 30 students strongly disagreed, 5 students disagreed, and 1 student agreed at the end of the course. In fact, all but 1 of the 36 students rated their skills more positively in 21 out of 24 statements on the CCAI at course end. To date, collaboration with the primary researcher of the CCAI is in progress to further analyze the students' responses on the CCAI (F. Balcazar, personal communication, July 9, 2012).

Course Assessment

Qualitative statements from the IDEA evaluation, the standard student course assessment used at Rush University College of Health Sciences (CHS), were also instructive in gaining insight about the students' reactions to the class (IDEA Center, 2012). Some of the comments from the students included

- "I definitely feel like I'm much more prepared to work with patients who are from different cultural backgrounds because of the activities we did in class and outside of class."
- "The idea of treating patients from other countries was scary to me when I first started this course, but I'm so much more comfortable because I realize that I don't have to agree with all their beliefs and values. I just have to respect them."
- "At first I wasn't sure why we were encouraged to partner with people from non-OT backgrounds, but after doing our service learning I can't emphasize enough how meaningful and instructive it was because it opened my eyes to how to work with people from way different backgrounds and circumstances than most of us have ever dealt with. I learned so much from the staff and clients' points of views."
- "I feel so fortunate that our class was given the opportunity to really actively get involved with these different community sites. It was an awesome experience!"

Determining Course Phases

The course was divided into five phases of learning and practice training that consisted of

- *Phase 1:* Self-reflection and imagining alternative values other than one's own. Learning how clinical reasoning serves as a strategic and reflective process to provide culturally responsive caring. Initial assessment of CCAI (Balcazar et al., 2008).
- *Phase 2:* Learning about different models and theories; focus on two specific models with direct "occupational therapy in community" relevance in preparation for community service activities.
- *Phase 3:* Preparation and development of community collaboration relationships.
- *Phase 4:* Service learning opportunities: community collaborative activities. Taking action: transitioning classroom learning to community; applying concepts to propose culturally sensitive occupational therapy programs of care in community sites.
- *Phase 5:* Establishment of **community partnerships** from class projects; ongoing relationships between occupational therapy students, faculty,

and community organization representatives. Reassessment of CCAI (Balcazar et al., 2008).

Detailed information pertaining to the five course phases is described in Appendix 24.A.

Classroom Learning

Classroom learning introduced students to the multiple ways of thinking about and defining culture, theoretical concepts, and theories of cultural responsiveness or competency. Students also considered how their backgrounds and values potentially influence their behaviors personally and professionally. Activities, class lectures, discussions (including reviews of the required readings), and guest speaker presentations also covered topics related to diversity of cultural values, beliefs, and behaviors, as well as how they are created and maintained. Additionally, discussions covered how Western occupational therapy values do not always reflect others' values and how this dissonance can negatively affect practice (Chiang & Carlson, 2003).

Students were then exposed to various models of cultural competence. The similar and unique components of each model were discussed in terms of their applicability to occupational therapy practice (Balcazar et al., 2009; Campinha-Bacote, 2001; Hammell, 2004; Muñoz, 2007; Nochajski & Matteliano, 2008; Purnell & Paulanka, 2003; Suarez-Balcazar et al., 2011).

Students were required to keep a reflective journal of their experiences through all stages of this course. Journal entries were shared in small-group discussions and with the instructor and were incorporated into written assignments. Bazyk et al. (2010) regard the keeping of a reflective journal as a way to facilitate students' self-understanding. Another benefit of journal writing is that instructors can gain insight on how students' experiences in the class are influencing their learning (Bazyk et al., 2010).

Cultural Competence Models

Following initial cultural awareness activities, the class learned about two models of cultural competence: (1) the Cultural Brokering Model (Jezewski, 1993; Jezewski & Sotnik, 2001) and (2) the Center for Capacity Building for Minorities with Disabilities Research (CCBMDR) Cultural Competence Model

(Balcazar et al., 2009; Suarez-Balcazar et al., 2011). These models were chosen for their direct relevance to occupational therapy and rehabilitation providers in general as well as for people with disabilities.

Reflection 24.3. Faculty Reflection: Developing Culturally Responsive Care

As health care professionals, we have a moral responsibility to incorporate culturally responsive care to engender improved quality of life for individuals with diverse life experiences.

- Think of 2 class activities or discussions that you could develop based on students' reflections written in their journals.
- Write 2 journal questions that stimulate students' reflections of how occupational therapy is uniquely positioned to provide culturally sensitive care for people in underserved communities.

These models were introduced through presentations by two faculty–researchers from UIC who specialized in or developed these models in their research and practice. Two doctoral-level students from the UIC nursing and public health schools contributed to the presentations by demonstrating how they were using each model in their community health practicum placements. Students discussed the two cultural competency models in class and participated in activities using the models to increase their skill in integrating these frameworks into their upcoming community projects.

Cultural Brokering Model

The *Cultural Brokering Model* is conceptualized as bringing together groups or individuals of different cultural backgrounds with the goal of producing positive change (Jezewski, 1993). This model consists of three hierarchical steps of intervention for health care providers and other stakeholders for the ultimate purpose of respecting and empowering underserved culturally or ethnically diverse groups or individuals. Its tenets include

- Advocating for clients,
- Serving as a liaison between client and others, and

- Intervening to minimize conflict or to promote change.

The model has three stages of intervention:

1. *Problem identification:* Recognize a problem between client and system (examination of situation from cultural perspective; understand clients' cultural meanings of views of disability and health care).
2. *Intervention phase:* Identify strategies (facilitate client staying connected and invested; establish trust and rapport). Mediate, negotiate, and advocate.
3. *Outcome:* Assess degree to which problem has been resolved (Jezewski & Sotnik, 2001).

CCBMDR Cultural Competence Model

The ***CCBMDR Cultural Competence Model*** is conceptualized within a framework that highlights the desire to know and understand people of different cultural backgrounds. The unique feature of this model is the emphasis on organizational support that is absent from many existing models (Balcazar, Suarez-Balcazar, Willis, & Alvarado, 2010). The components of the model include

- *Willingness to engage:* Assume that service providers seeking cultural competence training must be willing to engage in the process.
- *Critical awareness:* Understand our personal biases toward people who are different from us, and critically examine our own position of privilege in society (class differences and experiences of oppression).
- *Cultural knowledge:* Familiarize ourselves with others' cultural characteristics, history, values, belief systems, and behaviors.
- *Skills development:* Develop ability to communicate effectively and empathically with clients and incorporate clients' beliefs, values, experiences, and aspirations into planning and intervention. Requires problem-solving skills and understanding of dynamics of oppression, racism, and other forms of discrimination.
- *Practice/application:* Apply all previous components in a particular context.
- *Organizational support:* Cannot work unless support is in place (Suarez-Balcazar et al., 2011).

Service Learning and Community Collaboration

Student preparation for service learning experiences was addressed preliminarily through writing, discussions about anticipating and finding meaning of service experiences, reflecting on what populations would likely most benefit, and planning the steps.

Initially, a few students expressed trepidation and raised questions regarding the nature of performing occupational therapy in nontraditional settings, such as homeless shelters or HIV/AIDS clinics. These concerns were addressed through class discussions and role playing related to required readings addressing occupational therapists and students' conceptualization of cultural competence (AOTA, 2014; Hammell, 2013; Murden et al., 2008; Pooremamali, Persson, & Eklund, 2011; Suarez-Balcazar et al., 2009) and synopses of health care professionals' experiences of providing therapy to people in non-Western societies (Bazyk et al., 2010; Kramer-Roy, 2012; Taff & Hoyt, 2012).

Community organizations, agencies, and health care facilities that provided services to underserved and culturally diverse populations expressed a desire to collaborate with students from the occupational therapy program. Collaborators were identified: the director of Multicultural Affairs and Community Services, the associate provost for Professional Education and Community Engagement, and the director and provost of the nursing department engaged in community health initiatives at Rush University Medical Center. These individuals acted as liaisons who connected the students to community organizations in the greater Chicago area. Students met with each of the liaisons through two class activities and by appointments outside of class.

Students prepared for community collaboration through a series of steps that reflected the components inherent in a service learning model (Jenkins & Sheehey, 2012). These steps involved identifying a need in the community, determining specific goals and objectives for service projects, establishing the skills necessary for community projects, and ensuring that needed resources and activities were available (Bazyk et al., 2010; Jenkins & Sheehey, 2012).

Reflection 24.4. Nontraditional Settings

Service learning is most effectively implemented when all parties appreciate the benefits and strengths of developing partnerships for their own organizations as well as the overall social contribution the relationships foster.

- Describe and present 2–3 examples of how implementing occupational therapy in non-traditional settings such as homeless shelters or drop-in centers fosters a richer contextual understanding of disability as a sociocultural as well as an individual condition.

Identifying Collaborative Sites

First, 9 groups of 4 students each identified potential community collaborative sites with which they desired to engage that fulfilled the components of the service learning framework (Jenkins & Sheehey, 2012). Then the groups practiced making professional contacts, creating community relationships, and brainstorming ideas for their weekly collaborative projects. The preliminary step was to select a site with which to develop a partnership.

The course offered three major community collaborative projects along with several smaller in-class activities. Several of the activities were adapted or inspired from *A Guide to Cultural Competence in the Curriculum Occupational Therapy* (CIRRIE, 2012; Nochajski & Matteliano, 2008), while numerous activities were created directly from the instructor's clinical experiences.

Obtaining Institutional Review Board Training

Before collaborating in community projects, the students completed Institutional Review Board (IRB) training in conducting research in human development and behavioral sciences, and they obtained IRB certification that prepared them for the initial steps of designing and implementing the health care interview assignment. Detailed verbal and written descriptions of the projects were communicated to the community partners and recipients of services, and written informed consent was obtained from the people involved. The instructor and fellow students provided feedback during group activities and on written assignments before finalizing any documents and letters.

Conducting Health Care Provider Interviews

The first community project involved all of the students, in groups of 4, conducting health care provider interviews at their selected community sites. Before the interviews, the students obtained informed consent from and approval by the instructor and organization representative. The provider interview project involved data collection and analysis using a qualitative methodology.

Students audiotaped and transcribed the 1-hour interviews, which enabled them to identify and describe the major themes in the discussion section of their assignments. The themes obtained from these interviews were used as the foundation to guide the second and third projects. This assignment and the preliminary steps gave students the opportunity to directly communicate with professionals to learn about their experiences working with culturally diverse clients and families.

Many of the providers were professionals from other disciplines in addition to occupational therapy. Such variety enabled students to gain an appreciation for other professionals' roles and responsibilities as well as the strategies they use in working with diverse populations. Opportunities to draft research proposals, consent forms, interview questions, and analysis of interviews were also instrumental in facilitating an in-depth understanding of the multitude of positive as well as challenging issues confronting people of diverse backgrounds and the organizations providing services. These activities exposed students to the process involved in designing and implementing qualitative inquiry.

Reflection 24.5. Classroom to Community Activities

- Prepare questions you might pose to health care providers who work in a community health care clinic in an inner city with a population that includes refugees and illegal immigrants. Questions should focus on how health care workers communicate with clients who might come from vastly different backgrounds from themselves.

Developing Community Experience

The second project involved developing a practical experience in the community that consisted of a weekly 2-hour engagement for 6 weeks. In the community experiences, groups of 4 students interacted with clients and families from diverse cultural and ethnic backgrounds and professionals from multiple disciplines.

This second project was an extension of the first one in which students developed a weekly 1- to 2-hour commitment with the organizations and providers where their interviews were conducted. The students gained permission from the directors or managers of each site to conduct these interviews, obtained the instructor's approval, and submitted a formal written plan of objectives and goals to be achieved as a result of their involvement.

Students gained ongoing exposure to agencies, organizations, or institutions that provided services to people of diverse ethnic, racial, disability, or other backgrounds. Students could then interact with staff, clients, and families under the direct supervision and guidance of an assigned supervisor. They also received consistent feedback and frequent site visits from the instructor. Students also increased their knowledge of service needs and the significance of occupational therapy practice.

With the instructor's guidance, students designed and implemented individualized activities for their groups such as teaching life skills, translating emergency phone numbers in people's native languages, or working with ethnically diverse older adults in a homeless shelter to self-advocate for access to health services.

Ongoing partnerships provided the groundwork for the third and final community project, which was the design, implementation, and presentation of culturally responsive occupational therapy interventions and programs.

Designing and Presenting Culturally Responsive Occupational Therapy

Experience the students gained from the first two community projects led to the final project that involved designing and presenting a culturally responsive occupational therapy program or intervention to the students' community sites (Nochajski & Matteliano, 2008). All the knowledge and skills the students developed throughout the course culminated in this project.

Students designed culturally responsive programs and interventions and then proposed them to their community supervisors, instructor, and visiting students and faculty–researchers. This assignment required students to comprehensively incorporate the theoretical and practical information they learned in the classroom and during their community experiences. Some groups identified potential cultural barriers or challenges that they observed as thwarting the achievement of meaningful client and family goals for their particular community site; other groups determined a need for culturally responsive interventions that were not available or accessible (e.g., transportation to the Mexican consulate for information on Hispanic health centers serving new immigrants with diabetes and high blood pressure).

Students constructed practical problem-solving strategies to address the challenges or lack of services and supports for their client population. Students were required to incorporate the Cultural Brokering Model (Jezewski, 1993) and the CCBMDR Cultural Competence Model (Balcazar et al., 2009; Suarez-Balcazar et al., 2011) as a culturally competent–oriented theoretical framework to justify their clinical decisions and program recommendations.

Assignment requirements included creating a professional PowerPoint presentation and paper describing organization characteristics, strengths, problems identified, and strategies proposed.

Approximately 75% to 80% of students continued their participation in their community collaborative partnerships after the class ended, and at least two community sites agreed to participate in the master's occupational therapy program as Level I and Level II fieldwork sites in 2014. Several of these partnerships simultaneously served as partial requirements for students' master's projects that involved the design and implementation of an occupational therapy intervention within a community organization. All students expressed their interest, apart from their master's requirements, in continuing their involvement with their community organizations.

Classroom-to-Community Learning Framework

I desired to have a multitude of interactive student-learning experiences based on the idea that optimal learning occurs when one is exposed to a variety of experiences and opportunities for active practice of skills (Bazyk et al., 2010). In fact, research that examines effective cultural competency training recommends combining traditional teaching techniques, such as lectures and class discussions, with experiential learning activities and community service participation (Svinicki & McKeachie, 2011).

This course also incorporated interdisciplinary collaboration through the participation of faculty–researchers and students from nursing and public health graduate programs in selected classes; their roles included brainstorming potential community projects and providing feedback to the students about their community assignments. Cultural responsiveness was also comprised of community organizations serving underserved ethnically diverse populations, faculty and students from other disciplines, and university administrators representing various professional backgrounds.

I chose to use aspects of a *service learning framework* for this course because of its effectiveness in exposing students to community organizations serving culturally diverse populations. Service learning in occupational therapy has been associated with preparing students for successful transition into practice (Bazyk et al., 2010; Braveman & Suarez-Balcazar, 2009) and providing opportunities for students to appreciate the complexities of disability as experienced by clients and families (Gitlow & Flecky, 2005; Phelan, 2011).

The experiential learning framework offered students opportunities to practice skills learned in the classroom so they could increase their confidence and competence and gain an appreciation for the value of occupational therapy intervention in nontraditional workplaces (Bazyk et al., 2010; Braveman & Suarez-Balcazar, 2009; Jenkins & Sheehey, 2012).

The students unanimously reported through written feedback on the course evaluation (IDEA Center, 2012) that collaborating with community organizations was a uniquely transformative experience. They lauded the meaningful relationships created with people from disparate life situations and cultural backgrounds, the application of the cultural competency models learned in class, and the numerous opportunities for multidisciplinary learning.

Responses collected from CCAI (Balcazar et al., 2009; Suarez-Balcazar et al., 2011) further supported the positive impact of this course on the students' increased confidence and preparedness in providing culturally sensitive interactions. The students also reported, through class discussions prompted by entries from their reflective journals, that their engagement with clients and staff in community organizations was illuminating; their interactions helped them appreciate the unique contributions of occupational therapy practice in nontraditional settings for people of various minority status with and without disabilities.

Reflection 24.6. Propose Services for Muslim Women

Design an occupational therapy intervention that you will propose to the directors of a shelter for Muslim women who have experienced sexual and other abuse. This shelter currently does not include occupational therapy services, so you will need to justify why occupational therapy reflects the values inherent in an organization that attempts to both protect and empower the people it serves.

- How will you ensure that your proposed intervention addresses the cultural beliefs and values of the people you are designing it for?

Outcomes Derived From the Course

Specific outcomes are outlined in each phase description in Appendix 24.A. In general, the course yielded these outcomes:

- Students gained practical skills and strategies they believed they would use during their clinical practicums and future clinical practice.
- The students unanimously reported they felt more skilled and confident in working with people who differed from their experiences with regard to ethnicity, socioeconomic, educational, and cultural aspects.
- Many of the students' proposal presentations relating to design and implementation of culturally sensitive care in different sites of care were subsequently submitted for upcoming conferences with the objective of informing current practice.
- Ongoing collaborative relationships between students and community organizations were implemented with students' direct application of culturally sensitive interventions and programs (e.g., training

modules working with translators and identification of community resources for Asian Americans with disabilities).

- Community partnerships established during the class continued, in many instances, beyond the time frame of the course.
- Students expressed their excitement in being able to apply their skills and knowledge gained in the course to the community and more traditional health care organizations.

Future Steps: Recommendations

The following steps are recommended in an effort to continue to refine culturally responsive programs:

- Develop an educational framework to refine current program development, implementation, and evaluation.
- Explore the feasibility of creating and implementing interdisciplinary and multi-university cultural competence training.
- Design and implement collaborative community research projects with occupational therapy students to explore the needs of community members with disabilities.
- Conduct qualitative in-depth interviews with recipients of community services as well as health care providers to gain firsthand perspectives of individuals' needs and goals.
- Create occupational therapy outreach to greater Chicago and other communities serving residents of ethnic backgrounds and other underserved minorities with disabilities. Develop clinical and research partnerships for community integration for people of minority backgrounds with disabilities (perhaps as collaboration with other geographic regions and settings [i.e., Boston-area universities, rehabilitation hospitals, and disability organizations]).
- Research the dissemination or publication of course outcomes using service learning and classroom-to-community models and opportunities for student co-authorship.

Summary

Occupational therapy educators face the challenge of imparting cultural competence training to students who often possess limited knowledge of the individuals with whom they will interact in an ever-changing cultural climate. A mission of present-day occupational therapy is to continue to provide services as well as to forge new services, in response to modern-day needs (i.e., access to the Internet for older adults) for individuals from diverse cultural and ethnic backgrounds, with both understanding and sensitivity.

To help students not only effectively gain cultural awareness but competently apply their knowledge in the community, the model proposed here breaks the barriers of traditional classroom learning to create a classroom as clinic and bridge the classroom-to-community gap. This interactive community outreach service learning model encourages students to reflect on their past experiences and belief systems and revise them as necessary based on new knowledge gained from a multitude of practical learning opportunities.

Students had an opportunity to engage in experiential learning with selected community organizations, many of which did not have occupational therapy services already in place. Through the success of the classroom-to-community bridge model, students reported an increased self–other awareness and understanding of diverse populations and settings. As an exciting outcome of this teaching process, the "bridge" concept has had far-reaching extensions: New relationships with diverse populations were developed and solidified, students continued their outreach projects after the class ended, and new proposals related to cultural competence were reflected in their involvement with research in this important area.

References

Abreu, B., & Peloquin, S. (2004). Embracing diversity in our profession. *American Journal of Occupational Therapy, 58*(4), 353–360. http://dx.doi.org/10.5014/ajot.58.3.353

Adichie, C. (2009). Chimamanda Adichie: The danger of a single story. *TED.* Retrieved from http://www.ted.com/talks/lang/eng/chimamanda_adichie_the_danger_of_a_single_story

American Occupational Therapy Association. (2014). Occupational therapy practice framework: Domain and process (3rd ed.). *American Journal of Occupational Therapy, 68*(Suppl. 1). http://dx.doi.org/10.5014/ajot.2014.682006

Balcazar, F., Suarez-Balcazar, Y., & Taylor-Ritzler, T. (2009). Cultural competence: Development of a conceptual framework. *Disability and Rehabilitation, 31,* 1153–1160. http://dx.doi.org/10.1080/09638280902773752

Balcazar, F., Suarez-Balcazar, Y., Taylor-Ritzler, T., & Keys, C. B. (Eds.). (2010). *Race, culture and disability: Rehabilitation science and practice.* Sudbury, MA: Jones & Bartlett.

Balcazar, F., Suarez-Balcazar, Y., Taylor-Ritzler, T., Rodakowski, J., Willis, C., & Portillo, N. (2008). *Cultural Competence Assessment Instrument (CCAI)* [Assessment instrument]. University of Illinois at Chicago, Chicago: Center for Capacity Building on Minorities with Disabilities Research. Provided by F. Balcazar, fabricio@uic.edu

Balcazar, F., Suarez-Balcazar, Y., Willis, C., & Alvarado, F. (2010). Cultural competence: A review of conceptual frameworks. In F. Balcazar, Y. Suarez-Balcazar, T. Taylor-Ritzler, & C. B. Keys (Eds.), *Race, culture, and disability: Rehabilitation science and practice* (pp. 281–305). Sudbury, MA: Jones & Bartlett.

Bass-Haugen, J. (2009). Health disparities: Examination of evidence relevant for occupational therapy. *American Journal of Occupational Therapy, 63*(1), 24–34. http://dx.doi.org/10.5014/ajot.63.1.24

Bazyk, S., Glorioso, M., Gordon, R., Haines, J., & Percaciante, M. (2010). Service learning: The process of doing and becoming an occupational therapist. *Occupational Therapy in Health Care, 24*(2), 171–187. http://dx.doi.org/10.3109/07380571003681194

Black, R. M. (2002). Occupational therapy's dance with diversity. *American Journal of Occupational Therapy, 56*(2), 140–148. http://dx.doi.org/10.5014/ajot.56.2.140

Black, R. M., & Wells, S. A. (2007). *Culture and occupation: A model of empowerment in occupational therapy.* Bethesda, MD: AOTA Press.

Braveman, B., & Suarez-Balcazar, Y. (2009). Social justice and resource utilization in a community-based organization: A case illustration of the role of the occupational therapist. *American Journal of Occupational Therapy, 63*(1), 13–23. http://dx.doi.org/10.5014/ajot.63.1.13

Campinha-Bacote, J. (2001). A model of practice to address cultural competence in rehabilitation nursing. *Rehabilitation Nursing, 26*(1), 8–11. http://dx.doi.org/10.1002/j.2048-7940.2001.tb02201.x

Center for International Rehabilitation Research Information & Exchange (CIRRIE). (2012). Buffalo, NY: University of Buffalo. Retrieved from http://cirrie.buffalo.edu/

Chiang, M., & Carlson, G. (2003). Occupational therapy in multicultural contexts: Issues and strategies. *British Journal of Occupational Therapy, 66*(12), 559–567. http://dx.doi.org/10.1177/030802260306601204

Gitlow, L., & Flecky, K. (2005). Integrating disability studies concepts into occupational therapy education using service learning. *American Journal of Occupational Therapy, 59*(5), 546–553. http://dx.doi.org/10.5014/ajot.59.5.546

Gupta, J. (2012). An issue of occupational (in)justice: A case study. *Disability Studies Quarterly, 32*(3), 1–19. Retrieved from http://dsq-sds.org/article/view/3280/3114

Hammel, J., Magasi, S., Heinemann, A., Whiteneck, G., Bogner, J., & Rodriguez, E. (2008). What does participation mean? An insider perspective from people with disabilities. *Disability and Rehabilitation, 30*(19), 1445–1460. http://dx.doi.org/10.1080/09638280701625534

Hammell, K. R. W. (2013). Client-centered practice in occupational therapy: Critical reflections. *Scandinavian Journal of Occupational Therapy, 20*(3), 174–181. http://dx.doi.org/10.3109/11038128.2012.752032

Hammell, K. R. W. (2004). Dimensions of meaning in the occupations of daily life. *Canadian Journal of Occupational Therapy, 71*(5), 296–305. http://dx.doi.org/10.1177/000841740407100509

IDEA Center. (2012). *Individual Development and Educational Assessment (IDEA)* [Data file]. Diagnostic Form Report, IDEA Center. Retrieved from http://ideaedu.org/services/student-ratings-of-instruction/

Jenkins, A., & Sheehey, P. (2012). A checklist for implementing service-learning in higher education. *Journal of Community Engagement and Scholarship, 4*(2). Retrieved from http://jces.ua.edu/a-checklist-for-implementing-service-learning-in-higher-education/

Jezewski, M. A. (1993). Culture brokering as a model for advocacy. *Nursing & Health Care, 14*(2), 78–85.

Jezewski, M. A., & Sotnik, P. (2001). Culture brokering: Providing culturally competent rehabilitation services to foreign-born persons. In J. Stone (Ed.), *The Rehabilitation Provider's Guide to Cultures of the Foreign-Born.* [Monograph]. Center for International Rehabilitation Research Information & Exchange. Retrieved from http://cirrie.buffalo.edu/culture/monographs/cb.php

Kirsh, B., Trentham, B., & Cole, S. (2006). Diversity in occupational therapy: Experiences of consumers who identify themselves as minority group members. *Australian Occupational Therapy Journal, 53*(4), 302–313. http://dx.doi.org/10.1111/j.1440-1630.2006.00576.x

Kramer-Roy, D. (2012). Supporting ethnic minority families with disabled children: Learning from Pakistani families. *British Journal of Occupational Therapy, 75*(10), 442–448. http://dx.doi.org/10.4276/030802212X13496921049581

Magasi, S., & Hammel, J. (2009). Women with disabilities' experiences in long-term care: A case for social justice. *American Journal of Occupational Therapy, 63*(1), 35–45. http://dx.doi.org/10.5014/ajot.63.1.35

Matteliano, M., & Stone, J. (2010). Cultural competence education in rehabilitation. In F. Balcazar, Y. Suarez-Balcazar, T. Taylor-Ritzler, & C. B. Keys (Eds.), *Race, culture, and disability: Rehabilitation science and practice* (pp. 207–228). Sudbury, MA: Jones & Bartlett.

Muñoz, J. P. (2007). Culturally responsive caring in occupational therapy. *Occupational Therapy International, 14*(4), 256–280. http://dx.doi.org/10.1002/oti.238

Murden, R., Norman, A., Ross, J., Sturdivant, E., Kedia, M., & Shah, S. (2008). Occupational therapy students' perceptions of their cultural awareness and competency. *Occupational Therapy International, 15*(3), 191–203. http://dx.doi.org/10.1002/oti.253

Neistadt, M. E. (1987). Classroom as clinic: A model for teaching clinical reasoning in occupational therapy education. *American Journal of Occupational Therapy, 41*(10), 631–637. http://dx.doi.org/10.5014/ajot.41.10.631

Nochajski, S. M., & Matteliano, M. A. (2008). A guide to cultural competence in the curriculum. In J. Stone & M. A. Matteliano (Eds.), *Curriculum guides.* Center for International Rehabilitation Research Information & Exchange. Retrieved from http://cirrie.buffalo.edu/culture/curriculum/guides/ot.php

Phelan, S. (2011). Constructions of disability: A call for critical reflexivity in occupational therapy. *Canadian Journal of Occupational Therapy, 78*(3), 164–172. http://dx.doi.org/10.2182/cjot.2011.78.3.4

Pooremamali, P., Persson, D., & Eklund, M. (2011). Occupational therapists' experience of working with immigrant clients in mental health care. *Scandinavian Journal of Occupational Therapy, 18*(2), 109–121. http://dx.doi.org/10.3109/11038121003649789

Purnell, L. D., & Paulanka, B. J. (2003). *Transcultural health care: A culturally competent approach.* Philadelphia: F. A. Davis.

Robertson, L. (2012). *Clinical reasoning in occupational therapy controversies in practice.* West Sussex, England: Wiley-Blackwell.

Stepnick, L., & Silow-Carroll, S. (2006). *Patient-centered care for underserved populations: Best practices: A case study of Massachusetts General Hospital.* Economic and Social Research Institute. Retrieved from http://www2.massgeneral.org/disparitiessolutions/z_files/massgen.pdf

Suarez-Balcazar, Y., Balcazar, F., Taylor-Ritzler, T., Portillo, N., Rodakowsk, J., Garcia-Ramirez, M., & Willis, C. (2011). Development and validation of the cultural competence assessment instrument: A factorial analysis. *Journal of Rehabilitation, 77*(1), 4–13. Retrieved from http://vlex.com/vid/of-cultural-competence-instrument-analysis-418444526

Suarez-Balcazar, Y., Rodawoski, J., Balcazar, F., Taylor-Ritzler, T., Portillo, N., Barwoski, D., & Willis, C. (2009). Perceived levels of cultural competence among occupational therapists. *American Journal of Occupational Therapy, 63*(4), 498–505. http://dx.doi.org/10.5014/ajot.63.4.498

Svinicki, M., & McKeachie, W. J. (2011). *McKeachie's teaching tips: Strategies, research, and theory for college and university teachers* (13th ed.). Belmont, CA: Wadsworth/Cengage Learning.

Taff, S., & Hoyt, C. (2012, November 26). Going global in Guatemala. Supporting emerging occupational therapy practice in developing nations. *OT Practice*, pp. 14–19. Retrieved from https://www.scribd.com/document/115934702/OT-Practice-November-26-Issue

Tervalon, M., & Murray-García, J. (1998). Cultural humility versus cultural competence: A critical distinction in defining physician training outcomes in multicultural education. *Journal of Health Care for the Poor and Underserved, 9*(2), 117–125. http://dx.doi.org/10.1353/hpu.2010.0233

Appendix 24.A. Course Phases

PHASE 1: SELF-REFLECTION

- Self-reflection and imagining alternative values other than one's own. Learning how clinical reasoning serves as a strategic and reflective process to provide culturally responsive caring.

Objectives: Understand one's own cultural backgrounds and biases through self-reflective activities and class discussions. Administer CCAI to establish baseline information of students' perception of their cultural competency abilities and opportunities (Balcazar et al., 2008).

Strategies: Explore clinical reasoning as a reflective process (Neistadt, 1987) and as a conscientious problem-solving approach to implement sound and respectful care (Robertson, 2012).

Students were required to keep a reflective journal to record their experiences, reactions to readings and class discussions, and observations in the community in terms of understanding interactions and behaviors in different ways (Abreu & Peloquin, 2004; Black, 2002; Pooremamali, Persson, & Eklund, 2011; Taff & Hoyt, 2012).

Outcomes: Students identified relevant cultural beliefs and values that have shaped who they are and potentially will affect their clinical practice. Students acknowledged how their own biases could negatively affect professional interactions and decisions through self-exploration of own values, beliefs, and biases. Students demonstrated appreciation of how one's beliefs may subtly create barriers to provision of care.

EXAMPLES OF STUDENT CLASSROOM ACTIVITIES

Class Activity 1: "Who am I?"

Explore your own cultural background. Try going back two or three generations. Describe your ancestors, including their country of origin, family, language(s) spoken, religion, education, occupation, and beliefs regarding health or disease, disability, and education. Describe family roles and rules, family support networks, music, food preferences

and eating styles, entertainment, clothing, and child-rearing practices. How have cultural influences been maintained, changed, or disappeared throughout time or generations?

Goal: To address beginnings of cultural awareness and sensitivity. Self-reflection exercises encourage students to start thinking about their own race, culture, and identities that they subscribe to (gender, sexual orientation, occupation, religion, marital status, age, geographic location, race, nationality, ethnicity, disability, family roles, and socioeconomic status).

Class Activity 2: Preliminary outreach to community partners

- Students are required to initiate and complete IRB training at Rush University Medical Center; must receive IRB approval for interview projects before embarking on interview assignment.
- Students work in small groups and identify potential service partners in the community who work with ethnically and otherwise culturally diverse populations.
- Make initial contacts to explore interest in partnering with students and faculty.

PHASE 2: MODELS AND THEORIES OF CULTURAL COMPETENCE

- Learning about different models and theories; focus on two specific models with direct "occupational therapy in community" relevance in preparation for community service activities.

Objectives: Focus on classroom lectures and discussion from readings, including learning about work occupational therapists have accomplished in cultural competency training and social justice interventions (Braveman & Suarez-Balcazar, 2009; Kirsh, Trentham, & Cole, 2006; Kramer-Roy, 2012; Magasi & Hammel, 2009).

Strategies: Visiting presenters introduced models (Balcazar et al., 2009; Jezewski & Sotnik, 2001), provided examples of how they are used, and explained benefits of implementing them with clinical examples.

Outcome: Students verbalized and demonstrated knowledge of two models, including the ability to apply principles and steps of models to case scenarios. Students initiated and planned steps for making contact with community partners. Students developed professional mentoring relationships with representative cultural experts and visiting students who collaborated in class.

EXAMPLES OF ACTIVITIES

Multidisciplinary classroom opportunities focused on two cultural competence models

1. Culture Brokering Model (Jezewski & Sotnik, 2001). Researchers and visiting professor (education program–UIC).
2. CCBMDR Cultural Competence Model (Balcazar et al., 2009; Suarez-Balcazar et al., 2011). CCBMDR, Department of Disabilities and Human Development; UIC.
   - PhD and master's students from UIC (nursing and public health programs) in training taught cultural competency models.

Activity 1: Case studies

Student projects in class incorporating models (e.g., case studies from instructors' clinical experiences and CIRRIE [2012]).

Activity 2: Conceptual model analysis activity

Students present paper about relevance of CCBMDR and Culture Brokering Models to occupational therapy practice (Jezewski & Sotnik, 2001; Suarez-Balcazar et al., 2011).

PHASE 3: DEVELOPING COMMUNITY COLLABORATIVE PARTNERSHIPS

- **Preparation and development of community collaboration relationships.**

Objectives: Identify and confirm community partners and selected sites of care to introduce occupational therapy cultural sensitivity strategies or programmatic proposals. Apply classroom knowledge to community organizations. Develop outreach relationships with

organizations serving people of ethnic and racial minorities with disabilities.

Strategies: Students were provided with opportunities to learn about community organizations serving multicultural populations through Rush University liaisons. Student groups, with approval of the instructor and agency personnel, established contracts with professionals of disability organizations or other clinical sites to conduct health care provider interviews and then develop ongoing partnerships.

Outcome: Students, in groups of 4, identified at least 4 potential sites or organizations to contact for interviews and eventual program proposals with one organization selected ultimately.

EXAMPLES OF ACTIVITIES

Activity 1: Community contact activities

Students worked closely with the director of Multicultural Affairs and Community Services and the associate provost for Professional Education and Community Engagement, both at Rush University, to make initial contacts, establish relationships, and practice writing proposals, contracts, and intervention programs.

Activity 2: Practice sessions for making community connections

Students wrote short introduction letters to potential community organizations or partners and described their role as occupational therapy students desiring to develop partnership in community.

Activity 3: Working with interpreters; working with families or caregivers

Students produced strategies and problem-solving steps, using clinical decision and problem-solving steps for working respectfully with families and caregivers of various ethnicities and other backgrounds.

PHASE 4: SERVICE LEARNING OPPORTUNITIES: TAKING ACTION

- **Service Opportunities: community collaborative activities. Taking Action: transitioning classroom learning to community; applying** concepts learned to propose culturally sensitive occupational therapy programs of care in community site.

Objective: Develop partnerships with community organizations.

Strategies: Students reviewed interview questions with professor and shared in class for discussion. Students reviewed transcripts and practiced synthesizing for major themes.

Outcome: Completed transcripts with interview themes were used for research projects and as preparatory steps to proposing and implementing culturally responsive care in community organizations.

EXAMPLES OF ACTIVITIES

Community Project 1: Multicultural health care provider interviews

Conduct health care provider interviews with occupational therapists, other professionals, or agency staff working with individuals from diverse cultural backgrounds in greater Chicago (Phase 3: Initial community contacts).

Community Project 2: 6-week (2 hours per week) community outreach participation

Students created culturally responsive intervention or program development project for their community outreach sites.

Community Project 3: Create a proposal and presentation for professional conference.

Examples of strategies and interventions students proposed to implement culturally competent occupational therapy care:

- **Implement regular follow-up care:** Home visits from members of health care team to increase understanding of family's culture, home and community environments, attitudes about health care and disability, and resource needs.
- **Education and empowerment:** Develop accessible disability learning center, providing materials about disabilities and health care in multiple languages, including videos and illustrations for patients and family members.

PHASE 5: ESTABLISHMENT OF LONG-TERM COMMUNITY PARTNERSHIPS

- Establishment of community partnerships from class projects; ongoing relationships among occupational therapy students, faculty, and community organizations.

Objectives: Demonstrate ability to establish effective written and verbal communication skills that contribute to long-term partnerships with community leaders. Re-administered CCAI (Balcazar et al., 2008) for assessment of students' experiences with service learning model of cultural responsive training.

Strategies: Reviewed and confirmed with collaborators that ongoing community outreach would transform into ongoing or long-term relationships. Written structure of collaborations submitted to organizations that simultaneously served as the site of some students' master's of occupational therapy projects.

Outcomes: Community collaborations from student projects. Course assessments and analyses of findings.

COMMUNITY PARTNERSHIPS, INTERVENTION PARTNERSHIPS, AND RESEARCH COLLABORATIONS PROVIDING OCCUPATION-BASED SERVICES TO UNDERSERVED POPULATIONS

Serving as students' master's research or intervention projects (requirement for occupational therapy entry-level master's students).

1. **Hamdard Center for Health and Human Services Domestic Violence Program (Chicago):** Agency for Asian, Bosnian, and Middle Eastern clients who are victims of domestic violence.
2. **Growing Home:** Organization operating urban farms offering transitional employment and job training for people with histories of incarceration, homelessness, or substance dependence in Chicago area.

References

Abreu, B., & Peloquin, S. (2004). Embracing diversity in our profession. *American Journal of Occupational Therapy, 58*(4), 353–360. http://dx.doi.org/10.5014/ajot.58.3.353

Balcazar, F., Suarez-Balcazar, Y., & Taylor-Ritzler, T. (2009). Cultural competence: Development of a conceptual framework. *Disability and Rehabilitation, 31,* 1153–1160. http://dx.doi.org/10.1080/09638280902773752

Balcazar, F., Suarez-Balcazar, Y., Taylor-Ritzler, T., Rodakowski, J., Willis, C., & Portillo, N. (2008). *Cultural Competence Assessment Instrument (CCAI).* [Assessment instrument]. University of Illinois at Chicago, Chicago: Center for Capacity Building on Minorities with Disabilities Research. Provided by F. Balcazar, fabricio@uic.edu

Black, R. M. (2002). Occupational therapy's dance with diversity. *American Journal of Occupational Therapy, 56*(2), 140–148. http://dx.doi.org/10.5014/ajot.56.2.140

Braveman, B., & Suarez-Balcazar, Y. (2009). Social justice and resource utilization in a community-based organization: A case illustration of the role of the occupational therapist. *American Journal of Occupational Therapy, 63*(1), 13–23. http://dx.doi.org/10.5014/ajot.63.1.13

Center for International Rehabilitation Research Information and Exchange (CIRRIE). (2012). Buffalo, NY: University of Buffalo. Retrieved from http://cirrie.buffalo.edu/

Jezewski, M. A., & Sotnik, P. (2001). Culture brokering: Providing culturally competent rehabilitation services to foreign-born persons. In J. Stone (Ed.), *The rehabilitation provider's guide to cultures of the foreign-born.* [Monograph]. Center for International Rehabilitation Research Information & Exchange. Retrieved from http://cirrie.buffalo.edu/culture/monographs/cb.php

Kirsh, B., Trentham, B., & Cole, S. (2006). Diversity in occupational therapy: Experiences of consumers who identify themselves as minority group members. *Australian Occupational Therapy Journal, 53*(4), 302–313. http://dx.doi.org/10.1111/j.1440-1630.2006.00576.x

Kramer-Roy, D. (2012). Supporting ethnic minority families with disabled children: Learning from Pakistani families. *British Journal of Occupational Therapy, 75*(10), 442–448. http://dx.doi.org/10.4276/030802212X13496921049581

Magasi, S., & Hammel, J. (2009). Women with disabilities' experiences in long-term care: A case for social justice. *American Journal of Occupational Therapy, 63*(1), 35–45. http://dx.doi.org/10.5014/ajot.63.1.35

Neistadt, M. E. (1987). Classroom as clinic: A model for teaching clinical reasoning in occupational therapy education. *American Journal of Occupational Therapy, 41*(10), 631–637. http://dx.doi.org/10.5014/ajot.41.10.631

Pooremamali, P., Persson, D., & Eklund, M. (2011). Occupational therapists' experience of working with immigrant clients in mental health care. *Scandinavian Journal of Occupational Therapy, 18*(2), 109–121. http://dx.doi.org/10.3109/11038121003649789

Robertson, L. (2012). *Clinical reasoning in occupational therapy controversies in practice.* West Sussex, England: Wiley-Blackwell.

Suarez-Balcazar, Y., Balcazar, F., Taylor-Ritzler, T., Portillo, N., Rodakowsk, J., Garcia-Ramirez, M., & Willis, C. (2011). Development and validation of the cultural competence assessment instrument: A factorial analysis. *Journal of Rehabilitation, 77*(1), 4–13. http://vlex.com/vid/of-cultural-competence-instrument-analysis-418444526

Taff, S., & Hoyt, C. (2012, November 26). Going global in Guatemala. Supporting emerging occupational therapy practice in developing nations. *OT Practice,* pp. 14–19. Retrieved from https://www.scribd.com/document/115934702/OT-Practice-November-26-Issue

Chapter 25.

BUILDING AN INCLUSIVE EDUCATIONAL ENVIRONMENT TO SUPPORT DIVERSITY

Leslie K. Roundtree, DHS, MBA, OTR/L; Regina T. Smith, DHS, OTR/L; and Elizabeth Wanka, DrOT, OTR/L

> *Culture consists of connections, not of separations.*
> **Carlos Fuentes (1988, p. 21)**

Chapter Highlights

- Diversity in Occupational Therapy Programs
- High-Context Culture
- Contextual Learning Experience: Example of an Urban University
- Building a High-Context Educational Culture
- Benefits and Challenges of a High-Context Culture

Key Terms and Concepts

- ✧ Coaching
- ✧ Diversity
- ✧ Explicit communication
- ✧ Group study
- ✧ High-context cultures
- ✧ Integrated curriculum design

- ✧ Low-context cultures
- ✧ Modeling
- ✧ Peer support
- ✧ Service learning
- ✧ Team-taught courses
- ✧ Universal design principles

The occupational therapy profession has been striving to develop a globally connected and diverse workforce (American Occupational Therapy Association [AOTA], 2007a, 2015). Occupational therapy educational programs play a crucial role in meeting this strategic objective. This chapter describes how one urban state university's occupational therapy program created a "high-context" culture to provide a transformative educational experience for its diverse student population.

Diversity in Occupational Therapy Programs

Historically, students in occupational therapy educational programs have been homogeneous, consisting primarily of Caucasian middle-class women. Although there has been some change in the last 20 years in the ratio of race/ethnicity and gender from 90% to 84% Caucasian and 10% to 12% male, diversity continues to be limited among entry-level occupational therapy students within the categories collected (AOTA, 1994, 2012). Diversity within American society is pluralistic and related to a wide variety of factors beyond those traditionally cited, such as race, ethnicity, and gender.

Diversity is far more complex than ethnicity or race (Black & Wells, 2007; Kosoko-Lasaki, Cook, & O'Brien, 2009). According to Black (2002), **diversity** "is defined in broad terms that include not only racial and ethnic characteristics, but also gender, age, ability, sexual orientation, and class" (p. 140). Therefore, occupational therapy programs must consider a variety of characteristics, including age, socioeconomic status, first-generation college, disability status, number of dependents, and marital status among the students enrolled. These characteristics define each student's personal context and greatly influence the success and difficulty in completing his or her education.

To understand diverse student populations, educators must acknowledge each student's unique contribution to the academic environment. Developing and maintaining diversity within educational programs for health professions present both a challenge and an opportunity. The challenges encountered arise from a wide range of personal contexts and environmental factors the students bring to the day-to-day educational experience; educators often perceive circumstances as a threat to quality education (Ghosh, 2012; Klinger & Murray, 2012). For example, a low-income student who is distraught during class due to having no heat in her home or a student who is a parent may be upset over not having child care on the day of a test creates decision-making dilemmas for both the student and the educator. Yet, the opportunity provided by diverse student populations creates an authentic multicultural environment in which to explore varied perspectives and contexts. The growing diversity requires educational programs to create learning environments that acknowledge student similarities and differences while simultaneously offering all students opportunities for success.

Occupational therapy's principles emphasize person–environment interaction, which acknowledges that environment greatly influences performance. Consequently, occupational therapy programs must create an environment and context that support learning for all students.

High-Context Culture

Edward Hall (1997), an anthropologist and pioneer cross-cultural researcher, described how communication and the use of time and space create what he termed "high- and low-context cultures." **High-context cultures** are those in which individuals are deeply involved with each other and information is shared both verbally and nonverbally to understand the expectations of the environment (Hall, 1997). High-context cultures have a great commitment to long-term relationships, a sense of cohesiveness, and an internal locus of control among members. In high-context cultures, credibility is based on relationships and trust. Individuals involved in a task focus on building relationships with each other before completing the task. The process of task completion can be lengthy as members work on developing trust and communication.

Low-context cultures, on the other hand, are more focused on verbal language and what is explicitly stated rather than on nonverbal and environment cues that add meaning. This type of culture exhibits low commitment to relationships, fragile bonds between people, and a more external locus of control. For example, proceeding quickly to task completion and developing credibility through performance is emphasized. The focus is on completing the task rather than on developing relationships with the individuals involved in completing the task.

Most minority populations tend to have high-context cultures, in which interdependence is greatly valued (Giddens, 2008; Hall, 1997; Ibarra, 1999).

Reflection 25.1. Context in Higher Education

Consider the educational environment.

- What components are most emphasized and valued?
- Are individual accomplishments highly valued?
- How much focus is given to the relationships between faculty, faculty and students, and students and students?

Contextual Learning Experience: Example of an Urban University

The changing demographics of diversity in higher education can be seen in one urban state university that has a combined bachelor and master entry-level occupational therapy program. This 150-year-old urban institution was once a predominately majority educational institution but has been transformed over the past 30 years to a comprehensive university that is now predominantly minority. As a result, the university's mission has emphasized the recruitment, education, and graduation of nontraditional learners and those of diverse backgrounds.

The mission of the occupational therapy program is congruent with the university mission in educating underrepresented students of diverse backgrounds to become occupational therapists who provide effective and competent care to meet the demands of a rapidly changing health care system. The mission of both the university and occupational therapy program generates the diverse student population envisioned in AOTA's (2007a) *Centennial Vision*. The diverse student population prompted the urban occupational therapy program to develop a culture that addresses a wide variety of student needs.

The student body in this program is unique in its diversity when compared to the majority of occupational therapy programs. In 2012, among a group of 70 students, 57% were African American, 8.5% Asian, 3% Native Hawaiian/Pacific Islander, 28% Caucasian, and 3% Other. In regard to ethnicity, 11% were Hispanic and 89% non-Hispanic. Fourteen percent (14%) of the students were male,

60% of the students were ages 30 or older, and 24% were married. Other diversity characteristics included 44% of the students were first-generation college students, 44% were socioeconomically disadvantaged, and at least 41% were working during the program. Twenty-seven percent (27%) of the students were parents of school-age or younger children, and of those parents, 50% were single or divorced. Additionally, 8.5% of the students had an identified disability.

To address the needs of a diverse student population, when this occupational therapy program transitioned from an undergraduate degree to a combined bachelor of science/master of occupational therapy degree in 2004, the faculty purposefully created a high-context culture by embedding four multifaceted approaches into the curriculum. This contextual learning experience emphasizes (1) intentional design for faculty teamwork, (2) explicit communication and self-reflection, (3) universal design of support for all learners, and (4) building a sense of community and family.

Building a High-Context Educational Culture

Creating a culture within a program requires the participation of all stakeholders. The following approaches engage faculty, students, and their families in the educational experience.

Intentional Design for Faculty Teamwork

Faculty roles and responses to students are crucial and set the tone for an educational experience. To support the inclusive environment, the occupational therapy program intentionally designed its organizational structures and the processes that facilitate collaboration and faculty teamwork. A team-teaching approach was implemented to emphasize ongoing communication among faculty.

Typically, in *team-taught courses* two faculty members are assigned and divide the content based on expertise. During any given class session, one or both faculty members may be present. Nevertheless, ongoing communication about the day's activities is crucial for cohesiveness and course continuity.

The program was built with an *integrated curriculum design* in which no one faculty member has ownership of any course; course design is a collaborative effort of all faculty. Faculty members use each other's strengths, and the collaboration supports individual and program development. This organizational structure creates a sense of cohesiveness among the faculty for the success or failure of the courses. Research on faculty development and leadership describes how the sense of community among faculty assists with ongoing change and innovations in teaching (Dee & Daly, 2009; Kezar & Lester, 2009).

The meetings held at the beginning and end of each semester are an example of this intentional organizational structure. Meetings are scheduled before classes begin and after finals. During these meetings, all faculty members discuss the strengths and weaknesses of each course and student feedback, as well as provide input on course design and curriculum fit. At the beginning-of-the-semester meeting, faculty members review and critique syllabi, instructional strategies, learning activities, and course schedules. At the end-of-the-semester meeting, the faculty members discuss grades for each course and student issues, and assess their own performance.

The meeting discussions are different from the required peer review of each faculty member. Team members can evaluate each other; however, to reduce partiality, the same peer cannot evaluate faculty members two semesters in a row. In conjunction with debates about pedagogy, faculty members have ongoing discourse regarding students' responses to the structure and demands of the curriculum. This discourse, along with student assessment data, allows the faculty to adjust course material or format in a timely manner. Thus, the success of each course hinges on the team and all faculty members taking responsibility for the outcomes.

As a team, faculty members are committed to building strong relationships to maintain cohesiveness and support the intentional design. For example, at the faculty meetings, a standing agenda item is Faculty Share. During this time, faculty members share personal and professional successes and challenges. Besides conducting the business of the department, college, and university, the Faculty Share segment creates a supportive environment that develops unity. Consequently, the faculty members create a culture among themselves that mirrors the interdependence that is asked of the students.

Reflection 25.2. Faculty Share

- How much sharing is done between faculty members about individual courses, assignments, and class learning activities?
- Do faculty members value each other's opinions, or is there competition?

The program structure and culture also affect faculty recruitment. Faculty must be comfortable working as a team and willing to build a cohesive structure for students with diverse learning needs and backgrounds. The program has been successful in recruiting a diverse faculty team that is reflective of the student body.

Explicit Communication and Self-Reflection

The second approach we used to create a high-context culture was explicit communication and self-reflection. Doolittle, Sudeck, and Rattigan (2008) highlight the need for ongoing and direct communication to build effective learning communities. When working with diverse populations, one cannot assume that communication styles and patterns are the same. Faculty and students must continually engage in *explicit communication* and self-reflection to ensure a mutual understanding of both overt and covert sociocultural norms. *Explicit communication* is clear and detailed to minimize confusion and doubt.

The program's approach to communication was designed to facilitate the development of students' intra- and interpersonal skills. Research has shown that academic success is positively affected when students reflect on their own attitudes and biases as well as their own performance (Bercher, 2012; Smith, 2011). In this occupational therapy program, students are challenged to reflect on and analyze their role and responsibility in their own learning and their interactions with peers and faculty; then they must determine how they would change or improve the outcome when confronted with a similar situation. The classroom and fieldwork are both venues in which students can explore skills and support an internal locus of control.

The program uses multiple strategies to facilitate explicit communication and self-reflection such as an adapted professional development tool that was developed by the department, individual advisement, coaching and role modeling, engagement in service activities, and an assigned buddy system. Additionally, throughout the curriculum, course assignments emphasize self-reflection such as self-assessments and reflective journaling. Many occupational therapy programs have initiated the use of professional development tools or behavior checklists as well as provide individual advisement to students.

Continuous Communication

This occupational therapy program maintains continuous communication with students to encourage and support inter- and intrapersonal skill development. Students are required to meet at least twice per semester with their advisors. Advisors share student professional development goals with instructors. In turn, instructors provide feedback to a student in class or individually regarding inter- and interpersonal development skills. For example, when a student is very quiet and has a goal to increase class participation, an instructor may approach the student at the end of a class session and provide feedback regarding the student's initiative.

Reflection 25.3. Communication Style

- Ask students or faculty to identify examples of explicit and implicit communication.
- Discuss the types of communication used within one's own family and community, how the messages are interpreted, and the impact on relationships.

Coaching and Modeling

Coaching and **modeling** are the common threads that link all of the strategies. *Coaching* involves the direct observation of performance with immediate feedback in both group and individual situations. Coaching, along with self-reflection, facilitates a collaborative relationship between the faculty and students. *Modeling* refers to faculty demonstrating the professional behaviors and performance that reflect best practice.

Faculty coaches and models professional behaviors within multiple contexts and encourage students to self-reflect on each experience. These contexts include faculty-supervised Level I fieldwork experiences, student–faculty meetings, and service activities, as well as unscheduled hallway encounters. All interactions are considered to be teachable moments.

For example, in faculty-supervised Level I fieldwork, the faculty member demonstrates how to interview facility staff to obtain information about the environment or how to interview clients about their individual needs. Students and faculty then process these experiences to discuss the effectiveness of the communication and interactions. Students are encouraged and challenged to comment on the faculty member's behavior and compare observations to their own behaviors.

Students also develop skills in coaching and role modeling for their peers and future student cohorts. They hold each other accountable to the norms of the program, encourage each other to participate, and challenge each other to examine their own behavior. For example, students often remind each other of the dress code or encourage a peer to talk to his or her advisor and seek out assistance when under stress. Coaching and modeling by faculty and students create an environment for building relationships and promote development of intra- and interpersonal skills.

Peer Support

Peer support is the social support provided by one's peer group. The Student Occupational Therapy Association (SOTA) organized a peer support program known as the Buddy System. This system offers support for incoming students and provides a venue for sharing challenges at a nonthreatening peer-to-peer level. The senior students share tips on how they organize themselves to study, manage their time, and work with peers to share information. The Buddy System also gives students an opportunity to develop their own skills in mentoring, coaching, and role modeling.

The effect of coaching and modeling in this program aligns with researchers' assertions that these techniques build enduring relationships and a sense of community (Budhoo & Spurgeon, 2012; Law & Aquilina, 2013). One can feel the sense of community during the comprehensive exam period when second-year students facilitate study groups for the first-year students or when students seek feedback on their attempts to imitate or design learning activities that they have seen faculty implement in class.

Reflection 25.4. Cultural Objects

- In a class or meeting, ask everyone to bring 2 objects or artifacts that represent their culture. Encourage members to share what aspect of their culture is represented in the object or artifact and the values, rituals, or norms reflected.

Service Learning

Service is another component that builds inter- and intrapersonal communication skills. ***Service learning*** experiences are embedded throughout the curriculum in several courses and grant projects. According to Flecky and Gitlow (2011), "Service learning engages faculty and students with community partners in structured opportunities to meet academic learning objectives while addressing acknowledged community needs" (p. 2). Beyond service learning assignments and projects that are connected to a grade or other obligation, the program encourages students to develop a heart for service. Throughout the year, faculty and students volunteer for a variety of activities in the department, college, university, and community.

For example, several public schools with high populations of students with special needs invite students to volunteer during their annual field days or Special Olympics. Approximately one-third of the occupational therapy students participate in the events, which typically occur when occupational therapy classes are not in session. Students have also initiated clothing drives for local homeless shelters and mental health facilities. Through various service activities, students have multiple opportunities to reflect on their ability to interact with others, assume leadership roles, and value the role of service in the community.

Universal Design of Support for All Learners

Best practices in teaching promote the use of a variety of pedagogical strategies within the classroom to address the different learning styles found among students (Hooper, 2006). Academic environments with diverse student populations have greater variability of needs and contextual issues that affect all aspects of students' learning (Chita-Tegmark, Gravel, Serpa, Domings, & Rose, 2011; Schwieger, Gros, & Barberan, 2010). Currently, all levels of education, from elementary to post-secondary, are considering ***universal design principles*** that involve making curricula flexible and adaptable to a variety of learning needs and styles (Lancaster, 2008; Rose, Harbour, Johnston, Daley, & Abarbanell, 2006).

Typically, the increasing diversity in student populations within higher education has raised concerns that these students may lack adequate academic preparation and do not fit into the academy milieu (Klinger & Murray, 2012). This urban institution embraces diversity and uses a variety of student learning needs and contextual issues to build a culture of inclusion. A rigorous process is used for admission to the occupational therapy program, and the diverse students admitted are highly qualified. Application processes that may limit applicants based on socioeconomic status or cultural differences are avoided, which helps to build a diverse pool. Given the rigor of occupational therapy education and the diversity of students, the occupational therapy program adopted the principles of universal design and academic support.

Student Success Workshops

To increase the ability to succeed, this program offers all students help to develop and incorporate additional skills and strategies rather than exclusively targeting support to students when they start to have difficulty. The program works closely with a variety of university resources to enhance student performance. Several mechanisms have been developed to structure academic support within the program such as an adapted version of AOTA's *Professional Development Tool* (AOTA, 2003), Student Success workshops, and group study activities.

A unique characteristic of this program is a series of Student Success workshops conducted in conjunction with university resources. Given the demands of occupational therapy education, the amount of content covered, the demand for application of concepts, and a national competency measure of the certification examination, the faculty has identified common areas of challenge for students. These areas include test taking, study strategies, concept mapping, and research writing.

Additionally, to assist incoming students in their transition to a professional program, other workshops such as stress management and time management are offered. Faculty and students discuss content and learning strategies shared during the Student Success workshops in the various courses. Individually and as a group, students and faculty reflect on the use of the strategies and their effectiveness. This iterative approach reinforces faculty teamwork, communication, and self-reflection needed to build an interdependent learning community.

Reflection 25.5. Academic Support Programs

- Are your academic support programs seen as a resource for all students or only select students?
- Who participates in the academic support programs?
- What is the message given to students when referred to the services?

Group Study

Group study is an informal gathering of students to exchange ideas on a subject and is a basic approach used for building learning communities (Yan & Kember, 2004). However, this occupational therapy program views a group study strategy as a means to reduce competition between students and promote success of the entire student body. Each student is encouraged to study with everyone in the cohort as well as across cohorts.

For example, second-year students have been observed leading study groups for first-year students. This is a beneficial situation for everyone. It helps refresh earlier content learned by the second-year students and helps the first-year students increase their comprehension of new concepts. The explicit communication is that the entire cohort is to be successful and that each student supports the others.

Building a Sense of Community and Family

To build a sense of community and family, faculty, staff, and students celebrate as a collective group. This shared ritual of celebration supports retention of the diverse student population. These celebrations start with the orientation of a new group and continue through graduation and beyond. Formal and informal celebrations recognize everyone's efforts and successes at various times throughout the year. Students, faculty, and staff recognize both personal and professional milestones such as birthdays, acknowledgments of presentations or publications, and the completion of each semester.

Celebrations enable all participants to contribute and build connections within the learning environment. Developing a sense of community encourages interdependence among students and promotes a sense of social responsibility toward and with others (Bettez, 2011). The program embraces the idea of community and acknowledges the role each person has in supporting others' efforts to achieve success; therefore, everyone has an active part to play in successes and celebrations.

At the beginning of each academic year, the department hosts Family Night. This event includes all students, faculty, staff members, and their families. Students are encouraged to bring anyone who is considered to be a support to them while they are in the program. Faculty and staff members do the same. This event includes parents, children, spouses, siblings, significant others, and friends. In addition, alumni and their families are invited.

The annual Family Night is designed for networking, sharing, and building support. The event is a potluck dinner where everyone contributes to the meal. Food-enhanced events enable the natural sharing of cultural customs and rituals (Twiss, 2012). Although there is no formal program, the program director welcomes everyone and instructs the guests to mingle, ask questions, and share experiences. Family members have the opportunity to meet everyone the students encounter in the program, including faculty, staff, and other students. The faculty and staff share more about what it means to be in a demanding professional program. Alumni provide encouragement and serve as role models for success. Some families come year after year to catch up with each other and reminisce about the successes and challenges they experienced while going through the program.

Reflection 25.6. Celebrations

- Discuss the types of formal and informal celebrations in your department. Reflect on the purpose of the event, who participates, and the level of interactions among the participants.

Multiple celebrations are held each year. Some celebrations are department traditions such as the student-sponsored graduation party; others are spontaneous such as welcoming back a peer from a military leave of absence. Whether the event is small or large, informal or formal, these celebrations create opportunities for bonding and building community.

Benefits and Challenges of a High-Context Culture

Benefits

The major benefits of this multifaceted approach to learning are in the retention, graduation, certification exam pass, and employment rates of the diverse student population. In terms of retention, student attrition rates due to academic issues have decreased. The faculty members have found a strong association between students who value, adopt, and actively participate in program activities and their academic status within the program. The success in student retention is significant; the program graduates the highest number of racial- and ethnic-minority occupational therapists in the state. Within the past 5 years, other master's programs in the state have graduated between 17% and 28% of racial and ethnic minorities in occupational therapy. In contrast, 75% of the graduates from this urban program represented racial- or ethnic-minority groups (Illinois Board of Higher Education, 2007–2011).

A primary measure for all occupational therapy education programs is the first-time pass rate on the National Certification Board of Occupational Therapy (NBCOT) certification examination. Although the first-time pass rate of this program's graduates has fluctuated over time, the pass rate has steadily increased to a 76% first-time pass rate and a 95% overall pass rate. Although the first-time pass rate is a significant measure for all programs, the emphasis remains on the group's success to reach the ultimate goal of receiving certification, even if all test takers do not pass the exam on the first attempt. The evidence of community and student cohesiveness without the guidance of faculty is seen as graduates continue to study and work together to ensure that the entire cohort passes the certification exam either on the first or subsequent attempts.

Given the shortage of occupational therapists nationwide, all of the graduates of this program who pass the NBCOT exam are fully employed.

According to the Institute of Medicine (2004) and the U.S. Department of Health and Human Services Health Resources & Services Administration Bureau of Health Professions (2006) reports on health care workforces, diversity research shows that African American, Hispanic, Native American, and other ethnic groups are likely to practice in underserved communities and provide services to large numbers of patients with low socioeconomic status. Aligned with this research, a high proportion (70%) of the program's graduates practice occupational therapy in diverse and underserved communities.

For many of these diverse students, becoming an occupational therapist has significantly influenced their lives. Many of those who complete the program are first-generation college graduates and receive the first graduate degree in their family. Entering the health care workforce offers new socioeconomic opportunities along with advancement, which boosts the individual and his or her family. The ongoing social events within this program foster an alumni network that continues to bring graduates back to the educational environment to share their experiences.

Challenges

Although this high-context occupational therapy program offers many benefits, it also faces challenges. This type of cultural context is not comfortable for all students, particularly those who are not accustomed to or do not embrace a high level of communication and interdependence. On a few occasions, newly admitted students have been surprised by the extent of diversity within the student and faculty groups and have had difficulty relating and adjusting to the program's culture and demands. During information sessions and inquiries from potential applicants, faculty members attempt to minimize culture shock by providing rich descriptions of the program's culture and diversity. It is difficult to assess how this information affects potential applicants. The program has not received any feedback to indicate that applicants who do not apply or accept an invitation for admission do so because of the program's culture or diversity.

Another challenge is the amount of faculty commitment and time needed for ongoing communication and teamwork to support this high-context culture. Because communication is highly valued, faculty members often engage with students outside of regular office hours and scheduled meetings. Faculty and staff work as a team to ensure that boundaries are maintained to avoid dependency among the students. Therefore, faculty must be organized, protect their time, and balance their university responsibilities while providing support to the students. Although advisement is part of the faculty workload, all other initiatives and activities are considered to be services within the faculty retention and evaluation process. During the faculty recruitment process, members of the occupational therapy department explicitly communicate that they desire faculty who are committed to serving the program's diverse population.

A newer challenge is an increase in the number of millennial students admitted to the program. This generation of students often requires a great deal of external reinforcement, has a low tolerance for challenge, and is easily stressed (Bland, Melton, Welle, & Bigman, 2012; Montag, Campo, Weissman, Walmsley, & Snell, 2012). The program's collective group effort corresponds well to the social style of the millennial generation; however, the emphasis on self-reflection and the demands of the program seem to conflict with this generation's approach to education. Self-reflection and self-monitoring are crucial skills in developing the self-efficacy necessary for academic learning and student success (Bercher, 2012; Kitsantas, Winsler, & Huie, 2008). The program faculty is currently exploring metacognition and self-regulation strategies that promote self-efficacy and self-reflection.

When a large, nontraditional, and diverse student population that has multiple roles and responsibilities is present, varied personal contexts directly impact attrition. This program has had challenges, especially in the past 2 years (2013–2014), with more students withdrawing due to family illness, financial crises, or deaths of loved ones. Researchers exploring the reason for attrition across professional education in medical and health disciplines have found personal and family reasons to be a major factor (Kruzicevic et al., 2012; Pryjmachuk, Easton, & Littlewood, 2009). Because most of these unfortunate events cannot be anticipated, the faculty must work closely with other university resources to provide necessary support to the students.

Summary

This chapter discussed one urban occupational therapy program's approach in creating an inclusive culture that embraces diversity. Simply having a large diverse student population does not guarantee retention and graduation of diverse students. Programs must welcome students from diverse backgrounds, accept the unique personal contexts that these students bring to the environment, and develop strategies to assist and support the needs of a diverse student population. This occupational therapy program has created a multifaceted approach that can serve as a model and assist in reaching the *Centennial Vision* for diversity in our profession to meet the needs of our changing society.

References

American Occupational Therapy Association. (1994). *Education Data Survey Final Report*. Rockville, MD: Author.

American Occupational Therapy Association. (2003). *Professional development tool*. Bethesda, MD: Author. Retrieved from http://www.aota.org/education-careers/advance-career/pdt.aspx

American Occupational Therapy Association. (2007). AOTA's *Centennial Vision* and executive summary. *American Journal of Occupational Therapy, 61,* 613–614. http://dx.doi.org/10.5014/ajot.61.6.613

American Occupational Therapy Association. (2012). *Academic Programs Data Report*, Academic Year 2011–2012. Retrieved from http://www.aota.org/-/media/Corporate/Files/EducationCareers/Educators/OTEdData/Annual%20Data%20Report%202011-2012.pdf?la=en

American Occupational Therapy Association. (2015). Philosophy of occupational therapy education. *American Journal of Occupational Therapy, 69*(Suppl. 3), 6913410052. http://dx.doi.org/10.5014/ajot.2015.696S17

Bercher, D. A. (2012). Self-monitoring tools and student academic success: When perception matches reality. *Journal of College Science Teaching, 41*(5), 26–32.

Bettez, S. C. (2011). Critical community building: Beyond belonging. *Educational Foundations, 25*(3–4), 3–19. Retrieved from http://files.eric.ed.gov/fulltext/EJ954978.pdf

Black, R. M. (2002). Occupational therapy's dance with diversity. *American Journal of Occupational Therapy, 56*(2), 140–148. http://dx.doi.org/10.5014/ajot.56.2.140

Black, R. M., & Wells, S. (2007). *Culture and occupation: A model of empowerment in occupational therapy*. Bethesda, MD: AOTA Press.

Bland, H. W., Melton, B. F., Welle, P., & Bigman, L. (2012). Stress tolerance: New challenges for millennial college students. *College Student Journal, 46*(2), 362–375. http://dx.doi.org/10.1111/j.2150-1092.2012.00045_41.x

Budhoo, M. R., & Spurgeon, P. (2012). Views and understanding of clinicians on the leadership role and attitude to coaching as a development tool for clinical leadership. *International Journal of Clinical Leadership, 17*(3), 123–129.

Chita-Tegmark, M., Gravel, J., Serpa, M., Domings, Y., & Rose, D. (2011). Using the universal design for learning framework to support culturally diverse learners. *Education, 192*(1), 17–22. Retrieved from http://gaia.flemingc.on.ca/~jmior/EDU705Web/Georgian/UDL/UDL%20to%20Support%20Culturall%20Diverse%20Learners.pdf

Dee, J., & Daly, C. (2009). Innovative models for organizing faculty development: Pedagogical reflexivity, student learning empathy, and faculty agency. *Human Architecture: The Journal of the Sociology of Self-Knowledge, 7*(1), 1–21. Retrieved from http://scholarworks.umb.edu/humanarchitecture/vol7/iss1/2/

Doolittle, G., Sudeck, M., & Rattigan, P. (2008). Creating professional learning communities: The work of professional development schools. *Theory into Practice, 47*(4), 303–310. http://dx.doi.org/10.1080/00405840802329276

Flecky, K., & Gitlow, L. (2011). *Service-learning in occupational therapy education: Philosophy and practice.* Sudbury, MA: Jones & Bartlett.

Fuentes, C. (1988). *Myself with others: Selected essays.* New York: Farrar, Straus & Giroux.

Ghosh, R. (2012). Diversity and excellence in higher education: Is there a conflict? *Comparative Education Review, 56*(3), 349–365. http://dx.doi.org/10.1086/666545

Giddens, J. F. (2008). Achieving diversity in nursing through multicontextual learning environments. *Nursing Outlook, 56*(2), 78–83. http://dx.doi.org/10.1016/j.outlook.2007.11.003

Hall, E. (1997). *Beyond culture.* Garden City, NY: Anchor Press/Doubleday & Co.

Hooper, B. (2006). Epistemological transformation in occupational therapy: Educational implications and challenges. *OTJR: Occupation, Participation and Health, 26*(1), 15–24. http://dx.doi.org/10.1177/153944920602600103

Ibarra, R. A. (1999). Multicontextuality: A new perspective on minority underrepresentation in SEM academic fields. *Research News on Minority Graduate Education. 1*(3). Retrieved from http://ehrweb.aaas.org/mge/Archives/3/Multi.html

Illinois Board of Higher Education. *Annual Data Book of Illinois Higher Education.* Retrieved from http://www.ibhe.state.il.us/Data%20Bank/DataBook/default.asp

Institute of Medicine. (2004). *In the nation's compelling interest: Ensuring diversity in the health care workforce.* Washington, DC: National Academies Press.

Kezar, A., & Lester, J. (2009). Supporting faculty grassroots leadership. *Research in Higher Education, 50*(7), 715–740. http://dx.doi.org10.1007/s11162-009-9139-6

Kitsantas, A., Winsler, A., & Huie, F. (2008). Self-regulation and ability predictors of academic success during college: A predictive validity study. *Journal of Advanced Academics, 20*(1), 42–68. http://dx.doi.org/10.4219/jaa-2008-867

Klinger, C. M., & Murray, N. (2012). Tensions in higher education: Widening participation, student diversity and the challenge of academic language/literacy. *Widening Participation and Lifelong Learning, 14*(2), 27–44. http://dx.doi.org/10.5456/WPLL.14.1.27

Kosoko-Lasaki, S., Cook, C. T., & O'Brien, R. L. (2009). *Cultural proficiency in addressing health disparities.* Sudbury, MA: Jones & Bartlett.

Kruzicevic, S., Barisic, K., Banozic, A., Esteban, C., Sapunar, D., & Puljak, L. (2012). Predictors of attrition and academic success of medical students: A 30-year retrospective study. *Plos ONE, 7*(6), 1–4. http://dx.doi.org/10.1371/journal.pone.0039144

Lancaster, P. (2008). Universal design for learning. *Colleagues, 3*(1), Article 5. Retrieved from http://scholarworks.gvsu.edu/colleagues/vol3/iss1/5

Law, H., & Aquilina, R. (2013). Developing a healthcare leadership coaching model using action research and systems approaches—A case study: Implementing an executive coaching programme to support nurse managers in achieving organisational objectives in Malta. *International Coaching Psychology Review, 8*(1), 54–71. Retrieved from http://www.academia.edu/7891544/Developing_a_healthcare_leadership_coaching_model_using_action_research_and_systems_approaches_a_case_study_Implementing_an_executive_coaching_programme_to_support_nurse_managers_in_achieving_organisational_objectives_in_Malta

Sullivan Commission. (2004). *Missing persons: Minorities in the health profession, a report of the Sullivan Commission on diversity in the healthcare workforce.* Retrieved from http://www.aacn.nche.edu/media-relations/SullivanReport.pdf

Montag, T., Campo, J., Weissman, J., Walmsley, A., & Snell, A. (2012). In their own words: Best practices for advising millennial students about majors. *NACADA Journal, 32*(2), 26–35. http://dx.doi.org/10.12930/0271-9517-32.2.26

Pryjmachuk, S., Easton, K., & Littlewood, A. (2009). Nurse education: Factors associated with attrition. *Journal of Advanced Nursing, 65*(1), 149–160. http://dx.doi.org/10.1111/j.1365-2648.2008.04852.x

Rose, D. H., Harbour, W. S., Johnston, C., Daley, S. G., & Abarbanell, L. (2006). Universal design for learning in postsecondary education: Reflections on principles and their application. *Journal of Postsecondary Education and Disability, 19*(2), 135–151. Retrieved from http://www.udlcenter.org/sites/udlcenter.org/files/UDLinPostsecondary.pdf

Schwieger, F., Gros, E., & Barberan, L. (2010). Lessons from the culturally diverse classroom: Intellectual challenges and opportunities of teaching in the American university. *College Teaching, 58*(4), 148–155. http://dx.doi.org/10.1080/87567555.2010.484033

Smith, E. (2011). Teaching critical reflection. *Teaching In Higher Education, 16*(2), 211–223. http://dx.doi.org/10.1080/1356 2517.2010.515022

Twiss, K. (2012). The archaeology of food and social diversity. *Journal of Archaeological Research, 20*(4), 357–395. http://dx.doi .org/10.1007/s10814-012-9058-5

U.S. Department of Health and Human Services Health Resources & Services Administration Bureau of Health

Professions. (2006, October). *The rationale for diversity in the health professions: A review of the evidence.* Rockville, MD: Author. Retrieved from http://bhpr.hrsa.gov/healthworkforce /supplydemand/usworkforce/rationalefordiversity.pdf

Yan, L., & Kember, D. (2004). Engager and avoider behaviour in types of activities performed by out-of-class learning groups. *Higher Education, 48*(4), 419–438. http://dx.doi.org /10.1023/B:HIGH.0000046710.58007.9c

Chapter 26.

FOSTERING CULTURAL AWARENESS THROUGH FIELDWORK EXPERIENCES WITH PEOPLE FROM A REFUGEE BACKGROUND

Yda J. Smith, PhD, OTR/L

[W]hat I learned . . . is how they work with one another and how they work in their own environments. Their expectations, rules . . . I learned when you sit on a chair, when you don't sit on a chair, when you shake hands, when you don't shake hands, when you look somebody in the eyes or don't, refuse food, so on and so forth . . . [Y]ou're in the home, you're in their work sites . . . places like that working with them and you're the one that's out of place when you're there, so you don't get that experience anywhere else.
Yda J. Smith, Erika Cornella, & Nyles Williams (2013, p. 5)

Chapter Highlights

- Refugees and Why They Migrate
- Refugees in the United States
- Common Problems Faced During Resettlement
- Description of Fieldwork Setting
- Cultural Considerations for Students Before Work Begins
- Resolving Communication Barriers
- Developing Trust
- Managing Time
- Understanding How Culture Affects Employment
- Working in Client Homes
- Outcomes: Students' Cultural Learning

Key Terms and Concepts

- ❖ Natural environment
- ❖ Refugee
- ❖ Resettlement
- ❖ Trust

Awareness of variations in cultural backgrounds, behaviors, and beliefs is critical in the field of occupational therapy, and much can be learned about this topic in a classroom setting. Guided self-reflection, readings, classroom discussions, and guest lecturers from a variety of cultural groups all provide opportunities for students to become more aware of worldviews that are different from their own. However, as valuable as these classroom activities are, nothing can replace the power of lessons learned through interactions with people from differing cultures within the context of their own community settings (Keen & Hall, 2009). Within these contexts, some students may learn for the first time what it is like to be a minority—to be the "other."

Rich, profoundly moving, and life-changing experiences are common when students are personally involved with individuals and families off campus in the *natural environment* of their homes and communities. The quote that opens this chapter was provided by an occupational therapy student after completing a 12-week University of Utah fieldwork placement working with former refugees in Salt Lake City. The Immigration and Refugee Resettlement Fieldwork Program, sponsored by the Division of Occupational Therapy, was initiated in 2004 and currently runs for 40 weeks a year, with an average of 10 full-time and 7 part-time fieldwork students each year. Students from a variety of U.S. occupational therapy programs participate.

This chapter briefly describes the program and provides examples of the types of cultural encounters students experience, issues that have occurred, approaches taken to resolve these issues, and the educational benefits derived from this fieldwork experience.

Refugees and Why They Migrate

The United Nations High Commissioner for Refugees (UNHCR, 2005) defines a *refugee* as a person who, "owing to a well-founded fear of being persecuted for reasons of race, religion, nationality, membership of a particular social group, or political opinion, is outside the country of his or her nationality and who is unable to, or unwilling to, return to the country of origin" (p. 5).

People become labeled as *refugees* when they are forced to migrate across international borders due to political unrest and when their own governments are incapable of protecting them from physical harm inflicted by others. According to UNHCR, the number of refugees worldwide in 2014 was 19.5 million (UNHCR, 2014). Final statistics for more recent years will, no doubt, be higher, with the number of Syrian refugees reaching 4 million in July 2015 (UNHCR, 2015). The U.S. Office of Refugee Resettlement (USORR, 2015) reports that 69,986 refugees were settled in the United States in 2014, with 1,085 of them placed in Utah. The majority of refugees arriving in Utah that year were from Burma, Iraq, Somalia, and the Democratic Republic of the Congo. Utah typically receives around 1,000 refugees per year.

Refugees in the United States

When refugees step foot on U.S. soil, they have entered a country willing to accept their presence and protect them from harm. After 1 year, they are expected to apply for permanent residence, and after 5 years, they can apply for U.S. citizenship (U.S. Citizenship and Immigration Services, 2008).

Many people with refugee backgrounds consider the term *refugee* inappropriate and offensive. For these individuals, they no longer identify as a refugee. Having arrived and no longer fleeing, they want to leave this label, and its connotation of lack of belonging to a nation-state, behind. Some resent the continued use of the term *refugee* after arrival in their host country and want to be called *new Americans, people with a refugee background,* or *people with refugee experience* (A. Mohamed, personal communication, August 30, 2013).

Similar issues regarding labels have come up in other countries, including Canada (Kumsa, 2006). For this reason, this chapter does not label people in the United States as *refugees,* although the term is commonly used by refugee resettlement service providers.

Common Problems Faced During Resettlement

Resettlement is a term used to describe the act of moving from a settled position in one location to another. In some cases, literature about refugees refers to relocation in a third country as an act of *settlement*, not resettlement, reflecting the perception that one cannot be truly settled in a refugee state. In the United States, the term *resettlement* is most commonly used. For refugees, resettlement in a new country, free from the stresses and violence of their homeland and the confinement of refugee camps, is an enormously positive event. When asked how life is different in the United States, many respond with statements such as "can sleep at night" or "safe here" (H. Sido, personal communication, 2005). Still, the transition to life in the United States has tremendous challenges.

Language barriers are prevalent and contribute to difficulties securing employment (Haines, 2010; Mitchell, 2009; Mitschke, Mitschke, Slater, & Teboh, 2011). Occupational restrictions, exacerbated by transportation and technological barriers, such as participation in education and community social events, can lead to occupational deprivation (McAllister, Penn, Smith, Van Dort, & Wilson, 2010; Whiteford, 2000) as access to occupations is denied.

People with refugee backgrounds, in particular those from developing countries, often come from agrarian or urban environments where written language and computer skills were not needed to provide for the basic necessities of life. In other cases, they are highly educated and held professional positions in their home countries, but their education and certifications are not accepted as legitimate in the United States. They must be formally recertified to practice their profession legally (Rabin, 2013).

Adapting to a new culture and environment can be extraordinarily stressful (Haines, 2010; Mitchell, 2009). Routines are disrupted, and former occupational roles may be lost (Whiteford, 2004). Many are unable to participate in cultural traditions and meaningful occupations they once found valuable.

> Men, women, and children with a refugee background have specific occupational needs that must be met to ensure quality of life, some of which include learning a new language, new ways of social interaction, new occupations, and new routines, as well as fulfilling new social and occupational roles. (Smith, Cornella, & Williams, 2013, p. 3)

Reflection 26.1. Establishing Evaluation Priorities

A 67-year-old Congolese man has just been admitted to your clinic with injuries from a motor vehicle accident. He has been in the United States for 2 months with refugee status. He speaks broken English.

• Given the information above, where would you begin with this man?
• What is the first thing you would want to address with him?

When addressing resettlement of people with refugee backgrounds who have recently arrived in their new country, an occupational perspective can facilitate resettlement work and enhance the adjustment process through individually targeted life skills training (Whiteford & Suleman, 2013). Although occupational therapy education provides the training to prepare students for work in this setting, occupational therapists are rarely employed by refugee service providers. To explore the benefits of occupational therapy services in work with people with a refugee background, an occupational therapy fieldwork program was developed in Salt Lake City, Utah.

Description of Fieldwork Setting

The University of Utah Division of Occupational Therapy Immigration and Refugee Resettlement Fieldwork Program began in 2004 with the intent to address the occupational needs of people of immigrant or refugee backgrounds. Students from the University of Utah (UU) and schools in other parts of the United States elect to participate in this fieldwork program under the supervision of an occupational therapist.

The program works as a collaboration between students, UU faculty, culturally diverse populations living in the local community, and community organizations, including University Neighborhood Partners–Hartland Partnership (UNP–Hartland), the International Rescue Committee, and Utah Health and Human Rights. UNP–Hartland is university and grant funded and provides a home base for the occupational therapy fieldwork program.

Supervision across all of the settings is provided by one occupational therapist employed by the UU. The settings (e.g., community center, refugee resettlement agency, nonprofit mental health service) vary in terms of their primary missions and funding sources, but all provide services for people who have come to the area with immigration or refugee backgrounds.

Occupational therapy students collaborate with social work students, neighborhood residents, and community organizations to determine youth and adult programming that provides individual and group sessions. Occupational therapy students provide classes and training in cultural orientation, rules of the road for driving, computer access, and completion of college and financial aid applications.

Running the PAR FORE Group

Occupational therapy students also run the PAR FORE group (a life skills and golf program for youth), which was founded by Alexander Lopez (Lopez & Block, 2011). Activities and discussions during the life skills portion of PAR FORE cover core values of the program (perseverance, accountability, resilience, fellowship, opportunity, respect, and empowerment), the importance of education, goal setting, verbal and nonverbal communication, stress management, and teamwork as well as golf etiquette.

Traditional Weaving

UNP provides space and support for a traditional weaving group, facilitated by occupational therapy, for women from Burma who are from the Karen and Karenni ethnic groups, providing the women with an opportunity to restore and maintain their participation in a deeply meaningful occupation (Smith, Stephenson, & Gibson-Satterthwaite, 2013; Stephenson, Smith, Gibson, & Watson, 2013).

Occupational Therapy in the Home and Community

The International Rescue Committee (IRC) is a refugee resettlement agency funded through federal funds and grants; it manages client cases and provides services for people with refugee backgrounds for their first 2 years. Occupational therapy students teach the predriving class at this location, but they do the majority of their work in the community with individuals who are learning how to live in a Western urban environment for the first time. Individual sessions vary greatly, depending on interests and needs, and include public transportation training

(see Figure 26.1), grocery shopping, and budgeting and money management, as well as home maintenance. Frequently, students are brought in on cases that are complicated by health issues such as diabetes, cognitive impairments, or physical disabilities.

Reflection 26.2. Measuring Your Comfort Level

Identify and highlight the numerous occupations that occupational therapy students may be involved in when working with people with refugee backgrounds who have recently arrived in the United States.

- How comfortable would you feel when engaged in these activities with former refugees who have vastly different cultural behaviors and expectations than your own?
- If uncomfortable, what action can you take to ease some of your discomfort?
- Can you think of other occupations you might want to engage in with this population?

Additional Home-Based Services

At times, students are asked by staff of partnering agencies to help adult residents understand how to clean their apartments to avoid the possibility of eviction. Western homes are different from the ones many new residents are accustomed to maintaining, and residents may need basic training to meet apartment management standards.

Working on home maintenance can also create opportunities to provide education on apartment leases, resident rights, and how to communicate with the apartment manager when home repairs are needed. Interacting with people with refugee backgrounds in their homes on such personal issues may present encounters with alternative belief and value systems. Students learn about these alternative perspectives by talking with their supervisor, with knowledgeable and experienced staff at the various organizations they work with, and with the clients themselves.

Working With Survivors of Torture

Occupational therapy students provide individual sessions with people accessing services at the Utah Health and Human Rights Project (UHHR), which is funded through grants that serve refugees and

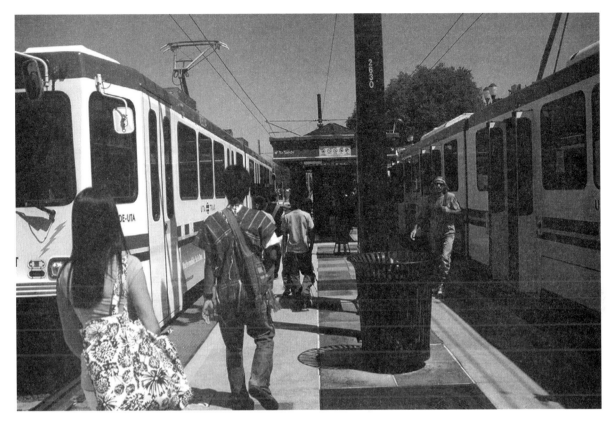

Figure 26.1. Public transport training.

asylum seekers who are survivors of torture. Therapists at UHHR provide mental health services for this population, most having been diagnosed with major depressive disorder, posttraumatic stress disorder (PTSD), generalized anxiety disorder, or a combination of these.

Sessions with students may include life skills training such as the ones mentioned above or may be more focused on mental health, facilitating engagement in meaningful occupations within the home or community. Occasionally occupational therapy cognitive assessments are requested because of the high incidence of mild to moderate brain trauma caused by injuries suffered during imprisonment or torture in their home countries.

Although some sections of Western-based cognitive assessments are culturally inappropriate for this population and results, in most cases, cannot be compared to a normed value, the assessments provide important information that informs treatment planning. Cognitive assessments addressing memory skills may be helpful during requests for disability funding or for access to U.S. citizenship by means of a path that takes the person's cognitive disability into consideration.

Students involved in this fieldwork program are assigned to multiple settings that provide a great deal of variety in the types of strategies needed to meet the occupational needs of the people who are assigned to them. The students organize their own schedules, provide their own transportation from one site to another, and communicate regularly with caseworkers, therapists, and other staff at the various organizations.

Meetings are held weekly with their occupational therapy supervisor, and supervision is provided during many of the classes and individual sessions. Students are required to write documentation in a format that includes objective observations, assessments, and goals. They also write critical practice audits and weekly activity summaries.

Cultural Considerations for Students Before Work Begins

To facilitate positive therapeutic relationships, students must be aware of many cultural considerations before starting their work with this population.

Appropriate Clothing

Discussing appropriate clothing and behavior in clients' homes is a good place to begin a conversation with students about cultural considerations. Many people coming to the United States are more modest in their dress and may be offended by some of the clothing typical of Westerners, especially during the summer. Students are given these guidelines:

- Avoid tops, such as those with spaghetti straps, that expose a lot of skin on the upper trunk and arms. Avoid short skirts and shorts.
- Keep dress, even if casual, neat and clean.
- Remove shoes just inside the front door when entering homes. (It is helpful to wear shoes that slip on and off easily.)
- Because a standard custom in the home is to sit on the floor rather than on furniture, students should be prepared to sit on the floor but may be offered a seat on a couch or chair. The student should determine if the most polite gesture is to sit on the furniture, or if residents of the home are clearly accustomed to sitting on the floor, it may be more appropriate to thank them for the offer but to sit on the floor with everyone else to demonstrate the desire to develop positive relationships and shift power away from students, who may be viewed as professionals by the people they are working with.

Food and Drink

Frequently, food and drink are offered as a gesture of appreciation for the presence of the students and their willingness to help with life skills training. It may be considered rude to refuse these offers. On the other hand, students are told by their occupational therapy supervisor that they are not expected to eat food or drink beverages that are not in line with their own food restrictions. For example, vegetarians are not expected to eat meat when it is offered to them. Often the offered drink is high in sugar content, which may also be an issue for the student. One strategy is to bring a bottle of water to the home session but demonstrate gratitude for the offer. Another option is to take the soft drink, do not open it, and when leaving, state gratefully that it will be consumed later.

In some cases, food is prepared each time the student visits, interfering with the student's treatment plan. If this occurs, the student should graciously let the person know that other activities need to take priority. All families that students work with have limited budgets, which should also be considered when deciding whether to accept offers of food and drink.

Gender Roles

Gender-based roles within the family, informed by religious beliefs or cultural traditions, often differ from family role expectations the student is accustomed to. Before a first visit, students should research common customs and beliefs of that person's cultural group and reflect on how these are the same or different from the student's personal cultural expectations.

Families from Islamic cultures may expect women to stay home, raise children, and care for the family. They may come from locations where women are not encouraged, or are not allowed, to drive cars. Issues around community access and driving can become a point of tension between a husband and wife. U.S. government programs for refugee resettlement may require that both a husband and wife work outside the home to receive government benefits such as food stamps and health care. Additionally, families may not be able to meet their expenses without both parents being employed.

Women often have an easier time securing employment because hotel housekeeping jobs are relatively abundant; work for men with limited English skills may be harder to locate. In some cases, women become the primary financial provider, which can significantly upset family dynamics.

In addition, when women come to the United States and see the many options that Westernized women have in terms of education, employment, and so forth, they may decide they would like to participate in activities outside of their traditional roles.

Occupational therapy students assigned to work with women from Islamic cultures have, on occasion, felt conflicted as to how to best offer occupational services. In one case, for example, the woman of the household wanted to learn how to drive and pass the written driver's license test. She also wanted to learn how to ride the bus, shop on her own, and use a credit card. Her husband did not approve of any of these activities, expecting her to stay home and to get help from male family members when shopping. She asked the students to work on these skills with her when her husband was not home.

This led to some discomfort for the students and to conversations with their supervisor about how to handle this dilemma. Students discussed their sense of unease with her and worked within her home for the next few sessions. As therapy progressed, she made the personal choice to comply with her husband's wishes.

Getting to Know Clients

An occupational therapist in any setting must get to know the people on their caseload in areas that go beyond the medical diagnosis, but it is particularly important when working with people from cultures where time is taken to get to know each another. As a general rule, health care professionals in the United States ask questions of their patients and clients, but they do not share much about themselves, maintaining a professional distance. When developing a therapeutic relationship with people with a refugee background, sharing something of yourself can be important. In addition, health care professionals generally do not ask about the person's traditional health care beliefs. When working with former refugees, students may need to take time to ask questions, listen, and learn about personal traditional approaches to healing if relationships built on trust are to be developed. Dedication to the well-being of a particular family or community can also be enhanced by attending events such as birthday parties, weddings, and cultural celebrations.

Reflection 26.3. Understanding Health Care Beliefs

List 3 questions you might ask people with a refugee background that would help you understand their traditional health care beliefs.

Resolving Communication Barriers

Most people with a refugee background that occupational therapy students interact with in this program speak little or no English when they arrive in the United States. The agencies referring people to occupational therapy have limited budgets, so interpretation services are frequently not available.

In some cases, clients' friends, family members, or even neighbors can assist.

However, depending on the sensitivity of the conversation, it may not be appropriate to ask a friend or family member to help (Refugee Health Technical Assistance Center, 2011). This is especially true when health care issues are being discussed. When setting up interpreter services, one cannot assume that because the interpreter speaks the same language, the service will be appropriate for that person. For example, members of Somali communities often avoid interpreters from their own cultural group for fear their private information will become a source of gossip (A. Mohamed, personal communication, November 26, 2013). People of the Karen ethnic group from Burma may refuse to work with Burmese interpreters (P. L. Eh, personal communication, September 7, 2013), and members of the Somali Bantu community may be uncomfortable with Somali interpreters because of their personal experiences of persecution in their home countries (Smith, 2011).

When topics that need to be discussed are complex, an interpreter may be necessary, but in most cases, the skills being addressed by the student do not require assistance in this area. Highly simplified English and gestures can go a long way in communicating how to accomplish daily activities. For example, learning how to ride public transportation can be taught by pointing out significant landmarks, demonstrating how to pay the fare, and showing how to pull the cord to alert the driver to stop. Color coding and drawings can be used to assist with occupation-based interventions such as medication management. Shopping for food in a grocery store can be done with little or no communication in English.

Developing Trust

For the most part, people with refugee backgrounds have little trouble developing a sense of ***trust*** in the occupational therapy student and her or his integrity and abilities. They are eager to learn and grateful for opportunities to spend time with students who are providing group or individual training. In most cases they willingly, and spontaneously, share personal information and private documents. The information and papers they share are helpful in development of appropriate intervention content, but new Americans must be made aware that personal information, such as Social Security numbers, need to be shared cautiously.

Working with people with significant histories of torture or trauma can result in challenges to the development of trust. Some refugees are survivors of physical or mental torture or both (Hollifield et al., 2002). PTSD and symptoms of depression are common and can result in complaints of "diffuse bodily pain, headaches, sleeplessness, nightmares, poor concentration, flashbacks, intrusive thoughts, shame, guilt, hopelessness, disorientation, and feelings of betrayal" (Black, 2011, p. 219). Such traumatic experiences can make it difficult to feel safe and develop relationships with others.

In addition, many people with refugee backgrounds have lost people very close to them, and they may avoid short-term relationships, such as those inherent in student–client relationships, to avoid sensations of loss or abandonment. In some cases, therapists in a position to refer people to an occupational therapy student may choose to protect their clients from what they perceive to be the potential threat of continued traumatization caused by this short-term association. However, if handled appropriately, these clients may be able to experience high-quality relationships that do not lead to further traumatization.

If the referring caseworker or therapist is reluctant to refer clients to occupational therapy because of a history of torture or PTSD, the potential value of occupational therapy should be pointed out. Occupational therapy can focus on life skills training, which can result in reduced levels of stress. It can also focus on engagement in meaningful activities that provide an opportunity for clients to focus on a task they find pleasurable, shifting their thoughts away from their recurring negative mental images. A referring case worker or therapist can be informed that occupational therapy education includes training in how to gather information about personal and environmental factors that affect participation in occupations, understanding that "symptoms need to be understood contextually and within the spiritual, cultural, and social traditions of each survivor" (Black, 2011, p. 219).

Students need to spend time listening and observing rather than rushing into treatment. Allowing the client to share information about cultural, social, and religious practices can provide valuable information for a comprehensive assessment that results in more appropriate treatment approaches.

The development of positive relationships can be enhanced by demonstrating an interest in cultural traditions, asking people questions about their country and family members, and learning a few words in their native language.

Managing Time

Management of daily appointments is an issue that comes up frequently. People coming to the United States with refugee status are often from cultures where relationships with people and human interactions take precedence over schedules. This can be frustrating for U.S. students who are from cultures where time compartmentalizes events and who expect appointments to start on time.

Participants may show up for classes well after they have started, which disrupts the smooth delivery of the lesson plan, or they may not show up at all. Students often arrive at someone's home at the mutually agreed upon time only to find that the person they are planning to work with is not there.

People not accustomed to writing down appointments or using a calendar may not demonstrate interest in suggestions as to how to remember appointments because this has never been part of their lifestyle. Teaching how to track appointments is particularly challenging when someone is illiterate, not only in English but also in her or his native language. Strategies that can be helpful for class attendance include calling participants before classes begin or knocking on participant doors before class starts to remind them to attend. Students can also work on strategies for remembering appointments. Keeping a monthly calendar in the home to track appointments is often helpful, but those new to using a calendar need to get accustomed to looking at it daily.

Reflection 26.4. Temporal Expectations

- Are you a person who is (1) Always on time? (2) Rarely on time? (3) Often early?
- How would you feel and what would you do if the new Americans you are working with do not adhere to U.S. cultural expectations for time management?
- What strategies might you use to help them adjust to U.S. temporal expectations?

Understanding How Culture Affects Employment

Numerous cultural issues affect access to employment opportunities in the United States. In many cultures, men work outside the home while women are at home cooking, cleaning, and raising children. Dress codes in work settings may create problems for women who are Muslim. In adherence to traditional Muslim dress standards, Muslim women often refuse employment in a setting where they are required to wear pants (A. Ibrahim, personal communication, January 14, 2013). People adhering to Muslim traditions may not be willing to handle pork products of any kind, even if they are canned. However, most entry-level jobs are in housekeeping and manufacturing where dress codes dictate that skirts or dresses are not allowed, and no options are offered for altering work duties to avoid pork products.

Occupational therapy students are not expected to locate employment options, but they can discuss possible compromises that Muslim women have used in the past, such as wearing a long apron over pants. Students also provide capacity-building opportunities while helping people fill out job applications, create a résumé, or role play interviewing skills. During this process, students become aware of the many cultural challenges women may face in relation to employment and the internal conflicts some must deal with while reconsidering or renegotiating their roles and responsibilities.

Working in Client Homes

Much of the work done by students in this program takes place in the home. One fieldwork occupational therapy student wrote the following in a reflection paper:

> The setting context significantly influences the way I do my work and how I interact with my clients. . . . During a home visit I tend to take more of a backseat . . . allowing them to welcome me into their home and show me how to behave in a culturally competent manner. . . . I also tend to be more observant during a home visit as I note and analyze how they behave, dress, decorate their home, etc., and how this may alter my impression of their strengths and needs.

There are advantages and disadvantages to working in the home environment, but when it comes to learning about cultural context, the advantages are tremendous. In the client's home environment, one can see the furnishings, photographs, and wall decorations that provide information about religious and cultural preferences, history, and values. These items can spark conversation and be used to demonstrate interest in the person's background. There is a noticeable shift in dynamics between the therapist and the client when the client is in her or his own space. Clients may appear more at ease and are often more willing to share their thoughts and concerns, and trust may be more easily developed.

Distractions, such as children making noise or interruptions caused by friends dropping by, can disrupt the session, but within the home, family dynamics are more apparent. One occupational therapy student commented, "Visiting clients in their natural environment is the quickest way to get a sense of how they spend their time, how well they are able to manage the home, and the dynamics between parents and children."

In the home, students can see how well the home is maintained and gain access to utility bills and other items that are needed for life skills training. People who come to the United States with refugee status are often confused by the mail they receive. They are unable to tell utility bills, health care statements, and other important documents apart from junk mail. Bill paying, home cleaning and management, communication with rental management, and other home-related tasks are best taught in the natural environment. Another student stated, "It is also very easy to implement change. The changes you implement are more durable because they are made with the person and their context in mind."

Outcomes: Students' Cultural Learning

To examine the educational benefits of fieldwork education working with people with a refugee background, 14 occupational therapy students who completed a 12-week full-time fieldwork experience with this program were interviewed to get their perspectives on the program. Several educational benefits were identified, but cultural awareness stood out as a major theme throughout all interviews (Smith et al., 2013). The following quotes from study participants demonstrate lessons learned:

> "I developed a cultural sensitivity that could not have been learned anywhere else . . . I am [now] able to put aside my own agenda or American perspective to really understand the occupational profile of an individual, which so often is incredibly influenced by culture, and use that information to develop meaningful treatment" (p. 5).

> "I am not afraid to work with someone who doesn't speak English, and that's a huge confidence booster for me . . . . It also helped me be more bold in incorporating their culture into the therapy" (p. 5).

> "[I] still feel like I have a long way to go in cultural competency. I think I see now that it's a process, not really, like an end goal" (p. 5).

> "I think when you're not exposed to these other groups you have some type of preconceived notion of who they are or who they're not, and this can impact how you interact with that person" (p. 5).

Direct involvement with people from other cultures can foster self-reflection on personal cultural beliefs and can lead to an awareness of biases and inaccurate assumptions. It can help students approach individuals with a more open and inquisitive mind-set and can cultivate more positive therapeutic relationships.

Since the initiation of the Immigration and Refugee Resettlement Fieldwork Program, students have consistently expressed their appreciation for an opportunity to work in an environment that reinforces the value of occupation-based practice in the client's natural setting. Along with experiences that teach invaluable lessons about culturally effective care, students have been able to practice foundational professional skills such as grading tasks and therapeutic use of self. Numerous educational advantages are inherent in this emerging practice setting while, at the same time, refugee resettlement service providers discover how occupational therapy can enhance the quality of resettlement work.

Summary

Thousands of refugees arrive in cities throughout the United States every year and need education and training in how to function within a society far different from the one they left behind. It is an honor and privilege to get to know these individuals and to have the chance to learn from them. This chapter briefly described an occupational therapy fieldwork program working with people with a refugee background that sets the stage for recognition and respect for diverse cultural beliefs, values, and lifestyles.

Culturally effective care can be developed within a setting of this nature, providing students with the opportunity to realize that what they have always considered "normal" may be only one version of normalcy, and culture, in all of its variations, is a part of each person as an occupational being.

References

Black, M. (2011). From kites to kitchens: Collaborative community-based occupational therapy with refugee survivors of torture. In F. Kronenberg, N. Pollard, & D. Sakellariou (Eds.), *Occupational therapies without borders: Towards an ecology of occupation-based practices* (Vol. 2, pp. 217–226). New York: Elsevier.

Haines, D. W. (2010). *Safe haven: A history of refugees in America.* Sterling, VA: Kumarian.

Hollifield, M., Warner, T. D., Nityamo, L., Krakow, B., Jenkins, J., Kesler, J., … Westermyer, J. (2002). Measuring trauma and health status in refugees: A critical review. *Journal of the American Medical Association, 288*(5), 611–621. Retrieved from http://www.healtorture.org/sites/healtorture.org /files/JAMA%202002.pdf

Keen, C., & Hall, K. (2009). Engaging with difference matters: Longitudinal student outcomes of co-curricular service-learning programs. *Journal of Higher Education, 80*(1), 59–79. Retrieved from https://muse.jhu.edu/article/256462

Kumsa, M. K. (2006). "No! I'm not a refugee!" The poetics of belonging among young Oromos in Toronto. *Journal of Refugee Studies, 19*(2), 230–255. http://dx.doi.org/10.1093/jrs /fel001

Lopez, A., & Block, P. (2011). PAR FORE: A community-based occupational therapy program. In F. Kronenberg, N. Pollard, & D. Sakellariou (Eds.), *Occupational therapies without borders: Towards an ecology of occupation-based practices* (Vol. 2, pp. 285–292). New York: Elsevier.

McAllister, L., Penn, C., Smith, Y., Van Dort, S., & Wilson, L. (2010). Fieldwork education in non-traditional settings or with non-traditional caseloads. In L. McAllister, M. Paterson, J. Higgs, & C. Bithell (Eds.), *Innovations in allied health fieldwork education: A critical appraisal* (pp. 39–47). Rotterdam, Netherlands: Sense.

Mitchell, A. (2009). Reflections on working with South Sudanese refugees in settlement and capacity building in regional Australia. In N. Pollard, D. Sakellariou, & F. Kronenberg (Eds.), *A political practice of occupational therapy.* London: Elsevier.

Mitschke, D. B., Mitschke, A. E., Slater, H. M., & Teboh, C. (2011). Uncovering health and wellness needs of recently resettled Karen refugees from Burma. *Journal of Human Behavior in the Social Environment, 21,* 490–501. http://dx.doi.org/10.1080 /10911359.2011.566466

Rabin, L. (2013). *Credential recognition in the United States for foreign professionals.* Washington, DC: Migration Policy Institute.

Refugee Health Technical Assistance Center. (2011). *Best practices for communicating through an interpreter.* Retrieved from http://refugeehealthta.org/access-to-care/language-access /best-practices-communicating-through-an-interpreter/

Smith, Y. J. (2011). *They bring their memories with them: Somali Bantu resettlement in a globalized world* (Doctoral dissertation). Ann Arbor, MI: Proquest.

Smith, Y. J., Cornella, E., & Williams, N. (2013). Working with populations from a refugee background: An opportunity to enhance the occupational therapy educational experience. *Australian Occupational Therapy Journal.* http://dx.doi.org /10.1111/1440-1630.12037

Smith, Y. J., Stephenson, S., & Gibson-Satterthwaite, M. (2013). The meaning and value of traditional occupational therapy practice: A Karen woman's story of weaving in the United States. *WORK: A Journal of Prevention, Assessment and Rehabilitation, 45*(1), 25–30. http://dx.doi.org/10.3233/WOR-131600

Stephenson, S. M., Smith, Y. J., Gibson, M., & Watson, V. (2013). Traditional weaving as an occupation of Karen refugee women. *Journal of Occupational Science, 20*(3), 224–235. http://dx.doi.org/10.1080/14427591.2013.789150

Suleman, A., & Whiteford, G. (2013). Understanding occupational transitions in forced migration: The importance of life skills in early refugee resettlement. *Journal of Occupational Science, 20*(2), 201–210. http://dx.doi.org/10.1080/14427591 .2012.755908

United Nations High Commissioner for Refugees. (2005). *Refugee status determination: Identifying who is a refugee.* Retrieved from http://www.unhcr.org/cgi-bin/texis/vtx/home/opendoc PDFViewer.html?docid=4d944d5b9&query=definition %20refugee

United Nations High Commissioner for Refugees. (2011). *Statistics and operational data.* Retrieved from http://www.unhcr .org/en-us/figures-at-a-glance.html

United Nations High Commissioner for Refugees. (2014). *World at War UNHCR Global Trends: Forced Displacement in 2014.* Retrieved from http://www.unhcr.org/556725e69.html

United Nations High Commissioner for Refugees. (2015). *Total number of Syrian refugees exceeds four million for first time.* Retrieved from http://www.unhcr.org/cgi-bin/texis/vtx/search ?page=search&docid=559d67d46&query=number%20syrian %20refugees

U.S. Citizenship and Immigration Services. (2008). *I am a refugee or aslyee: How do I become a U.S. permanent resident?* Retrieved from http://www.uscis.gov/sites/default/files/USCIS /Resources/D3en.pdf

U.S. Office of Refugee Resettlement. (2015). *Fiscal year 2014 refugee arrivals.* Retrieved from http://www.acf.hhs.gov/programs /orr/resource/fiscal-year-2014-refugee-arrivals

Whiteford, G. (2000). Occupational deprivation: Global challenge in the new millennium. *British Journal of Occupational Therapy, 63,* 200–205. http://dx.doi.org/10.1177 /030802260006300503

Whiteford, G. (2004). Occupational issues of refugees. In M. Molineux (Ed.), *Occupation for occupational therapists* (pp. 183–199). Malden, MA: Blackwell.

Section V.

CULTURE AND COMMUNITY, POPULATION-BASED PRACTICE

Chapter 27.

OCCUPATION-BASED COMMUNITY PRACTICE: UNTAPPED OPPORTUNITIES

Jyothi Gupta, PhD, OTR/L, FAOTA

Chapter Highlights

- Health Care Spending
- Health Inequities
- Defining Community
- Community Practice
- Occupational Therapy in Primary Care
- Community-Built Practice: Health Beyond Health Care
- Occupational Needs of Underserved Communities

Key Terms and Concepts

- ✧ Chronic diseases
- ✧ Chronic poverty
- ✧ Community
- ✧ Community practice
- ✧ Community-based practice
- ✧ Community-based rehabilitation
- ✧ Community-built practice
- ✧ Emerging paradigm
- ✧ Emerging practice
- ✧ Employer-sponsored wellness programs

- ✧ Habilitation
- ✧ Habilitation services
- ✧ Health inequities
- ✧ Interprofessional teams
- ✧ Mechanistic paradigm
- ✧ Occupation paradigm
- ✧ Primary care
- ✧ Rehabilitation services
- ✧ Teen pregnancy
- ✧ Triple Aim

Occupational therapy can offer individuals, families, and communities its unique perspective of the influences of everyday occupational lives on health and well-being. Culturally effective programming on primary prevention and health promotion can curtail rapidly rising health care costs, preventing the burden of chronic diseases and reducing health inequities. This chapter discusses opportunities in the community for occupation-based programming that can meet the occupational needs of many and, in doing so, also address some of the challenging health and social issues confronting society and curb the escalating cost of health care.

Health Care Spending

Health spending in the United States was about 17% of the nation's gross domestic product (GDP) in 2012. This spending is 1.5 times higher and 2.5 times more than the average spending of any of the 34 member countries of the Organisation for Economic Co-operation and Development (OECD). When it comes to health spending and pharmaceutical expenditure, the United States holds the top spot. This kind of spending on health care is unsustainable in the long run.

Despite this spending, the United States ranks 24th of 30 for health indicators such as life expectancy, immunization, and infant mortality. The United States has the highest rate of obesity among all countries, with nearly 64% of people 15 years or older being obese. Obesity is preventable and is a risk factor for many chronic conditions such as cardiovascular diseases and cancer (OECD, 2014).

Chronic diseases are noncommunicable pathologies that develop over a period of time. They are a leading cause of disability and death (Centers for Disease Control and Prevention [CDC], 2014). Chronic disease and multimorbidity, common among the elderly, cost 7 times more to treat compared to a treating a single condition (CDC, 2014). Health care spending is disproportionate: 5% of the population accounts for 49% of health care spending, and 20% of the population accounts for 80% of health care spending (Ehrlich, Kofke-Egger, & Udow-Phillips, 2010).

Approximately 75 cents of every health care dollar is spent treating chronic diseases, but only 3 cents is spent on prevention. The five most costly and preventable chronic conditions are (1) cardiovascular conditions, (2) cancer, (3) chronic obstructive pulmonary disease (COPD) or asthma, (4) diabetes, and (5) hypertension. These chronic diseases cost the United States nearly $347 billion—30% of total health spending in 2010 (American Public Health Association, 2013).

Early modification of the risk factors for chronic diseases can prevent the occurrence of these medical conditions and consequent disability. Billions of dollars can be saved in health spending. Chronic diseases such as obesity, diabetes, hypertension, and heart disease are disproportionately represented in the poor and in people of color.

Health Inequities

Health inequities are avoidable differences in health status between different population groups that are a result of unfair or unjust distribution of health determinants (World Health Organization, 2015). As of 2014, 42 million Americans (i.e., 1 of 6 Americans younger than age 65) were uninsured (Congressional Budget Office, 2014). Although health inequities related to income and access to coverage exist across demographic lines, the persistent disproportionate population-based inequities can no longer be ignored. Furthermore, the Institute of Medicine ([IOM], 2003) reported that racial and ethnic minorities are less likely to receive routine medical procedures and experience a lower quality of health services even when insurance status, income, age, and severity of conditions are comparable.

There is growing pressure for health research and services that demonstrate "greater sensitivity to communities' perceptions, needs, and unique circumstances" (Green & Mercer, 2001, p. 1926). Addressing health promotion at the community level in culturally effective ways can mitigate health inequities.

Defining Community

At its broadest, *community* includes residents of a local area, practitioners, service agencies, and policy makers. Typically *community* has been defined geographically—a group of people living in a particular area or locality—but this is a limited view of a community because it does not account for groups based on other dimensions such as shared characteristics or interests. In the literature, ideas of community are based on different assumptions because there is no accepted definition.

One evidence-based participatory study on the meaning and characteristics of community defines *community* as a "group of people with diverse characteristics who are linked by social ties, share common perspectives, and engage in joint action in geographical locations or settings" (MacQueen et al., 2001, p. 1936). This study identified the following five core elements of community:

1. *Locus, a sense of place:* Community can be located or situated in a place or setting. This encompasses *specific areas* like neighborhood, block, zip code, and city; *specific settings,* such as household, organization, coffee shop, grocery store, church, school, and community center; and the *general area* where people live.
2. *Sharing, common interests and perspectives:* Communities form when people create groups based on shared values, beliefs, interests, likes, dislikes, identity, and history.
3. *Joint action, a source of cohesion and identity:* Community emerges when people do things together such as hang out, socialize, discuss, and take action around social issues. Examples include forming a Neighborhood Watch, cleaning up the neighborhood, participating in charity drives, and so forth.
4. *Social ties, the foundation of community:* Interpersonal relationships are the foundation for community. These relationships are built on trust, safety, understanding, and familiarity.
5. *Diversity, social complexities within communities:* Intergroup differences in community emerge as a result of depth and types of interpersonal relationships, stratification based on class or expertise, differing abilities, stigmatization or marginalization, and those with multiple group affiliations within the community. Cultural and ethnic diversity is not included in this dimension of community.

The concept of community is challenging because of its complexity and variety, and the nested identities of its members. For instance, people of color who are gay or have mental health issues may be confronted with issues on two counts: (1) those that are relevant to their race or ethnicity and (2) others that pertain to their sexual identity or mental illness. Such challenges require these individuals to navigate competing allegiances and identity in terms of their communal identity. Understanding the motivations that bind the members of any community is the first step for exploring a relationship that is mutually beneficial for the community and occupational therapy.

Reflection 27.1. Community

- In your own words, define *community.*
- Create a list of all the communities you belong to.
- What characteristics of communities make you feel connected to them?

Community Practice

The term **community practice** refers to practice in settings that are not traditional or mainstream occupational therapy settings such as hospitals, rehabilitation facilities, and schools. Community practice spans a wide array of services from "prevention and health promotion, acute and chronic medical care, habilitation and rehabilitation, and direct and indirect service provision" in community settings (Scaffa, 2014, p. 5).

The various levels of care that capture the range of health services are described in Table 27.1. With the exception of school-based therapy that includes rehabilitation and habilitation services, traditional occupational therapy is primarily involved in rehabilitation at the secondary and tertiary levels of care.

The philosophical approach to practice in community differentiates the nature of community practice and relationships with the community members. The main differences in approaches are whether the change is top down (professional experts) versus bottom up (the community) and whether the community is viewed from a strengths or deficits perspective. These attitudes influence the nature and extent of relationship between service providers and community.

Community-based practice refers to health services provided locally and outside of larger institutions such as hospitals and medical centers. Such services are driven by the medical paradigm that places the power and control in the hands of the practitioners. The focus of intervention is on remediation of medical issues treated by various health professions (Stewart & Law, 2003).

In contrast, ***community-built practice*** is a collaborative biopsychosocial approach that is based on the community's strengths and is wellness oriented (Wittman & Velde, 2001). This approach is better aligned with occupational therapy's client-centered focus and is necessary to build trust with historically marginalized and oppressed communities.

Table 27.1. Classification of Levels of Health Care

Levels of Care and Prevention	Description
Primary care: Prevention of injury or disease occurrence by risk reduction	• Emphasizes prevention, health promotion, and health maintenance • Provides more general care than specialized care • Patients reside in community and are ambulatory • Addresses minor health issues or the early stages of potentially complex health issues • Care typically occurs in outpatient office setting • Least expensive form of care
Secondary care: Interrupts disease progression by early detection and intervention	• Emphasizes addressing health problem • More specialized care that includes routine surgery • Patients are partially nonambulatory, typically bedridden for part of the day • Hospital-based inpatient settings • More expensive than primary care
Tertiary care: Limits the physical and social consequences of disease, disability, or death	• Focuses on more complex health problems that require intensive and complex care • Hospital-based or medical center–based care that may require care in settings such as skilled nursing facilities • Requires advanced personnel, methods, techniques, and equipment • Most expensive type of care

Sources. Baird & Haas, 2011; Katz & Ali, 2009.

Intervention focuses on community-identified issues. Practitioners share their professional knowledge and facilitate problem solving, and solutions emerge through a collaborative process based on mutual respect for professional and community expertise. This win–win situation elicits buy-in from the community. This approach is also more conducive to culturally effective programming and empowering community members to take charge of their health and well-being.

Community-Based Rehabilitation

Community-based rehabilitation (CBR) involves culturally compatible rehabilitation services in the community that are inclusive of community stakeholders, including individuals with disability, and uses local resources (Fransen, 2005). Although CBR has no clear definition or specific description of how it should be conducted, it is philosophically aligned with health promotion and occupational therapy because it promotes empowerment, enablement, meaningful and active lifestyles, social justice, and respect for diversity (Thibeault & Hébert, 1997).

Rehabilitation services are aimed at helping individuals retain, relearn, or improve skills for daily living and functioning in society that were lost or impaired because of illness or injury. *Habilitation* helps with skills development for reasons other than injury or disease.

Habilitation services help individuals retain, learn, and improve skills needed for optimal functioning in everyday environments across the lifespan.

They also include maintenance and preventing further deterioration of functioning (Brown, 2014). For example, children experiencing developmental delays in writing, talking, or play can benefit from in-context occupational therapy services in schools.

Re-Emerging Practice and Community Practice

Health care spans primary, secondary, and tertiary levels of care (see Table 27.1). Traditional occupational therapy practice that is reimbursement driven and associated with biomedical settings is classified at secondary and tertiary levels of care, but this chapter contends that community practice is not merely an extension of medical practice in the community. Therefore, traditional occupational therapy practice tied to reimbursement by health insurance in the community (e.g., home care, outpatient services) will not be discussed here; this chapter will instead focus on what is referred to as *emerging practice* or nontraditional practice such as community reintegration of people who were incarcerated, services in homeless shelters, services in the foster care system, and the like (Scaffa & Reitz, 2014; Thew, Edwards, Baptiste, & Molineux, 2011).

It seems more accurate to call practice in community "re-emerging" practice because it is not a new idea and many practitioners have historically been engaged in community practice. The historical beginning of occupational therapy records occupation-based programs in the community aimed to promote social integration through productive and meaningful use of time (McColl, Law, Doubt, Pollock, & Stewart, 2002; Quiroga, 1995; Scaffa, 2014; Whittman & Velde, 2001).

Emerging Trends in Community Practice

Kielhofner (2007) discussed three points of crisis within the occupational therapy profession that triggered major shifts in the practice paradigm. The crisis in the 1950s shifted practice from its original holistic *occupation paradigm* into the biomedical *mechanistic paradigm.* During the occupation paradigm (1900s–1940s), holistic practice embraced occupation as the central concept of practice and included work, self-care, play, and rest. During the mechanistic paradigm (1950s–1970s), the profession opted to align with medicine to be recognized as a scientific profession and focused on disease and impairments and moved away from occupation. A second crisis occurred in the 1970s when therapists saw the reductionist approaches of medicine that occupational therapy had adopted during the mechanistic paradigm as inadequate. This dissatisfaction ushered in the *emerging paradigm* (1980s–present) that has re-embraced the original holistic philosophy of occupational therapy and sees humans as occupational beings.

However, it remains unclear how much current practice actually reflects this shift; perhaps the emerging paradigm shift is still evolving in the direction of occupation-based practice. Two intraprofessional trends have also brought focus to community-based and population-based practice: (1) the expanding knowledge from occupational science and (2) the inclusion of nontraditional practice settings in educational curriculum.

Expanding Knowledge

First, advances in the conceptual and theoretical knowledge base for justification of occupational therapy in community practice with individuals and specific communities have grown. Literature has emerged that is attempting to build evidence for as yet untested assumptions of the profession and others that challenge some of these assumptions. Examples of such research include studies that show the link among occupation, health, and well-being (Clark et al., 1997; Wilcock, 2006); environment and occupation (Dickie, Cutchin, & Humphrey, 2006;

Thompson & Kent, 2014); social structures and occupation (Galvaan, 2012; Prodinger & Turner, 2013; Rudman, 2013; Stadnyk, Townsend, & Wilcock, 2010; Whiteford & Townsend, 2011); and occupational injustices and community-based rehabilitation (Kronenberg & Pollard, 2006; Kronenberg, Pollard, & Salkellariou, 2010; Kronenberg, Fransen, & Pollard, 2005).

Nontraditional Community Settings

Second, many professional education curriculums have created learning opportunities in nontraditional community sites for coursework, projects, or fieldwork placements. Examples of community sites are homeless shelters, prison systems, and centers for refugees. Communities are places where occupations occur and students learn occupation-based practice in context. In biomedical settings, the range of occupations available is typically limited to basic activities of daily living, whereas in the community there is a diverse and wide range of occupations. Perhaps occupations in natural environments are more meaningful because they occur in the familiar everyday context of living and have deeper associations to lived experiences. For instance, preparing a meal for one's family has more dimensions to it than the task of meal preparation in a rehabilitation setting. The latter is functional, whereas the former has social significance.

Community practice is also more amenable to enact client-centered occupational therapy whose philosophy is based on empowerment through sharing of information and power and through collaborative decision making (Canadian Association of Occupational Therapists [CAOT], 2013b). Unlike the power and prestige of the professional experts in medical settings, the clients are the experts of their lives and their communities.

Occupational Therapy in Primary Care

Primary care is community practice that provides integrated, accessible, and accountable personal health care services by clinicians (IOM, 1994; Patient Protection and Affordable Care Act, 2010). U.S. society is aging, and advances in medical interventions have meant that large numbers of individuals are dealing with chronic diseases and their management. Older adults and those with chronic conditions often experience episodic crises requiring costly interventions in hospitals. The *Triple Aim* of cutting costs, improving population health, and improving individual care experience is the reason for recent health policy changes to provide services to this population in primary care settings (Berwick, Nolan, & Whittington, 2008).

Primary care practice is an example of community-based practice. It is both the first point of entry into the health care system and the site of continuing care for the diagnosis and treatment of acute and chronic illnesses. Other health services provided are health promotion, disease prevention, health maintenance, counseling, and patient education (American Association of Family Physicians, 2014).

Occupational therapy's role on *interprofessional teams* in primary care settings has been described in position papers (American Occupational Therapy Association [AOTA], 2014; CAOT, 2013a). Occupational therapy practitioners are well qualified to educate clients on the importance of incorporating health-sustaining occupational habits and routines for continued functioning despite injury or chronic disease. The overall goal for occupational therapy in primary care is maximizing occupational engagement and participation for individuals to satisfy basic necessities and to fulfill social roles and responsibilities to promote meaningful living, well-being, and a high quality of life. Roles and services that occupational therapists can provide on the primary care team are listed in Table 27.2.

Primary care practice is still a part of the health services continuum that is tied to medical health insurance. However, as change shifts cost to prevention and health promotion, this is an opportunity that must not be missed by occupational therapy practitioners.

Community-Built Practice: Health Beyond Health Care

Several professional leaders have advocated for practice to address broader health and occupational needs of the community (e.g., Finn, 1971/2005; Grady, 1994/2005; Reilly, 1971; West, 1967/2005), but occupational therapy practice has largely remained connected to health insurance–supported practice in biomedical settings (AOTA, 2015). For example, a historical timeline that traces community practice in occupational therapy demonstrates the scarcity of community involvement with sporadic programs for pregnant teens and for the elderly (Scaffa, 2014). Why has the profession been hesitant to move practice beyond the health care industry to the community context where everyday occupations happen and clients live their daily lives?

Barriers to Community-Built Practice

Some of the challenges noted by Laukaran (1977) and elaborated on by Scaffa (2014) reflect current barriers to occupational therapy community practice:

Table 27.2. Occupational Therapy Roles, Skills, and Services in Primary Care

Occupational Therapy Roles and Skills	Occupational Therapy Services Examples

Counseling
Consultation
Education
Coaching
Advocate
Coordinate
Adapt
	• Self-management of conditions such as diabetes or arthritis
	• Adapt ways of doing occupations by incorporating energy conservation and joint protection techniques for managing pain and fatigue
	• Self-management of addictions and mental health issues
	• Home modifications for accessibility and safety
	• Fall risk screening and falls prevention
	• Prevention, health promotion, and lifestyle redesign
	• Safety and injury prevention
	• Caregiver education and support
	• Palliative and end-of-life care
	• Resources for social integration and participation
	  ◦ Adult day programs
	  ◦ Driving, transportation, and community mobility
	  ◦ Employment services
	  ◦ Work transition and retirement planning services
	  ◦ Volunteering
	  ◦ Other social services

Sources. AOTA, 2014; CAOT, 2013a.

- The profession is perceived as a medical profession.
- Practitioners historically have been associated with work in medical institutions, particularly psychiatry.
- Educational programs typically emphasize practice in medical settings and have been slow to shift their attention to community practice.
- Knowledge gaps in theories and framework for community practice hinder expansion to the community.
- Practitioners have limited opportunity for community practice.

As long as occupational therapy practitioners are visible in acute, subacute, outpatient, and home-care rehabilitation settings, they will be seen as allied to biomedicine. Occupational therapists continue to be present in these practice settings, which are deemed as traditional practice, because the profession continues to remain primarily dependent on health care insurance reimbursement that favors a biomedical approach to health.

Energy expended on advocacy goes into maintaining the scope of practice in the medical environment and preventing encroachment by other professions. Although many community positions (e.g., community nonprofits that provide social services to various groups such as the homeless, refugees, parolees, and unemployed) may not call for an occupational therapist, practitioners need to pursue these positions (Scaffa, 2014).

Community practice can occur only if alternate sources for funding, outside of health insurance, are explored.

Occupation-Based Community Practice

Occupational therapy can enhance occupational engagement for healthy people and populations across different age groups in occupational categories of self-care, leisure, or productivity, and systems such as education, urban development, or social services.

Lifestyle Redesign

The best-known model for working with a healthy group is the Well Elderly Study Program (Clark et al., 2015; Jackson, Carlson, Mendel, Zemke, & Clark, 1998). Studies demonstrated the health benefits and cost-effectiveness of occupational therapy group interventions aimed at maintaining healthy occupational habits and routines among older adults (Clark et al., 2012).

Employer-Sponsored Wellness Programs

Many health insurance companies support participation in **employer-sponsored wellness programs,** generally referred to as *corporate health and wellness.* These offer great opportunities for occupational therapy to address issues of workplace health, older workers, injury prevention, and stress (Gupta & Sabata, 2010; Gupta & Lughermo, 2009; Hall, 2011; Spangler, 2013; Thew, 2011). These programs are successful when they are developed as culturally effective programs that take into consideration the workplace's unique organizational culture.

Community Health Centers

Community health centers are also suitable venues to organize community health education groups such as senior wellness groups, self-esteem groups for women, mental health support groups, and children's activity groups (Trentham & Cockburn, 2011). Many community nonprofit organizations offer programming to meet the many gaps in social services and often rely on lay volunteers to develop and implement these programs. This is another area that can easily be fulfilled by occupational therapy practitioners. The nature of services can vary depending on the needs of the individual or groups, and many of these needs typically include learning skills for performing daily occupations.

Occupational Needs of Underserved Communities

In the spirit of the AOTA's (2007) *Centennial Vision's* commitment "to meet society's occupational needs" (p. 613), it is worth identifying where the occupational needs exist in society. Groups with occupational needs in the community can be identified by understanding broad and current social issues that challenge or disrupt the occupational lives. Examples of social issues and opportunities and roles for community occupational therapy practice are presented in Table 27.3.

Table 27.3. Examples of Programming for Community Health and Well-Being

Community Issue	Examples of Community Program Opportunities and Suitable Topics	Select References
Health disparities	• Culturally effective health education on use of daily life occupations to develop habits and routines to manage life stressors, make lifestyle changes, access health services and resources	Dieterle, 2014

Chronic unemployment	• Welfare-to-work program (for individuals living on welfare assistance):
	  ○ Develop programs addressing workplace interpersonal skills, behaviors, interests, work habits and routines, communication, time management, organizational skills, work–life balance, etc.
	• Ticket-to-work programs (for individuals with disability):
	  ○ Empower clients to access rehabilitation services, vocational services, and paid employment. Practitioners can facilitate best-match job options and appropriate level of accommodation at work.
		Wilson-Mowrey & Riels, 2014
		Nochakski & Reitz, 2014

Chronic poverty	• Occupational groups for at-risk children: Basic life skills, healthy habits and routines, group work, emotional self-regulation, conflict resolution, physical activity, bullying, etc. • Youth after-school programs: Healthy relationships, violence, bullying, health education, career planning, study habits, stress management, anger management, community service, etc. • Teen pregnancy: School–life balance, health education, parenting, healthy relationships, assertive communication, self-esteem, building support network, stress management, life skills, career planning, etc. • Adults: Healthy habits and routines, managing chronic stress, emotional health, budgeting, leisure, social support, parenting, etc.	Centers for Disease Control and Prevention (CDC), 2014. http://bit.ly/JKUHk3 Anderson et al., 2003. http://bit.ly/29UIwQx
Incarceration	• Community reintegration programs ○ Work programs, community living skills, anger management, stress management, communication skills, social support groups, leisure and recreation, physical activity, health education, etc.	Eggers, Muñoz, Sciulli, & Crist, 2006. http://bit.ly/29OtGKv Molineaux & Whitford, 1997. http://bit.ly/2aatjNk Casteneda & Reitz, 2014
Homelessness	• Programs that address basic life skills, community resources, mental health counseling, vocational services, substance abuse, etc.	Thomas, Gray, McGinty, & Ebringer, 2011. http://bit.ly/29OwaJ9 VanLeit, Starrett, & Crowe, 2006. http://bit.ly/2d6gDGr
Asylum seekers, refugees, new immigrants	• Programs to assist with starting a new life in a new context in all areas of daily living, work, school, leisure, etc.	Gupta & Sullivan, 2008, 2013. http://bit.ly/2adBsyY Burchett & Matheson, 2010. http://bit.ly/2aapfNf
Domestic violence and other forms of abuse	• Occupation-based therapeutic groups to facilitate emotional healing, psychosocial well-being, interpersonal communication skills, resiliency and coping mechanisms, social support, etc.	Javaherian, Krabacher, Andriacco, & German, 2007. http://bit.ly/2a1A0km

Chronic Poverty

Chronic poverty is a complex and multidimensional social phenomenon in which poverty is experienced over long durations, perhaps over the course of one's lifetime, and sometimes intergenerationally. Individuals who are chronically poor often lack assets and are not part of mainstream society. Additionally, contextual factors, including socioeconomic and sociopolitical policies and structures, underlie chronic poverty (Shepherd et al., 2014).

Chronic poverty is a particular risk factor for poor health and well-being as individuals experience chronic stress toxicity and occupational injustices. Chronic poverty is often associated with cumulative adverse childhood experiences such living in an unstable home environment; with food insecurity, family turmoil, neglect, or abuse; and in unsafe neighborhoods (Evans & Kim, 2011).

Early-life adversity related to chronic poverty affects health during childhood and continues into adulthood. It is a risk factor for chronic disease. Chronic diseases such as diabetes, hypertension, cardiovascular disease, depression, addictions, and mental health issues are a tremendous social burden because they affect productivity, quality of life, and the overuse of health care services. Extensive evidence supports prevention programs as a means to alter this health trajectory and consequently reduce the social and economic burdens of illness (Center on the Developing Child at Harvard University, 2010).

Children who grow up experiencing chronic poverty are exposed to cumulative and multiple adverse events that negatively affect their social, emotional, and cognitive development (Jensen, 2009). Examples of health risks include alcohol abuse, illicit drug use, depression, risk for intimate partner violence, multiple sexual partners, sexually transmitted diseases, smoking, early sexual activity, and unintended pregnancies (CDC, 2014).

Haskins (2014) reports on successful social programs that are tackling some of these difficult social issues. A majority of these programs are based in the community and educate, support, and coach individuals and groups. Occupational therapy practitioners are trained in developing and implementing such programs in partnership with other community stakeholders.

Teen Pregnancy

Despite some decrease in *teen pregnancy,* pregnancy in girls 13–19, the United States still has the highest rates of teen pregnancy among all industrialized nations (Kearney & Levine, 2012). Chronic poverty is a risk factor for teen pregnancy, which has negative consequences for the adolescent, the child, and society. Teen pregnancy drains societal resources through public assistance payments, lost tax revenue, and greater expenditures for public health care, foster care, and criminal justice services (U.S. Department of Health and Human Services, 2014). Hispanic and Black adolescents are at a greater risk for teen pregnancy compared to their White peers, as are teens in foster care systems or welfare systems and teens growing up in poor neighborhoods (CDC, 2014).

Some of the contextual factors for teen pregnancy include low levels of family education and income, neighborhood segregation, lack of positive youth involvement, and low-income neighborhood inequality (Boonstra, 2014). There are examples of evidence-based comprehensive programs that have succeeded in preventing teen pregnancy through activities and educational programs (Philliber, Williams-Kaye, Herrling, & West, 2002).

Reflection 27.2. Serving Underserved Communities

Identify strategies to advance practice in the community.

- What are some of the action steps needed to advocate for occupational therapy in underserved communities?

Summary

Health inequities lead to loss of productivity, disability, and costly secondary- and tertiary-level care. Particularly for low-income groups that may not have health insurance, community health promotion educational programs can increase awareness of risk factors and help with lifestyle changes.

The health care industry is challenged to cut spending levels that cannot be sustained, and recent policy changes reflect a shift toward enhanced primary and preventive care in the community to reduce chronic diseases and health inequities. Occupational therapy practitioners have a timely opportunity to be a part of the health care solution. The CDC (2014) has identified public health priorities that include teen pregnancy, physical activity, nutrition and obesity, motor vehicle injury, and HIV/AIDS. This presents a great opportunity for occupational therapy to engage in interprofessional community-based programming that addresses these priority public health issues.

The profession can contribute by providing a wide range of culturally effective services, including health and wellness programs for diverse and underserved populations. Community- and occupation-based practice in the natural contexts of clients' daily lives can provide a broad range of services to individuals and groups with occupational needs within and outside of the health care system.

References

American Association of Family Physicians. (2014). *Primary care.* Retrieved from http://www.aafp.org/about/policies/all/primary-care.html#5

American Occupational Therapy Association. (2007). AOTA's *Centennial Vision* and executive summary. *American Journal of Occupational Therapy, 61,* 613–614. http://dx.doi.org/10.5014/ajot.61.6.613

American Occupational Therapy Association. (2014). The role of occupational therapy in primary care. *American Journal of Occupational Therapy, 68*(Suppl. 3), 25–33. http://dx.doi.org/10.5014/ajot.2014.686S06

American Occupational Therapy Association. (2015). *2015 AOTA Salary and Workforce Survey.* Retrieved from http://www.aota.org/education-careers/advance-career/salary-workforce-survey.aspx

American Public Health Association. (2013). *Prevention and public health fund: Dedicated to improving our nation's public health.* Retrieved from http://healthyamericans.org/health-issues/wp-content/uploads/2015/02/150219_PPHF.pdf

Anderson, C. A., Berkowitz, L., Donnerstein, E., Huesmann, L. R., Johnson, J. D., Linz, D., . . . Wartella, E. (2003). The influence of media violence on youth. *Psychological Science in the Public Interest, 4*(3), 81–110. http://dx.doi.org/10.1111/j.1529-1006.2003.pspi_1433.x

Baird, R., & Haas, M. (2011). Introduction to public health, public health agencies and the APHA. In M. T. Haneline & W. T. Meeker (Eds.), *Introduction to public health for chiropractors* (pp. 1–34). Sudbury, MA: Jones & Bartlett.

Berwick, D. M., Nolan, T. W., & Whittington, J. (2008). The triple aim: Care, health, and cost. *Health Affairs, 27,* 759–769. http://dx.doi.org/10.1377/hlthaff.27.3.759

Boonstra, H. (2014). What is behind the declines in teen pregnancy rates? *Guttmacher Policy Review, 17*(3), 15–21. Retrieved from https://www.guttmacher.org/about/gpr/2014/09/what-behind-declines-teen-pregnancy-rates

Brown, D. (2014). Health policy perspectives—Habilitative services: An essential health benefit and an opportunity for occupational therapy practitioners and consumers. *American Journal of Occupational Therapy, 68,* 130–138. http://dx.doi.org/10.5014/ajot.2014.682001

Burchett, N., & Matheson R. (2010). The need for belonging: The impact of restrictions on working on the well-being of an asylum seeker. *Journal of Occupational Science, 17*(2), 85–91. http://dx.doi.org/10.1080/14427591.2010.9686679

Canadian Association of Occupational Therapists. (2013a). *CAOT position statement: Occupational therapy in primary care.* Retrieved from https://www.caot.ca/pdfs/positionstate/PS_PrimaryCare.pdf

Canadian Association of Occupational Therapists. (2013b). *Enabling Occupation II: Advancing an occupational therapy vision for health, well-being, and justice through occupation* (2nd ed.). Ottawa, ON: CAOT Publications ACE.

Castaneda, R., & Reitz, M. (2014). Forensic mental health practice within the community. In M. E. Scaffa & M. Reitz (Eds.), *Occupational therapy in community-based practice settings* (pp. 309–320). Philadelphia: F. A. Davis.

Centers for Disease Control and Prevention. (2014). *Chronic disease prevention and health promotion.* Retrieved from http://www.cdc.gov/chronicdisease/overview/index.htm

Center on the Developing Child at Harvard University. (2010). *The foundations of lifelong health are built in early childhood.* Retrieved from http://developingchild.harvard.edu/resources/the-foundations-of-lifelong-health-are-built-in-early-childhood/

Clark, F., Azen, S. P., Zemke, R., Jackson, J., Carlson, M., Mandel, D., . . . Lipson, I. (1997). Occupational therapy for independent-living older adults. A randomized controlled trial. *Journal of the American Medical Association, 278*(16), 1321–1326. http://dx.doi.org/10.1001/jama.1997.03550160041036.

Clark, F., Blanchard, J., Sleight, A., Cogan, A., Floríndez, L., Gleason, S., . . . Vigen, C. (2015). *Lifestyle Redesign: The intervention tested in the USC well elderly studies* (2nd ed.). Bethesda, MD: AOTA Press.

Clark, F., Jackson, J., Carlson, M., Chou, C., Cherry, B. J., Jordan-Marsh, M., . . . Azen, S. P. (2012). Effectiveness of a lifestyle intervention in promoting the well-being of independently living older people: Results of the well elderly 2 randomised controlled trial. *Journal of Epidemiology and Community Health, 66,* 782–790. http://dx.doi.org/10.1136/jech.2009.099754

Congressional Budget Office. (2014). *Insurance coverage provisions of the Affordable Care Act—CBO's April 2014 baseline.* Retrieved from https://www.cbo.gov/sites/default/files/51298-2014-04-ACA.pdf

Dickie, V., Cutchin, M. P., & Humphry, R. (2006). Occupation as transactional experience: A critique of individualism in occupational science. *Journal of Occupational Science, 13*(1), 83–93. http://dx.doi.org/10.1080/14427591.2006.9686573

Dieterle, C. (2014). Lifestyle redesign programs. In M. E. Scaffa & M. Reitz (Eds.), *Occupational therapy in community-based practice settings* (pp. 377–389). Philadelphia: F. A. Davis.

Eggers, M., Muñoz, J., Sciulli, J., & Crist, P. (2006). The community reintegration project: Occupational therapy at work in a county jail. *Occupational Therapy In Health Care, 20*(1), 17–37. http://dx.doi.org/10.1080/J003v20n01_02

Ehrlich, E., Kofke-Egger, H., & Udow-Phillips, M. (2010). *Health care cost drivers: Chronic disease, comorbidity, and health risk factors in the U.S. and Michigan.* Ann Arbor, MI: Center for Healthcare Research & Transformation. Retrieved http://www.chrt.org/publication/health-care-cost-drivers-chronic-disease-comorbidity-health-risk-factors-u-s-michigan/

Evans, G., & Kim, P. (2011). Childhood poverty and health. Cumulative risk exposure and stress dysregulation. *Psychological Science, 18*(11), 953–957. http://dx.doi.org/10.1111/j.1467-9280.2007.02008.x

Finn, G. L. (1971/2005). The occupational therapist in prevention programs. In R. Padilla (Ed.), *A professional legacy: The Eleanor Clarke Slagle lectures in occupational therapy, 1955–2004* (2nd ed., pp. 177–189). Bethesda, MD: AOTA Press.

Fransen, H. (2005). Challenges for occupational therapy in community-based rehabilitation: Occupation in a community approach to handicap in development. In F. Kronenberg, S. S. Algado, & N. Pollard (Eds.), *Occupational therapy without borders: Learning from the spirit of survivors* (Vol. 1, pp. 166–182). Oxford, England: Elsevier/Churchill Livingstone.

Galvaan, R. (2012). Occupational choice: The significance of socio-economic and political factors. In G. E. Whiteford & C. Hocking (Eds.), *Occupational science: Society, inclusion, participation* (pp. 152–162). Chichester, West Sussex, England: Blackwell.

Grady, A. (1994/2005). Building inclusive community: A challenge for occupational therapy. In R. Padilla (Ed.), *A professional legacy: The Eleanor Clarke Slagle lectures in occupational therapy, 1955–2004* (2nd ed., pp. 493–511). Bethesda, MD: AOTA Press.

Green, L. W., & Mercer, S. L. (2001). Can public health researchers and agencies reconcile the push from funding bodies and the pull from communities? *American Journal of Public Health, 91*(12), 1926–1938. Retrieved from https://www.fhi360.org/sites/default/files/webpages/sp/RETC-CR/nr/rdonlyres/eckb3vszm3kqtshj36kytmomaijqw4x42jgrsvsgmziwvncg3aopn3wd4d43hljxixq22kjba6aqhf/retccrWhatisCommunity.pdf

Gupta, J., & Lughermo, T. (2009, April). *Improving employee health and work performance: A corporate wellness program model.* Presented at the AOTA Annual Conference & Expo, Houston, TX.

Gupta, J., & Sabata, D. (2010). Maximizing occupational performance of older workers: Applying the person–environment–occupation model [Continuing education article]. *OT Practice, 15*(7), CE1–CE8. Retrieved from http://search.ebscohost.com/login.aspx?direct=true&db=rzh&AN=2010642270&site=ehost-live

Gupta, J., & Sullivan, C. (2008). Enabling immigrants to overcome participation challenges. *OT Practice, 13*(5), 25–32.

Gupta, J., & Sullivan, C. (2013). The central role of occupation in the doing, being and belonging of immigrant women. *Journal of Occupational Science, 20*(1), 23–35. http://dx.doi.org/10.1080/14427591.2012.717499

Hall, S. (2011). An occupational perspective of a disability-focused employment service. In M. Thew, M. Edwards, S. Baptiste, & M. Mollineux (Eds.), *Role emerging occupational therapy: Maximising occupation-focused practice* (pp. 83–96). Oxford, England: Wiley-Blackwell.

Haskins, R. (2014, December). *Social programs that work.* Retrieved from http://www.brookings.edu/blogs/up-front/posts/2014/12/01-show-me-evidence-haskins

Institute of Medicine. (1994). *Defining primary care: An interim report.* Washington, DC: National Academies Press. Retrieved from http://www.nap.edu/read/9153/chapter/1

Institute of Medicine. (2003). *Unequal treatment: Confronting racial and ethnic disparities in health care.* Washington, DC: National Academies Press.

Jackson, J., Carlson, M., Mendel, D., Zemke, R., & Clark, F. (1998). Occupation in lifestyle redesign: The well-elderly study occupational therapy program. *American Journal of Occupational Therapy, 52*(5), 326–336. http://dx.doi.org/10.5014/ajot.52.5.326

Javaherian, H., Krabacher, V., Andriacco, K., & German, D. (2007). Surviving domestic violence: Rebuilding one's life. *Occupational Therapy in Health Care, 21*(3), 35–59. http://dx.doi.org/10.1080/J003v21n03_03

Jensen, E. (2009). How poverty affects behavior and academic performance. In E. Jensen (Ed.), *Teaching with poverty in mind: What being poor does to kids' brains and what schools can do about it* (pp. 13–45). Alexandria, VA: ASCD.

Katz, D. L., & Ali, A. (2009, February). *Preventive medicine, integrative medicine & the health of the public.* Commissioned paper for Institute of Medicine of the National Academies presented at the Summit on Integrative Medicine and the Health of the Public. Retrieved from https://www.nationalacademies.org/hmd/~/media/Files/Activity%20Files/Quality/IntegrativeMed/Preventive%20Medicine%20Integrative%20Medicine%20and%20the%20Health%20of%20the%20Public.pdf

Kearney, M. S., & Levine, P. B. (2012). Why is the teen birth rate in the United States so high and why does it matter? *Journal of Economic Perspectives, 26*(2), 141–166. http://dx.doi.org/10.1257/jep.26.2.141

Kielhofner, G. (2007). *Conceptual foundations of occupational therapy* (4th ed.). Philadelphia: F. A. Davis.

Kronenberg, F., & Pollard, N. (2006). Political dimensions of occupation and the roles of occupational therapy. *American Journal of Occupational Therapy, 60*(6), 617–625. http://dx.doi.org/10.5014/ajot.60.6.617

Kronenberg, F., Fransen, H., & Pollard, N. (2005). The WFOT position paper on community-based rehabilitation: A call upon the profession to engage with people affected by occupational apartheid. *World Federation of Occupational Therapists Bulletin, 51*(1), 5–13. http://dx.doi.org/10.1179/otb.2005.51.1.002

Kronenberg, F., Pollard, N., & Sakellariou, D. (Eds.). (2010). *Occupational therapies without borders: Towards an ecology of occupation-based practices* (Vol. 2, pp. 65–84). London: Elsevier.

Laukaran, V. H. (1977). Toward a model of occupational therapy for community health. *American Journal of Occupational Therapy, 31*(2), 71–74.

MacQueen, K. M., McLellan, E., Metzger, D. S., Kegeles, S., Strauss, R. P., Scotti, R., . . . Trotter II, R. T. (2001). What is community? An evidence-based definition for participatory public health. *American Journal of Public Health, 91*(12), 1929–1938. http://dx.doi.org/10.2105/AJPH.91.12.1929

McColl, M. A., Law, M. C., Doubt, L., Pollock, N. & Stewart, D. (2002). *The theoretical basis of occupational therapy* (2nd ed.). Thorofare, NJ: Slack.

Molineaux, M., & Whitford, G. (1997). Prisons: From occupational deprivation to occupational enrichment. *Journal of Occupational Science, 6*(3), 124–130. http://dx.doi.org/10.1080/14427591.1999.9686457

Nochakski, S. M., & Reitz, M. (2014). Work and career transitions. In M. E. Scaffa & M. Reitz (Eds.), *Occupational therapy in community-based practice settings* (pp. 1–18). Philadelphia: F. A. Davis.

Organisation for Economic Co-operation and Development. (2014). *OECD health statistics 2014: How does the US compare?* Retrieved from http://www.oecd.org/unitedstates/Briefing-Note-UNITED-STATES-2014.pdf

Patient Protection and Affordable Care Act, Pub. L. 111–148, 42 U.S.C. §§ 18001-18121 (2010).

Philliber, S., Williams-Kaye, J., Herrling, S., & West, E. (2002). Preventing pregnancy and improving health care access among teenagers: An evaluation of the Children's Aid Society–Carrera program. *Perspectives on Sexual and Reproductive Health, 34*(5), 244–251.

Prodinger, B., & Turner, S. M. (2013). Using institutional ethnography to explore how social policies infiltrate into daily life. *Journal of Occupational Science, 20*(4), 357–369. http://dx.doi.org/10.1080/14427591.2013.808728

Quiroga, V. (1995). *Occupational therapy: The first 30 years 1900–1930.* Bethesda, MD: American Occupational Therapy Association.

Reilly, M. (1963). Occupational therapy can be one of the great ideas of 20th century medicine. *American Journal of Occupational Therapy, 16,* 1–9.

Rudman, D. L. (2013). Enacting the critical potential of occupational science: problematizing the 'individualizing of occupation'. *Journal of Occupational Science, 20*(4), 298–313. http://dx.doi.org/10.1080/14427591.2013.803434

Scaffa, M. E. (2014). Community-based practice: Occupation in context. In M. E. Scaffa & M. Reitz (Eds.), *Occupational therapy in community-based practice settings* (pp. 1–18). Philadelphia: F. A. Davis.

Scaffa, M. E., & Reitz, M. (2014). *Occupational therapy in community-based practice settings* (2nd ed.). Philadelphia: F. A. Davis.

Shepherd, A., Scott, L., Mariotti, C., Kessy, F., Gaiha, R., da Corta, L., . . . Sen, B. (2014). *The chronic poverty report 2014–2015: The road to zero extreme poverty.* London: Overseas Development Institute. https://www.odi.org/sites/odi.org.uk/files/odi-assets/publications-opinion-files/8834.pdf

Stadnyk, R., Townsend, E., & Wilcock, A. (2010). Occupational justice. In C. Christiansen & E. Townsend (Eds.), *Introduction to occupation: The art and science of living* (pp. 329–358). Upper Saddle River, NJ: Pearson Education.

Stewart, D., & Law, M. (2003). The environment: Paradigms and practice in health, occupational therapy and inquiry. In L. Letts, P. Rigby, & D. Stewart (Eds.), *Using environments to enable occupational performance* (pp. 3–16). Thorofare, NJ: Slack.

Thew, M. (2011). Promoting well-being in a large organization: Challenges and opportunities. In M. Thew, M. Edwards, S. Baptiste, & M. Mollineux (Eds.), *Role emerging occupational therapy: Maximising occupation-focused practice* (pp. 66–82). Oxford, England: Wiley-Blackwell.

Thew, M., Edwards, M., Baptiste, S., & Molineux, M. (2011). *Role emerging occupational therapy: Maximising occupation-focused practice.* West Sussex, England: Blackwell.

Thibeault, R., & Hébert, M. (1997). A congruent model for health promotion in occupational therapy. *Occupational Therapy International, 4*(4), 271–293. http://dx.doi.org/10.1002/oti.60

Thomas, Y., Gray, M., McGinty, S., & Ebringer, S. (2011). Homeless adults engagement in art: First steps towards identity, recovery and social inclusion. *Australian Occupational Therapy Journal, 58*(6), 429–436. http://dx.doi.org/10.1111/j.1440-1630.2011.00977.x

Thompson, S., & Kent, J. (2014). Healthy built environments supporting everyday occupations: Current thinking in urban planning. *Journal of Occupational Science, 21*(1), 25–41. http://dx.doi.org/10.1080/14427591.2013.867562

Trentham, B., & Cockburn, L. (2011). Promoting occupational therapy in the community health center. In M. Thew, M. Edwards, S. Baptiste, & M. Mollineux (Eds.), *Role emerging occupational therapy: Maximising occupation-focused practice* (pp. 97–110). Oxford, England: Wiley-Blackwell.

U.S. Department of Health and Human Services. (2014). *Negative impacts of teen childbearing.* Retrieved from http://www.hhs.gov/ash/oah/adolescent-health-topics/reproductive-health/teen-pregnancy/health-impact.html#_ftn2

VanLeit, B., Starrett, R., & Crowe, T. (2006). Occupational concerns of women who are homeless and have children: An occupational justice critique. *Occupational Therapy in Healthcare, 20*(3–4), 47–62. http://dx.doi.org/10.1080/J003v20n03_04

West, W. (1967/2005). Professional responsibility in times of change. In R. Padilla (Ed.), *A professional legacy: The Eleanor Clarke Slagle lectures in occupational therapy, 1955–2004* (2nd ed., pp. 141–151). Bethesda, MD: AOTA Press.

Whiteford, G., & Townsend, E. (2011). Participatory Occupational Justice Framework (POJF 2010): Enabling occupational participation and inclusion. In F. Kronenberg, N. Pollard, & D. Sakellariou. (Eds.), *Occupational therapies without borders: Towards an ecology of occupation-based practices* (2nd ed., pp. 65–84). New York: Elsevier.

Wilcock, A. A. (2006). *An occupational perspective of health* (2nd ed.). Thorofare, NJ: Slack.

Wilson-Mowrey, E., & Riels, L. A. (2014). Welfare to work and ticket to work programs. In M. E. Scaffa & M. Reitz (Eds.), *Occupational therapy in community-based practice settings* (pp. 257–270). Philadelphia: F. A. Davis.

Wittman, P. P., & Velde, B. P. (2001). Occupational therapy in the community: What, why, and how. *Occupational Therapy in Health Care, 13*(3–4), 1–5. http://dx.doi.org/10.1080/J003v13n03_01

World Health Organization. (2015). *Health impact assessment: Glossary of terms.* Retrieved from http://www.who.int/hia/about/glos/en/index1.html

Chapter 28.

DEVELOPING A HANDWRITING INSTRUCTION PROGRAM FOR ADULTS LEARNING ENGLISH AS A SECOND LANGUAGE

Victoria Nackley, MS, OTR/L; Cora Bruns, MS, OTR/L; and Nancy Hollins, PhD, OTR/L

Chapter Highlights

- Integrating Into the United States: Case Example of Ahado
- Handwriting and Occupational Therapy
- Description of Handwriting Program
- Cultural Adaptations and Considerations
- Impact of the Handwriting Instruction Program

Key Terms and Concepts

- ✧ Callirobics
- ✧ Compositional skills
- ✧ Cultural integration
- ✧ English as a Second Language
- ✧ Evaluation Tool of Children's Handwriting–Manuscript

- ✧ Handwriting
- ✧ Handwriting Instruction Program
- ✧ Handwriting Without Tears
- ✧ Refugee

Difficulty in handwriting can present a challenge for people integrating into American culture. When an individual seeks medical attention, a medical history form needs to be completed. When a child is sick and stays home from school, a note needs to be written to explain the child's absence. When a bill needs to be paid, the individual may need to write a check. When an individual applies for a job, a job application must be completed. When an individual seeks to rent an apartment, a lease agreement needs to be signed.

This chapter describes the development of an occupational therapy intervention that transformed a commonly accepted handwriting program for children, *Handwriting Without Tears* (Olsen, 2003a), into a culturally appropriate handwriting program for adult immigrants and refugees.

Integrating Into the United States: Case Example of Ahado

Ahado, a 40-year-old refugee from Somalia, labors to print her name and demographic information on a job application. At a rate of only eight letters per minute, she spends a significant amount of time completing the application. Because her native language does not have a written form, Ahado's handwriting does not reflect her age but rather resembles the script of a 6-year-old. Although Ahado has made great strides toward seeking gainful employment in her new country by learning to speak, understand, and read English, the manager bypasses her application because of her handwriting. This experience was common for many refugees in upstate New York and served as an impetus for development of the *Handwriting Instruction Program (HIP)*.

To achieve the goal of independent living and full employment, adult refugees like Ahado must learn to speak, comprehend, read, and write the English language. *Cultural integration* to life in the United States also entails securing housing, seeking employment, navigating the education system, accessing medical care, and managing finances, which require using English in all its forms.

Reflection 28.1. Communicating in a New Country

Consider that you have relocated to a new country whose residents speak a language different from your own native language. You need to find housing, secure employment, and integrate your children into the education system.

- How would written, verbal, and nonverbal communication challenges affect your integration into daily life activities within that new country?

Handwriting and Occupational Therapy

Handwriting entails graphic creation of letters, numbers, words, and sentences to convey meaning. Acquisition of handwriting develops from specific instruction but also emerges through foundational skills in areas such as motor control, cognition, visual perception, and visual–motor integration.

Occupational therapy practitioners are frequently considered handwriting experts in various contexts, from schools to rehabilitation centers to community programs. Practitioners are well versed in evaluation and intervention with respect to handwriting. Many programs exist for handwriting instruction for children, which have been found to be effective in improving handwriting skill, legibility, and speed. They have also greatly affected language skills.

Promoting skill in handwriting requires that individuals have at least 20 sessions of handwriting instruction. Handwriting instruction programs can thus be provided twice weekly across a 10-week period, with the component of practice being essential to skill acquisition (Hoy, Egan, & Feder, 2011).

Graham (2009–2010) indicated that handwriting directly affects *compositional skills* (Medwell & Wray, 2007), which involve the individual's ability to convey meaning in a written format through the construction of sentences, paragraphs, and larger written works such as essays. Because effective handwriting improves word production and composition quality, handwriting instruction should be considered as a component to teaching compositional writing (Peverley, 2006). Handwriting instruction of adults may serve as a critical element in *English as a Second Language (ESL)* education to foster development of reading and writing skills, thereby assisting in the integration process.

Reflection 28.2. Timed Writing

- Have a stopwatch available to measure the amount of time it takes you to write your first, middle, and last name; address; and telephone number. Record the time that it took for that writing task.
- Count how many characters were used.
- Considering a rate of 8 letters per minute (not uncommon for the adult refugee), how long would it take you to write that information?
- Reflect on what it might be like to complete a form at a physician's office.
- To experience the frustration of using a new writing script, complete the same task in a right-to-left fashion.
- Identify your thoughts and feelings while engaged in that activity.

Description of Handwriting Program

Context

The handwriting program described in this chapter is supported by the Adult Learning Center of the Mohawk Valley Resource Center for Refugees (MVRCR) in Utica, New York. The greater Utica area, known as "The Town That Loves Refugees" (United Nations High Commissioner for Refugees, 2005), welcomes individuals of various cultures and ethnicities. This agency provides extensive services to refugees and immigrants to assist in the process of integration, including an education program that addresses ESL. Because various factors influence the immigration of individuals to the United States and to the Utica area, the population at the MVRCR is variable. Adult learners range from age 18 years to older adulthood.

Cora Bruns, the academic fieldwork coordinator for Utica College's occupational therapy program, was appointed to the position of coordinator for Project SHINE (Students Helping in the Naturalization of Elders) on the Utica College campus in 2004. Her role was to place college students working for Project SHINE in volunteer positions at the Adult Learning Center.

As Bruns placed college students in these classrooms, she decided that the best way to understand the volunteer role would be for her to become a volunteer. In this role, using her observational skills as an occupational therapist, she recognized that the learners were struggling to understand the marks on the whiteboard and how those marks translated into language. Many of the learners had no formal education in their native language, so handwriting was not familiar to them. She also noted that many of these learners lacked such foundational handwriting components as left-to-right progression, top-to-bottom orientation, effective pencil grasp, appropriate spatial orientation, and size concepts.

As a volunteer, Bruns could address handwriting of some individuals, but she knew that a more structured approach was necessary to address the needs of this population in general. Teachers at the Adult Learning Center expressed frustration in addressing the basics of handwriting while being stretched to address the other basic needs of the learner within the ESL curriculum, including reading, writing, speaking, and understanding English, along with other, often numerous needs. With approximately 25 students of varying levels in each class, the teachers did not have the resources to provide the attention to handwriting that was needed. Further concerns were voiced by teachers that the learners' difficulty with handwriting acquisition frequently prohibited them in daily activities, such as completing job applications or writing a note to a child's teacher.

Bruns recruited Victoria Nackley, an occupational therapy faculty member at Utica College, to help her explore current practices for teaching handwriting to adults learning ESL. Their inquiry led them to search literature in the adult basic education and ESL areas. They found that the literature emphasized learning language through the process of writing (e.g., Azevedo & Goncalves, 2012; Pour-Mohammadi, Abidin, & Fong, 2011; Sheen, Wright, & Moldawa, 2009) but did not address the process of learning to write. No literature was found that described a systematic, curricular approach to teaching handwriting to adult learners.

This lack of literature seemed to reflect that handwriting instruction was not a common concern for adults learning ESL who had already acquired a written script in their native language or had learned to write proficiently in English prior to coming to the United States. Yet, a need existed for those individuals who had not yet achieved handwriting fluency, whether in their own native language or in English.

Reflection 28.3. Refugees and Occupation

Research the definition of a *refugee,* and describe it in your own words.

- What occupations might be most challenging for an adult refugee trying to assimilate to life in the United States?
- What differences might the individual encounter in the United States compared with the individual's native country?

Consider the skill set of the occupational therapist.

- What skill sets are unique to the occupational therapist that could be applied to assisting individuals with the assimilation process?

Developing the Handwriting Instruction Program

With support of the local agency, Bruns and Nackley undertook the task of developing a handwriting instruction program. Because adult handwriting programs were not reported in published literature, they turned to handwriting programs for children. After comparing programs, Bruns and Nackley selected the Handwriting Without Tears (HWT) approach to inform program development.

Bruns and Nackley identified four characteristics of the HWT program that would address the needs of adult learners. The following program characteristics led them to select HWT:

1. The HWT approach begins with uppercase letters, emphasizing simple lines and curves. It was believed these simple strokes would be easier to use initially for learners without experience in written language.
2. HWT incorporates kinesthetic awareness of letter formation that would assist learners who had limited experience with gripping a pencil.
3. HWT reinforces spatial orientation, which would assist adult learners who have difficulty with spatial aspects of letter formation and placing letters appropriately on the paper.
4. HWT has a strong emphasis on practice, which was not only important but also possible, given the structure of the educational program.
5. Bruns and Nackley titled their program *Handwriting Instruction Program (HIP)*. It was developed as a 10-week course, held twice weekly for 1 hour. With Bruns and Nackley as primary instructors, HIP has evolved into a program assisted by student volunteers, occupational therapy students, and classroom teachers. The program has been adopted and is currently conducted by a lead teacher at the agency who works with learners who are new to ESL.

How the Handwriting Instruction Program Works

Now in existence for 11 years, HIP typically enrolls up to 20 adult learners at one time, an optimal number to manage the class effectively. Participation of the refugees and immigrants in HIP is voluntary for the learners and based on teacher recommendation. Participants' attendance does vary because of various factors, including family obligations, health concerns, and time involved in looking for work.

Preparing for Handwriting

To prepare for handwriting, learners engage in sensorimotor activities for alertness, writing readiness, and community building. Drawing from principles of sensory processing and self-regulation, instructors lead the learners in whole-body activities, such as running in place, doing chair push-ups, and engaging in arm squeezes. These exercises cause smiles and laughter to erupt among the learners. The whole-body warm-up exercises are followed by whole-arm activities in which the students move their arms bilaterally to directional instructions, such as down, across, curve, and slant, to reinforce concepts for use later during handwriting instruction (see Figure 28.1).

Wrist, hand, and finger preparatory activities follow, such as wrist circles, hand squeezes, and thumb-to-finger touching. Next, actual gripping activities with a pencil ensue, using a "pinch, flip, and write" approach to properly grasp the pencil, followed by finger-shifting or pencil rotation exercises. While repeating the oral instructions to promote language acquisition, the instructors have the learners practice the letter pattern in the air with their fingers, then on paper with pencils.

Handwriting Instruction

Next, each session proceeds with instruction in individual letter or number formation, approximately three letters per session. As with the HWT approach, the instructors begin with uppercase letters and progress to lowercase letters (see Figure 28.2).

The instructors follow the HWT sequence of letter instruction, which introduces letters from simple to complex, related to the pencil movements required. The instructor introduces each letter while pointing to the alphabet mural on the wall. The learners are then encouraged to suggest words that begin with that letter. The instructors have created their own instruction sheets for the learners to practice each letter, choosing words for their contextual relevance to the learner. The instruction sheets contain pictures of words that begin with the particular letter. The instruction sheets allow the learners to correctly practice each letter numerous times for mastery.

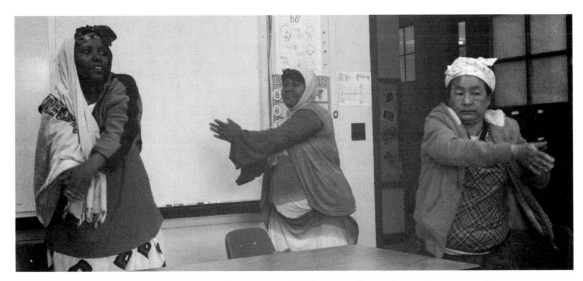

Figure 28.1. Whole-body exercises to reinforce directional concepts.
Source. Photo by Laurence P. Pacilio, Utica College. Used with permission.

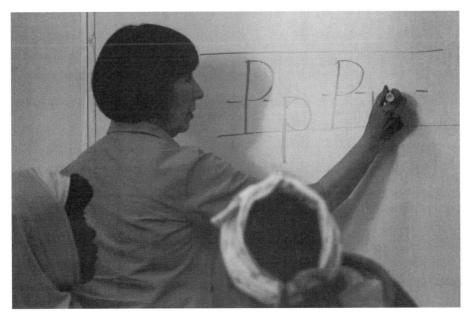

Figure 28.2. Demonstration of uppercase and lowercase letter formation.
Source. Photo by Laurence P. Pacilio, Utica College. Used with permission.

The sequence of each session follows a consistent format. The instructor begins by projecting the instruction sheet onto a whiteboard and demonstrating letter or number formation while repeating the directions. Then the instructor assists learners to repeat the directions while forming the letters in the air with their fingers to encourage kinesthetic awareness of letter formation.

With demonstrations provided as needed, learners proceed to writing the letter on the instruction sheet with the premise that practice makes perfect. Individual assistance is provided until the learner

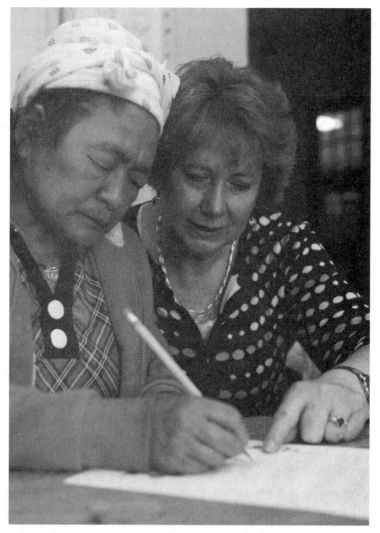

Figure 28.3. Individual instruction to promote accurate letter formation.
Source. Photo by Laurence P. Pacilio, Utica College. Used with permission.

acquires the correct pattern of letter formation (see Figure 28.3). While teaching how to combine letters into written words and how to write a sequence of words, the instructor reinforces appropriate spacing between individual letters and words.

Throughout the instructional process, the learners are given numerous opportunities to practice previously learned letters. The instructor frequently poses questions such as "How do I make a little *h?*" Learners then respond verbally using the same directional terms as given during the instructions. This process assists the learners not only in language

acquisition but also in gaining consistency in letter formation.

Once learners can write sufficient letters, they are instructed to write contextually relevant words. Using a basic dictionary for American English (Gadsby, 1999), instructors have chosen words for the instruction sheets that seem pertinent to the process of the learners' assimilation to mainstream American culture (e.g., *key, school, table*). When possible, instructors provide examples of the words to reinforce understanding. For example, if the word on the instruction sheet is *sit,* then the instructor would demonstrate sitting.

Reflection 28.4. Observation and Interview

Observation and interview serve as vital tools in uncovering challenges for individuals who show a poor fit between their skills and their lived context.

- Where in your community could you observe and interview individuals from other cultures and countries who may need assistance in integrating into the community?

Cultural Adaptations and Considerations

HIP was adapted to address adults' multicultural needs and promote a comfortable, friendly learning environment. To date, the program has served individuals from Somalia, Myanmar, Afghanistan, Nepal, Vietnam, former Soviet countries, and various Spanish-speaking countries.

Acknowledging the Oral Language Barrier

One of the first steps the instructors took when creating HIP involved acknowledging the oral language barrier. Bruns and Nackley simplified the language that they used when giving instructions or conveying information. Although the instructors used the foundational elements of HWT to inform program development, they screened each word from the HWT curriculum, eliminating any word they felt was irrelevant or difficult for an ESL learner to understand. They eliminated the use of idioms as much as possible. They also attempted to provide words that would apply to their students' daily lives. When making these adaptations, they also minimized the child-oriented components of the HWT curriculum to make the program more relevant to the adult learner.

For example, HWT uses a worksheet with the following dialogue to teach a child how to write a lowercase "a": "*Magic C, up like a (picture of a helicopter is displayed to the child), up, slide down, bump (picture of bumper cars)*" (Olsen, 2003b, p. 14). Acknowledging that the words *magic, helicopter, slide,* and *bumper*

cars would be challenging for the ESL adult learner to comprehend, the instructors decided to alter the directions in their instruction sheets. Consequently, they modified and simplified the instructions for the lowercase "a" to "*around, up, down, stop.*" Rather than having pictures of an alligator (which is not contextually relevant for a refugee new to the United States) and the words *at, sat, as,* and *was* (the meanings of which are difficult to describe in simple terms), the instructors included realistic pictures of an *arm, apple, airplane, animal(s), ant,* and *America,* complemented by the words *April* and *August.*

Other examples of language adaptations include

- The terms *big letters* and *little letters* were substituted for *capital* and *lowercase.*
- Spatial concepts of *top/bottom, up/down, big/little, across, around, curve, line,* and *circle* were selected for use with all letter formation for simplicity and consistency. A dilemma arose when choosing the most appropriate word for a diagonal line such as in the letter *K* or *V.* HWT uses the word *slide,* with a picture of a child's slide to direct the child to draw a diagonal line for the letters *K* or *V.* The instructors chose to use the word *slant* because a child's slide had little relevance to the adults' daily lives and could reflect a cultural bias.
- Emphasis was placed on nouns and verbs that could be easily depicted and would assist in language acquisition. The following copying words were eliminated: *as, of, with, are, it,* and *to* because they could not be readily described for the learners in simple English terms.

See Table 28.1 for a comparison of the HWT program with the HIP.

Adapting Instruction

Emphasizing Writing Direction

Another key part of culturally adapting the program involved emphasizing writing direction. Instructors identified the need to reinforce a top down, left–right progression to writing. This was accomplished by orienting the learners to the instruction sheet projected on the board, stressing the left-to-right/top-to-bottom sequence, and providing individual instruction as

Table 28.1. Comparison of Handwriting Programs

Handwriting Without Tears by Olsen (2003b)	Handwriting Instruction Program by Bruns & Nackley
Terminology entails child-oriented language and idioms, such as "frog jump back to the starting corner."	Idioms were eliminated to promote language comprehension.
Directional concepts are expressed in idioms such as "up like a helicopter."	Directional concepts were simplified to include the following terms: *down, across, slant, around,* and *curve.*
Common English words are used for writing practice that can be difficult for the ESL learner to comprehend because of their abstract nature (e.g., *as, like, too, of, if, with, luck*).	Concrete nouns and verbs that are applicable to the ESL adult were selected from the *Longman Basic American Dictionary* for letter practice (Gadsby, 1999).
Letter descriptions entail the terms *capital* and *lowercase.*	Terminology was simplified to the terms *big letters* and *little letters.*
Words appealing to children yet irrelevant to adult ESL learners are used in the program: *snowman, alligator, igloo,* and *koala.*	Words with contextual relevance for the adult ESL learner were chosen: *key, table, money,* and *bus.*
Directions for letter formation can have long descriptions. For the letter "e," the directions are "start, hit the ball, run the bases, stop."	Brief directions were simplified for each letter. For the letter "e," the directions are "across, around, stop."
Several practice words are not able to be depicted in visual format, such as *to, with,* or *like.*	Each practice word was chosen that could be depicted visually to assist the learner in language acquisition.

needed. Some individuals at the Adult Learning Center had handwriting experience using a right-to-left direction. Others had no experience with a starting point for their writing. Many of the adult students would simply start at the bottom of the page and haphazardly write letters anywhere on the page.

Facilitating Speed and Rhythm

One of the observations made early in the program development process was that besides poor legibility, learners were noted to be slow and labored in their writing. Consequently, the instructors began using music to facilitate speed and rhythm when writing. The learners copied various pencil patterns (e.g., across, down, slant, curve, circle) and letters to instrumental music to improve handwriting speed. The learners enjoyed the relaxing rhythms, which in turn assisted in developing rhythmicity in handwriting.

Promoting Accurate Letter Formation

The instructors recognized that promoting accurate letter formation often required them to correct the learners' handwriting. They acknowledged that this correction process might stifle the learners who were giving their best attempts to learn. Thus, the instructors would purposely form a letter incorrectly on the projected instruction sheet, asking the

learners, "Is this one good?" The process empowered the learners to discern accurate letter formation and verbally correct the instructors. The process also provided comic relief within the classroom, relaying the sentiment that it was OK to make mistakes and subsequently correct them.

Writing Signatures

Many of the refugees and immigrants were observed to misspell their names or write their names using all uppercase letters, with incorrectly formed letters. A key feature of HIP became an emphasis on the adult learners' ability to sign their names. Each learner was provided with a sheet of paper with his or her name written correctly and was encouraged to practice copying the name on a regular basis. Once the learners were able to easily write their name, they were given the option of transitioning to a cursive signature. Practice continued with demonstration by the instructors. One of the successes of HIP was that, at the end of the sessions, many learners were able to sign important monthly documents in cursive. Teachers within the education program were thrilled, and learners proudly displayed their newly acquired skill.

Maintaining a Relaxed, Fun Atmosphere

Many of the learners have been apprehensive and reserved and therefore hesitant to participate. To address this issue, the instructors have made efforts to keep the sessions relaxed, intentionally providing opportunities for laughter and enjoyment. Through these efforts, the instructors have found they can build a supportive community of learners, which in turn increases motivation to participate.

For example, finger-shifting and rotation activities on the pencil during the preparatory work usually yield a chuckle. As the adults move their fingers up and down or around on the pencil in unison, one or more pencils tend to drop, often by the instructors. Another technique that has been found useful is to have the adult learners' critique the instructor's spacing of letters and words on the whiteboard accompanied by a friendly banter.

Reflection 28.5. Pro Bono Work

The *Occupational Therapy Code of Ethics* (American Occupational Therapy Association, 2015) supports pro bono work to contribute to the occupational performance needs of others. It also supports advocacy to promote occupational engagement.

- Where and how could you as an occupational therapist donate your time to benefit others who are new to the United States in your community?
- How could you advocate for opportunities for the adult refugee to promote greater assimilation within the adult's new context?

Impact of the Handwriting Instruction Program

Program evaluation on the HIP is limited at this point. Bruns and Nackley collected pre–post data on 15 learners in Fall 2005 and 8 learners in Spring 2006. The *Evaluation Tool of Children's Handwriting–Manuscript (ETCH–M)* was used as a measure of letter legibility and letters written per minute (LPM). The learners made 13.7% gains in letter legibility, with posttest results approaching accepted standards for legibility. Gains in LPM were 6.4% for the combined group. As an example of the change and improvement noted in letter formation, readers are directed to Figures 28.4 and 28.5, where changes in letter legibility and writing speed of one learner are illustrated.

Banus, Jennings, and Carr (2007) used the ETCH–M in a pretest–posttest study to measure the effect of HIP on word legibility, letter legibility, number legibility, and LPM. They reported an increase in the mean scores of 15 HIP participants on all dependent variables, although only letter legibility improvement reached significance ($p = .007$).

A primary limitation to improvement has been inconsistent attendance of the learners, a limitation that has been noted during all sessions of the program. In both groups of data reported, the degree of improvement was noted to be related to attendance: The more times learners attended sessions, the more they improved. Inconsistent attendance does not appear to reflect learner satisfaction with the program but is an artifact of the varied demands placed

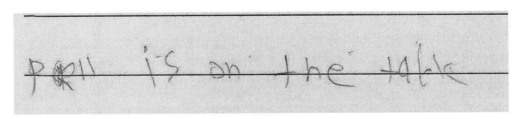

Figure 28.4. Example of pretest writing for HIP participant H.K. (3 minutes, 50 seconds).

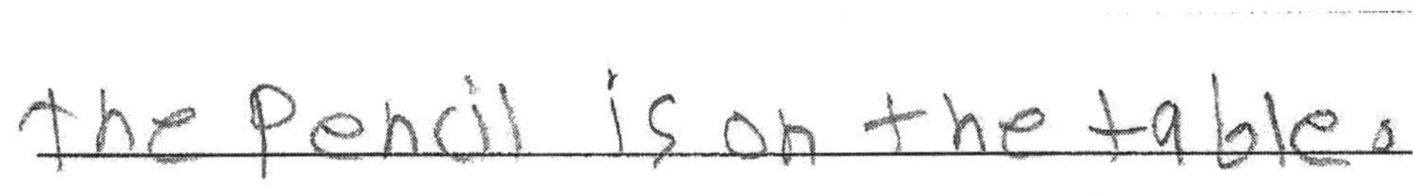

Figure 28.5. Example of posttest writing for HIP participant H.K. (30 seconds).

on this population in terms of assimilating to a new country and unfamiliarity with American systems of employment, housing, and schooling.

HIP is constantly evolving. For example, occupational therapy students introduced **Callirobics,** a program of handwriting exercises and patterns that are set to music (Laufer, 2006). The instructors found the program to be too structured for the needs of the group, and while they still use music, they no longer use Callirobics. Because of this evolving nature, perhaps the best evidence of effectiveness is the anecdotal evidence that provides the motivation to continue by all involved, including the learners and instructors at the Adult Learning Center.

Educators at the Adult Learning Center overwhelmingly welcomed the HIP. Teachers reported (1) improvement in the learners' attention and concentration, (2) learners' pride in their individual progress, and (3) knowledge of letter formation improved overall learning. Unsolicited comments from educational staff indicated the learners are faster at handwriting and have more confidence in their handwriting. Learners consistently indicated their gratitude throughout each session.

Utica College students have benefited from this multicultural experience. HIP began serendipitously as a service learning opportunity for college students through Project SHINE but has evolved into a vital community alliance for the college and the occupational therapy program. This multicultural experience, reflective of the uniqueness of the Utica area, also provides an innovative practice model for occupational therapists and students. It has served as a research project for the benefit of HIP and graduate occupational therapy students.

Summary

HIP provides an example of meeting an occupational need for individuals attempting to integrate into life in the United States. The program description offers occupational therapists a mechanism for adapting current occupational therapy practices to meet the occupational performance needs of adult refugees. These adaptations take into consideration the unique nature of an individual learning English as a second language, requiring a certain skill set and specific instructional practices.

Respectful, culturally sensitive practices that address this skill set have served as hallmarks of the program's success. Although research and anecdotal evidence provide support for the program, further assessment of the program's impact is needed.

References

American Occupational Therapy Association. (2015). Occupational therapy code of ethics (2015). *American Journal of Occupational Therapy, 69*(Suppl. 3), 6913410057p1–6913410057p6. http://dx.doi.org/10.5014/ajot.2015.696S03

Azevedo, N. R., & Goncalves, M. J. (2012). Writing and reading with art: Adult literacy, transformation, and learning. *Adult Learning, 23*(2), 69–75.

Banus, A. R., Jennings, A. M., & Carr, L. M. (2007). *The effectiveness of Handwriting Without Tears and Callirobics with an adult immigrant population.* Unpublished thesis, Utica College, Utica, NY.

Gadsby, A. (1999). *Longman basic dictionary of American English.* Harlow, UK: Pearson.

Graham, S. (2009–2010). Want to improve children's writing: Don't neglect their handwriting. *American Educator, 33*(4), 20–27.

Hoy, M. M. P., Egan, M. Y., & Feder, K. P. (2011). A systematic review of interventions to improve handwriting. *Canadian Journal of Occupational Therapy, 78*(1), 13–25. http://dx.doi.org/10.2182/cjot.2011.78.1.3

Laufer, L. (2006). *Handwriting exercises to music.* Charlottesville, VA: Callirobics.

Medwell, J., & Wray, D. (2007). Handwriting: What do we know and what do we need to know? *Literacy, 41*(1), 10–15. http://dx.doi.org/10.1111/j.1467-9345.2007.00453.x

Olsen, J. (2003a). *Handwriting Without Tears kindergarten teacher's guide.* Cabin John, MD: Handwriting Without Tears.

Olsen, J. (2003b). *My printing book.* Cabin John, MD: Handwriting Without Tears.

Peverley, S. (2006). The importance of handwriting speed in adult writing. *Developmental Psychology, 39*(1), 197–216. http://dx.doi.org/10.1207/s15326942dn2901_10

Pour-Mohammadi, M., Abidin, M. J. Z., & Fong, C. L. (2012). The effect of process writing practice on the writing quality of form one students: A case study. *Asian Social Science, 8*(3), 88–99. http://dx.doi.org/10.5539/ass.v8n3p88

Sheen, Y., Wright, D., & Moldawa, A. (2009). Differential effects of focused and unfocused written correction on the accurate use of grammatical forms by adult ESL learners. *System, 37,* 556–569. http://dx.doi.org/10.1016/j.system.2009.09.002

United Nations High Commissioner for Refugees. (2005). The town that loves refugees. *Refugees, 1*(138), 1–31.

Chapter 29.

THE LIVING WELL PROGRAM: A COMMUNITY-BASED PARTICIPATORY WELLNESS PROGRAM

Jyothi Gupta, PhD, OTR/L, FAOTA

Chapter Highlights

• Health Care: Access, Prevention, and Primary Care
• Health Disparities
• Community-Based Programs
• Program Implementation Strategies
• Living Well Program

Key Terms and Concepts

✧ Aging Gracefully program
✧ Community-based participatory research
✧ Cycle of frailty
✧ Healthy Body Healthy Spirit
✧ Healthy Changes program
✧ Health disparities

✧ Living Well Program
✧ Primary care
✧ Primary prevention
✧ Triangulation
✧ Well Elderly Study
✧ Wellness in Tillery program

How people live their daily lives in safe communities and have access to basic necessities such as stable housing, education, and work greatly affect their health, well-being, and reduction of risk for developing chronic disease. The *Living Well Program (LWP),* a community-based primary prevention program, was developed to address health inequities in a predominantly African American low-income, urban community that was reported as one of the worst for health inequities in the state of Minnesota (Shomer, 2005). This chapter discusses the process used to identify the needs of a community, the development and implementation of LWP, and program evaluation. Challenges encountered during this process are also addressed.

Health Care: Access, Prevention, and Primary Care

The spiraling costs of health care in the United States coupled with widening income gaps have made access to health care out of reach for millions of Americans. The Patient Protection and Affordable Care Act ([ACA], 2010) was meant to make health insurance accessible to millions of Americans who are uninsured or underinsured. Although access to health care is an important element for health, its contribution is not proportionally large compared with other health determinants, including genes and biology, health services, health behaviors, physical environment, and social environment (Centers for Disease Control and Prevention [CDC], 2014).

Attention has been directed to primary prevention and primary care as a means to health care cost reduction with the mandatory coverage for preventive services under the ACA (Cassidy, 2010). *Primary prevention* refers to risk reduction for injury or disease, whereas *primary care* refers to general care for minor health issues, health maintenance, and routine preventive procedures (Katz & Ali, 2009). Expanding preventive services across the board will not reduce health care spending; in fact, in some instances, preventive screening can increase spending (Cohen, Neumann, & Weinstein, 2008).

It appears that reducing health care costs depends on *where* prevention services are delivered and *who* the service targets are. It has been suggested that prevention programs delivered outside of a doctor's office or a clinic (e.g., community site, patient's home) and strategically targeted to those who are vulnerable for developing chronic diseases are expected to reduce health care spending (Cohen & Neumann, 2009).

Health Disparities

Health disparities are differences in the health status, morbidity, and mortality of groups based on factors such as race, ethnicity, income, geography, immigrant status, and sexual orientation (U.S. National Library of Medicine, 2015). In the United States, significant health disparities exist due to gender, age, race, education, income, disability, and geographic location (CDC, 2013). Evidence suggests that provider bias, prejudice, and stereotyping may contribute to differences in care, access to care, quality of life, physical function, and overall health (Smedley,

Stith, & Nelsen, 2003). African Americans comprise 13% of the U.S. population, making them the second largest minority population after Hispanics/Latinos, who are about 17% of the population (U.S. Census Bureau, 2015).

The Office of Minority Health (2014) reported that the death rate for African Americans was generally higher than White individuals for heart diseases, stroke, cancer, asthma, influenza and pneumonia, diabetes, HIV/AIDS, and homicide. African American adults were 70% more likely than White adults to be diagnosed with diabetes, nearly twice as likely to die from diabetes, 40% more likely to have high blood pressure, and 50% more likely to die from a stroke. Stuber, Galea, Ahern, Blaney, and Fuller (2003) identified health disparities in four low-income Latino and African American neighborhoods that were associated with poor self-assessed mental health and racial discrimination, although they were unable to discern the directionality of this relationship.

Hueston and Hubbard (2000) examined access and utilization of preventive health care services among African Americans and reported that individual differences in educational level, marital status, or insurance status were not associated with the use of preventive services. Moreover, when health care services are accessible, African American patients across most socioeconomic classes in both rural and urban settings follow up with recommended preventive services.

Aging Population

Older Americans account for more than three-quarters of the health expenditures in the United States (CDC, 2014). The number of individuals ages 65 or older will reach 83.7 million by the year 2050 (Ortman, Velkoff, & Hogan, 2014). The cost of providing health care to someone age 65 or older is three to five times greater than the cost for someone younger.

One explanation for increased health care expenses is the high incidence of chronic conditions and pathologies that occur in the older population. The average 75-year-old American has three diagnosed chronic conditions and takes 4.5 different medications. In addition, nearly 50% of older adults are diagnosed with hypertension, roughly 20% are diagnosed with heart disease, and 20% are diagnosed with cancer. More than 65% of older Americans have some form of cardiovascular disease, and half of all older men and two-thirds of all older women have arthritis (CDC, 2014).

Physical activity is a key component in keeping older adults healthy, allowing them to maintain the highest level of function and independence. Currently, only 25% of men and 20% of women ages 65 years or older meet the recommended guidelines for regular physical activity. Among adults ages 65 to 74 years, 28%–37% of women and 18%–33% of men reported no participation in regular physical activity. Finally, among adults age 75 years or older, 38%–54% of women and 27%–38% of men reported no participation in any leisure time physical activity (Stewart et al., 2001).

Age-related changes that affect multiple body systems contribute to a continuum of decline, which may result in impairment, functional limitation, or disability. The *cycle of frailty* describes the relationships between the various components of the biologically aging human body and subsequent decline in function (Fried & Watson, 1998). For example, age-related musculoskeletal changes, such as loss of muscle mass, can lead to decreased strength and power, leading to impaired balance, decreased walking speed, and eventual falls and injuries. This can then lead to decreased activity, decreased total energy expenditure, and result in further loss of muscle mass, thus completing the cycle.

The older adult population has complex and expensive medical needs. As this growing population continues to age, the demand on the health care system will only become greater. Intervention to improve the health of this population is essential to combat the increasing demands on the health care system.

Low-Income At-Risk Populations

African American older adults residing in inner cities demonstrated an increased level of dependency in activities of daily living (ADLs) and an increased prevalence of depression compared with a racially diverse control group (Miller et al., 1996). The inner-city group also demonstrated an increased prevalence of worsening health and a tendency toward poorer self-rated health.

Decline in ADLs varies among older adults from different ethnic groups, with African American older adults associated with an increased risk of ADL decline (Moody-Ayers, Mehta, Lindquist, Sands, &

Covinsky, 2005). Socioeconomic status and cognitive function were found to be the largest factors affecting the ADL decline in African Americans ages 70 to 79 years old. Moody et al. (2005) concluded that the etiology of Black–White health disparities related to unexplained differences in cognitive function was likely due to the difference in quality education, economic standing, and inadequate treatment of comorbidities.

In the Twin Cities metropolitan area in Minnesota, disparities were reported in education, income, wealth, and health on the basis of race, class, and place disparities (Shomer, 2005). Shomer's (2005) study showed that high rates of high school dropouts put individuals at risk for unemployment or low-skilled and low-wage jobs. Moreover, there is a mismatch of job availability and skill set between lower skilled residents of central cities and the high-skilled jobs available in the central cities.

African American median household income was reported at $29,404, which is half the median household income for the total population in the area. Nearly 23% of the Twin Cities population lives in the poor neighborhoods in the metro area, of which 54% are racial minorities and 46% are foreign born. More than 40% of the central city neighborhoods are households living at or below the poverty level, compared with relatively none in the suburban areas. Increased levels of poverty correlate with an increase in violent crime (Shomer, 2005).

Community-Based Programs

Efforts at reducing and eliminating health disparities have led to various program initiatives in specific communities and populations, particularly for older adults, such as evidence-based programs targeting independent-dwelling older adults that focus on physical activity, fall prevention, nutrition, and mental health (Gillespie et al., 2003). In a systematic review, Gillespie et al. identified four effective strategies to reduce falls in older adults by 14%–39% with intervention using one or more of the following:

1. Exercises,
2. Reduction of in-home hazards,
3. Discontinuation of certain psychotropic medications, and
4. A multifactorial risk assessment with targeted management.

Prescription of specific balance or strength exercise programs was identified as an effective community-based strategy to reduce falls and fall risk by 29%–49%.

Well Elderly Study

The *Well Elderly Study* showed that preventive group occupational therapy was effective in improving health, quality of life, and function in a population of multiethnic, urban, independent-living older adults (Clark et al., 1997). Costs for the 9-month program averaged $548 per subject. Post-intervention health care costs were lower for the occupational therapy group ($967) than for the active control group ($1,726), the passive control group ($3,334), or a combination of the control groups ($2,593; Hay et al., 2002).

Chronic Disease Self-Management Programs

Chronic disease self-management programs also resulted in health care cost savings of $714 per person in emergency room visits and hospital utilization. Potential savings of about $6.6 billion are projected from this program reaching just 10% of Americans with one or more chronic conditions (National Council on Aging [NAC], 2014). Participants of the NAC's *Healthy Changes program* designed to assist older adults in daily self-management of diabetes reported that the social interactions and friendships established from the community-based group setting were as valuable as the information and resources provided.

Health Promotion Programs for African Americans

Community-based programs in low-income, urban areas where African Americans are more represented are sparse but documented in the literature. The *Aging Gracefully program* is an enrichment program developed by nursing practitioners that aims to promote social support, coping with aging, and enhancing self-care among independent-living African American older adults in inner-city public housing in Baltimore (Gerson, Dorsey, Berg, & Rose, 2004). Group leaders noted that participation and social interaction were facilitated by scheduling sessions in the morning, conducting sessions at the participants' site of residence, and focusing on the positive as opposed to the negative aspects of aging.

A second study, titled the *Wellness in Tillery program,* was a community-based intervention conducted by occupational therapy students (Barnard et al., 2004). The participants in this program were predominantly African Americans over 65 years old. This study reported the benefit of participants' input in program design that was thought to have enhanced perceived wellness, maintenance of meaningful activities, and improved quality of life. Finally, the *Healthy Body Healthy Spirit* trial that was targeted to socioeconomically diverse African American populations noted that churches are very effective venues for culture-specific health promotion activities (Resnicow et al., 2005).

Program Implementation Strategies

Research provides valuable insights for reducing participation barriers, improving program effectiveness, and minimizing participant dropout rates in programs developed in the community.

Reducing Barriers

Identified barriers to community program participation include a lack of basic knowledge or motivation to address health problems, a lack of social support, challenges in accessing health promotion programs, and existing corporate and public policies that promote unhealthy practices (Nied & Franklin, 2002).

Marrongiello and Gottlieb (2004) identified logistic issues such as transportation, safety, time, and interest as common barriers to participation in community-based programs. Using a central location, such as a neighborhood community center, may help prevent transportation barriers.

Safety concerns in community-based programs include neighborhood crime, limited mobility, fear of falling, and poor accessibility at program sites. Logistics of scheduling around participants' conflicting appointments, family commitments, and daily routines may decrease program enrollment. Additionally, it has been shown that a general lack of interest in the program topic may be linked to a lack of perceived need for change, or discrepancy between actual need and perceived need (Cohen-Mansfield & Frank, 2008). This reinforces the importance of topic selection to maximize behavior modification.

Improving Program Effectiveness

To increase a program's effectiveness, tailoring wellness programs to the specific needs of the community is essential, especially with a racially or ethnically diverse population. To accomplish this, it is critical to establish relationships with the community prior to initiating the program (Gerson et al., 2004).

Incorporating the religion, traditions, political perspectives, and daily routines of the target population has been suggested (Barnard et al., 2004). The community-based program must also stress the importance of balancing didactic communication and open dialogue between participants and facilitators in creating an environment where participants feel safe when sharing valuable life experiences and knowledge. These insights, drawn from previous health and wellness programs in the research literature, guided the conceptualization of the LWP used in the present study.

Maximizing Retention and Minimizing Program Dropout Rates

Shriner and Stack-Cutler (2012) reported that the five most often used and most effective strategies are (1) convenient location, (2) reminders about sessions, (3) linguistic resources, (4) snacks or meals provided, and (5) diversity of team members.

Living Well Program

The LWP is a grant-funded health promotion program designed for and with participation by African American residents in a low-income urban neighborhood in a Midwest city. The program evolved to address maintaining health while coping with poverty-associated stress. Exhibit 29.1 describes the program's overarching goal and objectives.

Method

The LWP was designed on some of the key principles of *community-based participatory research (CBPR),* which is an equitable and participatory approach to research that is inclusive of research participants and key community members in the research process (Minkler, 2005). The principles of CBPR encompass the following: The community's identity was defined by a specific geographical neighborhood; a strengths-focused approach recognized the assets and resources within the community; empowering community members through education was the motivation for program development; and the program focused on local social determinants of health and their impact on health and well-being (Israel et al., 2008). The community work was conducted in three phases:

1. Finding out the needs of the community,
2. Developing a framework for a program informed by the community-identified needs, and
3. Evaluating the program to understand ways to improve the program to better serve the community.

Exhibit 29.1. The Living Well Program: Overarching Goal and Objectives

Goal: To develop and implement a culturally responsive, interprofessional health and wellness promotion program for a low-income urban community using a community-based participatory research approach.

1. To empower participants to be full partners in the process that will promote their health.

2. To enable participants to identify the information they need to develop meaningful strategies for health improvement, maintenance, and management of chronic disease.

3. To facilitate participants to identify the barriers to achieving, maintaining, or regaining health and ways to overcome those barriers.

4. To facilitate participants' identification of and involvement in meaningful occupations.

5. To educate participants to identify strategies to incorporate the information learned in the program into their everyday lives.

6. To provide participants with information regarding community resources that can help sustain participation, wellness, and health following the discontinuation of the wellness program.

Phase I: Needs Assessment of the Community

The LWP was designed to be community driven and participatory in nature. Building trust is key to CBPR, particularly in communities that have experienced historical exploitation and oppression and consequently mistrust "outsiders" (Minkler & Wallerstein, 2008).

The first step was to identify a community liaison who was known and trusted by the community to assist with the identification, facilitation, and recruitment of participants for the program. The liaison's role was instrumental in gaining access to the community. The identified liaison was a long-term resident of 35 years, an active community member in the local church and organizations, and a public health school nurse. The liaison's endorsement of the LWP as a community member and a collaborator made it possible to gain entry into the community.

The community liaison provided feedback on the needs assessment survey and distributed and collected the survey. The content of the survey included general demographics, medical history, health perceptions, barriers to accessing the community, and personal interests. The survey focused on topics related to health and wellness. A total of 100 surveys were distributed in the community, and completed surveys were collected, analyzed, and used as a guide for program topics that the community identified as important to them.

Phase II: Curriculum Development and Program Implementation

The results of the needs assessment guided LWP development. Given the program's participatory nature, it was designed with flexibility so that the community-driven nature was upheld throughout the process of development and implementation. The program content was divided into 10 individual sessions (see Exhibit 29.2).

Each 2-hour session was delivered in a group format on a weekly basis. The sessions were held at two different sites in the same zip code: (1) a government-subsidized high-rise and (2) a community center. These sites were identified with the help of the community liaison as central locations for the targeted population.

The sessions were led by two licensed occupational therapists and assisted by student researchers. The sessions comprised this outline:

- Introduction of session objectives
- Quick recap of concepts presented in the previous sessions
- Topic presentation
- Large-group discussion
- Breakout group activity and discussion
- Resources to participants relevant to the session topic

The 36-item Short Form Health Survey (SF–36) is a tool that has been validated to measure quality of life (Finch, Brooks, Stratford, & Mayo, 2002).

Exhibit 29.2. The Living Well Program: Session Topics Addressing Health and Well-Being

Session	Topics
1.	Health, well-being, and quality of life occupations: Everyday activities, health, and well-being
2.	Partnering in community-based participatory research; occupations, habits, and routines for health and well-being
3.	Physical activity, health, and well-being
4.	Nutrition, health, and well-being (eating healthy on a limited budget)
5.	Safety, health, and well-being (falls risk and prevention)
6.	Community mobility (transportation)
7.	Volunteering and community excursions
8.	Active mind and memory
9.	Emotional wellness and mental health (stress management and depression)
10.	Social participation and spiritual wellness

It was administered to the participants prior to the initiation of the LWP. The SF–36 was not used for monitoring change but rather to get a baseline summary of the participants' perceptions of their health and wellness status.

Phase III: Program Evaluation

To evaluate the LWP, the researchers obtained quantitative data using a program evaluation questionnaire with 12 questions designed to assess the relevance of the session topics to the participants and identify behavioral change and barriers to change. In addition, there were questions regarding future topics of interest.

The qualitative component of the program consisted of two semi-structured interviews. The first interview was to gain a deeper understanding of each participant's life experience and occupational history. The second interview was to obtain each participant's perspective regarding the LWP. Each interview was audio recorded and transcribed verbatim.

The content was organized, and each researcher familiarized themselves with the data. Following this, a thematic framework was identified to develop a codebook. The data were coded, charted, and mapped to assist in the interpretation.

Multiple forms of ***triangulation*** were used to ensure the validity and reliability of the data. The five types of triangulation that were used for improving the validity included data, investigator, theory, methodological, and environmental (Guion, Diehl, & McDonald, 2011).

Data triangulation was achieved by interviewing multiple participants. To accomplish investigator triangulation, multiple investigators were used to analyze the data. Theory triangulation was achieved by the use of multidisciplinary perspectives, specifically, physical therapy and occupational therapy. The combination of qualitative and quantitative methods of evaluation assured methodological triangulation. Finally, environmental triangulation was achieved by the use of participants from multiple settings, namely a high-rise complex and a community center.

Results

Phase I: Needs Assessment

The needs assessment survey had a response rate of 79%. The average age of the participants was 69 years, 75% of participants were women, and the majority lived below the federal poverty level. In addition, 63% of the survey respondents stated they felt they would benefit from more information regarding their medical conditions (e.g., diabetes, hypertension, arthritis), and 78% felt they needed more information on how to maintain and improve their health.

Participants also indicated that a community-based wellness program would improve their quality of life. Of the participants, 86% stated they would be happier if they had the opportunity to share their personal stories, 75% stated they would be happier if they had the opportunity to exercise in a group, and 87% stated they would be happier if they had more opportunities to learn about things that were of interest to them. These findings were used to guide the design and inform the content and process of program development and implementation.

Phase II: Program Implementation

Although all sessions had an average of 20 participants, only 14 participants consistently participated with 100% attendance in all the LWP sessions across both sites. Attendance was more consistent in the community center although these participants had to get to the site from their homes. Many of these participants car-pooled or used public transportation. Despite offering sessions on-site, the public high-rise building had very sporadic participation and more people came in randomly to sessions.

With the exception of one Latina who was a long-term resident of the community, the participants were all African American; the average age of participants between the two sites was 55 years. The program evaluation data were obtained only from the 14 participants who attended all the sessions, although all other participants' feedback was collected throughout the duration of the program implementation.

Phase III: Program Evaluation

The quantitative results from Phase III were from a program evaluation questionnaire, which was distributed to the 14 participants and completed at the end of the final session.

- A majority of participants (94%) rated each session at the highest level of interest and helpfulness.
- The sessions that received the highest rating from the largest percentage of participants were physical activity, stress management, and healthy eating.

- A majority of participants (83%) also identified a need for more classes on all 10 topics, particularly stress management and depression.
- 83% of participants reported having a great deal of influence over their state of health, and 75% reported having made a great deal of change in their effort to improve their state of health or prevent disease.
- 69% of participants reported their level of daily physical activity had changed a great deal.
- 100% of participants reported their level of daily physical activity had improved since the start of the program.

Participants also identified strategies to improve their current health situation. Ninety-two percent of participants reported having made a concrete plan after completion of the program. In addition, participants identified specific barriers to maintaining, managing, or improving their personal health. Participants' key areas of concern were limited finances and transportation challenges that restricted their ability to participate in their community.

The qualitative results of Phase III were from interviews of participants from both sites. The four overarching topics that emerged were (1) chronic stress, (2) inescapable poverty, (3) mistrust of the health care system, and (4) perceived lack of social support.

Chronic Stress. Chronic stress was overwhelmingly prevalent at the high-rise site and experienced to a certain degree by some at the community center site. **Chronic stress** is extensive and unrelenting stress persisting over long periods of time with serious health consequences (American Psychological Association, 2015). Purely by serendipity, most of the participants at the community center site lived in their own homes, had the support of their spouses or other family members, and had access to transportation to get to the community center. They had established relationships among themselves over the years as participants in ceramic classes and other craft activities and had developed a system of carpooling or giving rides to each other.

In contrast, participants at the high-rise site were in subsidized housing and received social assistance either through welfare payments or through disability benefits. They were living alone, and most had no family nearby. Only one participant had a car.

Limited finances were a major source of stress for many participants who had to live on limited income.

My financial situation is so chaotic that I don't know if I'm coming or going . . . you know I can't work a job, I'm too stressed, I'm in too much pain . . . right now I am not doing anything I'm too disabled . . . so I'm behind in my mortgage, I don't have enough to make a mortgage anyway. I owe everybody.

Inescapable Poverty. For many participants, particularly those in the high-rise site who experienced chronic poverty and had not worked for various reasons, a sense of hopelessness prevailed.

By the time you get a minimum wage job and have to deal with people and their attitudes. And then you have to worry about transportation, go to get to a job, got to worry about uniform, you're not coming out with much of anything. And then you have taxes. So you're not coming out with anything. You got a job for $5/hour and you actually come out with $1/hour. And you've put in all this time for $1/hour . . . you don't have time, you have to work, and then you end up just surviving. Not to get rich, just surviving.

Mistrust of the Health Care System. Participants reported poor experiences in their interactions with systems including health care. Tuskegee was mentioned during sessions, and for these participants, it was part of their living memory and not a mere historical event. They had family who were affected, and they spoke about Tuskegee in ways that it was very real and recent in their lives. *Tuskegee* refers to the untreated syphilis study that started in 1932 and lasted 40 years. The study used more than 600 Black men as subjects and is a classic case of breach in biomedical research ethics, including not obtaining informed consent and withholding treatment in order to understand the natural progression of the disease.

The participants of the LWP program also discussed poor treatment by service providers. One participant who had hip replacement was in a great deal of pain and said that her physician did not give her strong pain medications despite her asking for them. When asked about her thoughts on this physician's behavior, she commented that "they think we are junkies or we will sell the drugs for money."

I have used it [health insurance] . . . I did use it . . . I have trouble with my digestive system. It was probably a couple of years ago. I went thinking they [doctors] could help me, but what they prescribed for me was what I was already taking, so I didn't go back . . . I didn't go back.

Perceived Lack of Social Support. Most of the participants lived alone and had no family or other social support. One participant said, "Some days I lay up there [in my room] and I'd be crying, wishing my mother was still here so I had someone to talk to. But I have a sister . . . and I don't hardly talk to her."

An indicator for the success of the program was that 92% of participants stated that they "formed a concrete plan to maintain, manage, and improve their current health status" at the conclusion of the program. The design of the LWP was such that every session included a discussion regarding perceived barriers specific to the session topic. Having participants self-identify their personal barriers and collectively come up with strategies to overcome these barriers was empowering for them. Often participants commented on how enjoyable it was to be able to share their experiences, because too often no one cared about their stories.

Discussion

At the conclusion of the LWP, most participants indicated that they were able to identify barriers to their health improvement, use strategies that they were taught to tackle perceived barriers to health in their lives, and be full partners in the process to promote their overall health. This finding is consistent with the literature that preventive group health promotion led by health care professionals was effective in improving the health of independent-living older adults in low-income, multiethnic, urban areas (Clarke et al., 1997; Gillespie et al., 2003). Participants in the LWP reported improved daily physical activity and described their efforts to make healthy behavioral changes. Because no follow-up studies were conducted, there is no evidence of sustained efforts.

The social support created by the participatory nature of the sessions may have had unanticipated benefits to the participants. In the early stages of the program implementation, it became obvious that the participants at the two sites were different in many ways. Those who resided in the high-rise site were economically, socially, physically, and mentally worse off than those who participated at the community center site. Participants at the community center

were very active and resourceful, had access to transportation, and were a long-standing social group with shared interests in ceramics and crafts. Participants at the high-rise site had lived in the same building for years, but they did not socialize or interact with one another initially.

Over the course of the program, however, the level of social interaction between the participants, particularly at the high-rise site, improved a great deal. Several of the participants at the high-rise site stated that they had formed a walking group following the conclusion of the physical activity session. The benefit of increased social interaction was also documented by other studies (Gerson et al., 2004; National Council on Aging, 2014).

The LWP encountered many of the same barriers reported in the literature. During informal discussions in multiple sessions, participants identified several environmental factors that posed a challenge to their level of participation. These included high crime in the neighborhood; limited income; limited access to transportation; and inability to afford prescription glasses, medicine, and suitable footwear for walking. Participants' statements reflect the link between social and contextual factors and health, and highlight the challenges programs such as LWP face in promoting a healthy lifestyle in populations living "in crisis." It appears that the focus of health promotion activities that solely target changes in individual behaviors is insufficient in addressing disparities and has to shift to addressing root causes in the social environment that predispose certain groups of individuals to health disparities (Link & Phelan, 1995).

Exhibit 29.3 lists the strengths, challenges, and lessons learned in the process of implementation of the LWP. Recognizing the community as a unit of identity, capitalizing on the strengths and assets within the community, using a collaborative and equitable approach to partnership building, learning with and from the community, and addressing local contextual barriers to health and identifying sustainable solutions were some of the guiding principles of CBPR that were incorporated into the LWP (Israel et al., 2008).

The author has 15 years of experience working with various underserved communities and understands the unique issues that exist for different communities. Even so, the extent of occupational deprivation and chronic stress experienced by the residents of the public high-rise site was unanticipated. This experience clearly highlighted the significance of the social health determinants and contextual factors on

> **Exhibit 29.3. Summary of the Strengths, Challenges, and Lessons Learned From the Living Well Program**
>
> **Strengths**
>
> - This community-based program was held at sites where participants lived and met in the community. Thus, the program was in their daily living context.
> - Providing the program at two locations within the community targeted two different groups of individuals of the same community.
> - Identifying a key community leader to serve as liaison for the author to meet with key community stakeholders helped her gain access into community.
> - The participatory nature of the program that was strengths-focused gave voice to people who are not often asked to share their stories and opinions.
> - Community building through an interactive group format helped group members form new relationships. For example, the public high-rise residents did not know each other until they participated in the program although they were long-term residents of the building.
> - The occupation-centered program was a novel approach to health and well-being and elicited active engagement of participants.
>
> **Challenges Encountered**
>
> - Partnership building and gaining the trust of community members take time.
> - Time constraints made scheduling very challenging, as participants were unable to meet during times that worked for most program implementers, who also had to coordinate around physical therapy and occupational therapy program schedules.
> - Consistent attendance of participants was a major challenge. Average session attendance was about 20, but only 14 were present for all sessions across two sites.
> - The chronic stress experienced by participants in the public high-rise site in particular was further exacerbated with local politics of the building that often percolated into program time. This did not occur at the community center site.
> - It was challenging to sustain the program and build community capacity.
>
> **Lessons Learned**
>
> - Flexibility in programming is key for success. For example, after participants requested that stress be covered as a topic in every session, we linked the session topic to stress. How can physical activity or healthy eating or healthy routines alleviate stress?
> - Be prepared for the time-intensive nature of community-based programming.
> - Literacy issues and lack of prescription glasses challenged some participation with some activities. Having a number of people on the programming team allowed for one-on-one working with these participants.
> - Rewards outweigh challenges: Empowering community residents with information on how to take charge and gain control of their health is a powerful experience for both participants and program implementers.
> - Data collection challenges are common issues in underserved communities and have to be factored in. Examples include getting sufficient numbers to participate consistently and the challenge of using standardized tools with participants with low educational levels and literacy.
> - Identifying ways in which the program can continue is essential for building capacity within the community. Identifying interested community members who can continue to implement the wellness program and collaborating with other community health agencies in the area to integrate wellness into their services are some ways to meet community needs.

an individual's or a community's ability to engage in meaningful occupations to sustain health and well-being.

Transportation was a critical challenge for participants at the high-rise public housing site. Most participants did not own a car, public transportation lacked frequency, and the bus stop near the building was eliminated during the course of the LWP. This problem of transportation in particular affected a planned community activity of taking residents to the local farmer's market, which by car is less than 10 minutes away. However, because the market is across a highway, taking a bus would involve going downtown and transferring to another bus route that would go across the highway, which under the best circumstances is an hour or two just for the commute. Similarly, accessing a grocery store is also a challenge. One strategy that was identified by the group, and supported by the one resident who owned a car, was to share the ride with those interested and willing to pay a fee to offset the cost of driving.

Listening to the everyday experiences of the participants in the program revealed how their lives had changed over the years. The neighborhood where the participants from the community center had raised their families changed for the worse over the years, and they no longer felt safe in their neighborhoods. One participant who loves to garden gave up this meaningful occupation after the targets of a random gang-related shooting were chased through her yard where she was gardening. On the positive side, the residents of the public high-rise have initiated a community garden in the building yard to grow vegetables in the summer.

Summary

The goal of the LWP was to develop a prototype model of community-based participatory programs for underserved inner-city populations. The qualitative research used in this study provided an in-depth perspective to some of the challenges faced by the target population. Despite the limitations created by a low number of participants, several valuable insights were gained by conducting the LWP. The positive results of the study demonstrate that a culturally responsive, interdisciplinary health and wellness promotion program has benefits for the underserved population residing in north Minneapolis. Further research is needed to determine whether these results are transferable to similar populations in other cities. The continued presence of wellness programs in this community is both warranted and desired.

Acknowledgments

This study was funded by a grant from the Medica Foundation. The author thanks Dr. Catherine Sullivan, PhD, OTR, for her valuable collaboration at all stages of the project. One aspect of the LWP was a faculty-led research project for the following students of the Doctor of Physical Therapy Program: Jennifer Gruenhagen, Cindy Michel, Marc Schultz, Jon Staiger, and Christie Thames. Thank you for your work on this project.

References

American Psychological Association. (2015). *Understanding chronic stress.* Retrieved from http://www.apa.org/helpcenter/understanding-chronic-stress.aspx

Barnard, S., Dunn, S., Reddic, E., Rhodes, K., Russell, J., Tuitt, T. S., . . . White, K. (2004). Wellness in Tillery: A community-built program. *Family and Community Health, 27*(2), 151–157.

Cassidy, A. (2010, December 28). Health policy briefs: Preventive services without cost sharing. *Health Affairs.* Retrieved from http://www.healthaffairs.org/healthpolicybriefs/brief.php?brief_id=37

Centers for Disease Control and Prevention. (2013). Health disparities and inequality report—United States, 2013. *MMWR, 62*(3), 1–189. Retrieved from http://www.cdc.gov/mmwr/pdf/other/su6203.pdf

Centers for Disease Control and Prevention. (2014). *Physical activity and good nutrition: Essential elements to prevent chronic diseases and obesity.* Retrieved from https://stacks.cdc.gov/view/cdc/7044/

Clark, F., Azen, S. P., Zemke, R., Jackson, J., Carlson, M., Mandel, D., . . . Lipson, L. (1997). Occupational therapy for independent-living older adults: A randomized controlled trial. *JAMA, 278*(16), 1321–1326. http://dx.doi.org/10.1001/jama.1997.03550160041036

Cohen, J. T., & Neumann, P. J. (2009). *The cost savings and cost-effectiveness of preventive care* (Robert Wood Johnson Synthesis Report No. 18). Retrieved from http://www.rwjf.org/content/dam/farm/reports/issue_briefs/2009/rwjf46045/subassets/rwjf46045_1

Cohen, J. T., Neumann, P. J., & Weinstein, M. C. (2008). Does preventive care save money? Health economics and the presidential candidates. *New England Journal of Medicine, 358*(7), 661–663. http://dx.doi.org/10.1056/NEJMp0708558

Cohen-Mansfield, J., & Frank, J. (2008). Relationship between perceived needs and assessed needs for services in community-dwelling older persons. *The Gerontologist, 48*(4), 505–516. http://dx.doi.org/10.1093/geront/48.4.505

Finch, E., Brooks, D., Stratford, P. W., & Mayo, N. (2002). *Physical rehabilitation outcome measures: A guide to enhanced clinical decision making* (2nd ed.). Hamilton, ON: BC Decker.

Fried, L. P., & Watson, J. (1998). Frailty and failure to thrive. In W. Hazard (Ed.), *Principles of geriatric medicine and gerontology* (pp. 1387–1402). Columbus, OH: McGraw-Hill.

Gerson, L. D., Dorsey, C., Berg, J., & Rose, L. E. (2004). Enhancing self-care in community dwelling older adults. *Geriatric Nursing, 25*(5), 272–276. http://dx.doi.org/10.1016/j.gerinurse.2004.08.008

Gillespie, L. D., Gillespie, W. J., Robertson, M. C., Lamb, S. E., Cumming, R. G., & Rowe, B. H. (2003). Interventions for preventing falls in elderly people. *Cochrane Database Systematic Reviews, 4.* http://dx.doi.org/10.1002/14651858.CD000340

Guion, L., Diehl, D. C., & McDonald, D. (2011). *Triangulation: Establishing the validity of qualitative studies.* Gainesville: University of Florida, Institute of Food and Agricultural Science.

Hay, J., LaBree, L., Luo, R., Clark, F., Carlson, M., Mandel, D., . . . Azen, S. P. (2002). Cost-effectiveness of preventive occupational therapy for independent-living older adults. *Journal of the American Geriatrics Society, 50*(8), 1381–1388. http://dx.doi.org/10.1046/j.1532-5415.2002.50359.x

Hueston, W. J., & Hubbard, E. T. (2000). Preventive services for rural and urban African-American adults. *Archives of Family Medicine, 9,* 263–266.

Israel, B. A., Schulz, A. J., Parker, E. A., Becker, A. B., Allen, A. J., & Guzman, R. (2008). Critical issues in developing and following CBPR principles. In M. Minkler & N. Wallerstein (Eds.), *Community-based participatory research for health: From process to outcomes* (pp. 47–66). San Francisco: Wiley.

Katz, D. L., & Ali, A. (2009, February). *Preventive medicine, integrative medicine and the health of the public.* Paper commissioned for the Institute of Medicine Summit on Integrative Medicine and the Health of the Public. Retrieved from https://www.nationalacademies.org/hmd/~/media/Files/Activity%20Files/Quality/IntegrativeMed/Preventive%20Medicine%20Integrative%20Medicine%20and%20the%20Health%20of%20the%20Public.pdf

Link, B. G., & Phelan, J. (1995). Social conditions as fundamental causes of disease. *Journal of Health and Social Behavior,* (Extra Issue), 80–94.

Marrongiello, B. A., & Gottlieb, B. H. (2000). Self-care among older adults. *Canadian Journal on Aging, 19*(1), 32–57. http://dx.doi.org/10.1017/S0714980800014641

Miller, D. K., Carter, M. E., Miller, J. P., Fornoff, J. E., Bentley, J. A., Boyd, S. D., . . . Coe, R. M. (1996). Inner-city older Blacks have high levels of functional disability. *Journal of the American Geriatrics Society, 44*(10), 1166–1173. http://dx.doi.org/10.1111/j.1532-5415.1996.tb01365.x

Minkler, M. (2005). Community-based research partnerships: Challenges and opportunities. *Journal of Urban Health, 82*(2, Suppl. 2), ii3–ii12. http://dx.doi.org/10.1093/jurban/jti034

Minkler, M., & Wallerstein, N. (2008). Introduction to community-based participatory research. In M. Minkler & N. Wallerstein, (Eds.), *Community-based participatory research for health: From process to outcomes* (pp. 5–23). San Francisco: Wiley.

Moody-Ayers, S. Y., Mehta, K. M., Lindquist, K., Sands, L., & Covinsky, K. E. (2005). Black–White disparities in functional decline in older persons: The role of cognitive function. *The Journals of Gerontology Series A: Biological Sciences and Medical Sciences, 60*(7), 933–939. Retrieved from http://citeseerx.ist.psu.edu/viewdoc/download?doi=10.1.1.560.3583&rep=rep1&type=pdf

National Council on Aging. (2014). *Chronic disease self-management program.* Retrieved from https://www.ncoa.org/healthy-aging/chronic-disease/chronic-disease-self-management-program/

Nied, R. J., & Franklin, B. (2002). Promoting and prescribing exercise for the elderly. *American Family Physician, 65*(3), 419–426. Retrieved from http://www.aafp.org/afp/2002/0201/p419.html

Office of Minority Health, U.S. Department of Health and Human Services. (2014). *Profile: Black/African Americans.* Retrieved from http://minorityhealth.hhs.gov/omh/browse.aspx?lvl=3&lvlid=61

Ortman, J. M., Velkoff, V. A., & Hogan, H. (2014). *An aging nation: The older population in the United States.* Retrieved from http://www.census.gov/prod/2014pubs/p25-1140.pdf

Patient Protection and Affordable Care Act, Pub. L. No. 111–148, § 3502, 124 Stat. 119, 124 (2010).

Resnicow, K., Jackson, A., Blissett, D., Wang, T., McCarty, F., Rahotep, S., & Periasamy, S. (2005). Results of the Healthy Body Healthy Spirit trial. *Health Psychology, 24*(4), 339–348. http://dx.doi.org/10.1037/0278-6133.24.4.339

Shriner, L., & Stack-Cutler, H. (2012). *Recruitment and engagement of low-income populations: Service provider and researcher perspectives.* Retrieved from http://www.cup.ualberta.ca/wp-content/uploads/2011/07/Recruitment-and-Engagement-of-Low-Income-Populations1.pdf

Shomer, R. (2005). *Mind the gap: Reducing disparities to improve regional competitiveness in the Twin Cities.* Retrieved from https://www.brookings.edu/wp-content/uploads/2016/06/20051027_mindthegap.pdf

Smedley, B. D., Stith, A. Y., & Nelsen, A. R. (2003). *Unequal treatment confronting racial and ethical disparities in healthcare.* Washington, DC: National Academy Press.

Stewart, A. L., Verboncoeur, C. J., McLellan, B. Y., Gillis, D. E., Rush, S., Mills, K. M., . . . Bortz, W. M. (2001). Physical activity outcomes of CHAMPS II: A physical activity promotion program for older adults. *Journals of Gerontology Series A: Biological Sciences and Medical Sciences, 56*(8), M465–M470.

Stuber, J., Galea, S., Ahern, J., Blaney, S., & Fuller, C. (2003). The association between multiple domains of discrimination and self-assessed health: A multilevel analysis of Latinos and Blacks in four low-income New York City neighborhoods. *Health Services Research, 38*(6, Part 2), 1735–1759. http://dx.doi.org/10.1111/j.1475-6773.2003.00200.x

U.S. Census Bureau. (2015). *State and country quick facts.* Retrieved from https://www.census.gov/quickfacts/

U.S. National Library of Medicine. (2015). *Health disparities.* Retrieved from https://www.nlm.nih.gov/hsrinfo/disparities.html

Section VI.

CULTURE AND RESEARCH

Chapter 30.

HEALTH RESEARCH AND ISSUES OF RACE, ETHNICITY, AND CULTURE

Shirley A. Wells, DrPH, OTR, FAOTA

> *Research has often failed to establish the effectiveness of interventions for diverse, racial, ethnic, and cultural populations.*
> **Victoria Stanhope, Phyllis Soloman, Anita Pernell-Arnold, Roberta G. Sands, & Joretha N. Bourjolly (2005, p. 226)**

Chapter Highlights

- Emic and Etic Perspectives
- Research Models
- Health Research

Key Terms and Concepts

- ✧ Community-based participatory research
- ✧ Content analyses
- ✧ Cross-culture research
- ✧ Cultural studies
- ✧ Emic
- ✧ Ethnicity
- ✧ Ethnographic techniques
- ✧ Etic
- ✧ Father rule
- ✧ Fine-grained categories

- ✧ Race
- ✧ Research
- ✧ Minority algorithm
- ✧ Minority rule
- ✧ Mother rule
- ✧ NIH Revitalization Act of 1993
- ✧ Notion of normality
- ✧ Multicultural model
- ✧ Systematic observations

Until recently, knowledge of the health status, characteristics, and behaviors of ethnic groups and women in the United States was based on a few epidemiological activities and data that were designed with a focus on the general population, not minority groups (Bhopal, 2006). Minority and ethnic populations and women were often inadequately or inaccurately represented in health research. Studies either excluded them completely or included them in numbers too small to provide an understanding of the context of health and illness for these groups (Burlew et al., 2011).

Although there is great interest in culture in health research, several methodological challenges exist, such as lack of standardized definitions for interventions, standardized evaluation measures, culturally appropriate instruments, and secondary data sources with uniform racial, ethnic, and language data (Burlew et al., 2011; Lau, Chang, & Okazaki, 2010; Walter, Burke, & Davis, 2013). An additional challenge is the large sample size that is required to prove that cultural interventions are more effective than traditional interventions alone (Mendoza, Williams, Chapman, & Powers, 2012).

Researcher bias and inadequate data collection instruments, research designs, theories, and methodologies have been cited as reasons for the lack of empirical, realistic, and useful information on racial, ethnic, gender, and cultural differences (Baer et al., 2013; Lau et al., 2010; Lequerica & Krch, 2014). This chapter provides a critical review of the research models and methodologies used in research on culture, gender, and health. Including culture in health research is essential in providing the scientific foundation for improving health care practices, reducing health disparities, and developing health policies.

Emic and Etic Perspectives

Conducting research can be dangerous. According to Milner (2007), unsuccessful research on cultural influences can occur when and if researchers do not engage in processes that can circumvent misinterpretations, misinformation, and misrepresentation of individuals, communities, institutions, and systems. To avoid such pitfalls, researchers must first understand the etic and emic approaches to studying human beings.

Insider Point of View

The *emic,* which is the native's (i.e., insider) point of view, is culture specific. This perspective typically represents the internal language and meanings of a defined culture (Merriam, 2009). An emic perspective "attempts to capture participants' indigenous meanings of real-world events" (Yin, 2010, p. 11) and "looks at things through the eyes of members of the culture being studied" (Willis, 2007, p. 100).

Taking the emic (culture-specific) approach says that each culture has unique ideas, behaviors, and concepts and that this uniqueness must be the focus of the study. However, the findings of the study cannot be generalized or used to make cultural comparisons (Lee, 2002; Olive, 2014; Wombles, 2010). An emic approach protects researchers against ethnocentrism, because "using a set of behavioral standards developed according to the norms of one culture to assess a client from another culture is a culture imposition based on ethnocentricity" (Kavanagh & Kennedy, 1992, p. 32). Anthropologists predominantly follow the emic approach.

Outsider Point of View

An *etic* approach, which is the researcher's (outsider) view, is oriented to the researcher's personal or professional culture. It encompasses an external view on a culture, language, meaning associations, and real-world events. It comprises the "structures and criteria developed outside the culture as a framework for studying the culture" (Willis, 2007, p. 100).

When a researcher takes an etic approach, he or she uses preexisting theories, hypotheses, and perspectives as constructs to see if they apply to a setting or culture. The etic approach enables comparisons to be made across multiple cultures and populations. Using the etic (i.e., general cultural) approach signifies that cultures have both specific and universal dimensions and that both dimensions should be studied, to allow generalizations about relationships among variables across cultures (Lee, 2002; Olive, 2014; Wombles, 2010). The etic approach is followed mainly by cross-cultural social scientists (e.g., sociologists, psychologists).

Using Emic and Etic Approaches

Both the emic and etic perspectives involve tradeoffs. The emic view provides the subjective experience but limits objectivity, whereas the etic view may be more objective but loses the insider knowledge (Olive, 2014; Wombles, 2010). The research methods used to study cultures depend on the research question, the investigators' knowledge, the cultural acceptability of various techniques, the sophistication of the respondents, and many other variables.

When they know little about the culture and seek to obtain a holistic picture, researchers should use emic approaches and qualitative research methodologies such as

- *Ethnographic techniques:* Includes observation, ethnographic interviewing, fieldnotes, population or sample survey, and network research;
- *Systematic observations:* Setting up the study to eliminate or reduce bias by establishing decision rules that reduce inferences prior to data collection; and
- *Content analyses:* Systematically evaluating texts and coding (e.g., documents, oral communication, graphics) and converting the qualitative data into quantitative data.

Experimental designs using etic approaches (e.g., surveys, questionnaires) are useful when the researcher has limited goals, knows a great deal about the culture, and has some well-developed theory to test.

Survey analyses tend to oversimplify many of the differences among population groups and subgroups, resulting in false homogeneity within the group (Creswell, Klassen, Plano Clark, & Smith, 2011; Kagawa-Singer, Dressler, George, & Elwood, 2012). Niblo and Jackson (2004) suggest that combined etic and emic approaches are the most useful. They envision that future cross-culture research would first validate their instruments (emic approach), followed by identification of similarities and differences among the cultural groups (etic approach).

Case Example 30.1 demonstrates how data could be interpreted based-on the perspective taken.

Research Models

Research is the systematic and rigorous process of enquiry that aims to describe processes and develop explanatory concepts and theories to contribute to a scientific body of knowledge. Research on race, ethnicity, and culture has evolved over the years. Historically, research models were based on the ***notion of normality*** in which racial and cultural groups are viewed as negative or inferior to the White majority (Milner, 2007). White majority, their beliefs, and their experiences are viewed as "the norm" by which others are compared, measured, assessed, and evaluated (Corbie-Smith, Thomas, & St. George,

---

Case Example 30.1. Etic and Emic Perspectives

A researcher's view of a situation from an etic or emic perspective will determine his or her interpretation of an occurring event. For example, the reaction of a Vietnamese woman who just delivered a beautiful healthy baby boy can shed light on the distinction between these perspectives. The mother's reaction puzzled the delivery nurse attendant. The new mother ignored the baby when the nurse presented the baby to her. On the hospital records, the nurse described the mother's response as "Bonding—O."

As a researcher, if you accept the nurse etic viewpoint, the interaction will be interpreted as a lack of caring and appreciation for the child, whereas if you use the mother's emic point of view, the interaction will be interpreted as a form of protecting the child. Culturally, many Asian people believe that a baby is in grave danger when first born. To recognize the baby's presence by fussing over it would bring too much attention that might place the baby in jeopardy, a concept related to the evil eye (Dresser, 1996).

2002; Le, 2015). This deficit orientation and context denies that other cultures have their own unique integrity and affixes the problem within the disadvantaged person. Such models resulted in a research base that perpetuated a view that racial and ethnic groups are inherently pathological, deficient, and disadvantaged.

New and conceptually different models of research have emerged that provide more realistic knowledge about nondominant cultures, including

- ***Cross-culture research,*** which involves comparison of cultural traits or relationships between traits across societies;
- ***Cultural studies,*** which investigates the ways in which culture creates and transforms individual experiences, everyday life, social relations, and power;
- ***Multicultural model,*** which encompasses studying and comparing various ethnic groups that have different languages, economies, social structures, behavior, and attitude patterns; and

- *Community-based participatory research,* which actively includes the community and people being studied in the research process and approach.

These models and approaches are grounded in premises from research, theory, and practices of other scholars (De Las Nueces, Hacker, DiGirolamo, & Hicks, 2012; Olatundun, 2009; Sullivan & Cottone, 2010). Culturally linked research outcomes enable service providers to build on the strengths of an individual's culture and to use the unique resources of that culture to create solutions.

Health Research

Changing demographics in the United States have brought culture to the forefront in health care. The U.S. health care delivery system and policies targeting racial and ethnic populations historically used harmful models of research in which race and gender were often downplayed or negated in health analysis. The deficient system also claimed that minorities experience poor health and premature death because of pathological behaviors.

Health scientists generally continue to conduct research focused on the nature of humankind from European American ways of thinking and viewing of reality (Henrich, Heine, & Norenzayan, 2010). According to Kawaga-Singer et al. (2012), culture is "an overlooked and misused concept" and the mode of measurement has been "poorly understood and operationalized in health research" (p. 20). Thus, integrating the concepts of *race, ethnicity,* and *culture* into health research is difficult.

Disparities in health, health care, and health outcomes have been extensively documented in the public health and biomedical literature. Researchers too often fail to consider culture as a variable and confuse the concepts of race and ethnicity (Baer et al., 2013). Lack of consensus on a definition of culture and how to operationalize it in health research has led to oversimplification and limits the capacity to explain variation and disparities (Kagawa-Singer et al., 2012; Milner, 2007).

Race and Ethnicity

The current practice of differentiating human population health status and culture is through race and ethnicity (Kagawa-Singer et al., 2012). The use of such groups to categorize data assumes that standard, reliable, and valid definitions of race and ethnicity exist and that these definitions are used consistently. The validity of information provided for racial and ethnic groups is often taken for granted. In health research, race, ethnicity, and gender are rarely studied, yet they are frequently cited as a causal factor for targeted populations (Baer et al., 2013; Bhopal, 2006).

Race is a social categorization that incorporates biological, social, and cultural characteristics imposed on people for the purpose of making hierarchical, power-based distinctions in social relations (Markus, 2008; Smedley & Smedley, 2005). Using race as a variable implies that a genetic reason may explain differences in the incidence, severity, or outcome of medical conditions. Many studies use race as a proxy for other socioeconomic factors not collected in the research effort. The question to ask is whether race is being used as a biogenetic variable or as a proxy variable for environmental variables.

Ethnicity is a social categorization based on shared cultural values, language, and customs that is self-claimed or developed in relation to feelings of belonging to a chosen community (Markus, 2008; Smedley & Smedley, 2005). If race suggests biological differences, then ethnicity suggests nonbiological differences. Ethnicity is important, but only as a marker of social, environmental, and cultural risks.

Researchers need to be aware that racial and ethnic categories are labels that are used to gain potentially important information. The National Institutes of Health's ([NIH's], 2001) standard measure of race and ethnicity may not accurately reflect individuals' self-identified race and ethnicity.

Measuring Race and Ethnicity

The constructs of race and ethnicity are used as proxy cultural markers that are collected as data and often only at intake (Kagawa-Singer et al., 2012). The modes of measurements for race and ethnicity have rarely been questioned. The literature indicates that health research identifies targeted population groups and codes them as nominal (numerical values applied to non-numerical variables) and dichotomous (two categories only) variables. The use of these variables assumes groups to be homogeneous and static.

These data are used with little attention to the underlying measurement problems or the appropriateness of how the data will be used. For example,

Eisenhower, Suyemoto, Lucchese, and Canenguez's (2014) research findings suggested that measuring ethnicity as only Hispanic/Latina(o) or non-Hispanic/Latina(o) was problematic. The option "Hispanic/Latina(o)" confounds race as ethnicity for some Hispanics/Latina(o)s experiencing inequities, thereby making it difficult to differentiate between the influence of race and ethnicity on their lives. Eisenhower et al. advocated that the standard ethnicity measurement misses more specific or nuanced ethnic identifications such as self-identified Puerto Ricans and Dominicans.

Operationalizing (defining and using) race and ethnicity in a dichotomous way prevents researchers from understanding differences within racial groups. Because all individuals have both racial and ethnic experiences, the lack of an inclusive ethnicity question prevents researchers from capturing participants' lived experiences in both race and ethnicity categories, potentially contributing to missing or inaccurate data.

For example, Waters (1994) found that second-generation Caribbean Black immigrants vary in their identification as Black (racial identity), immigrant, or ethnic-specific (e.g., Jamaican, Haitian) and that these identities relate to different attitudes about opportunities and responses to racism. Eisenhower et al. (2014) suggested that Caribbean immigrants may check "Black or African American" as the closest available race option, or they may skip the question because the specific inclusion of "African American" in the Black category does not reflect their understanding of themselves as Black and the ethnicity question does not allow for an ethnic identity specification that makes this distinction clearer.

Current measures continue to confound race and ethnicity (Afshari & Bhopal, 2002; Kaplan & Bennett, 2003). This makes it difficult to accurately assess whether ethnic or racial aspects are underlying identified health disparities. According Eisenhower et al. (2014), using a measure that conceptually separates race and ethnicity and that provides respondents with adequate flexibility to identify themselves both racially and ethnically may decrease misclassification and increase validity.

Categories of Race and Ethnicity

Because the measurement of race and ethnicity is not scientific, rules are needed to guide assignment to categories so that the resulting statistics can be understood. Using race as a means of classifying the population has a long statistical tradition in the United States. The Office of Management and Budget's ([OMB's], 1997) Statistical Policy Directive No. 15, Race and Ethnic Standards for Federal Statistics and Administrative Reporting (Exhibit 30.1), has provided a common language for uniformity and comparability in the collection and use of data by federal agencies. Racial and ethnic categories are required in all federally sponsored data collection and reporting activities involving questions on race and ethnicity.

In 1997, OMB revised the standards for classification of race and ethnicity in federal data to include five categories for race:

1. American Indian or Alaska Native
2. Asian
3. Black or African American
4. Native Hawaiian or Other Pacific Islander
5. White—and two categories for ethnicity—Hispanic or Latino and Not Hispanic or Latino (OMB, 1997).

Exhibit 30.1. Office of Management and Budget Standards for the Classification of Federal Data on Race and Ethnicity

Race
- Black or African American
- White
- Asian
- American Indian or Alaska Native
- Native Hawaiian or Other Pacific Islander
- Some other race

Hispanic Ethnicity
- Hispanic or Latino
- Not Hispanic or Latino

Source. From Office of Management and Budget, 1997, *Revisions to the Standards for the Classification of Federal Data on Race and Ethnicity.* Retrieved from http://www.whitehouse.gov/omb/fedreg_1997standards

The 1997 OMB standards allowed individuals to report more than one race. With interracial marriage, the question of how to classify people whose parents are of different races was debated. Multiracial people and parents of multiracial children were asked to choose a single racial category, which forced people to deny the racial heritage of one parent when they must choose one race, adversely affecting self-esteem, sense of family, pride, and psychological well-being.

However, users of health data argued that a multiracial category would result in data that are not useful in analyzing the health status of population groups historically at risk for certain diseases, such as hypertension in the African American population. Furthermore, a multiracial category with no races indicated would become increasingly problematic for the offspring of parents who are themselves multiracial.

However, using the OMB standards may mask major differences within racial or ethnic populations. General grouping of ethnic populations does not allow researchers to identify subgroups that may be at risk, leaving its members underserved. For example, the OMB categories do not capture whether a Hispanic child has a Mexican or Cuban background or whether an Asian adult is of Vietnamese or Chinese ancestry.

The Institute of Medicine ([IOM], 2009) recommended adding more "granular" ethnicity categories, which were referred to as *fine-grained categories* and based on one's ancestry. According to the IOM, opportunities should be available for individuals who want to self-identify their ethnicity and language on local data collection instruments. The categories collected and analyzed need to reflect the population served. Local categories should be selected from a national standard set of granular ethnicities.

The IOM also recommended collecting data on spoken language. When possible and applicable, data collectors (individuals or institutions) should collect information on the primary language spoken at home for insight into a person's culture, or learn the preferred language of their subjects to receive written material from them. The IOM favors the collection and retention for analysis of specific multiple-race combinations rather than losing that detail by only offering the more general category of "multiracial," whenever possible.

Reflection 30.1. Granular Ethnicities Question and Example

- What is the participant's ancestry or ethnic origin?
- Ask the participant, "I would like you to describe your race or ethnic background. You can use specific terms such as Korean, Mexican, Haitian, Somali."

Assigning Race and Ethnicity Categories

Another problem with measuring cultural data that affects the quality of data involves errors in the reporting of race and ethnicity. Race and ethnicity are assigned through either self-identification or assignment by another person based on his or her perceptions, and both methods can present risks for reliability of data. Methodological research has revealed inaccuracies in the classification and coding of race and ethnicity on vital records.

Birth Certificates. Births recorded through birth certificates serve as the primary source for determining the size of each native-born birth cohort. Birth certificates in the United States have never listed the race of the child but record the race(s) of the mother and father. This information is then used to assign race to each child (Mason, Nam, & Kim, 2014).

Before 1989, the National Center for Health Statistics (NCHS) used a *minority algorithm* based on the race of the mother and father to determine the race of a newborn. In 1989, the NCHS moved to an algorithm based primarily on the race of the mother to tabulate birth data. By 2000, race was assigned to births based on the race of the father. In 2003, the NCHS implemented new standards to include the option of selecting more than one race on birth and death certificates; however, not all states have adopted this standard (Devine, Sink, DeSalvo, & Cortes, 2010). The ethnicity of a child, both before and after 1989, is determined by the ethnicity of the mother (Guarneri & Dick, 2012).

The NCHS approach to assigning a race to the child used the race of the mother, father, or both reported on the child's birth certificate:

- *Minority rule:* Uses the race of the minority parent,
- *Mother rule:* Uses the race of the mother, and
- *Father rule:* Uses the race of the father.

The minority rule, as used by the NCHS prior to adopting the use of the race of the mother, determines the race of the child based on the following:

1. When of the same race, the race of the child is the same as the race of the parents.
2. When of different races and one parent is White, the child is assigned the race of the minority parent.
3. When the parents are of different races and neither parent is White, the child is assigned the father's race, unless either parent is Hawaiian; then the child is assigned Hawaiian.
4. If the race was missing from one parent, the child is assigned the race of the other parent.
5. Items 1 and 4 also apply to both the Mother and Father rules (Devine et al., 2010).

Reflection 30.2. What Race Would Be Assigned?

Prior to 1989,

- If both parents are White, the child was considered _____.
- If the father is White and mother belongs to a different race, the child was given the race of the _____.
- If the father is non-White, the child was assigned the race of the _____.

What race will be assigned to your child?

Death Certificates

Death certificates are the basis of many key indicators used for the comparison of health among populations. Errors and inaccuracies can lead to problems in health research that rely on these data (Arias, Schauman, Eschbach, Sorlie, & Backlund, 2008).

Misclassification on death certificates can occur because the deceased does not have the option to self-report. Reporting is typically the responsibility of officials such as funeral directors, medical examiners, and coroners who complete these forms, who must gather information from next of kin or rely on personal observation. Often they make a decision on the basis their own judgment without necessarily ascertaining the race of the deceased from the next of kin. The last name of the individual commonly is used to determine ethnicity of the deceased (Arias et al.,

2008; Noymer, Penner, & Saperstein, 2011; Pierce & Denison, 2006).

Noymer et al. (2011) explored the role of cause of death in racial classification on death certificates. They examined the 22,905 death certificates of U.S. residents from the 1993 Current Mortality Sample. The proxy respondent was the decedent's next of kin. Noymer and colleagues found that Americans whose underlying cause of death was chronic liver disease or cirrhosis were more likely to be classified as American Indian on their death certificate, even if they were not classified as American Indian by their next of kin. This pattern was also found between dying of homicide and the likelihood of being classified as Black. Noymer et al. concluded that "stereotypes about who is likely to die a particular kind of death may color our official vital statistics" (Section 3, para 1).

Affordable Care Act

The Patient Protection and Affordable Care Act of 2010 (Pub. L. 111-148), Section 4302, contains provisions to implement new health data collection and analysis strategy by requiring that all national federal data collection efforts collect information on race, ethnicity, sex, primary language, and disability status (Civic Impulse, 2015). The law also provides the U.S. Department of Health and Human Services (DHHS) with the opportunity to collect additional demographic data to further improve our understanding of health care disparities (Office of Minority Health, 2015).

Data categories for Asian American and Pacific Islander populations have been expanded to include Asian Indian, Chinese, Filipino, Japanese, Korean, and Vietnamese. Mexican American and Chicano/a, Puerto Rican, and Cuban have been added to the Hispanic ethnic group. The law requires that data collection standards for these measures be used, to the extent that it is practical, in all national population health surveys. It applies to self-reported information only. The law also requires that any data standards published by the DHHS comply with standards created by the OMB.

Methodological Challenges

Research on ethnicity and health poses significant ethical and methodological challenges, including how samples are drawn, how participants are recruited, how researchers engage with minority ethnic individuals and groups, and how findings are interpreted.

Methodological Errors in Population Sampling

In selecting a sample, researchers should be concerned about the representativeness of the people they choose to interview or study. It is difficult in epidemiological studies of racial and ethnic groups to defend the selection of respondents using less than scientifically rigorous sampling methods and still obtain the critical approval of statisticians who are accustomed to using conventional sampling schema. The underrepresentation of racial and ethnic minorities in health research limits researchers' ability to conduct valid studies to enhance understanding of measuring and reducing health disparities.

The issue of sampling from small populations is one reason that no large-scale epidemiological study has been conducted with racial or ethnic minorities. Most large-scale studies include only small samples of minority group members. Large-scale studies usually weight the data to the population figures of the community or geographic region or the nation as whole. Such weighting may disguise the fact that the ethnic samples actually are quite small.

Small samples do not provide sufficient statistical power to detect significant health needs or conduct complex multivariate analyses to identify high-risk subgroups. When a large sample includes Asian Americans, Hispanics, and American Indians, they often are collapsed into one category (Keppel et al., 2005; Lau et al., 2010). Because numbers of minority group members may be limited and highly dispersed in any given geographic area, existing sampling frames can misidentify or misrepresent members of some minority groups.

Generally, in health research, the sample includes only individuals who are receiving health services. Data based on clinic populations offer insight into the health problems of the individuals who use the services but no information on how representative the clinic population is of the ethnic community (Foster, 2006). It also is well documented that ethnic groups delay seeking professional care for their health problems (DHHS, 2001), and because of this pattern of behavior, researchers often conclude that ethnic populations underuse health services. Instead, they should be asking,

- Why do certain groups use or not use health services?

- Are there differences in need among ethnically diverse groups?
- Why are services underutilized?
- Is there a cultural mismatch between those in need and the service strategies used?

To ensure representation of racial and ethnic minorities in research studies, Congress passed the ***NIH Revitalization Act of 1993.*** It requires the inclusion of racial and ethnic minorities and women in all studies conducted or supported by the NIH (DHHS, 2002). In the literature, strategies to bolster inclusion range from involving the community to adapting recruitment and retention procedures (Foster, 2006; Mendoza et al., 2012). Oversampling racial and ethnic minorities and partnering with primary care, schools, faith-based organizations, and other community agencies may be needed (Lau et al., 2010).

Researcher Bias

Researchers often are unaware of the racial, gender, and cultural misperceptions they bring to research. Inaccurate perceptions and associated ethnocentric biases influence what research questions are asked; how studies are designed; what research is funded; and how results are interpreted, disseminated, and applied.

Researchers who are members of dominant groups may not reflect on the effects of their racial, ethnic, gender, and cultural identities and consciousness on what they see and interpret in their studies. By constructing what they believe to be value methods of data collection and interpretation, they unwittingly rationalize and legitimatize their claims rather than acknowledge the intrusions of their life histories and cognitive styles in the research process (Milner, 2007; Zea, Reisen, & Diaz, 2003).

Researchers may selectively exclude participants they believe would be poor candidates on the basis of beliefs that minorities may dropout prematurely, be unable to follow directions properly, or fail to follow study rules and procedures (Mendoza et al., 2012). Researchers' bias against enrolling minorities in studies may be a contributing factor to their underrepresentation.

Low Participation

With the need to improve the generalizability of research findings, to achieve equitable distribution of the benefits and burdens of research, and to determine possible differences in treatment by race/ ethnicity and ensure accurate data about response to intervention, increasing representation of ethnic minorities in health research and especially in clinical trials is vital (Corbie-Smith, Miller, & Ransohoff, 2004; Corbie-Smith et al., 2002; Walter et al., 2013). To achieve this outcome, federal agencies are mandated to include ethnic minorities' representation in all clinical research (NIH, 1994). Despite this awareness, reasons for underrepresentation of minorities are not well described or understood and continue to be a concern for research investigators.

Mistrust. Mistrust of the health system and White researchers has accounted for some of the underrepresentation of racial and ethnic minorities in health research. Studies have suggested that trust is a factor in participation in research (Cooper et al., 2004; Suite, La Bril, Primm, & Harrison-Ross, 2007; Ulrich et al., 2013). Many minority participants have concerns about receiving inadequate treatment or misdiagnosis due to discrimination (Mendoza et al., 2012).

For example, the Tuskegee Syphilis Study involved conducting research on 600 Black men on the natural history of untreated syphilis without the benefit of patients' informed consent. The men were never given adequate treatment for their disease even when penicillin became the drug of choice for syphilis in 1947 (Centers for Disease Control and Prevention, 2016). Another example relates to the health consequences associated with the use of Diethylstibestrol (DES) and thalidomide by pregnant women from 1938 until 1971, in which exposure led to greater risk for breast cancer in DES mothers; rare vaginal cancer, abnormal reproductive organs, infertility, and high-risk pregnancies in DES daughters and an increased risk for breast cancer in DES daughters after age 40; and possible risk for testicular cancer in DES sons. This incident affected the attitude of women toward participation in research (Russell et al., 2007).

Most recently, the Baltimore Lead Paint Study, which recruited healthy children and their families to live in Baltimore houses with varying amounts of lead contamination, disproportionally affected minorities. The study was conducted in the early 1990s to test how well different levels of repair in Baltimore rental housing worked to reduce lead in the blood of inner-city children. The Maryland Court of Appeals ruled that the researchers failed to warn the parents about the risks of the study and the danger that their children could be poisoned by

lead in the houses. The court also ruled that parents cannot consent to the participation of a child in nontherapeutic research. Several of the children developed lead poisoning and neurological problems (Buchanan & Miller, 2006; Spriggs, 2004).

These examples have created biases and barriers against medical research for many Americans, especially members of minority populations and women. Corbie-Smith et al. (2002) recommended ongoing community involvement, engagement, and dialogue as a way to build trust and better understand the challenges and barriers specific to the community.

Financial Barriers. Another reason for low racial and ethnic minorities' participation in research is financial barriers (Mendoza et al., 2012; Ulrich et al., 2013). In a study by Ulrich and colleagues (2013), fear of having to pay for research treatment was found among Hispanics, indicating misinterpretation of what biomedical research entails. Ulrich and colleagues suggested that researchers should clearly describe the requirements of participation.

Although providing financial incentives to increase participation by minorities and underrepresented groups is an acceptable research practice, the poor may be unduly influenced to participate by even modest payments. Walter et al. (2013) found that low-income and racial or minority groups are susceptible to payment for participation. Their data indicated that low-income individuals request payment for participation similar to higher income peers, which makes proportional representation by socioeconomic status achievable. And higher payment may be necessary to increase Hispanics' participation in research and to achieve higher public participation overall.

Researchers' Cultural Knowledge and Identity. Researchers' lack of understanding of cultural values and expressions of racial and ethnic minority populations has been cited as a reason for low participation by these groups. Some studies note that investigators are more effective when they reside in the study neighborhoods, or at least share the culture under study (Fisher et al., 2002). Other studies have found that investigators' ethnicity significantly affected responses to racially sensitive questions (Burlew et al., 2011). Researchers' beliefs and values shape the answers to questions more than any objective data that might be collected and analyzed (Zea et al., 2003), because researchers may unintentionally alter the measurement of cultural context based on

Table 30.1. Recommended Wording for Questions Regarding Gender and Sexual Behavior

	Standard	Recommended
Gender	Male Female	1. What sex were you assigned at birth, on your original birth certificate? Female Male 2. How do you describe yourself? (check one) Female Male Transgender Do not identify as female, male, or transgender
Sexual behavior	In the past (time period, e.g., year) who have you had sex with?	In the past (time period, e.g., year) who have you had sex with? a. Men only, b. Women only, c. Both men and women, d. I have not had sex.

their perceptions. Also, the definitions of terms and constructs used in a study may convey the intended meaning to their participants (IOM, 2013). For instance, is the measure of sexual orientation questions socially acceptable when expressed in the language of the researcher or lesbian, gay, bisexual, and transgender communities? The Sexual Minority Assessment Research Team (2009) and GenIUSS Group and Herman (2014) recommend wording questions as shown in Table 30.1.

Misinterpretation of Findings

Misinterpretation of differences among racial and ethnic populations raises barriers to the development of new knowledge and more effective services. Cultural standards of data generalization are the basis of researcher presumptions about nondominant racial, ethnic, and female populations. It has been the norm to assume that male Eurocentric empirical realities can be generalized to explain the realities of racial and ethnic minorities and women. For decades, researchers using Eurocentric norms have applied Eurocentric concepts of family, deviance, social movements, psychological development, behavior, stratification, health, and even spirituality to the experiences of racial and ethnic minorities (Dillard, 2000; Milner, 2007).

Burlew et al. (2011) found in their study of multiple clinical trials in the National Institute on Drug Abuse Network that the conclusions in several studies would have been misleading for racial and ethnic groups if the researchers had used a data plan that assumed that the overall findings applied to racial and ethnic minorities. On the basis of the results, they recommended that researchers

- Establish data-analytic plans that examine rather than assume that their overall findings apply to specific racial and ethnic groups,
- Avoid combining racial and ethnic groups for data analyses, and
- Add within-group analyses to detect key subgroup differences.

Inadequate Measurement Instruments

Researchers often use standardized instruments without assessing the reliability and validity of these instruments for specific ethnic, racial, or gender populations. These instruments need to be culturally acceptable and appropriately translated to be valid (Cha, Kim, & Erlen, 2007). If the study population does not speak the same primary language as the researcher or interviewer (usually English), the instrument must be translated into another language. Because of the existence of diverse languages and dialects within languages, researchers must pay attention to regional and ethnic differences in language usage when translating instruments. It is important to use appropriate translation procedures and to use combined translation techniques based on the research environment and questions (Jones, Lee, Pillips, Zhang, & Jaceldo, 2001).

When translating and applying an instrument across cultures, researchers should be aware of potential difficulties or bias. Bias can threaten the validity of the comparison. Poor item translations, inappropriate item content, and lack of standardization in administrative procedures can lead to cultural bias (Kao, Hsu, & Clark, 2004). Sources of bias in construct, measurement, items, and scores can be introduced. Researchers need to ensure that the same concept is being measured in each culture (Lee & DukYoo, 2006).

Reflection 30.3. Translating Instruments

In one major health study, an instrument was translated from English to Spanish (Yu & Liu, 1994). In field use of the Spanish instrument, the researchers noted that respondents were scoring very low on the question, "How often do you kiss your child?" After checking and double-checking the original questionnaire, someone checked the translation and found that the translated question read, "How often do you kiss your puppy?"

- What would you do to ensure clarity when designing questionnaires for cross-cultural equivalence?

Summary

The radical demographic changes in the United States and global society require that occupational therapy practitioners and occupational therapy assistants become proactive in establishing new models of research for the study of nondominant racial, ethnic, and gender groups to encourage refreshing and more adequate logic of inquiry. Lack of relevant research and data contributes to imprecise explanation for health disparities among different populations.

Distrust of research efforts is common in many racial and ethnic communities (Corbie-Smith et al., 2002; Ulrich et al., 2013). Without adequate representation of racial and ethnic individuals in health research, health care providers cannot successfully understand or treat across groups. Including racial- and ethnic-minority participants without careful development of research instruments, procedures, and protocol can be detrimental to the development of inclusive health research that can help in addressing and reducing health disparities.

Researchers should reflect on the research process and interpretation. They should acknowledge the multiple roles, identities, and positions that researchers and participants bring to the research process. Researchers' development of cultural knowledge is also critical to the research process.

Reflection 30.4. Measurement Across Cultures

Develop a working plan for how you would involve clients from a culture other than your own in the development of a clinical research project.

Select at least 2 cultural intervention strategies or activities.

- How would you compare their effectiveness in delivering culturally effective care?
- What criteria would you use to measure their effectiveness?

References

Afshari, R., & Bhopal, R. S. (2002). Changing pattern of use of 'ethnicity' and 'race' in scientific literature [Letters to the editor]. *International Journal of Epidemiology, 31*(5), 1074. http://dx.doi.org/10.1093/ije/31.5.1074

Arias, E., Schauman, W. S., Eschbach, K., Sorlie, P. D., & Backlund, E. (2008). The validity of race and Hispanic origin reporting on death certificates in the United States. *Vital Health Statistics, 2*(148), 1–23. Retrieved from https://www.cdc.gov/nchs/data/series/sr_02/sr02_148.pdf

Baer, R. D., Arteaga, E., Dyer, K., Eden, A., Gross, R., Helmy, H., . . . Reeser, D. (2013). Concepts of race and ethnicity among health researchers: Patterns and implications. *Ethnicity and Health, 18*(2), 211–225. http://dx.doi.org/10.1080/13557858.2012.713091

Bhopal, R. (2006). Race and ethnicity: Responsible use from epidemiological and public health perspectives. *Journal of Law, Medicine and Ethics, 34*(3), 500–507. http://dx.doi.org/10.1111/j.1748-720X.2006.00062.x

Buchanan, D. R., & Miller, F. G. (2006). Justice and fairness in the Kennedy Krieger Institute lead paint study: The ethics of public health research on less expensive, less effective interventions. *American Journal of Public Health, 69*(5), 781–787. http://dx.doi.org/10.2105/AJPH.2005.063719

Burlew, A. K., Weekes, J. C., Montgomery, L., Feaster, D. J., Robbin, M. S., Rosa, C. L., . . . Wu, L. (2011). Conducting research with racial/ethnic minorities: Methodological lessons from the NIDA Clinical Trials Network. *American Journal of Drug and Alcohol Abuse, 37*(5), 324–332. http://dx.doi.org/10.3109/00952990.2011.596973

Centers for Disease Control and Prevention. (2016). *The Tuskegee timeline.* Retrieved from http://www.cdc.gov/tuskegee/timeline.htm

Cha, E. S., Kim, K. H., & Erlen, J. A. (2007). Translation of scales in cross-cultural research: Issues and techniques. *Journal of Advanced Nursing, 58*(4), 386–395. http://dx.doi.org /10.1111/j.1365-2648.2007.04242.x

Civic Impulse. (2015). *H.R. 3590—111th Congress: Patient Protection and Affordable Care Act.* Retrieved from https:// www.govtrack.us/congress/bills/111/hr3590

Cooper, S. P., Heitman, E., Fox, E. E., Quill, B., Knudson, P., Zahm, S. H., . . . Ryder, R. (2004). Ethical issues in conducting migrant farmworker studies. *Journal of Immigrant and Minority Health, 6*(1), 29–39. http://dx.doi .org/10.1023/B:JOIH.0000014640.64905.02

Corbie-Smith, G., Miller, W., & Ransohoff, D. (2004). Interpretations of 'appropriate' minority inclusion in clinical research. *American Journal of Medicine, 116*(4), 249–252. http://dx .doi.org/10.1016/j.amjmed.2003.09.032

Corbie-Smith, G., Thomas, S. B., St. George, D. M. (2002). Distrust, race, and research. *Archives of Internal Medicine, 162*(21), 2458–2463. http://dx.doi.org/10.1001/archinte .162.21.2458

Creswell, J. W., Klassen, A. C., Plano Clark, V. L., & Smith, K. C. (2011). *Best practices for mixed methods research in the health sciences.* Retrieved from https://obssr.od.nih.gov /wp-content/uploads/2016/02/Best_Practices_for_Mixed _Methods_Research.pdf

De Las Nueces, D., Hacker, K., DiGirolamo, A., & Hicks, L. S. (2012). A systematic review of community-based participatory research to enhance clinical trials in racial and ethnic minority groups. *Health Services Research, 47*(3, Part II), 1363–1386. http://dx.doi.org/10.1111/j.1475-6773.2012.01386.x

Devine, J., Sink, L., DeSalvo, B., & Cortes, R. (2010). *The use of vital statistics in the 2010 demographic analysis estimates* (Census Bureau Working Paper No. 88). Washington, DC: U.S. Census Bureau. Retrieved from https://www.census .gov/population/www/documentation/twps0088/twps0088 .pdf

Dillard, C. B. (2000). The substance of things hoped for, the evidence of things not seen: Examining an endarkened feminist epistemology in educational research and leadership. *International Journal of Qualitative Studies in Education, 13*(6), 661–681. http://dx.doi.org/10.1080/09518390050211565

Dresser, N. (1996). *Multicultural manners: New rules of etiquette for a changing society.* New York: Wiley.

Eisenhower, A., Suyemoto, K., Lucchese, F., & Canenguez, K. (2014). "Which box should I check?" Examining standard check box approaches to measuring race and ethnicity. *Health Research and Educational Trust, 49*(3), 1034–1055. http://dx.doi.org/10.1111/1475-6773.12132

Fisher, C. B., Hoagwood, K., Boyce, C., Duster, T., Frank, D. A., Grisso, T., . . . Zayas, L. H. (2002). Research ethics for mental health science involving ethnic minority children and youths. *American Psychologist, 57*(12), 1024–1040. http://dx.doi.org /10.1037/0003-066X.57.12.1024

Foster, M. W. (2006). Analyzing the use of race and ethnicity in biomedical research from a local community perspective. *Journal of Law, Medicine, & Ethics, 34*(3), 508–512. http://dx.doi .org/10.1111/j.1748-720X.2006.00063.x

GenIUSS Group, & Herman J. L. (Ed.). (2014). *Best practices for asking questions to identify transgender and other gender minority respondents on population-based surveys.* Los Angeles: Williams Institute.

Guarneri, C. E., & Dick, C. (2012). *Methods of assigning race and Hispanic origin to births from vital statistics data.* Washington, DC: U.S. Census Bureau, Population Division.

Henrich, J., Heine, S. J., & Norenzayan, A. (2010). The weirdest people in the world? *Behavioral and Brain Sciences, 33*(2–3), 61–83. http://dx.doi.org/10.1017/S0140525X0999152X

Institute of Medicine. (2009). *Race, ethnicity, and language data: Standardization for health care quality improvement.* Washington, DC: National Academies Press.

Institute of Medicine. (2013). *Collecting sexual orientation and gender identity data in electronic health records: Workshop summary.* Washington, DC: National Academies Press.

Jones, P. S., Lee, J. W., Pillips, L. R., Zhang, X. E., & Jaceldo, K. B. (2001). An adaptation of Brislin's translation model for cross-cultural research. *Nursing Research, 50,* 300–304.

Kagawa-Singer, M., Dressler, W. W., George, S. M., & Elwood, W. N. (2012). *The cultural framework for health.* Bethesda, MD: National Institutes of Health.

Kao, H., Hsu, M., & Clark, L. (2004). Conceptualizing and critiquing culture in health research. *Journal of Transcultural Nursing, 15*(4), 269–277. http://dx.doi.org/10.1177 /1043659604268963

Kaplan, J. B., & Bennett, T. (2003). Use of race and ethnicity in biomedical publication. *JAMA, 289*(20), 2709–2716. http://dx.doi.org/10.1001/jama.289.20.2709

Kavanagh, K. H., & Kennedy, P. H. (1992). *Promoting cultural diversity: Strategies for healthcare professionals.* Newbury Park, CA: Sage.

Keppel, K., Pamuk, E., Lynch, J., Carter-Pokras, O., Kim, I., Mays, V., . . . Weissman, J. S. (2005). Methodological issues in measuring health disparities. *Vital Health Statistics, 2*(141), 1–16.

Lau, A. S., Chang, D. F., & Okazaki, S. (2010). Methodological challenges in treatment outcome research with ethnic minorities. *Cultural Diversity and Ethnic Minority Psychology, 16*(4), 573–580. http://dx.doi.org/10.1037/a0021371

Le, C. N. (2015). *"The model minority image" Asian-Nation: The Landscape of Asian America.* Retrieved from http://www .asian-nation.org/model-minority.shtml

Lee, C. J. (2002). Aspects of emic and etic measurement: Lessons from Mary Poppins. *American Journal of Occupational Therapy, 56,* 214–216. http://dx.doi.org/10.5014/ajot.56.2.214

Lee, J., & DukYoo, J. (2006). Measurement issues across different cultures. *Journal of Korean Academy of Nursing, 36*(8), 1295–1300. Retrieved from http://www.kan.or.kr/new/kor/sub3/filedata/200608/1295.pdf

Lequerica, A., & Krch, D. (2014). Issues of cultural diversity in acquired brain injury (ABI) rehabilitation. *Neuro Rehabilitation, 34*(4), 645–653. http://dx.doi.org/10.3233/NRE-141079

Markus, H. R. (2008). Pride, prejudice, and ambivalence: Toward a unified theory of race and ethnicity. *American Psychologist, 63,* 651–670. http://dx.doi.org/10.1037/0003-066X.63.8.651

Mason, L. R., Nam, Y., & Kim, Y. (2014), Validity of infant race/ethnicity from birth certificates in the context of U.S. demographic change. *Health Services Research, 49*(1), 249–267. http://dx.doi.org/10.1111/1475-6773.12083

Mendoza, D. B., Williams, M. T., Chapman, L. K., & Powers, M. (2012). Minority inclusion in randomized clinical trials of panic disorder. *Journal of Anxiety Disorders, 26,* 574–582. http://dx.doi.org/10.1016/janxdis.2012.02.011

Merriam, S. B. (2009). *Qualitative research: A guide to design and implementation* (3rd ed.). Hoboken, NJ: Jossey-Bass.

Milner, R. H. (2007). Race, culture, and researchers positionality: Working through dangers seen, unseen, and unforeseen, *Educational Researcher, 36*(7), 388–400. http://dx.doi.org/10.3102/0013189X07309471

National Institutes of Health. (2001). *Toward higher levels of analysis: Progress and promise in research on social and cultural dimensions of health* (Publication No. 21-5020). Bethesda, MD: Author.

National Institutes of Health Revitalization Act of 1993, Pub. L. 103-43.

Niblo, D. M., & Jackson, M. S. (2004). Models for combining the qualitative emic approach with the quantitative derived etic approach. *Australian Psychologist, 39*(2), 127–133. http://dx.doi.org/10.1080/00050060410001701843

Noymer, A., Penner, A. M., & Saperstein, A. (2011). Cause of death affects racial classification on death certificates. *PLoS ONE, 6*(1), e15812. http://dx.doi.org/10.1371/journal.pone.0015812

Office of Management and Budget. (1997). *Race and ethnic standards for federal statistics and administrative reporting* (Statistical Policy Directive No. 15, revised). Washington, DC: Author.

Office of Minority Health. (2015). *Data collection standards for race, ethnicity, primary language, sex, and disability status.* Retrieved from http://minorityhealth.hhs.gov/omh/browse.aspx?lvl=2&lvlid=23

Olive, J. L. (2014). Reflecting on the tensions between emic and etic perspectives in life history research: Lessons learned. *Forum Qualitative Sozialforschung/Forum: Qualitative Social Research, 15*(2), Art. 6. http://nbn-resolving.de/urn:nbn:de:0114-fqs140268

Olatundun, O. I. (2009). What is cross-cultural research. *International Journal of Psychological Studies, 1*(2), 82–96. http://dx.doi.org/10.5539/ijps.v1n2p82

Patient Protection and Affordable Care Act, 42 U.S.C. § 18001 (2010).

Pierce, J. R., & Denison, A. V. (2006). Place-of-residence errors on death certificates for two contiguous U.S. counties. *Population Health Metrics, 4,* 1–6. http://dx.doi.org/10.1186/1478-7954-4-6

Russell, S. L., Katz, R. V., Kressin, N. R., Claudio, C., Green, B. L., Wang, M. Q., . . . Tzvetkova, K. (2007). Knowledge of DES and thalidomide: Relationship to attitudes to participation of women in biomedical research. *Annals of Epidemiology, 17*(9), 749–750. http://dx.doi.org/10.1016/j.annepidem.2007.07.080

Sexual Minority Assessment Research Team. L. Badgett & N. Goldberg (Eds.). (2009). *Best practices for asking questions about sexual orientation on surveys.* Los Angeles: Williams Institute.

Smedley, A., & Smedley, B. D. (2005). Race as biology is fiction, racism as a social problem is real: Anthropological and historical perspectives on the social construction of race. *American Psychologist, 60,* 16–26. http://dx.doi.org/10.1037/0003-066X.60.1.16

Spriggs, M. (2004). Canaries in the mines: Children, risk, non-therapeutic research, and justice. *Journal of Medical Ethics, 30*(2), 176–181. Retrieved from http://jme.bmj.com/content/30/2/176.full

Stanhope, V., Soloman, P., Pernell-Arnold, A., Sands, R. G., & Bourjolly, J. N. (2005). Evaluating cultural competence among behavioral health professionals. *Psychiatric Rehabilitation Journal, 28,* 225–233. http://dx.doi.org/10.2975/28.2005.225.233

Suite, D. H., La Bril, R., Primm, A., & Harrison-Ross, P. (2007). Beyond misdiagnosis, misunderstanding and mistrust: Relevance of the historical perspective in the medical and mental health treatment of people of color. *Journal of the National Medical Association, 99*(8), 879–885. Retrieved from https://www.researchgate.net/publication/6117012_Beyond_misdiagnosis_misunderstanding_and_mistrust_Relevance_of_the_historical_perspective_in_the_medical_and_mental_health_treatment_of_people_of_color

Sullivan, C., & Cottone, R. R. (2010). Emergent characteristics of effective cross-culture research: A review of the literature. *Journal of Counseling and Development, 88,* 357–362. http://dx.doi.org/10.1002/j.1556-6678.2010.tb00033.x

Ulrich, A., Thompson, B., Livaudais, J. C., Espinoza, N., Cordova, A., & Coronado, G. D. (2013). Issues in biomedical research: What do Hispanics think? *American Journal of Behavior, 37*(1), 80–85. http://dx.doi.org/10.5993/AJHB.37.1.9

U.S. Department of Health and Human Services. (2001). *Mental health: Culture, race and ethnicity* (Suppl. to Mental health: A report of the Surgeon General). Rockville, MD: Substance Abuse and Mental Health Services Administration, Center for Mental Health Services.

Walter, J. K., Burke, J. F., & Davis, M. M. (2013). Research participation by low-income and racial/ethnic minority groups: how payment may change the balance. *Clinical and Translational Science, 6*(5), 363–371. http://dx.doi.org/10.1111/cts.12084

Waters, M. C. (1994). Ethnic and racial identities of second-generation Black immigrants in New York City. *International Migration Review, 28*(4), 795–820. Retrieved from https://dash.harvard.edu/bitstream/handle/1/3686134/Waters_EthnicRacial.pdf?sequence=3

Willis, J. W. (2007). *Foundations of qualitative research: Interpretive and critical approaches.* Thousand Oaks, CA: Sage.

Wombles, K (2010). The emic and the etic in cross-cultural research. *Science 2.0.* Retrieved from http://www.science20.com/science_autism_spectrum_disorders/blog/emic_and_etic_crosscultural_research

Yin, R. K. (2010). *Qualitative research from start to finish.* New York: Guilford Press.

Yu, E. S., & Liu, W. T. (1994). Methodological issues. In N. Zane, D. Takeuchi, & K. Young (Eds), *Confronting critical health issues of Asian and Pacific Islander Americans* (pp. 22–50). Thousand Oaks, CA: Sage.

Zea, M. C., Reisen, C. A., & Diaz, R. M. (2003). Methodological issues in research on sexual behavior with Latino gay and bisexual men. *American Journal of Community Psychology, 31*(3/4), 281–291. http://dx.doi.org/10.1023/A:1023962805064

Chapter 31.

CULTURAL COMPETENCE AND THE RESEARCH PROCESS: A STUDY COMPARING MEXICAN AMERICAN AND EUROPEAN AMERICAN OLDER ADULTS' STRATEGIES FOR PROMOTING FUNCTIONAL INDEPENDENCE

Hon K. Yuen, PhD, OTR/L, and Angela E. Scoggin, PhD, OTR, FAOTA

I continue to work every day, and as long as I can do it I will continue to work. I try eating right and take care of myself so that I can be healthy and have the energy to continue working.
Study participant

Chapter Highlights

- Older Adults and Independence
- Studies of Middle-Class, White Older Adults
- Study of Mexican American Older Adults

Key Terms and Concepts

✧ Actions
✧ Cultural competence
✧ Hispanic culture

✧ Independence
✧ Personal attributes

For many older adults in the United States, being able to live independently in their home environment in the community and remain in control of their lives is extremely important (Wilken, Walker, Sandberg, & Holcomb, 2002). Maintaining independence is a universal indicator of successful aging across different cultures in modern society (Hilton, Gonzalez, Saleh, Maitoza, & Anngela-Cole, 2012). This chapter describes strategies used by working-class Mexican American community-dwelling older adults on maintaining independence and compares their actions and personal attributes with those used by middle-class, European American older adults to maintain independence.

Older Adults and Independence

Independence is the ability of a person to manage one's own household and affairs with minimal financial, physical, intellectual, or psychosocial reliance on others (Yuen, Gibson, Yau, & Mitcham, 2007). Independence enables older adults to continue living in their preferred environment without the need for formal community and home care services or institutionalization (Gignac, Cott, & Badley, 2000). Therefore, independence is regarded as an essential element of successful aging (Bowling & Dieppe, 2005).

Studies of Middle-Class, White Older Adults

Early studies on exploring the issue of independence among older adults predominantly used White or European Americans as the participants (Schwanen, Banister, & Bowling, 2012). In a study seeking insights into older adults' experience of health care service, Brown, McWilliam, and Mai (1997) interviewed 24 community-dwelling, primarily White older adults in Ontario, Canada, through focus groups on the question, "What part do you play in maintaining your own independence?" Respondents identified positive attributes and attitudes toward aging as major facilitators to their independence. Positive attitudes such as having a bright outlook, determination, and caring for others, coupled with positive attributes such as being active and involved and thinking ahead, promoted their independence (Brown et al., 1997).

Subsequently, a study investigated strategies used by 163 community-dwelling, primarily older European Americans to maintain independence. Yuen, Gibson, Yau, and Mitcham (2007) found that older adults used a set of complex interrelated *actions,* including engagement in various productive activities in their daily routine to promote health, to maintain adequate social support networks and resources, and to manage finances wisely. These actions seemed directly modified through *personal attributes* (i.e., attitudes and beliefs about aging), which included views

of aging, self-reliance, and perceived efficacy (Yuen et al., 2007). The overarching themes that emerged from these two studies are comparable, and the samples of these two studies were composed of mainly middle-class, White older adults.

Study of Mexican American Older Adults

Culture

Little is known about the strategies that low-income Hispanic older adults use to maintain independence. Hispanic older adults are one of the fastest growing population groups in the United States (Passel & Cohn, 2008). Low-income Hispanics, especially Mexican American older adults, are characterized by high rates of chronic health and disabling conditions, such as diabetes, obesity, heart disease, stroke, arthritis, hip fracture, and cancer, which are associated with functional or activities of daily living impairment (Bastida, Cuellar, & Villas, 2001; Centers for Disease Control and Prevention, 2004; Markides et al., 1996). Multiple chronic conditions and functional limitations certainly have a negative effect on maintaining independence.

Although Hispanic and European American cultures share the same religious heritage of Western tradition (Iannone, 1987), *Hispanic culture* has several unique characteristics that distinguish it from European American culture. For example, in general, European Americans tend to place more value on individualism and independence, whereas Hispanics tend to value collectivism and interdependence, with family as the core unit (Oyserman, Coon, & Kemmelmeier, 2002; Vargas & Kemmelmeier, 2013). The social structures and values system such as familial traditions of Hispanic culture may influence how Hispanic older adults maintain independence.

Study Objectives

The aims of this study are to explore strategies described by community-dwelling Mexican American older adults on maintaining independence and to compare their actions and personal attributes with those used by European American older adults to maintain independence. Understanding Hispanic older adults' actions and personal attributes to maintain independence can enable occupational therapy practitioners to pave ways for developing culturally and linguistically appropriate and realistic health services and interventions that assist these older adults to maintain their independence. Findings from this study will not only inform practice but also cultivate cultural competence in the health services sector and can assist policy and program development in community health care delivery that addresses disparities in this vulnerable population.

Reflection 31.1. Gaining Understanding Through Observation and Interaction

- How could observing and documenting community-dwelling older Mexican Americans' daily routine in their home environment, as well as interviewing and interacting with them, help one to understand the complexity of their daily lives?

Method

Design and Participants

A cross-sectional, qualitative research design was used for this study. Students in an introductory occupational therapy research course at the University of Texas–Pan American were asked to locate community-dwelling older adults of their choice who met the study's selection criteria. The selection criteria included participants who

- Lived at home in the Lower Rio Grande Valley, Hidalgo County, Texas, community;
- Identified themselves as Mexican American;
- Were ages 65 years or older;
- Were cognitively alert (i.e., oriented to time, place, person, and purpose);
- Were functionally communicative (i.e., able to carry on daily conversation); and
- Were not members of interviewers' immediate families or close relatives.

Study Setting

The Lower Rio Grande Valley in South Texas, of which Hidalgo County is a part, is located on the United States–Mexico border. An epidemiology study conducted between 2006 and 2008 for the U.S.–Mexico border region (Ghaddar, Brown, Pagán, & Diaz, 2010) revealed the following

statistics for Hidalgo County: 89.3% of the population was Hispanic/Mexican American compared with 14.7% of the general U.S. population; 32.9% of families lived below the poverty level compared with 9.8% of the general U.S. population, 30.4% were without health insurance compared with 15.9% of the general U.S. population; and 82.5% spoke a language other than English at home compared with 19.5% of the general U.S. population.

Another population survey study conducted between 2002 and 2003 on Mexican American adults living in the same region reported that 12% of the respondents were at least 60 years old, 45% had less than an 8th-grade education, and almost 20% had at least three coexisting chronic health problems (Mier et al., 2008). This region is disproportionately affected by a higher prevalence of diabetes compared with the national rate of 9% (Blackwell, Lucas, & Clarke, 2014), with 23.2% of the Mexican American residents ages 45 or older reported to have a diagnosis of diabetes (Bastida et al., 2001). Other high prevalence (self-reported) chronic health problems in this population were joint and bone problems (39.3%), hypertension (27.5%), cardiovascular disease (15.3%–24.5%), and cataracts (19.2%; Bastida et al., 2001).

Procedure

Students received the study package in class, along with detailed instructions on how to interview the participants. Principles and stages of the interview process were reviewed, and students were trained and practiced in administering the interviews. Each student was responsible for conducting 1 interview with one Mexican American older adult who met the study selection criteria. Students contacted participants to arrange the time and place of the interview. The student interviewer obtained informed consent from each participant after a discussion of the purpose and voluntary nature of the study and an assurance of confidentiality. The Institutional Review Board at the University of Texas–Pan American approved the study.

The method of data collection in this study was one-on-one, face-to-face, semistructured interviews. The study package, including the informed consent form and interview questions, was written in either English or Spanish. The interview questions were adopted from our previous study and written in English (Yuen et al., 2007); the questions were translated into

Spanish. A back-translation of the Spanish version to English was also conducted. The original English questions and the English back-translation version were compared for accuracy and equivalence. Any discrepancies in the Spanish version were negotiated and resolved among the translators. The primary translator was an occupational therapy faculty member who is a native Spanish speaker.

The data collection instrument consisted of a series of questions related to participants' sociodemographic background, including age, gender, marital status, living situation, educational level, employment, and mobility status. Six open-ended questions related to the meaning of independence, the participants' perceived independence, and their strategies for promoting independence. The sequence of these questions was designed to explore the meaning and issues related to functional independence prior to discussing specific strategies for maintaining and promoting independence. Students followed the sequence of the six questions as in our previous study (Yuen et al., 2007).

The interviews were conducted in either English or Spanish, depending on the choice of the participant and the language proficiency of the student interviewer. The responses to these questions were audiotaped with the participants' permission. Students offered to let participants listen to the tape or view the interview notes and correct or delete information. Student interviewers transcribed their interviews verbatim, removing all identifying information, and translated them into English if necessary. Students who did not have permission to audiotape the interview organized and typed their interview notes. Students turned in their notes and transcribed interviews (Spanish and English, if the interview was conducted in Spanish) to the course instructor. Students also turned in their interview tapes. Completion of the interview was part of a course requirement for the student interviewers.

Data Analysis

The study was carried out over 4 consecutive years, using new occupational therapy student interviewers each year. By the conclusion of the 4th year, 66 participants had been interviewed. One participant was from a nursing home, and 3 did not have any sociodemographic information collected. These 4 participants were excluded from the analysis.

Of the 62 interviews, 14 were conducted in Spanish. More than half (35) of the student interviewers

were given permission to audiotape. On the basis of the detailed sociodemographic information, it was concluded that no 2 students interviewed the same participant.

The study focused on responses to the interview question "What do you do to help yourself be more independent in the future?" Data were analyzed using content analysis to identify strategies used by Mexican American older adults to maintain and promote independence (Morse & Field, 1995).

The content analysis was completed in the following manner. We independently reviewed and coded all 62 transcripts. Initial codes were manually assigned to phrases and sentences; they were closely associated with the original text in order to maintain the participants' meaning. The occurrence of each coded text segment was recorded on the same Excel spreadsheet that was used in our previous study on European American older adults (Yuen et al., 2007). New codes were added when new topics emerged. Quotations with related codes (similar events and concepts) were grouped together to create categories, then collapsed into distinctly different themes and subthemes (Morse & Field, 1995).

To enhance credibility of the analysis, we reviewed each other's data interpretation and theme categorization, and compared and contrasted our findings. When there were disagreements, we reviewed transcripts, then discussed and resolved disagreements. We achieved perfect agreement for the themes, supporting the credibility of the data analysis. We then compared the similarities and differences in actions and personal attributes between Mexican American and European American older adults on maintaining and promoting independence.

Reflection 31.2. Avoiding Stereotypes

Although there were some differences between the older European Americans in Yuen et al.'s study and older Mexican Americans of the current study in the actions and personal attributes they adopted to maintain independence, there were more similarities in the identified themes.

- How might this remind occupational therapy practitioners of the importance of avoiding stereotypes when working with older adults from any cultural background?

Results

Of the 62 participants, 40 were women and 22 were men. The mean age of participants was 69.7 years (*SD* = 5.0, range = 65–87 years); the majority of participants (87%) were between 65 and 75 years old. More than 80% of them were living with their spouse or children and relatives, 56.5% were married, and most (87%) reported ambulating without the use of an assistive device. More than one-third of participants (35.5%) were working either part-time or full-time, about half (48.4%) had less than a Grade 9 education, and about a quarter (24.2%) had received a high school education or high school certificate or diploma. Detailed demographic information of the participants is shown in Table 31.1.

Given that the responses from the participants were very similar to those from the European American counterparts in our previous study (Yuen et al., 2007), we used the same conceptual framework of our previous study to categorize the data. We identified the same two overarching and interrelated domains: (1) actions and (2) personal attributes. The main themes and subthemes that emerged from the data are presented in Table 31.2, with specific quotations from participants.

Study Conclusion

Participants in this study verbalized the same types of strategies the European American older adults in our previous study (Yuen et al., 2007) used to promote independence. Despite the similarities, there are differences that may be due to the difference in cultural traditions between the two groups.

Health

"Stay physically active" and "eat healthy" were the two most common ways to promote health. Despite the high percentage of participants reported to have diabetes (27.4%) and cardiovascular disease (high blood pressure and high cholesterol; 22.6%), no single participant mentioned weight loss as a strategy to maintain health. The Mexican American participants only mentioned reduction in fat consumption or amount/portion of food intake, and eating more fish and chicken and less tortillas (as

Table 31.1. Demographic Information of the European American (*N* = 149)[a] and Mexican American (*N* = 62) Participants

Characteristic	European Americans *n*[b] (%[c])	Mexican Americans *n* (%)
Gender		
Female	109 (73.2%)	40 (64.5%)
Age[d]		
≤ 75 years	92 (62.2%)	54 (87.1%)
> 75 years	56 (37.8%)	8 (12.9%)
Marital status		
Married	71 (48.3%)	35 (56.5%)
Living situation		
Alone	56 (37.6%)	12 (19.4%)
With children/others	20 (13.4%)	15 (24.2%)
With spouse and children	6 (4.0%)	18 (29.0%)
Educational level		
College and beyond	61 (40.9%)	17 (27.4%)
Vocational or nursing school	6 (4.0%)	
High school/GED/high school graduate	66 (44.3%)	15 (24.2%)
Below high school	15 (10.1%)	30 (48.4%)
Employment status		
Work (full-time/part-time)	33 (22.1%)	22 (35.5%)
Mobility status		
Unaided	136 (91.3%)	54 (87.1%)

Note. [a]Data from the study by Yuen et al. (2007). [b]Total number may vary because of missing data. [c]Valid percentage. [d]Mean age for European American sample = 73.5 ± 6.2 years, range = 64–90; mean age for Mexican American sample = 69.7 ± 5.0 years, range = 65–87.

Table 31.2. Emerging Themes and Subthemes From Participants Describing Their Strategies to Promote Functional Independence

		Actions
Theme	**Subtheme**	**Example**
Promote health	Eat healthy	"Well, when I first got sick from the high blood pressure the doctor told me that I had to start eating better. . . . [The doctor] told her [my wife] I had to eat more fish and chicken and less tortillas" (67-year-old man).
		"I eat healthy sometimes because I have to cook healthy for my husband and my family" (67-year-old woman).
		"As far as food goes, I do not follow the same diet from before. My dinners are now not that heavy, and I cannot eat as much" (80-year-old woman).
	Practice health care management and preventive practice	"I keep my health the best, the best I can by going to the doctor frequently, doing all the necessary checkups (66-year-old man).
		"It's been 25 years since I quit smoking and drinking" (74-year-old man).
		"I watch my diet. I try to be more careful when I walk. I need to think about things carefully before doing something. I look at how much salt and sugar I take in every day. I've become more conscious about my health" (69-year-old man).
		"I take my medication on a daily basis, I take my preventative medication for diabetes" (65-year-old woman).
	Stay physically active	"I try to stay active. I don't like to sit at home all day. I get out of the house and run errands or visit with people" (67-year-old widow).
		"Well, I try to stay active. We walk every day if we have the time, two to three miles at a time. We go to the dances. We still have sex . . . sometimes" (66-year-old man).
	Keep the mind active	"I do crossword puzzles . . . I get involved with people, try to help people" (74-year-old woman, lives alone).
		"I try to use my mind, I try to concentrate, and I like to pray before I start doing something" (80-year-old woman).
	Enhance emotional health and spiritual well-being	"Keep active, volunteering, babysitting, and helping others that are less fortunate" (75-year-old woman).
		"Look, prayer will help you also to be independent because it's a lot of load for when one has a disability like mine, but if you're with God he will help you. I am always with God" (65-year-old woman with mobility problem).
		"I try to stay motivated by listening to the radio that makes me more happy and energetic " (82-year-old woman).
Maintain adequate social support networks and resources		"The neighbors will invite me here or there. That's when I take advantage on doing my errands" (71-year-old woman, lives alone).
		"When I see them outside, I just talk to the neighbor [lady] that I go over or she comes over and we talk" (68-year-old woman, lives alone).
		"I also have great friendships with everyone and with my cleaning lady" (65-year-old woman with mobility problem).
Manage finances wisely		"Work and save" (73-year-old woman, lives alone).
		Personal Attributes
Views on aging	Resistance	"I try not to allow myself to let my illness rule me. Okay. It's a mind game that we're in. But I feel that, uh, you can't afford to let yourself give in, and unfortunately a thing about diabetes . . . I have to rule it, instead of it ruling me. Just keep on going and so forth" (74-year-old man).

(Continued)

Table 31.2. Emerging Themes and Subthemes From Participants Describing Their Strategies to Promote Functional Independence *(Cont.)*

		Actions
Theme	**Subtheme**	**Example**
	Adjustment/ accommodation	"I keep myself busy around the house but I have a lady come by to help me" (65-year-old woman, lives alone).
	Positive thinking	"I continue to work every day, and as long as I can do it I will continue to work. I try eating right and take care of myself so that I can be healthy and have the energy to continue working" (68-year-old woman).
Self-reliance		"I am very independent, and I feel that as far as I need their [children's] love and care, but as far as financial, I don't need their financial part in it" (75-year-old woman).
		"I try not to depend too much on my children" (65-year-old woman).
Perceived efficacy		"Since I can't walk very much because of my knee. I cook for myself if I am hungry. . . . And I can do a lot of things on my own" (65-year-old woman).

Note. Adapted from Bowling & Dieppe (2005); Schwanen, Banister, & Bowling (2012).

per doctor's advice); few mentioned consumption of more fruits, vegetables, and whole grains or fibers. This may indicate a lack of nutritional knowledge of food items in participants for eating healthy.

Integrating physical, emotional–mental, and spiritual aspects was reported to be an important category for older Hispanics to maintain health (Alfinger & Causey, 1995). Although few participants explicitly verbalized integrating body–mind–spirit as a strategy to promote independence, several mentioned the importance of God as part of their view of life. Participants drew on spiritual strength through prayer and maintained a close relationship with God as a way to cope with stress. Using such a coping mechanism is vital for the maintenance and restoration of physical and mental health well-being (Jurkowski, Kurlanska, & Ramos, 2010; McCarthy, Ruiz, Gale, Karam, & Moore, 2004; Musgrave, Allen, & Allen, 2002).

Reflection 31.3. Importance of Family

Mexican American participants verbalized the importance of "orienting toward family" or "spending time with family" as a way to maintain health, and they enjoy being a part of their extended family life.

- How might their focus on sharing the relationships with their children and grandchildren, rather than seeking emotional and physical support, help to support their health?

Relationships

Consistent with the literature on health maintenance and successful aging in older Hispanics, our Mexican American participants verbalized the importance of "orienting toward family" or "spending time with family" as a way to maintain wellness (Alfinger & Causey, 1995; Collins, Decker, & Esquibel, 2006; Hilton et al., 2012). This is reflected by the extended family tradition of Mexican Americans, with the majority of the participants living with their adult children, grandchildren, and even family of their children (i.e., in-laws).

In contrast, very few European American older adults were enthusiastic about the idea of living with their children or other family members, except as a last resort (Theve-Gibbons, 2001). The fact that less than 20% of the Mexican American participants live alone compared with 38% of the European American sample of our previous study (Yuen et al., 2007) confirms that extended family tradition is part of the Mexican American culture (see Table 31.1). As explained by Hilton et al. (2012), Hispanic older adults enjoy being a part of the extended family life, focusing on sharing and participating in relationships with their children and grandchildren rather than seeking emotional and physical support.

Similar to European American older adults in our previous study (Yuen et al., 2007), the Mexican American participants have strong sources of social and emotional support and instrumental assistance, especially for those women who lived alone. They developed and nurtured good relationships with neighbors. As one 65-year-old woman who lived alone stated, "My neighbors are very good to me, they are always looking after me. So I cook and like to take them a plate to eat." A few participants also described strategies such as taking advantage of offers for help from neighbors as a way to get the assistance they needed without being dependent on their children.

Work

More than one-third of the participants work either part-time or full-time compared with only 22% of the European American sample of our previous study (Yuen et al., 2007; see Table 31.1). Several participants said they went back to work after they retired from one job, which was never mentioned by the European American sample of our previous study. The reasons for higher proportion of the participants working are unclear; it may relate to the economic reason of maintaining financial independence.

On the other hand, a 67-year-old woman said, "I still work but mostly because I want to; if you just stay home you lose your edge and you become a couch potato." To her, work may serve as a means to sustain body and mind. Overall, these participants considered the inclusion of family, community, God, and strong religious beliefs as important aspects of promoting independence.

Attitude

Several studies reported that Hispanic older adults typically hold positive attitudes and keep a positive outlook toward aging (Collins et al., 2006; Orellano, Mountain, Varas, & Labault, 2014). The following quote from a 68-year-old woman illustrated the positive views on aging: "I continue to work every day, and as long as I can do it I will continue to work. I try eating right and take care of myself so that I can be healthy and have the energy to continue working."

Practice Implications

Although there were some differences between the European American and Mexican American older adults in the actions and personal attributes they adopted to maintain independence, there were more similarities in the identified themes. This serves to remind occupational therapy practitioners of the importance of avoiding stereotypes when working with older adults from any cultural background (Collins et al., 2006). *Cultural*

competence is an important component to be incorporated when designing programs aiming to improve physical activity and diabetes self-management for socioeconomically disadvantaged, Spanish-speaking Mexican Americans (Mier et al., 2011; Peña-Purcell, Boggess, & Jimenez, 2011).

With almost 80% of the participants attending church on a regular basis, occupational therapy practitioners can work with church members and leaders to incorporate and deliver health education (physical activity, nutritional knowledge, and food choices) and health-related preventive and promotional programs at church to promote independence (Patel, Frausto, Staunton, Souffront, & Derose, 2013). In addition, occupational therapy practitioners should partner with other health care professionals such as dietitians to help Mexican American older adults develop healthy eating routines and habits through participation in valued activities in the church community.

Reflection 31.4. Church Attendance and Health Education

- With almost 80% of the participants attending church on a regular basis, how might occupational therapy practitioners work with church members and church leaders to incorporate and deliver health education (physical activity, nutritional knowledge, and food choices) and health-related prevention and promotion programs at church to promote independence?

Limitations

Because of the nature of the research design, we cannot claim the information we collected from the participants was theoretically saturated (i.e., no new insights seem to be coming from the data being collected). To gain a more in-depth understanding of the strategies that Mexican American older adults used to promote independence, researchers might have to stay in these older adults' homes for a short period of time and observe and document their daily routine as well as interact with them.

Summary

Findings from this study alert occupational therapy practitioners to the resourcefulness of many

Mexican American older adults and the kinds of functional independence strategies they adopt. Occupational therapy practitioners may have a role in advocating for and locating acceptable, accessible, and affordable community activities and resources to help Mexican American older adults with disability who experience barriers to participating in their community (Andonian & MacRae, 2011). Overall, this study could assist occupational therapy practitioners to design, develop, and implement health promotion and preventive program planning to meet the cultural needs of Mexican American older adults, as these programs are based on the older adults' plans of action and ways of thinking to promote independence.

Acknowledgments

We would like to acknowledge the older adults who agreed to be interviewed and the graduates of the University of Texas–Pan American occupational therapy program for their participation in this project. We also would like to thank Arturo Pecina, Jr., Christina Barrera, Alma Cavazos, Nancy Garcia, Celena Elizondo, Adhara Morales, Arnold Pecina, Silia Rodriguez, and Veronica Rodriguez-Reyna for their assistance with organization of the data for analysis. We would especially like to thank Alicia Balda, MEd, OTR, for her contribution in the translation of the questionnaire.

References

Alfinger, R. L., & Causey, M. E. (1995). Health concept of older Hispanic immigrants. *Western Journal of Nursing Research, 17*(6), 605–613. http://dx.doi.org/10.1177/019394599501700603

Andonian, L., & MacRae, A. (2011). Well older adults within an urban context: Strategies to create and maintain social participation. *British Journal of Occupational Therapy, 74*(1), 2–11. http://dx.doi.org/10.4276/030802211X12947686093486

Bastida, E., Cuellar, I., & Villas, P. (2001). Prevalence of diabetes mellitus and related conditions in a south Texas Mexican American sample. *Journal of Community Health Nursing, 18*(2), 75–84. http://dx.doi.org/10.1207/S15327655JCHN1802_01

Blackwell, D. L., Lucas, J. W., & Clarke, T. C. (2014). Summary health statistics for U.S. adults: National Health Interview Survey, 2012. *Vital Health Statistics, 10*(260), 1–171.

Retrieved from http://www.cdc.gov/nchs/data/series/sr_10/sr10_260.pdf

Bowling, A., & Dieppe, P. (2005). What is successful ageing and who should define it? *British Medical Journal, 331*(7531), 1548–1551. http://dx.doi.org/10.1136/bmj.331.7531.1548

Brown, J. B., McWilliam, C. L., & Mai, V. (1997). Barriers and facilitators to seniors' independence: Perceptions of seniors, caregivers, and health care providers. *Canadian Family Physician, 43*, 469–475. Retrieved from https://www.ncbi.nlm.nih.gov/pmc/articles/PMC2255330/

Centers for Disease Control and Prevention. (2004). Health disparities experienced by racial/ethnic minority populations. *Morbidity and Mortality Weekly Report, 53*(33), 755–756. Retrieved from https://www.cdc.gov/mmwr/preview/mmwrhtml/mm5333a1.htm

Collins, C. A., Decker, S. I., & Esquibel, K. A. (2006). Definitions of health: Comparison of Hispanic and African-American elders. *Journal of Multicultural Nursing and Health, 12*(1), 14–19.

Ghaddar, S., Brown, C. J., Pagán, J. A., & Diaz, V. (2010). Acculturation and healthy lifestyle habits among Hispanics in United States–Mexico border communities. *Revista Panamericana de Salud Publica, 28*(3), 190–197. http://dx.doi.org/10.1590/S1020-49892010000900009

Gignac, M. A., Cott, C., & Badley, E. M. (2000). Adaptation to chronic illness and disability and its relationship to perceptions of independence and dependence. *Journal of Gerontology Series B: Psychological Sciences and Social Sciences, 55*(6), P362–P372. http://dx.doi.org/10.1093/geronb/55.6.P362

Hilton, J. M., Gonzalez, C. A., Saleh, M., Maitoza, R., & Anngela-Cole, L. (2012). Perceptions of successful aging among older Latinos, in cross-cultural context. *Journal of Cross-Cultural Gerontology, 27*(3), 183–199. http://dx.doi.org/10.1007/s10823-012-9171-4

Iannone, M. (1987). A cross-cultural investigation of occupational role. *Occupational Therapy in Health Care, 4*(1), 93–101. http://dx.doi.org/10.1080/J003v04n01_08

Jurkowski, J. M., Kurlanska, C., & Ramos, B. M. (2010). Latino women's spiritual beliefs related to health. *American Journal of Health Promotion, 25*(1), 19–25. http://dx.doi.org/10.4278/ajhp.080923-QUAL-211

Markides, K. S., Stroup-Benham, C. A., Goodwin, J. S., Perkowski, L. C., Lichtenstein, M., & Ray, L. A. (1996). The effect of medical conditions on the functional limitations of Mexican-American elderly. *Annals of Epidemiology, 6*(5), 386–391. http://dx.doi.org/10.1016/S1047-2797(96)00061-0

McCarthy, M., Ruiz, E., Gale, B., Karam, C., & Moore, N. (2004). The meaning of health: Perspectives of Anglo and Latino older women. *Health Care for Women International, 25*(10), 950–969. http://dx.doi.org/10.1080/07399330490508730

Mier, N., Ory, M. G., Zhan, D., Conkling, M., Sharkey, J. R., & Burdine, J. N. (2008). Health-related quality of life among Mexican Americans living in colonias at the Texas–Mexico border. *Social Science and Medicine, 66*(8), 1760–1771. http://dx.doi.org/10.1016/j.socscimed.2007.12.017

Mier, N., Tanguma, J., Millard, A. V., Villarreal, E. K., Alen, M., & Ory, M. G. (2011). A pilot walking program for Mexican-American women living in colonias at the border. *American Journal of Health Promotion, 25*(3), 172–175. http://dx.doi.org/10.4278/ajhp.090325-ARB-115

Morse, J. M., & Field, P. A. (1995). *Qualitative research methods for health professionals* (2nd ed.). Thousand Oaks, CA: Sage.

Musgrave, C. F., Allen, C. E., & Allen, G. J. (2002). Spirituality and health for women of color. *American Journal of Public Health, 92*(4), 557–560. http://dx.doi.org/10.2105/AJPH.92.4.557

Orellano, E. M., Mountain, G., Varas, N., & Labault, N. (2014). Occupational competence strategies in old age: A mixed-methods comparison between Hispanic women with different levels of daily participation. *OTJR: Occupation, Participation and Health, 34*(1), 32–40. http://dx.doi.org/10.3928/15394492-20131205-01

Oyserman, D., Coon, H. M., & Kemmelmeier, M. (2002). Rethinking individualism and collectivism: Evaluation of theoretical assumptions and meta-analyses. *Psychological Bulletin, 128*(1), 3–52. http://dx.doi.org/10.1037//0033-2909.128.1.3

Passel, J., & Cohn, D. (2008). *U.S. population projections: 2005–2050.* Retrieved from Pew Hispanic Center website: http://www.pewhispanic.org/2008/02/11/us-population-projections-2005-2050

Patel, K. K., Frausto, K. A., Staunton, A. D., Souffront, J., & Derose, K. P. (2013). Exploring community health center and faith-based partnerships: Community residents' perspectives. *Journal of Health Care for the Poor and Underserved, 24*(1), 262–274. http://dx.doi.org/10.1353/hpu.2013.0016

Peña-Purcell, N. C., Boggess, M. M., & Jimenez, N. (2011). An empowerment-based diabetes self-management education program for Hispanic/Latinos: A quasi-experimental pilot study. *The Diabetes Educator, 37*(6), 770–779. http://dx.doi.org/10.1177/0145721711423319

Schwanen, T., Banister, D., & Bowling, A. (2012). Independence and mobility in later life. *Geoforum, 43*(6), 1313–1322. http://dx.doi.org/10.1016/j.geoforum.2012.04.001

Theve-Gibbons, S. (2001). Supported independence: Older women care-receivers. *Issues on Aging, 24*(1), 11–16.

Vargas, J. H., & Kemmelmeier, M. (2013). Ethnicity and contemporary American culture: A meta-analytic investigation of horizontal–vertical individualism–collectivism. *Journal of Cross-Cultural Psychology, 44*(2), 195–222. http://dx.doi.org/10.1177/0022022112443733

Wilken, C. S., Walker, K., Sandberg, J. G., & Holcomb, C. A. (2002). A qualitative analysis of factors related to late life independence as related by the old-old and viewed through the concept of locus of control. *Journal of Aging Studies, 16*(1), 73–86. http://dx.doi.org/10.1016/S0890-4065(01)00035-4

Yuen, H. K., Gibson, R. W., Yau, M. K., & Mitcham, M. D. (2007). Actions and personal attributes of community-dwelling older adults to maintain independence. *Physical and Occupational Therapy in Geriatrics, 25*(3), 35–53. http://dx.doi.org/10.1300/J148v25n03_03

Section VII.

EVALUATING CULTURAL EFFECTIVENESS

Chapter 32.

STRATEGIES AND TOOLS FOR ASSESSING CULTURAL COMPETENCE

Juleen Rodakowski, OTD, OTR/L, and Yolanda Suarez-Balcazar, PhD

Chapter Highlights

- Defining Cultural Competence
- Standards for Cultural and Linguistic Competence
- Assessing Cultural Competence
- Process of Assessing Cultural Competence

Key Terms and Concepts

✧ Chart reviews
✧ Cultural competence
✧ Cultural humility

✧ Cultural knowledge
✧ Culturally and linguistically appropriate services
✧ Organizational support

Despite the fact that professionals in the field of occupational therapy are not very diverse, these practitioners are likely to serve very diverse clients. The clients may have diversity in terms of race, ethnicity, religion, language spoken, and cultural values, among other factors typical of a diversifying society (Suarez-Balcazar & Rodakowski, 2007). This suggests that occupational therapy practitioners may be working not only with clients who may have differing habits, routines, and values but also with clients who may have a different understanding of the nature of basic activities of daily living, instrumental activities of daily living, rest and sleep, education, work, play, leisure, and social participation (Wells &

Black, 2000). Due to these differences, tensions may arise when the client is in need of culturally relevant services.

One of the core principles of occupational therapy practice is that practitioners use a client-centered perspective that matches skilled services to the cultural context of the client to obtain optimal outcomes; however, occupational therapy practitioners need to understand and implement culturally competent strategies to minimize potential tensions. This chapter defines cultural competence, discusses standards for cultural competence in health care, and introduces strategies and tools to assess cultural competence.

Defining Cultural Competence

A universally accepted definition of *cultural competence* is not available (Bonder, Martin, & Miracle, 2004), in part, because cultural competence is a complex, ongoing process (Balcazar, Suarez-Balcazar, & Taylor-Ritzler, 2009). Campinha-Bacote (1999), however, has developed one of the most commonly used definitions of cultural competence in health care. Within Campinha-Bacote's definition, cultural competence is displayed when a practitioner: (1) recognizes differences in culturally determined health beliefs and behaviors, (2) respects variations that occur within and among cultural groups, and (3) alters practice to provide effective services for clients from diverse backgrounds.

While considering this definition, Suarez-Balcazar and Rodakowski (2007) asserted that cultural competence requires personal growth and first-hand experience. They suggested that occupational therapy practitioners need to consider each client relationship as a unique cultural encounter to effectively obtain optimal outcomes for clients who are different from them (Suarez-Balcazar & Rodakowski, 2007).

Standards for Cultural and Linguistic Competence

The U.S. Department of Health and Human Services, Office of Minority Health ([OMH], 2011) developed standards for implementing cultural and linguistic competence in health care. OMH requires that the standards for *culturally and linguistically appropriate services (CLAS)* be integrated in organizations that receive federal funds. These standards were set with the recognition that health care professionals, including occupational therapy practitioners, will be required to serve more people who may not share a language, culture, or belief system with them, and related to the fact that expansion of client cultural backgrounds may cause tensions when clients need culturally and linguistically relevant services.

There are 15 CLAS standards organized in 1 principal standard and 14 others under the themes of Governance, Leadership, and Workplace (3 standards); Communication and Language Assistance (4 Standards); and Engagement, Continues Improvement and Accountability (7 Standards). **Standard 10** directly addresses assessing measuring cultural competence and says that health care

organizations should "Conduct ongoing assessments of the organization's CLAS-related activities and integrate CLAS-related measures into measurement and continuous quality improvement activities" (OMH, 2011, p. 1).

Reflection 32.1. Becoming Culturally Competent

- How do we know that cultural competence is happening?
- How do we know a practitioner is becoming culturally competent and that clients perceive the practitioner to be culturally competent?

Assessing Cultural Competence

One of the challenges encountered by practitioners and researchers alike is how to measure cultural competence, especially after acknowledging that it is a dynamic and ongoing process. Several options are available to assess cultural competence, and they include the following: (1) engaging in self-reflection, (2) rating self-perceived cultural competence, (3) client ratings of the practitioner's cultural competence, and (4) examining client outcomes.

Self-Reflection

Developing cultural competence begins with engaging in self-reflection. Occupational therapy practitioners are uniquely qualified to develop a culturally appropriate client–practitioner relationship given their expertise in therapeutic use of the self and use of a client-centered *Occupational Therapy Practice Framework* (American Occupational Therapy Association [AOTA], 2014). Nonetheless, self-reflection provides a first step to enhance one's cultural competence.

Self-reflection involves questioning the degree of knowledge about the client's culture, readiness to learn about cultural differences, and practicing *cultural humility* (i.e., accepting that we do not know enough about the client's culture and are ready to learn). Sue et al. (1998) argued that, to be culturally competent, one needs to possess specific information and cultural knowledge about particular social groups with whom one is working. Sawyer et al. (1995) defined *cultural knowledge* as the professional's knowledge of behavioral patterns that are seen in cultural groups. Areas of consideration include how members of a cultural group talk, think, behave, and feel and what their values are.

Exhibit 32.1 provides useful self-reflection questions in the process of developing cultural competence. Some of these questions have been adapted from Suarez-Balcazar, Balcazar, and Willis (2012) and Calzada and Suarez-Balcazar (2014).

Self-reflection fosters an understanding of the practitioner's and the client's worldviews. Suarez-Balcazar, Muñoz, and Fisher (2006) suggested that culturally competent occupational therapy practice requires a comprehensive knowledge base. That base facilitates occupational therapy practitioners to understand the perspective of clients from diverse backgrounds. This ongoing process of personal growth and self-reflection implies that one is learning about his or her own culture and that of others, engaging in multicultural experiences, and developing an understanding of others who are different from oneself.

Self-Ratings of Perceived Cultural Competence

The second strategy to assess cultural competence is to use available tools designed to help practitioners rate their perceived level of cultural competence.

Widely Used Assessment Tools

A literature review of assessment tools that measure cultural competence found 13 assessment tools, of which 9 included psychometric properties and were validated.

One example of a widely used tool for culturally competent serve care delivery is Campinha-Bacote's (1999) tool, the Process of Cultural Competence in the Delivery of Healthcare Services, which is often used in nursing. It measures the following four factors: (1) cultural awareness, (2) cultural knowledge, (3) cultural skills, and (4) cultural encounters.

Kim, Cartwright, Asay, and D'Andrea (2003) developed the Multicultural Awareness, Knowledge, and Skills Survey, which is often used in counseling and rehabilitation psychology. It measures three factors: (1) cultural awareness, (2) cultural knowledge, and (3) cultural skills.

Sodowsky (1996) developed the Multicultural Counseling Inventory, which is used in psychological counseling. It measures four factors: (1) multicultural counseling skills, (2) cultural awareness, (3) multicultural relationships, and (4) cultural knowledge.

Exhibit 32.2 provides useful self-reflection questions to consider in the process of developing cultural competence when considering assessment tools.

Exhibit 32.1. Self-Reflection Questions to Assess One's Readiness to Engage in Culturally Competent Practice

- What are my own cultural values and beliefs?
- Who am I as a cultural being?
- Am I prepared to meet the needs of my client, who is very different from me or other clients?
- Do I know enough about the client's cultural values, norms, and family patterns?
- Do I have any biases about the client's culture, race, ethnicity, religion, gender preferences, sociocultural background, beliefs, and values that can get in the way of providing care? If I do, what are those biases? And, what can I do to overcome my biases?
- Is there information I don't know about the client that might help me understand him or her better?
- Can I communicate with the client directly or via a translator? If I need to use a translator, how do I secure one at my clinical setting, and how do I know the quality of the translator?
- Does the client understand the purpose of occupational therapy, therapeutic goals, and what we are trying to accomplish together?
- Can I benefit from participating in cultural immersions, reading, or talking to others about my client's ethnic and cultural background?

Exhibit 32.2. Self-Reflection Questions to Use When Considering Cultural Competence Assessment Tools

- What assessment tools are available to rate my cultural competence?
- Do they measure aspects of cultural competence that I want to assess?
- Do they measure aspects of cultural competence that I need to assess?
- How would I use the information yield from the assessment tool?

Cultural Competence Assessment Instrument

The only tool available to measure cultural competence validated with occupational therapy practitioners is the Cultural Competence Assessment Instrument from the University of Illinois at Chicago (CCAI–UIC) developed by Suarez-Balcazar and colleagues (2009, 2011). Appendix 32.A provides a copy of the CCAI–UIC.

The CCAI–UIC validation study was conducted with a random sample of occupational therapists who were members of AOTA (Suarez-Balcazar et al., 2009). One thousand occupational therapy practitioners randomly selected from the AOTA directory of members were invited to participate in the study. A 47% response rate was received with the one-time mailing, resulting in sufficient statistical power to conduct a factor analysis and structural equation modeling.

The CCAI–UIC is the first psychometrically validated tool for measuring cultural competence in occupational therapists and measures three basic factors: (1) awareness and knowledge, a cognitive component; (2) skills development, a behavioral component; and (3) organizational support, a contextual component. Suarez-Balcazar et al. (2011) found that a three-factor model obtained strong psychometric properties.

An interesting finding of the study validating the CCAI–UIC is that *organizational support* arose as a necessary factor in the measurement of cultural competence. Organizational support is speaks to the organizational context and readiness to engage in culturally competent practice. This support directly influences practitioners' ability to implement culturally competent occupational therapy services (Suarez-Balcazar et al., 2009). This factor was not included in previously discussed tools. This may be because many tools emphasized the client–practitioner relationship without considering the environmental context.

Client Ratings of Practitioner's Cultural Competence

The third strategy to assess cultural competence is to use clients' ratings of a practitioner's cultural competence. Few studies have asked clients to rate a practitioner's level of cultural competence or the use of proxy measures such as comfort in relating and communicating with the practitioner. Most commonly the measures include questions about satisfaction with services or the practitioners.

Occupational therapy practitioners should assess the client's degree of satisfaction with therapy and degree of perceived level of cultural competence of the practitioner to examine delivery of culturally competent services from the client perspective. If this is done, areas for improvement in the delivery of culturally competent services can be identified and strategies implemented. Continuous improvement in the delivery of culturally competent services may minimize health disparities and ensure that client's needs are being met.

Several factors may bias the types of responses practitioners obtain. First, verbal or written questions of how comfortable clients felt with the practitioner or whether the practitioner was sensitive to their culture may elicit positive responses from clients for fear of losing services or in their efforts to be respectful (e.g., in some cultures, it is disrespectful to disagree or say no to a health professional, who is seen as a person of authority).

Second, paper surveys may not be returned by participants and, if used, need to include very informal simple language to adapt to the literacy level of the clients. Depending on practice setting, survey questions may need to be translated into the client's primary language. Given these scenarios, we recommend brief exit in-person interviews to assess clients' satisfaction conducted by bilingual and bicultural staff and not necessarily by the practitioner.

Client Outcomes

Another potential way to assess cultural competence is to examine client outcomes. Evidence, although limited, is beginning to emerge that suggests a relationship between practitioner cultural competence and client outcomes. Hasnain et al. (2011) conducted a systematic review of cultural competent interventions in health care and found that, indeed, cultural competence affected client outcomes. It is with caution that we recommend this given that client outcomes can be achieved because of many other reasons, not necessarily because of the level of competence of the practitioner. Client outcomes can be influenced by the client-centered approach of the practitioner and the achievement of therapeutic goals. However, issues such as cultural mistrust, challenges in developing client–practitioner rapport due to cultural misunderstandings, client attrition from services, and clients' lack of compliance may be outcomes worth examining.

Chart reviews of client characteristics and outcomes provide an opportunity to observe themes in the practitioner's practice. Chart reviews entail extracting information from clients' clinical charts and looking for similarities and differences in client characteristics (e.g., age, race, ethnicity, religion, and gender) and outcomes achieved (e.g., level of independence).

Several themes throughout the documentation can be explored. First, develop a profile of the types of clients who are seen in the practice, including ethnicity, language, and other demographic characteristics; referral course; compliance with occupational therapy treatment; absenteeism; and specific needs and challenges. Second, themes related to goal achievement may provide the opportunity to analyze the client outcomes.

Information captured may include goals that are frequently set, goals that are frequently achieved, and goals that are not achieved. Information gleaned in this process can be used to explore what aspects of the therapeutic relationship facilitated goal achievement. The practitioner may be able to explore attempts to understand the culture of the client and align that understanding with goal achievement. Ultimately, themes in a practitioner's narrative may provide insight into the strengths and areas for improvement in one's practice and cultural competence.

Process of Assessing Cultural Competence

Figure 32.1 depicts the process of assessing cultural competence. The process includes assessing practitioners' cultural competence, clients' perspective and outcomes, and organizational support. The willingness of an organization to engage in culturally competent practice directly influences practitioners' ability to implement culturally competent occupational therapy services (Suarez-Balcazar et al., 2009). If there are supports and services available and strong leadership at the clinical setting committed to providing culturally competent services, then the professional will be better able to provide culturally competent care. Thus, health care professionals have the opportunity to integrate cultural competence into their practice, but it requires the ongoing process of reflection, increasing knowledge, practicing skills, and assessing important client outcomes. Additional resources can be found through

- American Evaluation Association Statement on Cultural Competence: http://bit.ly/1J5NW8N
- Center of Excellence for Cultural Competence, New York Psychiatric Institute: http://nyculturalcompetence.org/

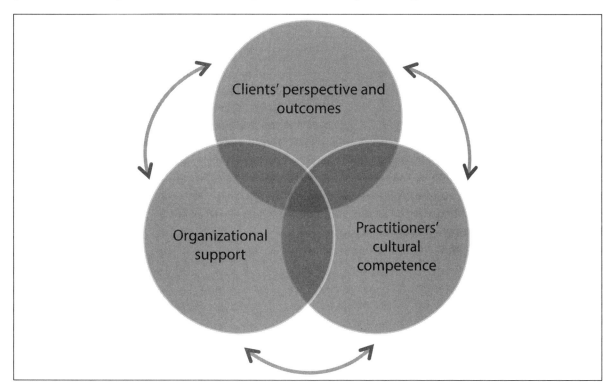

Figure 32.1.   Ongoing process of assessing cultural competence.

Summary

To provide culturally competent therapy, the practitioners need to be ready and open to different and new ways of intervening. This might include communicating through a translator, allowing family members to attend intervention sessions (but not using family members as translators—always request one, if needed), identifying resources in the language of the client, and understanding a client's cultural world in order to help the client manage his or her environment.

Cultural competence is an opportunity to better serve clients who have different values, norms, and patterns from those of the practitioner. Working with clients from diverse backgrounds requires a commitment for values and strategies that promote cultural competence. When serving clients from diverse backgrounds, cultural competence should be considered critical to provide services that allow clients to obtain optimal outcomes.

Despite a great deal of interest across disciplines, the integration of cultural competence in health care practice has been minimal due to limited research linking strategies to client-centered outcomes. Thus, one of the challenges for health professionals is to know how to measure cultural competence.

The guidelines in this chapter provide a way to measure cultural competence through self-reflection from the practitioner's perspective, from the client's perspective, and from the client's outcomes. Measuring and developing cultural competence will ultimately need to include the practitioner's openness to engage in the following activities: examining personal and organizational biases, accepting individuals from other cultures, developing and implementing nontraditional interventions, altering standard routines to better understand the unique cultural needs of clients, and acknowledging and refuting oppression when it is identified. Measuring cultural competence will be an ongoing process.

References

American Occupational Therapy Association. (2014). Occupational therapy practice framework: Domain and process (3rd ed.). *American Journal of Occupational Therapy, 68*(Suppl. 1), S1–S48. http://dx.doi.org/10.5014/ajot.2014.682006

Balcazar, F., Suarez-Balcazar, Y., & Taylor-Ritzler, T. (2009). Cultural competence: Development of a conceptual framework. *Disability and Rehabilitation, 31,* 1153–1160. http://dx.doi.org/10.1080/09638280902773752

Bonder, B. R., Martin, L., & Miracle, A. W. (2004). Culture emergent in occupation. *American Journal of Occupational Therapy, 58,* 159–168. http://dx.doi.org/10.5014/ajot.58.2.159

Calzada, E., & Suarez-Balcazar, Y. (2014). *Enhancing cultural competence in service agencies: A promising approach to serving diverse children and families.* Washington, DC: Department of Health and Human Services, Office of Planning, Research and Evaluation, Administration for Children and Families.

Campinha-Bacote, J. (1999). A model and instrument for addressing cultural competence in health care. *Journal of Nursing Education, 38(5),* 203–207. http://dx.doi.org/10.3928/0148-4834-19990501-06

Hasnain, R., Kondratowicz, D. M., Borokhovski, E., Nye, C., Balcazar, F., Portillo, N., . . . Gould, R. (2011). *Do cultural competency interventions work? A systematic review on improving rehabilitation outcomes for ethnically and linguistically diverse individuals with disabilities* (FOCUS: Technical Brief No. 31). Retrieved from http://ktdrr.org/ktlibrary/articles_pubs/ncddrwork/focus/focus31/Focus31.pdf

Kim, B., Cartwright, B., Asay, P., & D'Andrea, M. (2003). A revision of the Multicultural Awareness, Knowledge, and Skills Survey—Counselor edition. *Measurement and Evaluation in Counseling and Development, 36*(3), 161–180.

Sawyer, L., Regev, H., Proctor, S., Nelson, M., Messias, D., Barnes, D., & Meleis, A. I. (1995). Matching versus cultural competence in research: Methodological considerations. *Research in Nursing and Health, 18*(6), 557–567. http://dx.doi.org/10.1002/nur.4770180611

Sodowsky, G. R. (1996). The Multicultural Counseling Inventory: Validity and application in multicultural training. In G. R. Sodowsky & J. Impara (Eds.), *Multicultural assessment in counseling and clinical psychology* (pp. 283–324). Lincoln, NE: Buros Institute of Mental Measurements.

Suarez-Balcazar, Y., Balcazar, F., Taylor-Ritzler, T., Portillo, N., Rodakowski, J., Garcia-Ramirez, M., & Willis, C. (2011). Development and validation of a cultural competence assessment instrument: A factorial analysis. *Journal of Rehabilitation, 77*(1), 4–13.

Suarez-Balcazar, Y., Balcazar, F., & Willis, C. (2012). Cultural considerations in MS rehabilitation. In M. Finlayson (Ed.), *MS rehabilitation* (pp. 527–548). Boca Raton, FL: Taylor & Francis.

Suarez-Balcazar, Y., Muñoz, J., & Fisher, G. (2006). Building culturally competent community–university partnerships for occupational therapy scholarship. In G. Kielhofner (Ed.), *Scholarship in occupational therapy: Methods of inquiry for enhancing practice* (pp. 632–642). Philadelphia: F. A. Davis.

Suarez-Balcazar, Y., & Rodakowski, J. (2007). Becoming a culturally competent occupational therapy practitioner. *OT Practice, 12*(17), 14–17.

Suarez-Balcazar Y., Rodakowski, J., Balcazar, F., Taylor-Ritzler, T., Portillo, N., Barwacz, D., & Willis, C. (2009). Perceived levels of cultural competence among occupational therapists. *American Journal of Occupational Therapy, 63,* 498–505. http://dx.doi.org/10.5014/ajot.63.4.498

Sue, D. W., Carter, R. T., Casas, J. M., Fouad, N. A., Ivey, A. E., Jensen, M., . . . Vasquez-Nutall, E. (1998). *Multicultural counseling competencies: Individual and organizational development.* Thousand Oaks, CA: Sage.

U.S. Department of Health and Human Services, Office of Minority Health. (2011). *CLAS and the CLAS Standards.* Retrieved from https://www.thinkculturalhealth.hhs.gov /Content/clas.asp

Wells, S. A., & Black, R. M. (2000). *Cultural competency for health professionals.* Bethesda, MD: American Occupational Therapy Association.

Appendix 32.A. Cultural Competence Assessment Instrument

Awareness/Knowledge Domain

1. I openly discuss with others issues I have in developing multicultural awareness.
2. I learn about different ethnic cultures through educational methods and/or life experiences.
3. I examine my own biases related to race and culture that may influence my behavior as a service provider.
4. I actively strive for an atmosphere that promotes risk-taking and self-exploration.
5. I am sensitive to valuing and respecting differences between my cultural background and my clients' cultural heritage.
6. I feel that I can learn from my ethnic-minority clients.
7. It is difficult for me to accept that religious beliefs may influence how ethnic minorities respond to illness and disability.
8. I consider the cultural backgrounds of my clients when food is involved.

Skills Domain

9. I have opportunities to learn culturally responsive behaviors from peers.
10. I am effective in my verbal communication with clients whose culture is different from mine.
11. I am effective in my nonverbal communication with clients whose culture is different from mine.
12. I would find it easy to work competently with ethnic-minority clients.
13. I feel that I have limited experience working with ethnic-minority clients.
14. It is difficult to practice skills related to cultural competence.
15. I feel confident that I can learn about my clients' cultural background.
16. It is hard adjusting my therapeutic strategies with ethnic-minority clients.
17. I do not feel that I have the skills to provide services to ethnic-minority clients.

Organizational Support Domain

18. Cultural competence is included in my work place's mission statement, policies, and procedures.
19. My organization provides ongoing training on cultural competence.
20. My workplace supports using resources to promote cultural competence.
21. My workplace supports my participation in cultural celebrations of my clients.
22. At work, pictures, posters, printed materials, and toys reflect the culture and ethnic backgrounds of ethnic-minority clients.
23. I receive feedback from supervisors on how to improve my practice skills with clients from different ethnic-minority backgrounds.
24. The way services are structured in my setting makes it difficult to identify the cultural values of my clients.

Chapter 33.

EVIDENCE SUPPORTING CULTURAL EFFECTIVENESS

Roxie M. Black, PhD, OTR/L, FAOTA; Shirley A. Wells, DrPH, OTR, FAOTA; and Jyothi Gupta, PhD, OTR/L, FAOTA

Chapter Highlights

- Evidence Base of Cultural Effectiveness in Education
- Evidence Base of Cultural Effectiveness in Practice
- Evidence Base of Cultural Effectiveness in Research

Key Terms and Concepts

✧ Community-based participatory research
✧ Critical incidents
✧ Cultural adaptation of intervention
✧ Cultural competency training

✧ Cultural humility
✧ Culturally effective research
✧ Ethnography
✧ Intercultural communication

When the first edition of this book, *Cultural Competency for Health Professionals,* was published in 2000 (Wells & Black, 2000), there was very little, if any, evidence of the effectiveness of cultural competence in occupational therapy practice. Furthermore, the profession of occupational therapy was just beginning to address the importance of evidence-based practice and in 1999 had established the Evidence-Based Forum as a regular column in the *American Journal of Occupational Therapy* (Bailey, Bornstein, & Ryan, 2007).

Because the editors of this book have introduced and defined the concept of *cultural effectiveness* within this book, there was not yet been any

research that can provide evidence for this practice concept. However, in the past 15 years, numerous research studies have examined the effectiveness of aspects of cultural competence. Because the notion of *culturally effective care* has been developed on a foundation of cultural competence, which includes the concepts of cultural *self-awareness and attitudes, cultural knowledge,* and *cultural skills,* this chapter examines evidence available on those concepts as well as that of cross-cultural interactions and critical reflection. The chapter is divided into the three foci of this text—education, practice, and research—with examples of the latest evidence available within each area.

Evidence Base of Cultural Effectiveness in Education

The *Standards of Practice for Occupational Therapy* (American Occupational Therapy Association [AOTA], 2015) and many other occupational therapy documents identify the need of occupational therapy practitioners to understand the culture of their clients in order to provide effective care. As a result, many occupational therapy education programs are including content on culture, diversity, and cultural competence, and some are examining the results of cultural competence through research. However, much of the evidence of the impact of cultural competence and its components is found in disciplines other than occupational therapy.

Current Evidence

Several current studies do indicate that diversity training improves health professionals' culturally competent behaviors, especially in the areas of cultural awareness, openness, and sensitivity (Caplan & Black, 2014; Noble, Nuszen, Rom, & Noble, 2013; Sanner, Baldwin, Cannella, Charles, & Parker, 2010) on culturally competent skill behaviors such as communication (Beck, Scheel, De Oliveira, & Hopp, 2013; Kratzke & Bertolo, 2013; Schim, Doorenbos, & Borse, 2005; Smith, 2001) and patient adherence (May & Potia, 2013). One study found that cultural immersion and culture classes resulted in a greater sense of student self- and transcultural efficacy (Larsen & Reif, 2011), whereas other programs resulted in students' increase in self-confidence in their clinical skills (Comer, Whichello, & Neubrander, 2013; Matteliano & Stone, 2014).

However, some research indicates that some training programs do not result in positive movement toward cultural competence, and gaps in knowledge and culturally competent behavior still exist (Seeleman et al., 2014). Flores, Gee, and Kastner (2000) found that medical schools in the United States and Canada "provide inadequate instruction about cultural issues, especially the specific cultural aspects of large minority groups" (p. 451). Most of the studies examined indicated a need for further research.

There have been concerns about the rigor of studies about cultural competence. Price and colleagues (2005) conducted a systematic review to examine the methodological rigor of 64 studies

evaluating cultural competence training of health professionals. The authors found a lack of methodological rigor in most of the studies and concluded that the findings limit "the evidence for the impact of cultural competence training on minority health care quality. More attention should be paid to the proper design, evaluation, and reporting of these training programs" (p. 578). Table 33.1 provides research evidence for specific topics in cultural competence.

Future Considerations in Education

Most of the studies that examine the efficacy of teaching about culture, diversity, and the characteristics of cultural competence indicate the need for further research and a systematic approach to educational programming. Although occupational therapy education programs may deliver content on culture within their curricula, each program does this in a unique and individual manner. Nochajski and Matteliano (2008) attempted to address this issue by developing "A Guide to Cultural Competence in the Curriculum," which focuses on the "integration of cultural competency into existing courses, rather than creation of new courses" (p. i) and provides multiple objectives and activities. This very useful and comprehensive document is a step in the right direction, but it addresses only one of the multiple ways cultural content can be delivered to students.

Because of the uniqueness of each occupational therapy academic program, one approach to help students become culturally competent or culturally effective is not the answer. "One size does not fit all" in this case. Yet, educating occupational therapy practitioners to be culturally effective is vital in our global environments. In addition to engaging in more research that provides evidence of the effectiveness of the educational strategies currently being used, we must have ways for faculty to communicate with others who are engaged in this work. One approach may include having occupational therapy programs and faculty share, exchange, and store ideas, strategies, curricula, research, and publications regarding culturally effective education and care. The better we communicate with others who are engaged in developing and teaching cultural curricula, the more effective the occupational therapy workforce will be.

Table 33.1. Research Evidence on Educating for Cultural Competence

Topic	Studies/Link
Cultural awareness	Caplan & Black (2014) http://bit.ly/2a8DD88
	Noble, Nuszen, Rom, & Noble (2013) http://bit.ly/2aiOoW1
	Sanner, Baldwin, Cannella, Charles, & Parker (2010) http://bit.ly/2a4MOWS
Cultural safety	Arieli, Friedman, & Hirschfeld (2012) http://bit.ly/2a4MzLA
	Gerlach (2012) http://bit.ly/2a3OEUH
	Gray & McPherson (2004) http://bit.ly/1UpIVbO
	Jull & Giles (2012) http://bit.ly/2ahaeYP
	Whiteford (1995) http://bit.ly/2a8ZEo9
Culturally competent skills	Beck, Scheel, De Oliveira, & Hopp (2013) http://bit.ly/2alZM1L
	Kratzke & Bertolo (2013) http://bit.ly/29SuwtD
	Schim, Doorenbos, & Borse (2005) http://bit.ly/2a1gOBR
	Smith (2001) http://bit.ly/2aD4k3j
Student self-efficacy and confidence	Comer, Whichello, & Neubrander (2013) http://bit.ly/2bUyOz4
	Larsen & Reif (2011) http://bit.ly/2aD4lE6
	Matteliano & Stone (2014) http://bit.ly/2a8EMge
Rigor of current studies	Flores, Gee, & Kastner (2000) http://bit.ly/2akpW8q
	Price et al. (2005) http://bit.ly/2ahbSJV
	Seeleman et al. (2014) http://bit.ly/29Wky5W
Reflection	Lie, Shapiro, Cohn, & Najm (2010) http://bit.ly/2a92Dgo
	Paterson & Chapman (2013) http://bit.ly/29WkUJR

Evidence Base of Cultural Effectiveness in Practice

With the goal of providing "effective, equitable, understandable and respectful quality care and services that are responsive to diverse cultural health beliefs and practices, preferred language, health literacy and other communication needs" (U.S. Department of Health and Human Services, Office of Minority Health, 2015, Principal Standard 1), cultural competence has been linked to effective health care delivery. As a tool, cultural competence has highlighted the complexity of interacting with diverse populations, such as health care publishers and practitioners conflating culture with race and ethnicity and failing to capture the diversity within groups (DeLilly, 2012; Rajaram & Bockrath, 2014; Thackrah & Thompson, 2013).

Table 33.2. Research Evidence on Health Outcomes

Topic	Study/Link
Cultural competency training/ programs	Lie, Lee-Ray, Gomez, Bereknyei, & Braddock (2010) http://bit.ly/2aD9iwZ
	Pooremamali, Persson, & Eklund (2011) http://bit.ly/29SB37t
	Renzaho, Romios, Crock, & Sønderlund (2013) http://bit.ly/2amaAwX
	Smith, Cornella, & Williams (2014) http://bit.ly/2a1nCPF
	Truong, Paradies, & Priest (2014) http://bit.ly/2aiZ1rU
Culturally targeted/adapted intervention	Attridge, Creamer, Ramsden, Cannings-John, & Hawthorne (2014) http://bit.ly/2aoFrfl
	Bailey et al. (2009) http://bit.ly/2a6oPEw
	Kim & Park (2015) http://bit.ly/2a3YGFn
	Nierkens et al. (2013) http://bit.ly/2akyDQa
	Stedman & Thomas (2011) http://bit.ly/2a3ZlGZ
	Suarez-Balcazar, Friesema, & Lukyanova (2013) http://bit.ly/29VSgJz
	Ulrey & Amason (2001) http://bit.ly/2aj0FcX
	Vesely, Ewaida, & Anderson (2014) http://bit.ly/2a403nl

An abundance of literature details the ability of individual providers and institutions to integrate cultural competence into health care delivery, but few empirical studies exist that demonstrate competence actually improves patient health outcomes (Renzaho, Romios, Crock, & Sønderlund, 2013; Truong, Paradies, & Priest, 2014). The target of this evidence-based review is to look at existing studies that focused on cultural competency aimed at patient/client-related outcomes (Table 33.2).

Cultural Competency Training

Cultural competency (CC) training is used as a way to improve patient outcomes. Training has ranged from workshops or programs for health providers, culturally specific education or programs, interpreter services, peer education, patient navigators, and exchange programs (Truong et al., 2014). The effectiveness of these training programs on client/patient outcomes has been measured in various ways, such as physiological changes, increased knowledge of the health condition, patients' behavior changes such as exercises or dietary changes, and patient satisfaction and trust.

Patient-focused interventions have also been used to assess CC training programs and activities. Lie, Lee-Ray, Gomez, Bereknyei, and Braddock (2010) conducted a systemic review of the effects of CC training on patient-centered outcomes. Of the seven studies they examined, the patient outcome assessed ranged from self-reported satisfaction, provider communication, and clinical measures to environmental changes. Lie and colleagues determined that a positive relationship between CC training and patient outcome is inconclusive because the patient factors were not adequately accounted for or consistently reported. They concluded that CC training alone is inadequate to improve patient outcomes but is a trend in the direction of a positive impact.

Renzaho and colleagues' (2013) systematic review examined the effectiveness of patient-centered models that incorporated a CC perspective. They found no evidence of any significant findings in terms of patient health outcomes.

Smith, Cornella, and Williams (2014) investigated the perspectives of 14 occupational therapy students who were provided opportunities to develop cultural awareness and competence through a fieldwork experience working with people of refugee background. They determined that this type of CC training could optimize patient outcomes along with occupation-based and client-centered practice.

A study by Pooremamali, Persson, and Eklund (2011) explored how 8 occupational therapists coped with their feelings and thoughts when working with immigrant psychiatric clients from the Middle East region. Having no prior CC training caused the therapists frustration and uncertainty about their abilities and skills to help their clients and contribute to changes in their lives. Their findings revealed a need for CC knowledge and training for the therapists to become culturally competent, build cultural bridges, choose culturally adapted techniques, and construct communication with their immigrant clients.

Further research on CC training and its effect on patient health outcomes needs to address the provider, patient, and the educational training or curriculum to demonstrate how such training affects patient outcomes and health disparities (Lie, Lee-Ray, et al., 2010). Research should examine the limitation of previous studies, such as lack of control groups, the variability of health outcome measures, and the patient–provider relationship (Nierkens et al., 2013).

Renzaho and colleagues (2013) found that it was difficult to generalize the effectiveness of CC training for patient or client outcomes because there is no uniform definition or framework of *cultural competence,* the many potential outcomes from CC training, and the lack of methodological rigor in conducting CC studies. Truong and colleagues (2014) concluded that further research was required to determine what types of training were most effective in relation to particular outcomes as well as the long-term outcomes of CC programs.

Despite the weak evidence and paucity of literature for improvements in patient or client outcomes, data have been found that support the effectiveness of CC training in increasing patient satisfaction, health care access, and utilization.

Cultural Intervention Effectiveness

Cultural adaptation of intervention and service is another area used to evaluate the effectiveness of cultural competence on patient or client outcomes. To reduce health disparities, health providers need to deliver culturally competent health care that "focus[es] on risk reduction, vulnerability reduction, and promotion and protection of human rights" (Flaskerud, 2007, p. 432). The literature acknowledges the importance of modifying practice and interventions for culture as a way to increase the appropriateness of services delivered to clients of diverse cultural backgrounds and to achieve equity in outcomes (Dong, Chang, Wong, & Simon, 2013; Nierkens et al., 2013; Stedman & Thomas, 2011; Suarez-Balcazar, Friesema, & Lukyanova, 2013). Cultural adaptation occurs when an intervention or program's design, delivery, and evaluation incorporates the targeted population ethnic or cultural characteristics, values, behavioral patterns, and beliefs as well as relevant environmental and social forces (Nierkens et al., 2013).

In their study of Indigenous clients in North Queensland, Australia, Stedman and Thomas (2011) explored 7 occupational therapists' views of effectiveness on modifying their intervention with elderly Indigenous clients. The therapists indicated that to practice in culturally safe ways requires some effort of intervention modification. The findings indicate that intervention modifications need to be mindful of the culture and its impact on interventions and occupational performance as well as the impact of the sociocultural and physical environments. The results also highlight the importance of reflection to inform views of effectiveness and evaluation of practice.

Suarez-Balcazar and colleagues (2013) conducted a systematic review of culturally competent strategies for addressing and preventing obesity among African American and Latino children and youth. Based on the analysis, they found that intervention strategies considered to be important and effective were related to the health professionals' cognitive and behavioral level of cultural competence and the incorporation of culture by the sponsoring organization. Health care providers' cultural awareness and knowledge, along with skills in communicating, developing a relationship, and delivering the program, were imperative in meeting the needs of these populations. Suarez-Balcazar and colleagues concluded that culturally competent interventions hold "promise for improving the delivery and effectiveness of obesity prevention targeting ethnically/racially diverse populations" (p. 116). Cultural relevance of health intervention was also found to be critical when providing services to Chinese older adults (Dong, Chang, Wong, & Simon, 2013).

Intercultural communication styles have also been mentioned as affecting intervention effectiveness and improving client health outcomes. Ulrey and Amason (2001) found a relationship among cultural sensitivity, effective intercultural communication, and anxiety of health care providers. Health care providers who perceive themselves as high in cultural sensitivity or effective at intercultural communication reported experiencing less anxiety in intercultural situations. Ulrey and Amason concluded that by enhancing and increasing cultural sensitivity and intercultural communication skills, providers not only can help their patients but also can ease their own anxiety and job stress when dealing with patients from other cultures.

Kim and Park's (2015) study of cultural adaptation and counseling effectiveness with Asian Americans indicated that Asian Americans viewed culturally incongruent communication (i.e., direct) style as more satisfying and more credible than congruent (i.e., indirect) communication. These styles' effectiveness depends on a participant's adherence to traditional cultural values. Direct communication style and maintenance of harmony may serve the purpose of protecting an Asian American client from embarrassment in counseling. They recommended that counselors should be flexible in how they communicate with Asian American clients based on the cultural differences among the individuals and their cultural backgrounds.

A growing body of literature is revealing that culturally targeted and adapted interventions have greater effects than traditional treatments (Walsh, 2003). Programs reflecting only Westernized models without taking into account cultural variables may compromise patient or client outcomes (Calzada, 2010).

Vesely, Ewaida, and Anderson (2014) examined the effectiveness of 13 parenting education programs used by Latino families. Many of the programs recognized and incorporated Latino cultural values and beliefs and experiences. All of the programs in the study had educators who spoke Spanish when working with the parents, provided translated materials, and had incorporated cultural knowledge. However, none of the programs enacted a continuous process of evaluation to assess the health outcomes.

Additionally, a review by Attridge and colleagues (2014) concluded that culturally appropriate health education has short-to-medium effects on blood sugar

control and on knowledge of diabetes and healthy lifestyles for people from ethnic-minority groups with Type 2 diabetes mellitus at 12 and 24 months after the intervention. Cultural health education could lead to clinically important health outcomes if sustained.

In terms of behavior changes, Bailey and colleagues (2009) found that culturally specific programs for adults and children from minority groups who have asthma are more effective than generic programs in improving knowledge, quality of life, and control but not in all asthma outcomes. In a review by Nierkens and colleagues (2013), culturally targeted behavioral interventions were found to be more effective if cultural adaptations such as using pictures of the targeted population, using language-specific material, and incorporating family and religious values are implemented as a package of adaptations (multiple levels).

Nierkens and colleagues reviewed 17 studies that targeted smoking cessation, diet, and physical activity among adults from ethnic minorities in the United States. The results indicated that effective cultural interventions should address family influences, health literacy, and characteristics such self-identity and cultural values. Programs designed to promote positive racial group identity may aid in the reduction of health disparities and improvement of health (Chae, Lincoln, Adler, & Syme, 2010; Delilly, 2012).

Future Considerations for Practice

Recognizing the power and influence of culture on patient or client outcome is needed not only to promote inclusion and equality but also to improve trust and cooperation between providers and consumers. Because CC training aims to improve health care quality, it can lead to increased knowledge and awareness, decreased anxiety and stress when interacting with patients or clients from diverse cultures, and improved communication. Yet, there is inadequate evidence that this translates to improved patient or client outcome.

There is no uniform definition or framework of cultural competence that is accepted across the health spectrum and literature, although there are several measures used to assess cultural competence. Most CC training and programs measure effectiveness in terms of the practitioner's knowledge and behavior and not patient or client health. More research is needed to examine the impact of, as well as complexities in, translating CC training and programs into health outcomes. Researchers should measure cultural competence as part of their efforts to deliver high-quality care.

Although there is evidence that culturally targeted and adapted intervention can improve patient or client outcomes, the existing body of literature is limited and lacks consensus on measuring outcomes. Future research is needed to define exactly what culturally targeted or adapted intervention is and to determine which types of interventions are most effective for whom, in what context, and why.

Multilevel interventions should also be considered. The process of developing cultural targeted intervention, the way the intervention is executed, the types of determinants addressed, and the environmental levels addressed by the intervention are all factors that should be examined. Insight into these characteristics will contribute to the effectiveness of an intervention.

Whether practice or research driven, culturally adapted interventions should not undermine the core components and effectiveness of the intervention. Thus, culturally adapted interventions should not be taken lightly but instead be responsive to and used to support improved health outcomes for people from culturally diverse backgrounds.

Evidence Base of Cultural Effectiveness in Research

Despite theoretical articulations on the importance of client centeredness (Gupta & Taff, 2015; Hammell, 2013a) and context, including space and place (Law et al., 1996; Rowles, 1991), research with diverse cultural groups, either in or out of their natural contexts, is sparse in occupational therapy literature. Increasing diversity coupled with increasing health inequities creates an urgency for culturally effective research (CER) in occupational therapy. Clients who are not from the dominant Western culture hold different values and beliefs about occupational choices and behaviors. Understanding these behaviors in context is necessary to develop client-centered and culturally effective assessments and interventions.

Culturally effective research "takes into account the culture and diversity of a population when developing research ideas, conducting research, and exploring applicability of research findings" (Harvard Catalyst, 2010, p. 6). In CER, close attention is given to the entire research process from conceptualization to implementation: the study design, recruitment, outreach, culturally congruent methods of data collection and analysis, and interpretation of findings (Harvard Catalyst, 2010).

Occupational Therapy and Race

The occupational therapy profession was started by White middle-class women—a group that is the majority group of the profession today. It was not until the early to mid-1990s that serious efforts were made regarding diversity initiatives within the profession (Black, 2002). In an editorial, Hasselkus (2002) stated that researchers who cite race as a variable in their study must provide justification of its relevance to the study and cautioned against using race as a proxy for sociocultural variables. The latter point is critical for occupational therapy research because often rehabilitation is focused on changing individual behaviors that may be analyzed without situating these behaviors in the larger sociocultural and sociopolitical contexts (Gupta & Taff, 2015).

Although other professional organizations such as the American Public Health Association (2001) and the American Anthropological Association (1998) have articulated their stance on race, AOTA has not done so. Cena, McGruder, and Tomlin (2002) noted the blatant inconsistencies in the manner in which race, ethnicity, and social class were documented in articles in the *American Journal of Occupational Therapy*, the flagship journal of the profession, which that makes it difficult to synthesize the literature across studies. A solution they proposed was to identify documentation standards to capture the data in the professional body of literature.

This may not be necessary; as Breland and Ellis (2012) noted, the absence of race and ethnicity as variables in research studies suggested that authors consistently follow the American Psychological Association (APA) guidelines that consider race and ethnicity as "minimum adequate reporting standard" (Breland and Ellis, 2012, p. 116). Guideline 1 for reducing bias in research and reporting results includes precision or *specificity;* for example, describing participants as Chinese Americans is far more precise than saying Asian Americans because the latter is not specific, referring to an entire continent with many nations. Guideline 2 is for sensitivity in describing people of different race and ethnicity and not using labels that objectify people.

Person-first language promoted in occupational therapy education is a good example, for instance, referring to clients as "individuals with schizophrenia" and not "schizophrenics" (APA, 2010).

Researcher Motivation and Point of View

Engaging in CER starts with the motivation of the researcher for doing research with particular diverse groups. Ideally, a researcher is motivated to gain deeper perspective and understanding of the phenomenon being studied in particular cultural contexts (Lee & Zaharlick, 2013). For occupational therapy, the core phenomenon of interest is occupation: its performance as a means to social participation. The *etic* or outsider perspective encompasses an external view on a culture, language, meaning associations, and real-world events, in contrast to the *emic* or insider perspective that is the internal view from within the culture (Olive, 2014). This is relevant because most researchers often are cultural outsiders, and by adopting a purely etic perspective or approach to a study, they risk overlooking the hidden, nuanced meanings and concepts within a culture that can be gleaned only through in-depth interviews, repeated observations, and interpretations of the findings from cultural insiders.

CER is possible with paradigms in which researchers view cultural groups as the experts of their daily lives and occupations; in other words, researchers consider the emic perspective alongside the etic perspective (Wahyuni, 2012). Additionally, researchers adopt a stance of **cultural humility,** seeing themselves not as experts but as learners who are open to collaborating with participants as co-researchers.

Immersion in Cultural Context

It is imperative that research be conducted in the actual context of occupational enactment, because cultural contexts influence meanings, motivations, and occupational behaviors. By doing so, the researcher is also immersed in the cultural milieu, gathers "data" in context, and is able to witness cultural behaviors unfolding in the dynamics of the transactional interplay between the Person–Environment–Occupation in the cultural context. Immersion in the cultural context allows for repeat observations of occupational behaviors over long periods of time, thus enhancing

the validity and clarity of the researcher's understanding of the behavior(s) under study. Critical to CER is the researcher's competency in culture-specific knowledge, use of culturally appropriate methods, and culturally sensitive interpretations of findings.

Cultural proficiency is a prerequisite to be culturally effective in conducting research with diverse groups. Participants are collaborators with researchers in CER as they are the experts of their cultural and occupational lives and can best explain the nuanced understanding of the transactional relationship among culture, occupations, and self.

Research Methods

Qualitative research methods appear to be better suited to capture the sociocultural lived experience and reality of daily occupations because they aim to understand complex human behaviors and life experiences from the perspectives of the study participants' lived experiences (Creswell, 2013). Moreover, qualitative data analysis is a powerful tool to understand seemingly mundane human experiences of everyday life (Becker, 1996), which, after all, is the focus of occupational therapy.

Narrating one's occupational life experiences is a qualitative data inquiry that resonates with many populations. In a study on new immigrants from non-Western countries, the authors found that participants reported difficulties in completing self-reported surveys and assessments that used simple scales (Gupta, Sullivan, Schwirtz, & Garber, 2011). *Ethnography* is a qualitative research method traditionally used to study people and culture in their natural setting. Lee and Zaharlick (2013) discussed the compatibility of ethnography as an overarching meta-framework for conducting culturally competent research. In ethnography, the researcher typically is immersed in the community being researched over a long period of time, collecting data by repeated observations, systematic and detailed note-taking, questioning participants, and examining other cultural artifacts.

Best Practices for Culturally Effective Research

Knowing the culture well and interpreting the findings through a cultural lens are critical for cultural effectiveness. Figure 33.1 shows interacting

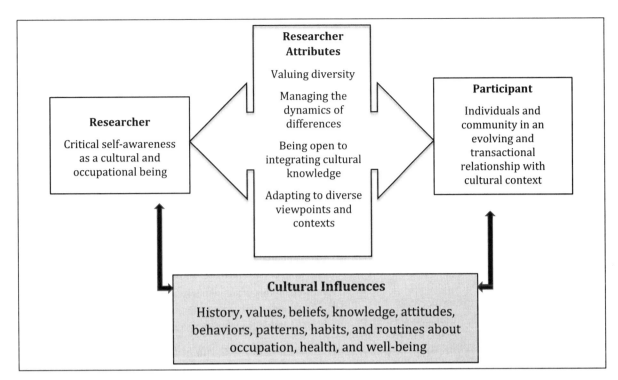

Figure 33.1.   A framework depicting the interacting concepts inherent in culturally effective research (CER).
Note. The model shows CER requires (1) the researcher be self-aware of his or her cultural identity that is influenced by both personal and professional cultures (shaded box); (2) the study participant is a cultural entity; and (3) both the researcher and the cultural community are influenced by their cultural history, values, beliefs, and such as shown in the shaded box. The researcher must value diversity and have skills to manage cross-cultural dynamics.

elements that are aspects of best practices for CER. In this framework, a researcher's understanding of self as a cultural and occupational being is important; furthermore, he or she understands that participants' occupational ways of doing, being, becoming, and belonging are in a dynamic and transactional relationship with their cultural context. Researchers commit to be culturally effective, value diversity, adapt to different cultural contexts, and open to differences in the understanding and interpretations of the phenomenon under study (Lee & Zaharlick, 2013).

Critical Cultural Self-Awareness

When researchers are cultural "outsiders," acquisition of cultural knowledge—histories, customs, beliefs, traditions, and practices—is necessary for effective cross-cultural communication and interpretation of data. Researchers are cautioned from interpreting findings from an outsider perspective to avoid

misrepresenting the results of the study (Fassinger & Morrow, 2013; Lee & Zaharlick, 2013).

Cultural humility is necessary for conducting CER because it requires researchers to acknowledge their position of power and be cognizant that their assumptions, beliefs, values, biases, and worldviews may be different, may not resonate, or may conflict with the cultural group of their study (Hammell, 2013b). The relevance and use of cultural safety while working with Indigenous populations is also recommended in occupational therapy literature (Gerlach, 2012).

Motivations for Research

Researchers should examine their own motivations for conducting research with a particular cultural group. The focus of research must be of value to the community being studied and not just an academic exercise. Fassinger and Morrow (2013) cautioned "outsider" researchers from dominant groups about conducting research with historically oppressed communities. Building trust and creating safe space needed for gaining deep and authentic insights from such communities may prove difficult because of issues of cultural safety.

Diverse Research Team

Having a diverse research team that includes cultural insiders and outsiders is helpful for effective recruitment of study participants, implementation, and critical data analysis. A few members of the research team members must be culturally and linguistically competent and genuinely interested in working with culturally diverse communities. Having team members who are from the cultural group, or are familiar with the culture and speak the language spoken by the participants, is helpful for building a relationship and trust with the community members so that the latter feel safe to be open in their conversations. A study of the caregiving experiences of Latino families that included bilingual and bicultural researchers on the team allowed for conducting interviews in the language preferred by participants, and perhaps these researchers were better able to navigate the cultural interface effectively as cultural insiders (Blanche, Diaz, Barretto, & Cermak, 2015).

Participatory Approaches

Including diverse participants in the study does not necessarily qualify the study as CER. An attitude of embracing study participants as research collaborators and engaging them in data analysis and interpretations of findings can provide researchers with authentic insights about the cultural influences on occupation. An approach such as **community-based participatory research** (CBPR) requires that community members be involved in all phases of the research process (Daley et al., 2010).

Moreover, studying a small subsection of a culture and overgeneralizing the findings for the entire cultural group must be avoided. Multiple perspectives and data triangulation are ways in which researchers can avoid misinterpreting results so rigor and validity of findings are ensured. Ideally, in CBPR, the researcher has an idea for study but enters the community with an open stance and is amenable to the focus of research to evolve based on participants' expressed interests, needs, and concerns of the community.

Cultural Mentors and Advisors

Using cultural advisors or a community advisory board can help researchers use culturally effective practices throughout the research process. Such community leaders can also serve as liaisons for recruitment purposes. Having a culturally diverse research team that includes cultural mentors and advisors from the community and being flexible and open to their feedback aids CER (Mohammadi, Jones, & Evans, 2008; Paskett et al., 2008; Reid & Chiu, 2011). Particularly for researchers who are cultural outsiders, having a consumer advisory board with members from the cultural group can "provide valuable insight regarding effective and efficient strategies for recruitment, retention, and intervention delivery" (Pyatak et al., 2013, p. 1197).

Diverse Methodological Competencies

Familiarity with quantitative, qualitative, and mixed-methods research and knowledge of core principles of CBPR (Israel et al., 2003) are optimal for CER. The knowledge allows the researcher flexibility in the choice of research design and methods that best fit with the cultural group or community and most suited to understanding the construct or phenomenon being investigated. Researchers should avoid using traditional methods, protocols, and instruments that have been developed using the majority cultural group as the normative group when studying another cultural group.

In a study with South Asian and Chinese mothers, Reid and Chiu (2011) cautioned researchers to be mindful that most research methods and instruments have been developed based on Western values and may be incongruent with certain cultural groups. They recommended using a culturally sensitive recruitment process, a research design that includes more interviews and focus groups, and culturally appropriate instruments.

Flexibility

Conducting research in any community involves the researcher contending with the real-life context of the study participants, which may pose challenges for the study. Particularly for populations from the low socioeconomic strata, many factors have serious impact on the integrity of the research study and must be considered in the study design and implementation. Some factors that have been identified include unstable living situations, which may result in unstable contact information that may affect retention; limited material and social resources that may affect consistent participation; criminal behaviors and subsequent incarceration; and conflicting personal and family goals (Pyatak et al., 2013).

Critical Reflexivity

Engaging in ongoing critical reflection has been suggested (Reid & Chiu, 2011). Creswell (2013) encouraged qualitative researchers to view themselves as instruments of research and to record and report their own biases, feelings, and thoughts as part of the research findings. Modifying practice through the use of a self-reflection tool has been suggested for working with Indigenous groups (Stedman & Thomas, 2011). Similarly, researchers are advised to engage in critical ongoing reflections throughout the research process (Thomas, Gray, McGinty, & Ebringer, 2011).

Addressing Power

Researchers are a product of the disciplinary or professional culture that influences their research paradigms. Simply put, a paradigm is the worldview that includes beliefs, assumptions, choice of methods, and criteria for rigor that have been accepted by the disciplinary community of scholars as a legitimate way of building knowledge (Denzin & Lincoln, 2011).

Despite the deeply held conviction of client-centered practice, occupational therapy research has not consistently been a collaborative endeavor, and the research agenda has often been driven by the researchers (Hammell, 2013a). Occupation and empowerment, rampant in the profession's discourse, triggered critical incidents for researchers working with Indigenous groups (Thomas et al., 2011). ***Critical incidents*** are cross-cultural situations in which researchers become aware of differences in communication and language and may be challenged to reexamine the beliefs and assumptions they have taken for granted. *Occupations* are the foundation of occupational therapy, and to practitioners they are goal-directed activities that people engage in their daily lives to take care of themselves and their families, fulfill roles and responsibilities, and a vehicle for social participation. However, to the Indigenous participants, *occupation* is associated with dispossession of their lands and loss of their cultural identity (Thomas et al., 2011).

Use of empowerment within the profession has been challenged by scholars such as Hammell (2013a, 2015), who contends that the use of empowerment implies the presumed power of the professional who, through interventions, can give power to clients who seek their services.

Future Consideration for Research

As the critical mass of scholars and researchers grows in the profession, it will benefit the professional community if best practices for CER are routinely incorporated in studies to obtain valid results. Deliberate efforts to recruit diverse participants that mirror the demographics of our society will make the research more applicable and relevant to a broad range of clients. CER is the way to develop culturally effective assessments and interventions to address occupational and health inequities.

Research with diverse populations and, particularly with historically marginalized and oppressed groups, is necessary for the profession. Research in non-dominant cultural communities requires researchers to approach participants from a culturally humble stance. Having representatives of the cultural group on the research team is helpful for build trust and rapport. Researchers also need to examine their own motivations for conducting research with cultural groups to become self-aware of themselves as cultural beings, to acknowledge their own biases and assumptions, and to exercise caution in interpreting findings from an outsider perspective.

Summary

As the editors of this book have noted, there are few empirical studies to help practitioners answer the question "Is it possible to deliver culturally effective care?" in the affirmative. Many educators, practitioners, and researchers have turned to cultural-effectiveness programs to present practitioners with a general approach to caring for patients or client and their families. Because of the uniqueness of each occupational therapy academic program, the better we engage in developing and teaching cultural curricula, the more effective the occupational therapy workforce will be. Giving students the clinical skills and tools to ask respectful questions and having opportunities to watch experienced clinicians model effective techniques are vital.

Most training programs have measured effectiveness in terms of the practitioner's knowledge and behavior instead of client health. The results of occupational therapy practitioners examining their practice and articulating culturally effective and adapted interventions would be improved quality of care, enhanced client satisfaction, better health outcomes, a stable and skilled workforce, and reduced health disparities. Having compelling occupational therapy evidence that measures cultural effectiveness would add to the delivery of high-quality care. Routinely incorporating cultural effectiveness to support and improve the rehabilitation outcomes of individuals with disabilities from diverse cultural and ethnic backgrounds would benefit the professional community. Delivering culturally effective care would also help reduce health disparities.

Research is needed to understand the multifaceted and multilayered processes and mechanisms through which education, practice, and research improve cultural effectiveness in the context of occupational therapy. The Model of Cultural Effectiveness presented in this book is just one important part of a broader occupational therapy response system that is continuously informed by structured feedback from literature, students, clinicians, clients, and the communities we serve.

References

American Anthropological Association. (1998). *American Anthropological Association's statement on "race."* Retrieved from http://www.americananthro.org/ConnectWithAAA/Content.aspx?ItemNumber=2583

American Occupational Therapy Association. (2015). Standards of practice for occupational therapy. *American Journal of Occupational Therapy, 69*(Suppl. 3), 913410057p1–6913410057p6. http://dx.doi.org/10.5014/ajot.2015.696S06

American Public Health Association. (2001). *Research and intervention on racism as a fundamental cause of ethnic disparities in health.* http://dx.doi.org/10.2105/AJPH.91.3.515

Arieli, D., Friedman V. J., & Hirschfeld, M. J. (2012). Challenges on the path to cultural safety in nursing education. *International Nursing Review 59*, 187–193. http://dx.doi.org/10.1111/j.1466-7657.2012.00982.x

Attridge, M., Creamer, J., Ramsden, M., Cannings-John, R., & Hawthorne, K. (2014). Culturally appropriate health education for people in ethnic minority groups with Type 2 diabetes mellitus. *Cochrane Database of Systematic Reviews 2014, 9,* CD006454. http://dx.doi.org/10.1002/14651858.CD006424.pub3

Bailey, D. M., Bornstein, J., & Ryan, S. (2007). A case report of evidence-based practice: From academia to clinic. *American Journal of Occupational Therapy, 61,* 85–91. http://dx.doi.org/10.5014/ajot.61.1.85

Bailey, E. J., Cates, C. J., Kruske, S. G., Morris, P. S., Brown, N., & Chang, A. B. (2009). Culture-specific programs for children and adults from minority groups who have asthma. *Cochrane Database of Systematic Reviews 2009, 2,* CD006580. http://dx.doi.org/10.1002/14651858.CD006580.pub4

Beck, B., Scheel, M. H., De Oliveira, K., & Hopp, J. (2013). Integrating cultural competency throughout a first-year physician assistant curriculum steadily improves cultural awareness. *Journal of Physician Assistant Education, 24*(2), 28–31.

Becker, H. S. (1996). The epistemology of qualitative research. In R. Jessor, A. Colby, & R. A. Shweder (Eds.), *Ethnography and human development: Context and meaning in social inquiry* (pp. 53–71). Chicago: University of Chicago Press.

Black, R. M. (2002). Occupational therapy's dance with diversity. *American Journal of Occupational Therapy, 56*(2), 140–148. http://dx.doi.org/10.5014/ajot.56.2.140

Blanche, E. I., Diaz, J., Barretto, T., & Cermak, S. A. (2015). Caregiving experiences of Latino families with children with autism spectrum disorder. *American Journal of Occupational Therapy, 69*(5), 6905185010p1–6905185010p11. http://dx.doi.org/10.5014/ajot.2015.017848

Breland, H. L., & Ellis, C. (2012). Is reporting race and ethnicity essential to occupational therapy evidence? *American Journal of Occupational Therapy, 66*(1), 115–119. http://dx.doi.org/10.5014/ajot.2012.002246

Calzada, E. J. (2010). Bringing culture into parent training with Latinos. *Cognitive and Behavioral Practice, 17,* 167–175. http://dx.doi.org/10.1016/j.cbpra.2010.01.003

Caplan, S., & Black, R. M. (2014). Evaluation of the cross-cultural health assessment as an interdisciplinary method of cultural competency education. *Journal of Nursing Education and Practice, 4*(4), 58–73. http://dx.doi.org/10.5430/jnep.v4n4p58

Cena, L., McGruder, J., & Tomlin, G. (2002). Representations of race, ethnicity, and social class in case examples in the American Journal of Occupational Therapy. *American Journal of Occupational Therapy, 56*(2), 130–139. http://dx.doi.org/10.5014/ajot.56.2.130

Chae, D. H., Lincoln, K. D., Adler, N. E., & Syme, S. L. (2010). Do experiences of racial discrimination predict cardiovascular disease among African American men? The moderating role of internalized negative racial group attitudes.

Social Science and Medicine, 7(6), 1182–1188. http://dx.doi.org/10.1016/j.socscimed.2010.05.045

Comer, L., Whichello, R., & Neubrander, J. (2013). An innovative master of science program for the development of culturally competent nursing leaders. *Journal of Cultural Diversity, 20*(2), 89–93.

Creswell, J. W. (2013). Research design: *Qualitative, quantitative, and mixed methods approaches.* Thousand Oaks, CA: Sage.

Daley, C. M., James, A. S., Ulrey, E., Joseph, S., Talawyma, A., Choi, W. S., . . . Coe, M. K. (2010). Using focus groups in community-based participatory research: Challenges and resolutions. *Qualitative Health Research, 20,* 697–706. http://dx.doi.org/10.1177/1049732310361468

DeLilly, C. R. (2012). Discrimination and health outcomes. *Issues in Mental Health Nursing, 33,* 801–804. http://dx.doi.org/10.3109/01612840.2012.671442

Denzin, N. K., & Lincoln, Y. S. (2011). *The Sage handbook of qualitative research.* Thousand Oaks, CA: Sage.

Dong, X., Chang, E. S., Wong, E., & Simon, M. (2013). Perceived effectiveness of elder abuse interventions in psychological distress and the design of culturally adapted interventions: A qualitative study in the Chinese community in Chicago. *Journal of Aging Research, 2013,* Article 845425. http://dx.doi.org/10.1155/2013/845425

Fassinger, R., & Morrow, S. (2013). Toward best practices in quantitative, qualitative, and mixed-method research: A social justice perspective. *Journal for Social Action in Counseling and Psychology, 5*(2), 69–83. Retrieved from http://psysr.org/jsacp/Fassinger-V5N2-13_69-83.pdf

Flaskerud, J. H. (2007). Cultural competence: What effect on reducing health disparities? *Issues in Mental Health Nursing, 28,* 431–434. http://dx.doi.org/10.1080/01612840701246628

Flores, G., Gee, D., & Kastner, B. (2000). The teaching of cultural issues in U.S. and Canadian medical schools. *Academic Medicine, 75*(5), 451–455. http://dx.doi.org/10.1097/00001888-200005000-00015

Gerlach, A. J. (2012). A critical reflection on the concept of cultural safety. *Canadian Journal of Occupational Therapy, 79*(3), 151–158. http://dx.doi.org/10.2182/cjot.2012.79.3.4

Gray, M., & McPherson, K. (2004). Cultural safety and professional practice in occupational therapy: A New Zealand perspective. *Australian Occupational Therapy Journal, 52,* 34–42. http://dx.doi.org/10.1111/j.1440-1630.2004.00433.x

Gupta, J., Sullivan, C., Schwirtz, T., & Garber, T. (2011, October). *Enhancing Participation and Health in New Immigrants: Translating Occupational Science into Occupational Therapy Practice.* Paper presented at the Annual Research Conference of the Society for the Study of Occupation, Park City, UT.

Gupta, J., & Taff, S. (2015). The illusion of client-centred practice. *Scandinavian Journal of Occupational Therapy, 4,*

244–251. http://dx.doi.org/10.3109/11038128.2015.1020866

Hammell, K. W. (2013a). Client-centred occupational therapy in Canada: Refocusing on core values. *Canadian Journal of Occupational Therapy, 80*(3), 141–149. http://dx.doi.org/10.1177/0008417413497906

Hammell, K. W. (2013b). Occupation, well-being, and culture: Theory and cultural humility. *Canadian Journal of Occupational Therapy, 80,* 224–234. http://dx.doi.org/10.1177/0008417413500465

Hammell, K. W. (2015). Client-centred occupational therapy: The importance of critical perspectives. *Scandinavian Journal of Occupational Therapy, 22*(4), 237–243. http://dx.doi.org/10.3109/11038128.2015.1004103

Hasselkus, B. R. (2002). The use of "race" in research. *American Journal of Occupational Therapy, 56*(2), 127–129. http://dx.doi.org/10.5014/ajot.56.2.127

Harvard Catalyst. (2010). *Cultural competence in research.* Retrieved from https://catalyst.harvard.edu/pdf/diversity/CCR-annotated-bibliography-10-12-10ver2-FINAL.pdf

Israel, B. A., Schulz, A. J., Parker, E. A., Becker, A. B., Allen, A. J., & Guzman, J. R. (2003). Critical issues in developing and following community based participatory research principles. In M. Minkler & N. Wallerstein (Eds.), *Community-based participatory research for health* (pp. 56–73). San Francisco: Jossey-Bass.

Jull, J. E. G., & Giles, A. R. (2012). Health equity, Aboriginal peoples and occupational therapy. *Canadian Journal of Occupational Therapy, 79,* 70–76. http://dx.doi.org/10.2182/cjot.2012.79.2.2

Kim, B., & Park, Y. S. (2015). Communication styles, cultural values, and counseling effectiveness with Asian Americans. *Journal of Counseling and Development, 93,* 269–279. http://dx.doi.org/10.1002/jcad.12025

Kratzke, C., & Bertolo, M. (2013). Enhancing students' cultural competence using cross-cultural experiential learning. *Journal of Cultural Diversity, 20*(3), 107–111.

Larsen, R., & Reif, L. (2011). Effectiveness of cultural immersion and cultural classes for enhancing nursing students transcultural self-efficacy. *Journal of Nursing Education, 50*(6), 350–354. http://dx.doi.org/10.3928/01484834-20110214-04

Law, M., Cooper, B., Strong, S., Stewart, D., Rigby, P., & Letts, L. (1996). The Person–Environment–Occupation model: A transactive approach to occupational performance. *Canadian Journal of Occupational Therapy, 63*(1), 9–23. http://dx.doi.org/10.1177/000841749606300103

Lee, M. Y., & Zaharlick, A. (2013). *Culturally competent research: Using ethnography as a meta-framework.* New York: Oxford University Press.

Lie, D. A., Lee-Ray, E., Gomez, A., Bereknyei, S., & Braddock, C., III. (2010). Does cultural competency training of health professionals improve patient outcomes? A systematic review and proposed algorithm for future research. *Journal of General Internal Medicine, 26*(3), 317–325. http://dx.doi .org/10.1007/s11606-010-1529-0

Lie, D., Shapiro, J., Cohn, F., & Najm, W. (2010). Reflective practice enriches clerkship students' cross-cultural experiences. *Journal of General Internal Medicine, 25*(Suppl. 2), S119–S125. http://dx.doi.org/10.1007/s11606-009-1205-4

Matteliano, M. A., & Stone, J. H. (2014). Cultural competence education in university rehabilitation programs. *Journal of Cultural Diversity, 21*(3), 112–118.

May, S., & Potia, T. A. (2013). An evaluation of cultural competency training on perceived patient adherence. *European Journal of Physiotherapy, 15*, 2–10. http://dx.doi.org/10.3109 /14038196.2012.760647

Mohammadi, N., Jones, T., & Evans, D. (2008). Participant recruitment from minority religious groups: The case of the Islamic population in South Australia. *International Nursing Review, 55*(4), 393–398. http://dx.doi.org/10.1111/j.1466 -7657.2008.00647.x

Olive, J. L. (2014). Reflecting on the tensions between emic and etic perspectives in life history research: Lessons learned. *Forum Qualitative Sozialforschung/Forum: Qualitative Social Research, 15*(2), Article 6. Retrieved from http://nbn-resolving .de/urn:nbn:de:0114-fqs140268

Nierkens, V., Hartman, M. A., Nicolaou, M., Vissenberg, C., Beune, E., Hosper, K., . . . Stronks, K. (2013). Effectiveness of cultural adaptations of interventions aimed at smoking cessation, diet, and/or physical activity in ethnic minorities: A systematic review. *PLOS One, 8*(10), e773373. http://dx .doi.org/10.1371/journal.pone.0073373

Noble, A., Nuszen, E., Rom, M., & Noble, L. M. (2013). The effect of a cultural competence educational intervention for first-year nursing students in Israel. *Journal of Transcultural Nursing, 25*, 87–94. http://dx.doi.org/10.1177/1043659613503881

Nochajski, S. M., & Matteliano, M. A. (2008). *A guide to cultural competence in the curriculum: Occupational therapy.* Buffalo, NY: Center for International Rehabilitation Research Information and Exchange. Retrieved from http:// cirrie.buffalo.edu/culture/curriculum/guides/ot.php

Paskett, E. D., Reeves, K. W., McLaughlin, J. M., Katz, M. L., McAlearney, A. S., Ruffin, M. T., . . . Gehlert, S. (2008). Recruitment of minority and underserved populations in the United States: The Centers for Population Health and Health Disparities experience. *Contemporary Clinical Trials, 29*(6), 847–861. http://dx.doi.org/10.1016/j.cct.2008.07.006

Paterson, C., & Chapman, J. (2013). Enhancing skills of critical reflection to evidence learning in professional practice. *Physical Therapy in Sport, 14*(3), 133–138. http://dx.doi .org/10.1016/j.ptsp.2013.03.004

Pooremamali, P., Persson D., & Eklund, M. (2011). Occupational therapists' experience of working with immigrant clients in mental health care. *Scandinavian Journal of Occupational Therapy, 18*, 109–121. http://dx.doi.org/10.3109 /11038121003649789

Price, E. G., Beach, M. C., Gary, T. L., Robinson, K. A., Gozu, A., Palacio, A., . . . Cooper, L. A. (2005). A systematic review of the methodological rigor of studies evaluating cultural competence training of health professionals. *Academic Medicine, 80*(6), 578–586. http://dx.doi .org/10.1097/00001888-200506000-00013

Pyatak, E. A., Blanche, E. I., Garber, S. L., Diaz, J., Blanchard, J., Florindez, L., & Clark, F. A. (2013). Conducting intervention research among underserved populations: Lessons learned and recommendations for researchers. *Archives of Physical Medicine and Rehabilitation, 94*(6), 1190–1198. http://dx.doi.org/10.1016/j.apmr.2012.12.009

Rajaram, S. S., & Bockrath, S. (2014). Cultural competence: New conceptual insights into is limits and potential for addressing health disparities. *Journal of Health Disparities Research and Practice, 7*(5), 82–89. Retrieved from http:// digitalscholarship.unlv.edu/cgi/viewcontent.cgi?article =1306&context=jhdrp

Reid, D. T., & Chiu, T. M. (2011). Research lessons learned: Occupational therapy with culturally diverse mothers of premature infants. *Canadian Journal of Occupational Therapy, 78*(3), 173–179. http://dx.doi.org/10.2182/cjot.2011 .78.3.5

Renzaho, A. M. N., Romios, P., Crock, C., & Sønderlund, A. L. (2013). The effectiveness of cultural competence programs in ethnic minority patient-centered health care: A systematic review of the literature. *International Journal for Quality in Health Care, 25*(3), 261–269. http://dx.doi.org/10.1093/intqhc/mzt006

Rowles, G. D. (1991). Beyond performance: Being in place as a component of occupational therapy. *American Journal of Occupational Therapy, 45*(3), 265–271. http://dx.doi.org /10.5014/ajot.45.3.265

Sanner, S., Baldwin, D., Cannella, K. A. S., Charles, J., & Parker, L. (2010). The impact of cultural diversity forum on students' openness to diversity. *Journal of Cultural Diversity, 17*(2), 56–61.

Schim, S. M., Doorenbos, A. Z., & Borse, N. N. (2005). Cultural competence among Ontario and Michigan healthcare providers. *Journal of Nursing Scholarship, 37*, 354–362. http://dx.doi.org/10.1111/j.1547-5069.2005.00061.x

Seeleman, C., Hermans, J., Lamkaddem, M., Suumond, J., Stronks, K., & Essink-Bot, M. (2014). A students' survey of cultural competence as a basis for identifying gaps in the medical curriculum. *BMC Medical Education, 14*, 216–226. http://dx.doi.org/10.1186/1472-6920-14-216

Smith, L. (2001). Evaluation of an educational intervention to increase cultural competence among registered nurses. *Journal of Cultural Diversity, 8*(2), 50–63.

Smith, Y. J., Cornella, E., & Williams, N. (2014). Working with populations from a refugee background: An opportunity to enhance the occupational therapy educational experience, *Australian Occupational Therapy Journal, 61,* 20–27. http://dx.doi.org/10.1111/1440-1630.12037

Stedman, A., & Thomas, Y. (2011). Reflecting on our effectiveness: Occupational therapy interventions with indigenous clients. *Australian Occupational Therapy Journal, 58,* 43–49. http://dx.doi.org/10.1111/j.1440-1630.2010.00916.x

Suarez-Balcazar, Y., Friesema, J., & Lukyanova, V. (2013). Culturally competent interventions to address obesity among African American and Latino children and youth. *Occupational Therapy in Health Care, 27*(2), 113–128. http://dx.doi.org/10.3109/07380577.2013.785644

Thackrah, R. D., & Thompson, S. C. (2013). Refining the concept of cultural competence: Building on decades of progress. *Medical Journal of Australia, 199*(1), 35–38. http://dx.doi.org/10.5694/mja13.10499

Thomas, Y., Gray, M., McGinty, S., & Ebringer, S. (2011). Homeless adults engagement in art: First steps towards identity, recovery and social inclusion. *Australian Occupational Therapy Journal, 58*(6), 429–436. http://dx.doi.org/10.1111/j.1440-1630.2011.00977.x

Truong, M., Paradies, Y., & Priest, N. (2014). Interventions to improve cultural competency in healthcare: A systematic review of reviews. *BMC Health Services Research, 14,* 99. http://dx.doi.org/10.1186/1472-6963-14-99

Ulrey, K. L., & Amason, P. (2001). Intercultural communication between patients and health care providers: An exploration of intercultural communication effectiveness, cultural sensitivity, stress, and anxiety. *Health Communication, 13*(4), 449–463. http://dx.doi.org/10.1207/S15327027HC1304_06

U.S. Department of Health and Human Services. Office of Minority Health. (2015). *The national CLAS standards.* Retrieved from http://minorityhealth.hhs.gov/omh/browse.aspx?lvl=2&lvlid=53

Vesely, C. K., Ewaida, M., & Anderson, E. A. (2014). Cultural competence of parenting education programs used by Latino families: A review. *Hispanic Journal of Behavioral Sciences, 36*(1), 27–47. http://dx.doi.org/10.1177/0739986313510694

Wahyuni, D. (2012). The research design maze: Understanding paradigms, cases, methods and methodologies. *Journal of Applied Management Accounting Research, 10*(1), 69–80.

Walsh, F. (2003). Family resilience: A framework for clinical practice. *Family Process, 42,* 1–18. http://dx.doi.org/10.1111/j.1545-5300.2003.00001.x

Wells, S. A., & Black, R. M. (2000). *Cultural competency for health professionals.* Bethesda, MD: American Occupational. Therapy Association.

Whiteford, G. E. (1995). Other worlds and other lives: A study of occupational therapy student perceptions of cultural difference. *Occupational Therapy International, 2*(4), 291–313. http://dx.doi.org/10.1002/oti.6150020407

SUBJECT INDEX

Note. Page numbers in *italics* indicate boxes, exhibits, figures, and tables.

CITATION INDEX

Note. Page numbers in *italics* indicate boxes, exhibits, figures, and tables.

Bennett, S., 16
Bennett, T., 391
Benson, P., 66, 67, 74, 174, 176, 178, 197, 198
Bentley, J. A., 373
Bercher, D. A., 324, 329
Bereknyei, S., 424, 425
Berg, C., 43
Berg, J., 374, 375, 379
Berggren, V., 27
Bergh, H., 235
Berlin, E., 151
Berry, J., 29
Bertolo, M., 67, 130, 132, 422
Berwick, D. M., 156, 207, 352
Betancourt, J. R., *53*, 67, 130
Bettez, S. C., 327
Beune, E., 425, 426
Beyers, M., 37
Bhatia, R., 37, 38
Bhembe, S., 105
Bhopal, R., 387, 390
Bhopal, R. S., 391
Bickell, N. A., 150
Bickmore, T., 156
Bickmore, T. W., 156
Bidani, R., 155
Bigby, J. A., 260
Bigman, L., 329
Biller, J., 207
Bishop, A., 194
Black, L. L., 95
Black, M., 339, 340
Black, M. M., 261
Black, R., 71, 85, 177, 180, 294, 298, 300, 301
Black, R. M., 52, 66, 84, 85, 142, 143, 144, 164, 219, 260, 262, 287, 304, 316, 322, 413, 421, 422, 427
Blackwell, D. L., 403
Blais, R., 184
Blake, J., 106
Blakeney, A. B., 43
Blanchard, J., 353, 430, 431
Blanche, E. I., 206, 430, 431
Bland, H. W., 329
Blas, E., 114, 123
Blissett, D., 374
Bluemel, J., 68, 69
Bobo, L., 153
Bockrath, S., 423
Bogan, K. E., 43
Boggess, M. M., 408

Bogner, J., 304
Bohan, K. D., 123
Bolorunduro, O., 207
Bonder, B., 4, 25, 52, 132, 141, 174, 414
Bonder, B. R., 25, 413
Bonilla-Silva, E., 68
Boninger, M. L., 207
Boone, M., 176
Boonstra, H., 355
Bornstein, J., 421
Borokhovski, E., 66, 67, 75, 416
Borse, N. N., 422
Bortz, W. M., 373
Boss, J. A., 193, *193*
Both, S., 97
Botorff, J. L., 9
Boud, D., 86, 106
Bound, J., 38
Bourjolly, J. N., 387
Bourke-Taylor, H., 179, 180, 182
Bowen, S., 140
Bowers, R., 286
Bowling, A., 402, *406–407*
Boyce, C., 395
Boyd, B. A., 24
Boyd, S. D., 373
Boyle, J. S., 179
Bracciano, A., 176, 282
Brach, C., 156
Braddock, C., III, 424, 425
Brady, D., 67
Braillie, H. W., 199
Branch, W. T., 67, 132
Brar, S. S., 270
Brascoupé, S., 56
Braveman, B., 312, 316
Braveman, P., 37
Breland, H. L., 427
Brezinkski, K. L., 54, 55
Bridges, D. R., 176
Bridges, M. W., 283
Brigden, D., 71, 76
Bringle, R. G., 296
Brobeck, E., 235
Brookover, C., 292
Brooks, D., 376
Brooks, J., 247, 250
Brooks, J. E., 68, 69
Brosco, J. P., 132
Brouwer, W., 155
Brown, C. J., 403